# Annual Update in Intensive Care and Emergency Medicine

The series *Annual Update in Intensive Care and Emergency Medicine* is the continuation of the series entitled *Yearbook of Intensive Care and Emergency Medicine* in Europe and *Intensive Care Medicine: Annual Update* in the United States.

Jean-Louis Vincent
Editor

# Annual Update in Intensive Care and Emergency Medicine 2023

Springer

*Editor*
Jean-Louis Vincent
Department of Intensive Care
Erasme University Hospital
Université libre de Bruxelles
Brussels, Belgium
e-mail: jlvincent@intensive.org

ISSN 2191-5709 ISSN 2191-5717 (electronic)
Annual Update in Intensive Care and Emergency Medicine
ISBN 978-3-031-23004-2 ISBN 978-3-031-23005-9 (eBook)
https://doi.org/10.1007/978-3-031-23005-9



This Springer imprint is published by the registered company Springer Nature Switzerland AG
The registered company address is: Gewerbestrasse 11, 6330 Cham, Switzerland

# Contents

# Abbreviations

| | |
|---|---|
| AKI | Acute kidney injury |
| APACHE | Acute physiology and chronic health evaluation |
| ARDS | Acute respiratory distress syndrome |
| COVID | Coronavirus disease |
| CPR | Cardiopulmonary resuscitation |
| CRP | C-reactive protein |
| CRRT | Continuous renal replacement therapy |
| CT | Computed tomography |
| CVP | Central venous pressure |
| ECMO | Extracorporeal membrane oxygenation |
| ED | Emergency department |
| GCS | Glasgow Coma Scale |
| ICU | Intensive care unit |
| IL | Interleukin |
| LV | Left ventricular |
| MAP | Mean arterial pressure |
| NIV | Non-invasive ventilation |
| PEEP | Positive end-expiratory pressure |
| RBC | Red blood cell |
| RCT | Randomized controlled trial |
| RRT | Renal replacement therapy |
| RV | Right ventricular |
| SARS-CoV-2 | Severe acute respiratory syndrome coronavirus-2 |
| SOFA | Sequential organ failure assessment |
| TBI | Traumatic brain injury |
| TNF | Tumor necrosis factor |
| VILI | Ventilator-induced lung injury |

# Part I

# Precision Medicine

# The Role of Transcriptomics in Redefining Critical Illness

1

T. M. Pelaia, M. Shojaei, and A. S. McLean

## 1.1 Introduction

Critical care medicine is rapidly evolving, with the approach to sepsis serving as a paradigmatic example. Our understanding of sepsis has been subject to decades of development and refinement, which reflects a continuous effort towards improving the management of this burdensome medical problem. Sepsis was recently redefined as "life-threatening organ dysfunction caused by a dysregulated host response to an infection", characterizing it as a syndrome that captures a vast heterogeneity of patients [1]. The updated definition is the first to emphasize the primacy of the non-homeostatic host response where the disruption of inflammatory, anti-inflammatory, metabolic, and circulatory processes is driven by a complex array of factors. Transcriptomics, the study of RNA transcripts in a specific cell or tissue, has dramatically progressed alongside critical care medicine, and while there is an inclination to associate key cellular pathways in sepsis with changes in gene expression derived from messenger RNA (mRNA) levels, the role of the transcriptome has expanded tremendously to non-coding RNAs (ncRNA) that possess dynamic regulatory functions.

Despite advancements in the comprehension of its pathophysiology, sepsis remains one of the leading causes of morbidity and mortality in critically ill patients [2]. As reinforced by the Surviving Sepsis Campaign, the current strengths in sepsis management rely on early identification of patients at risk, initial fluid resuscitation,

T. M. Pelaia (✉) · A. S. McLean
Department of Intensive Care Medicine, Nepean Hospital, Kingswood, NSW, Australia
e-mail: tpel0110@alumni.sydney.edu.au

M. Shojaei
Department of Intensive Care Medicine, Nepean Hospital, Kingswood, NSW, Australia

Centre for Immunology and Allergy Research, Westmead Institute for Medical Research, Westmead, NSW, Australia



J.-L. Vincent (ed.), *Annual Update in Intensive Care and Emergency Medicine 2023*, Annual Update in Intensive Care and Emergency Medicine,
https://doi.org/10.1007/978-3-031-23005-9_1

prompt antimicrobial therapy, as well as quickly identifying and controlling the infection source [3]. Yet due to the notoriety of its heterogeneous manifestations, there is a strong conviction for moving the current treatment paradigm toward a more personalized approach [4–6]. The ultra-sensitivity of transcriptomic profiling systems, such as RNA-sequencing (RNA-Seq), quantitative polymerase chain reaction (qPCR), and microarrays, means that interindividual variability in the host response is provided with a high level of molecular detail. While important insights can be drawn from these tools, the fundamental question is whether they translate to clinical utility. This includes strengthening the existing approach to sepsis that rests on timely intervention, as well as fostering a growing potential to redefine sepsis through the lens of precision medicine. In this chapter, we provide an overview of how RNA participates in sepsis pathophysiology, and give an update on the potential of transcriptomics to uncover new tools in the early detection and treatment of sepsis.

## 1.2 Transcriptomes: An Indispensable Player in Unraveling the Mechanisms of Sepsis

The growing body of data on sepsis pathophysiology has revealed an unprecedented level of molecular complexity. Such intricate analyses may initially appear to be far removed from the observable clinical characteristics of the critically ill patient. However, it is at this mechanistic level where a profound source of heterogeneity is discovered, providing a fresh outlook on developing rapid and precise methods for managing septic patients. While it is outside the scope of this chapter to investigate the pathophysiology in detail, highlighting the key cellular processes involved assists in understanding the governing role of transcriptomes.

### 1.2.1 Overview of the Molecular Pathophysiology of Sepsis

The host response to sepsis begins with detecting the invading microorganism via pathogen-associated molecular patterns (PAMPs). These foreign antigens interact directly with pattern recognition receptors (PRRs) present at the cell surface or intracellularly. This recognition event transduces the pathogenic signal to the cell nucleus through multiple pathways. A core example involves nuclear factor kappa B (NF-κB) signaling, which regulates the transcription of early-activation genes that code for a myriad of pro-inflammatory cytokines. This inflammatory network is crucial for the activation of innate immune cells and subsequent signaling cascades that ultimately serve to eliminate invading pathogens from the host. During early sepsis, however, this response is abruptly upregulated, leading to systemic inflammation that can beget endothelial damage, increased vascular permeability, hypercoagulation and metabolic dysfunction [7]. Reciprocal damage-associated molecular patterns (DAMPs) released from dying cells perpetuate the inflammatory and innate immune response. The secretion of inflammatory mediators is therefore amplified, resulting in sustained tissue inflammation and injury from excessive leukocyte infiltration. End organ dysfunction manifests consequently, with complications like acute respiratory distress syndrome (ARDS), acute kidney injury (AKI), cardiomyopathy, and encephalopathy commonly experienced. Many patients also develop secondary immunosuppression, typically characterized by a concurrent production of anti-inflammatory cytokines to compensate for the overwhelming pro-inflammatory response. An enhanced anti-inflammatory response is regulated by molecular pathways that result in widespread loss of immune cells and an impaired capacity for antigen presentation [7]. Thus, immunosuppressed patients are subservient to ongoing primary infection, the development of secondary infection, and viral reactivation.

### 1.2.2 Messenger RNA: The Driving Force of Transcriptomics

Inherent in the central dogma is the explicit role of mRNAs in sepsis pathophysiology. PRRs, cytokines, signal transducers, and immune cells are all composed of proteins that are coded, and thereby modulated, by mRNA expression. In this way, coding RNA transcripts have substantially informed our understanding of the dysregulated host response, and methods to investigate gene expression have evolved from microarrays that detect a predefined set of sequences, to RNA-Seq that covers the expression of the entire transcriptome. Dynamic gene expression profiles can now be analyzed at the tissue or cellular level, where differentially expressed genes that are up- or down-regulated between defined populations or time points are identified and cataloged to specific biological pathways and functions. In sepsis, transcriptomic studies are typically poised towards analyzing mRNA profiles from peripheral blood leukocytes, but have encompassed cecal ligation and puncture (CLP) animal models, tightly controlled human endotoxemia experiments with healthy volunteers, and clinical studies with critically ill patients that evidently encounter more complexity. The consensus is that the transcriptional response to sepsis is complex and highly protean, with up to thousands of differentially expressed genes emerging simultaneously and progressively [8–10]. Indeed, the transcription of PRR genes, notably those of the Toll-like receptor (TLR) family are upregulated during sepsis, as well as pro-inflammatory cytokines such as tumor necrosis factor α (TNF-α), interleukins (IL)-1α, -1β, -6, and -12, and type-I interferons (IFN) [8, 9]. Pathways associated with signal transduction are also enriched, including NF-κB, mitogen activated protein kinase (MAPK), janus kinase (JAK), and signaling transducer and activator of transcription (STAT) [8–10]. RNA transcripts related to mitochondrial dysfunction, protein synthesis, T helper cell differentiation, endotoxin tolerance, cell death, apoptosis, necrosis, and T-cell exhaustion are also profoundly modulated during sepsis [8, 11]. Novel transcriptional patterns are observed in the dysfunction of various organs, as well as among patients of different sex, age groups, and medical comorbidities [12].

### 1.2.3 MicroRNA: The Master Regulators of Gene Expression

There is increasing acknowledgement that a transcriptome-level understanding of sepsis exceeds mRNA expression, with ncRNAs emerging as a prominent feature. In particular, microRNAs (miRNAs) are identified as 'master regulators' of gene expression that primarily act post-transcriptionally by interacting with mRNAs to induce mRNA degradation and inhibit translation, and can act intra- and extracellularly [13]. The intricate crosstalk between miRNA and cellular pathways combined with its systemic influence has prompted much research into the involvement of miRNAs in sepsis. Transcriptomic profiling technologies, notably RNA-seq, have been applied to analyze the sepsis-induced effect on miRNAs, and have documented the differential expression of various miRNAs in multiple cell types [13, 14]. These findings have been corroborated with numerous *in vitro* studies to elucidate the function of miRNAs in the immunoinflammatory response, where they are shown to exhibit dynamic pro-inflammatory and anti-inflammatory activities. For example, miR-146a can negatively regulate the TLR4/NF-κB pathway, highlighting its involvement in endotoxin tolerance and attenuating the inflammatory response, thus its downregulation during sepsis worsens inflammation [14]. On the other hand, miR-135a has a pro-inflammatory effect on cardiomyocytes by activating the p38 MAPK/NF-κB pathway, and its expression is elevated in the serum of patients with sepsis-induced cardiac dysfunction [15].

### 1.2.4 Long Non-coding RNA: The miRNA Sponges

Long ncRNAs (lncRNAs) were once regarded as transcriptional noise, but their novel roles in gene regulation are now canonical. They have been classified as 'miRNA sponges' that bind to and sequester miRNAs, thereby reducing their regulatory effect on mRNAs. This adds another intricate dimension to the transcriptomic mechanisms underpinning sepsis where many lncRNAs are aberrantly expressed [16]. For example, the lncRNA THRIL is upregulated in human bronchial epithelial cells in sepsis and sponges miR-19a, which resulted in increased expression of TNF-α and promoted lung cell apoptosis [17]. Circular RNAs (circRNA) are a novel member of the lncRNA family, with a circular conformation that affords stability and resistance. They too hold the putative function as miRNA sponges, but also as 'miRNA reservoirs' that store and transport miRNAs to subcellular locations. Recent studies have elucidated the role of circRNAs in sepsis-induced organ failure via their sponging effects, but this research is still at an early stage [18].

## 1.3 From Transcriptomics to Clinical Tools

Advances in transcriptomics have illuminated three major sources of heterogeneity at the molecular level. First, the cellular functions involved in sepsis are governed by extensive gene regulatory networks involving intricate interactions between mRNAs, miRNAs, and lncRNAs, with the potential to produce a variety of outcomes. Second, expression patterns are highly dependent on the specialized functions of the cell type. Third, the transcriptional response undergoes large dynamic changes as sepsis progresses through different phases, thus giving rise to temporal heterogeneity. The influence of demographic factors and other clinical features adds to this mixed picture, and presents a huge challenge to translate this complexity into clinical practice. Yet with improvements in technologies and clinical trial design, this transcriptomic understanding of sepsis can be sensibly harnessed to address and possibly redefine two fundamental goals of critical care medicine: early identification and effective therapeutic intervention (Fig. 1.1).

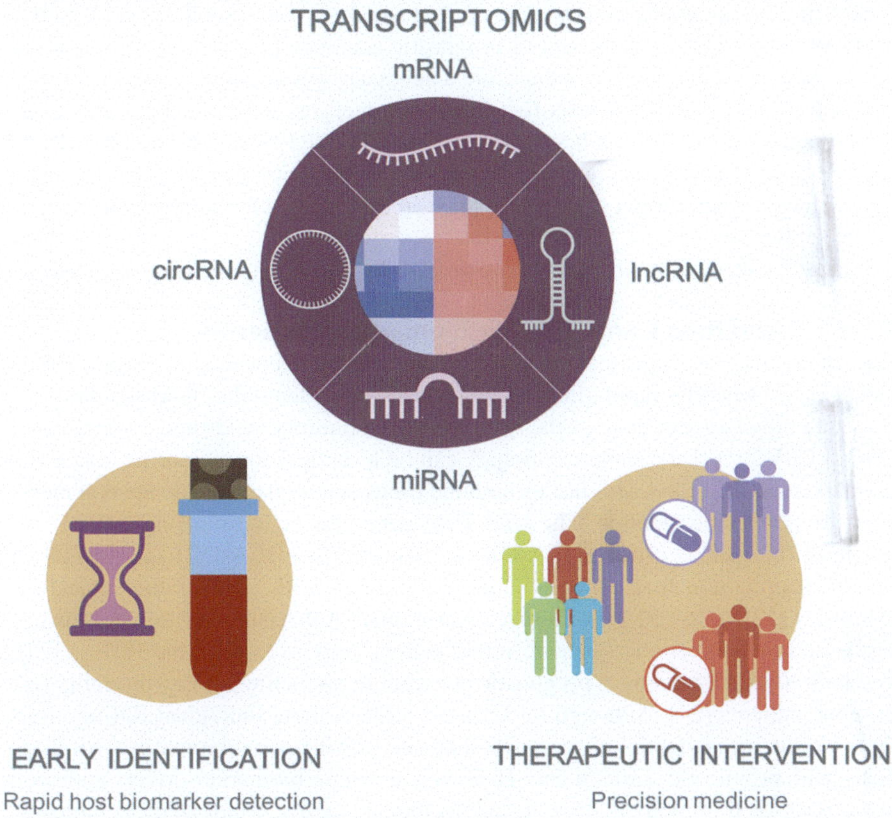


**Fig. 1.1** The role of transcriptomics in the early detection of sepsis by developing rapid host biomarkers, and in therapeutic intervention by facilitating a precision medicine approach

### 1.3.1 Time Is Critical: Current Challenges in the Early Detection of Sepsis

Sepsis is associated with an increasing risk of mortality for every hour it goes unrecognized, so an early diagnosis is crucial [19]. Ideally, a diagnosis of sepsis should answer the questions that are drawn from its definition: identifying the type of infection, measuring the host response, and predicting the likelihood of organ dysfunction. Identifying the causative pathogen is currently achieved with blood culture, yet a major limitation of this method is the delay to results (typically 48–72 h), which are also frequently read as a false negative [20]. Initial screening tools like the sequential organ failure assessment (SOFA) score can be laborious to calculate in a time-critical emergency, and the use of simplified versions, such as quick SOFA (qSOFA), can be to the detriment of prognostic accuracy [21]. The development of precise and rapid diagnostics is therefore a necessary yet arduous feat in the critical care setting, but biomarker tests for sepsis are emerging as promising candidates. Well established markers such as C-reactive protein (CRP) and procalcitonin (PCT) provide prompt and valuable glimpses into the host response, but discordances in their diagnostic and prognostic performance create the need for a more holistic view of the septic patient [20]. The transcriptomics approach proposes that novel RNA biomarkers can expedite the diagnostic process by harnessing the host response.

#### 1.3.1.1 Rapid Host Transcriptomic Biomarkers for Sepsis

The emergence of molecular diagnostics has garnered considerable attention in recent years, whereby rapid qPCR techniques are considered the 'gold standard' for detecting novel viruses such as the severe acute respiratory syndrome coronavirus 2 (SARS-CoV-2), yet the same technology can be leveraged for measuring host RNA biomarkers in the blood with fast turnaround times and high accuracy. Several markers warrant specific mention. The *HLA-DRA* gene may be a promising mRNA surrogate of the surface protein HLA-DR on monocytes (mHLA-DR) as a marker of immunosuppression that can be routinely measured with qPCR rather than flow cytometry [22]. miR-150 is a well-investigated miRNA that can discriminate between sepsis and non-infectious systemic inflammatory response syndrome (SIRS) [23]. The lncRNA GAS5 displays prognostic potential in predicting 28-day mortality risk in septic patients [24]. Although far from exhaustive, these individual RNAs reflect the wide-ranging potential of transcriptomics in deriving novel biomarkers for diagnosis and prognostic enrichment. However, a single-biomarker-driven approach towards sepsis is unlikely to be achieved in clinical practice. Many of these biomarkers are only effective at a specific time, in a certain population, or even in a particular tissue or cell, which underscores the perplexity of the sepsis response. Measuring a panel of biomarkers has been advocated to provide greater accuracy and generalizability. As an example, the *IFI27* gene is a well-characterized host biomarker for viral infection [25], but incorporating other viral-induced mRNAs (*JUP* and *LAX1*), as well as mRNAs that are upregulated in bacterial infections (*HK3*, *TNIP1*, *GPAA1*, and *CTSB*) can yield a gene signature that robustly evaluates whether an infection is likely to be of bacterial or viral origin [26]. This 7-mRNA "Bacterial-Viral Metascore" has recently formed part of a composite test alongside an 11-mRNA "Sepsis Metascore" and an 11-mRNA "Stanford Mortality Score" to further affirm the presence of an acute infection and to predict the risk of 30-day mortality (Table 1.1) [26, 29, 30]. The resultant 29-Host-Immune-mRNA panel called InSep™ (Inflammatix, Bulingame, CA) integrates rapid transcriptomic profiling with advanced machine learning to guide early clinical decisions in the emergency room about administering antibiotics, the need for further diagnostic workup, and the likelihood of an intensive care unit (ICU) transfer [33]. Other groups have reported similar advances in host mRNA expression signatures that have been summarized in Table 1.1 using areas under the curve (AUCs). Notably, SeptiCyte® RAPID (Immunexpress, Seattle, WA), the first FDA-cleared test to differentiate sepsis from non-infectious SIRS in 1 h, uses host response mRNA expression that is quantified with real time qPCR [28]. It has been clinically validated in retrospective and prospective studies (ClinicalTrials.gov Identifiers NCT01905033, NCT02127502, and NCT05469048). The development of qPCR for host mRNA detection has advanced towards point-of-care devices with the potential to address the unmet need of rapid

**Table 1.1** Host mRNA signatures for the diagnosis and prognosis of sepsis

| Setting [Ref] | Transcriptomic score | Performance (validated AUC) | Commercial platform |
|---|---|---|---|
| Sepsis vs. non-infectious SIRS on ICU admission in adults [27] | 4-mRNA classifier (SeptiCyte™ LAB SeptiScore™) | 0.82–0.89 | SeptiCyte™ LAB (Immunexpress, Seattle, WA) |
| Sepsis vs. noninfectious SIRS in patients with malignancy or treated with antineoplastic/immunosuppressant [28] | Simpler version of SeptiCyte™ LAB (SeptiCyte® RAPID SeptiScore®) | Adult: >0.88<br>Pediatric: >0.96 | SeptiCyte® RAPID (Immunexpress, Seattle, WA) |
| Sepsis vs. non-infectious SIRS [29] | 11-mRNA classifier (Sepsis MetaScore) | 0.83 (0.73–0.89) | Component of the InSep™ test (Inflammatix, Bulingame, CA) |
| Bacterial vs. viral infection [26] | 7-mRNA classifier (Bacterial-Viral MetaScore) | 0.91 (0.82–0.96) | Component of the InSep™ test (Inflammatix, Bulingame, CA) |
| 30-day mortality prediction in sepsis patients [30] | 12-mRNA classifier (Stanford Score) | 0.87 (0.64–1.0) | Component of the InSep™ test (Inflammatix, Bulingame, CA) |
| 28-day mortality prediction in pediatric septic shock [31] | 4-mRNA + 12-protein classifier (PERSEVERE-XP) | 0.96 (0.91–1.0) | |
| Abdominal sepsis vs. post-op gastrointestinal surgery control on ICU admission [32] | 3-mRNA classifier (sNIP score) | 0.91 (0.84–0.97) | |

*AUC* area under the curve, *SIRS* systemic inflammatory response syndrome, *ICU* intensive care unit and early detection of sepsis. Such technologies could also transform the approach to other critical illnesses where a sense of urgency is essential in their management. While the commercial availability of transcriptomic biomarker panels represents an important interface between the bench and the bedside, continued external clinical validation is required to ensure that reproducibility is upheld across heterogeneous populations. The emergence of ncRNA signatures for sepsis diagnosis, including the 14-lncRNA "SepSigLnc", also gives rise to the possibility of measuring a mixed panel of circRNA, lncRNA, miRNA, and mRNA markers for a more complete and interactive picture of the immuno-inflammatory status [34].

### 1.3.2 Trials and Tribulations: Current Challenges in the Treatment of Sepsis

In a similar vein to diagnosis, therapeutic approaches to sepsis are guided by its definition: controlling the infection, modulating the host response, and ameliorating organ dysfunction. Broad-spectrum antimicrobial therapy is prioritized due to its association in reducing mortality when administered early [3]. Fluid resuscitation and vasoactive agents are essential for the hemodynamic support of vital organ functions. Yet given that the dysregulated host response, rather than the infection itself, is the driver of adverse outcomes, host-directed-therapies have been long-sought-after. After decades of clinical trials, immunomodulatory agents that target PRRs, PAMPs, and pro-inflammatory cytokines have so far proven unsuccessful [35]. This emphasizes the difficulty for preclinical models to fully predict therapeutic efficacy at the bedside where tremendous heterogeneity exists. Attempts have been made to circumvent this challenge by recruiting more homogeneous groups of patients [7]. One study used decreased mHLA-DR levels to stratify sepsis patients for granulocyte-macrophage colony-stimulating factor (GM-CSF) administration, which was found to restore monocyte immunocompetence and shorten mechanical ventilation duration and length of ICU stay [36]. This study, among several others of a similar nature, represent the emergence of a core component of the precision medicine dogma where enrichment strategies are used to identify critically ill patients who could benefit from tailored therapies [6]. Once again, these examples rely on a single biomarker to define patient subsets, which may not capture a holistic view of the complex sepsis response. This is where transcriptomic profiling may facilitate with a more accurate identification of such discrete groups.

### 1.3.3 Deriving Transcriptomic Endotypes for Sepsis

As opposed to the top-down prognostic enrichment approach where a clinical feature drives the discovery of transcriptomic signatures associated with it, 'predictive enrichment' is a bottom-up approach that is mechanistically driven [6]. Distinct transcriptomic signatures, known as endotypes, are clustered based on shared biological processes that enable the targeted selection of patients who might benefit from targeted host-directed therapies. Several sepsis endotypes have been comprehensively validated and reviewed elsewhere [37], but include the immunosuppressed SRS1 and immunocompetent SRS2 endotypes [11]. Even though they are solely defined by transcriptomic mechanisms, these endotypes show significant differences in clinically relevant characteristics such as 30-day mortality. A post-hoc analysis of the VANISH randomized trial revealed that hydrocortisone administration was associated with higher mortality in the immunocompetent SRS2 endotype compared to the immunosuppressed SRS1, thus serving as an important consideration when designing future prospective trials [38]. While these endotypes were defined according to blood samples collected in the ICU, a recent addition was made to the literature with a multicohort study on emergency room patients with suspicion of sepsis [39]. Patients were stratified into five mechanistically diverse endotypes containing unique ~200-gene signatures denoted as neutrophilic-suppressive (NPS), inflammatory (INF), innate host defense (IHD), interferon (IFN), and adaptive (ADA). Patients with the NPS and IFN endotypes had higher SOFA scores, longer hospital stays, and higher 28-day organ failure. The study employs a theragnostic approach with dual benefit, allowing for the early detection and prognostication of sepsis, and the potential selection of a personalized therapeutic regime. External validation and simpler derivations of these ~200-gene endotypes will be required to improve their clinical utility, before their potential role in informing prospective clinical trial design is realized.

## 1.4 Challenges of Applying Transcriptomics in Critical Care

Several challenges lie ahead in realizing the full potential of transcriptomics in redefining sepsis and critical care. Peripheral blood has been the pragmatic choice for examining expression patterns, but these profiles may not be accurately extrapolated to other relevant cells involved in sepsis, and important information about specialized cell populations within this mixture may be lost. While methods such as CIBERSORT have been developed to account for leukocyte subtypes in bulk data [40], analyzing a single cell population, whether it be in the blood, the endothelium or from the dysfunctional organ, may be more sensible. The advent of single-cell RNA-seq can help to address this, having to date led to the discovery of novel signatures in monocytes associated with the various immune states [41]. Another challenge involves using transcriptomics to inform and enhance clinical trial design. Personalized approaches that combine prognostic and predictive enrichment strategies have been proposed, whereby patients are stratified based on transcriptomic signatures associated with the likelihood of developing adverse outcomes such as mortality and organ dysfunction (prognostic enrichment), followed by the low-risk patients receiving standard care and the high-risk patients being treated based on their underlying endotype (predictive enrichment) [6]. This leads to another challenge in defining subtypes and signatures that are clinically relevant, molecularly precise, and uniformly applicable. When addressing this, it may be important to realize that transcriptomics is just one dimension of an entire range of modalities that can facilitate a more holistic understanding of the biological pathways in sepsis. An 'integrated omics' approach combines data from genomics, epigenomics, transcriptomics, proteomics, lipidomics, metabolomics, and mircobiomics, and can help to build multimodal platforms for diagnosis, prognosis, and drug-discovery. These datasets are open to findings that may address more formidable challenges, particularly in dealing with the rapidly evolving pathophysiology of sepsis. Technological advances that provide clinicians with real-time data at the bedside will also help address this temporal heterogeneity. Importantly, interdisciplinary collaborations between investigators, clinicians, and industry are required to embrace new strategies driven by machine learning and high dimensional data, and to develop cost-effective, rapid technologies that are clinically feasible.

## 1.5 Conclusion

In this chapter, we have demonstrated the powerful roles of coding and ncRNAs in modulating the septic response. We have highlighted advances in transcriptomics that have enabled the identification of rapid host RNA biomarkers and clinically meaningful endotypes. Early recognition and treatment are the key tenets of current sepsis management, but transcriptomics holds the capacity to view these approaches from a revised angle—one that could facilitate a new era in critical care medicine.

## References


1. Singer M, Deutschman CS, Seymour CW, et al. The third international consensus definitions for sepsis and septic shock (Sepsis-3). JAMA. 2016;315:801–10.
2. Rudd KE, Johnson SC, Agesa KM, et al. Global, regional, and national sepsis incidence and mortality, 1990–2017: analysis for the Global Burden of Disease study. Lancet. 2020;395:200–11.
3. Evans L, Rhodes A, Alhazzani W, et al. Surviving sepsis campaign: international guidelines for management of sepsis and septic shock 2021. Crit Care Med. 2021;49:e1063–143.
4. Maslove DM, Tang B, Shankar-Hari M, et al. Redefining critical illness. Nat Med. 2022;28:1141–8.
5. McLean AS, Shojaei M. Transcriptomics in the intensive care unit. Lancet Respir Med. 2022;10:824–6.
6. Stanski NL, Wong HR. Prognostic and predictive enrichment in sepsis. Nat Rev Nephrol. 2020;16:20–31.
7. Gotts JE, Matthay MA. Sepsis: pathophysiology and clinical management. BMJ. 2016;353:i1585.
8. Calvano S, Xiao W, Richards R, et al. A network-based analysis of systemic inflammation in humans. Nature. 2005;437:1032–7.
9. Talwar S, Munson P, Barb J, et al. Gene expression profiles of peripheral blood leukocytes after endotoxin challenge in humans. Physiol Genomics. 2006;25:203–15.

10. Tang BM, Huang SJ, Mclean AS. Genome-wide transcription profiling of human sepsis: a systematic review. Crit Care. 2010;14:R237.
11. Davenport EE, Burnham KL, Radhakrishnan J, et al. Genomic landscape of the individual host response and outcomes in sepsis: a prospective cohort study. Lancet Respir Med. 2016;4:259–71.
12. Maslove DM, Wong HR. Gene expression profiling in sepsis: timing, tissue and translational considerations. Trends Mol Med. 2014;20:204–13.
13. Antonakos N, Gilbert C, Théroude C, Schrijver IT, Roger T. Modes of action and diagnostic value of miRNAs in sepsis. Front Immunol. 2022;13:951798.
14. Quinn SR, O'Neill LA. A trio of microRNAs that control toll-like receptor signaling. Int Immunol. 2011;23:421–5.
15. Zheng G, Pan M, Jin W, Jin G, Huang Y. MicroRNA-135a is up-regulated and aggravates myocardial depression in sepsis via regulating p38 MAPK/NF-κB pathway. Int Immunopharmacol. 2017;45:6–12.
16. Hashemian SMH, Pourhanifeh MH, Fadaei S, Velayati AA, Mirzaei H, Hamblin MR. Non-coding RNAs and exosomes: their role in the pathogenesis of sepsis. Mol Ther Nucl Acids. 2020;21:51–74.
17. Liu T, Liu J, Tian C, Wang H, Wen M, Yan M. LncRNA THRIL is upregulated in sepsis and sponges miR-19a to upregulate TNF-α in human bronchial epithelial cells. J Inflamm. 2020;17:31.
18. Wei L, Yang Y, Wang W, Xu R. Circular RNAs in the pathogenesis of sepsis and their clinical implications: a narrative review. Ann Acad Med. 2022;51:221–7.
19. Kumar A, Roberts D, Wood KE, et al. Duration of hypotension before initiation of effective antimicrobial therapy is the critical determinant of survival in human septic shock. Crit Care Med. 2006;34:1589–96.
20. Iskander KN, Osuchowski MF, Stearns-Kurosawa DJ, et al. Sepsis: multiple abnormalities, heterogeneous responses, and evolving understanding. Physiol Rev. 2013;93:1247–88.
21. Seymour CW, Liu VX, Iwashyna TJ, et al. Assessment of clinical criteria for sepsis: for the Third International Consensus Definitions for Sepsis and Septic Shock (Sepsis-3). JAMA. 2016;315:762–74.
22. Cajander S, Bäckman A, Tina E, Strålin K, Söderquist B, Källman. Preliminary results in quantitation of HLA-DRA by real-time PCR: a promising approach to identify immunosuppression in sepsis. Crit Care. 2013;17:R223.
23. Ma Y, Vilanova D, Atalar K, et al. Genome-wide sequencing of cellular microRNAs identifies a combinatorial expression signature diagnostic of sepsis. PLoS One. 2013;8:e75918.
24. Zhang W, Chen B, Chen W. LncRNA GAS5 relates to Th17 cells and serves as a potential biomarker for sepsis inflammation, organ dysfunctions and mortality risk. J Clin Lab Anal. 2022;36:e24309.
25. Tang BM, Shojaei M, Parnell GP, et al. A novel immune biomarker IFI27 discriminates between influenza and bacteria in patients with suspected respiratory infection. Eur Respir J. 2017;49:1602098.
26. Sweeney TE, Wong HR, Khatri P. Robust classification of bacterial and viral infections via integrated host gene expression diagnostics. Sci Transl Med. 2016;8:346ra91.
27. Miller RMI, Lopansri BK, Burke JP, et al. Validation of a host response assay, SeptiCyte LAB, for discriminating sepsis from systemic inflammatory response syndrome in the ICU. Am J Respir Crit Care Med. 2018;198:903–13.
28. Davis R, Krupa N, van der Poll T, et al. SeptiCyte® RAPID in sepsis cases with malignancy or treated with antineoplastics/immunosuppressants. Crit Care Med. 2021;49:643 (abst).
29. Sweeney TE, Shidham A, Wong HR, Khatri PA. A comprehensive time-course-based multicohort analysis of sepsis and sterile inflammation reveals a robust diagnostic gene set. Sci Transl Med. 2015;7:287ra71.
30. Sweeney TE, Perumal TM, Henao R, et al. A community approach to mortality prediction in sepsis via gene expression analysis. Nat Commun. 2018;9:694.

31. Wong H, Cvijanovich NZ, Anas N, et al. Improved risk stratification in pediatric septic shock using both protein and mRNA biomarkers. PERSEVERE-XP. Am J Respir Crit Care Med. 2017;196:494–501.
32. Scicluna BP, Wiewel MA, van Vught LA, et al. Molecular biomarker to assist in diagnosing abdominal sepsis upon ICU admission. Am J Respir Crit Care Med. 2017;197:1070–3.
33. He YD, Wohlford EM, Uhle F, Buturovic L, Liesenfeld O, Sweeney TE. The optimization and biological significance of a 29-host-immune-mRNA panel for the diagnosis of acute infections and sepsis. J Pers Med. 2021;11:735.
34. Zheng X, Leunk KS, Wong MH, Cheng L. Long non-coding RNA pairs to assist in diagnosing sepsis. BMC Genomics. 2021;22:275.
35. Marshall JC. Why have clinical trials in sepsis failed? Trends Mol Med. 2014;20:195–203.
36. Meisel C, Schefold JC, Pschowski R, et al. Granulocyte-macrophage colony-stimulating factor to reverse sepsis-associated immunosuppression: a double-blind, randomized, placebo-controlled multicenter trial. Am J Respir Crit Care Med. 2009;180:640–8.
37. Leligdowicz A, Matthay MA. Heterogeneity in sepsis: new biological evidence with clinical applications. Crit Care. 2019;23:80.
38. Antcliffe DB, Burnham KL, Al-Beidh F, et al. Transcriptomic signatures in sepsis and a differential response to steroids: from the VANISH randomized trial. Am J Respir Crit Care Med. 2018;199:980–6.
39. Baghela A, Pena OM, Lee AH, et al. Predicting sepsis severity at first clinical presentation: the role of endotypes and mechanistic signatures. EBioMedicine. 2022;75:103776.
40. Newman AM, Liu CL, Green MR, et al. Robust enumeration of cell subsets from tissue expression profiles. Nat Methods. 2015;12:453–7.
41. Reyes M, Filbin MR, Bhattacharyya RP, et al. An immune cell signature of bacterial sepsis. Nat Med. 2020;26:333–40.

# 2 Metagenomic Sequencing in the ICU for Precision Diagnosis of Critical Infectious Illnesses

L. P. A. Neyton, C. R. Langelier, and C. S. Calfee

## 2.1 Introduction

Infectious diseases, in particular respiratory and bloodstream infections, are a leading cause of intensive care unit (ICU) admission and death worldwide [1]. Identifying the underlying pathogens responsible for infectious critical illness remains a major challenge and delays timely and effective treatment. Indeed, pathogens remain undetected in up to 60% of cases of pneumonia [2] and over 30% of cases of sepsis [3, 4]. Appropriate antibiotic therapy is essential for effective management of critical infectious diseases; however, in most cases, treatment is empiric because existing microbiologic diagnostics are unable to identify an etiologic pathogen. This approach also contributes to antimicrobial resistance, opportunistic pathogens such as *Clostridium difficile*, and leads to other avoidable adverse drug effects [5, 6]. Rates of antimicrobial-resistant infections have markedly increased during the coronavirus disease 2019 (COVID-19) pandemic due in part to the overuse of broad-spectrum antibiotics from clinicians suspecting secondary bacterial infections but lacking diagnostics to confidently determine their existence [7, 8]. Thus, improvement in diagnostics for pathogens causing infectious illness in critically ill patients remains a major unmet need.

Metagenomics, the study of nucleotide sequences from all organisms in biological samples, offers an unprecedented opportunity to rapidly identify and characterize

L. P. A. Neyton (✉) · C. S. Calfee
Division of Pulmonary, Critical Care, Allergy and Sleep Medicine, Department of Medicine, University of California San Francisco, San Francisco, CA, USA
e-mail: lucile.neyton@ucsf.edu

C. R. Langelier
Division of Infectious Diseases, Department of Medicine, University of California San Francisco, San Francisco, CA, USA

Chan Zuckerberg Biohub, San Francisco, CA, USA



J.-L. Vincent (ed.), *Annual Update in Intensive Care and Emergency Medicine 2023*, Annual Update in Intensive Care and Emergency Medicine,
https://doi.org/10.1007/978-3-031-23005-9_2

infectious disease-causing pathogens, such as bacteria, viruses, and fungi, in a single test without a need for culture. The term metagenomics traditionally refers to DNA sequencing, whereas metatranscriptomics refers to RNA sequencing. However, the term metagenomics is commonly used to refer to DNA *and* RNA sequencing, both of which can be used for pathogen detection, with important differences and associated considerations. In this review, we will use the term metagenomics to refer to both DNA and RNA sequencing.

This chapter begins with providing an overview of the current metagenomic approaches used to identify pathogens. Next, we will describe examples of metagenomics applications and examine how the technique might be employed more widely to study and treat infectious diseases in the ICU.

## 2.2 Current Standards in Pathogen Detection

Historically, the gold standard for identification of bacterial and fungal pathogens has been culture [9]. Despite simplicity and low cost, the turnaround time for culture-based methods can extend up to several days or even weeks [10], leading to delayed diagnoses, inappropriate antimicrobial use, and in some cases excess disease transmission in the hospital due to missed infections [11]. While standard blood and respiratory cultures are relatively inexpensive compared to many medical diagnostic tests, in some countries, such as the USA, the cost of labor and routine use of mass spectrometry for taxonomic identification have led to per-patient costs of several hundred US dollars. Viral pathogens and some bacterial pathogens, such as *Mycoplasma pneumoniae* or *Legionella pneumophila*, may be difficult to detect with traditional culture-based methods [12]. Because empirical antibiotic treatment is typically administered as early as possible in patients presenting with infection-related symptoms, the use of culture-based identification might also lead to false negative results as antibiotics can sterilize microbial cultures.

Immunological methods, such as serology, can also be used to determine the presence of antibodies directed at the pathogen of interest. The major drawback of using immunological assays for the detection of pathogens is that antibody production requires several days to weeks following exposure to a pathogen, leading to false negative tests during the period of acute illness [13]. Antigen tests directly detect pathogen proteins and do have utility during acute illness; however, they are only available for a limited number of organisms and in many cases have limited sensitivity and/or specificity [13].

Viral detection, and increasingly *Mycobacterium tuberculosis* detection, is carried out using polymerase chain reaction (PCR) assays. Many pathogen genomes have been sequenced and are publicly available, which allows the design of species-specific probes that can be used to find and amplify microorganism-specific nucleic acid sequences, thus allowing the targeted detection of a set of pre-defined microorganisms, often within just a few hours [14]. However, despite the availability of many Food and Drug Administration (FDA)-approved microbial tests [15] allowing the identification of a range of different pathogens (bacteria, viruses, fungi, and parasites), only a handful of PCR-based assays are clinically accepted and available in routine practice, and less common organisms, novel emerging pathogens, or pathogen variants may be undetectable using such approaches.

All these methods are targeted, meaning that they focus on a pre-selected set of organisms. In many cases, only common pathogens are sought, thus limiting the chances of identifying less common pathogens of interest.

## 2.3 Principles of Metagenomics for Infectious Disease Diagnosis

The potential of metagenomics to improve infectious disease diagnosis in the ICU, where time to effective treatment is paramount [11], is significant. Metagenomics allows the unbiased detection, quantification, and characterization of genetic material from any organism within biological samples in a relatively short timeframe (Table 2.1).

**Table 2.1** Characteristics of commonly used pathogen identification strategies

| Identification method | Principle | Cost | Microbial detection | Additional considerations | Turnaround |
|---|---|---|---|---|---|
| Culture | Growth and isolation of species present in a sample | Low-moderate | Some species are difficult to culture or cannot be cultured (e.g., atypical organisms, viral, fungal pathogens) | • Medium-dependent<br>• Prior use of antimicrobial agents will affect sensitivity | Days to weeks |
| Immunological methods | Detection via antibodies | Low-moderate | Determined by the choice of antibody/antigen | • Antibody testing may not be useful during acute disease | Minutes to days |
| | Detection via antigens | | | • Limited by sensitivity/specificity | |
| PCR | Targeted amplification of specific pathogens | Moderate | Limited by PCR primer panel | • Detects only a few pre-selected microbes<br>• Some species might be preferentially amplified | Minutes to days |
| Metagenomics | Nucleotide sequences capture and amplification | High | Unbiased | • Host background will be dominant<br>• Contamination will greatly affect utility | Hours to days |

*PCR* polymerase chain reaction

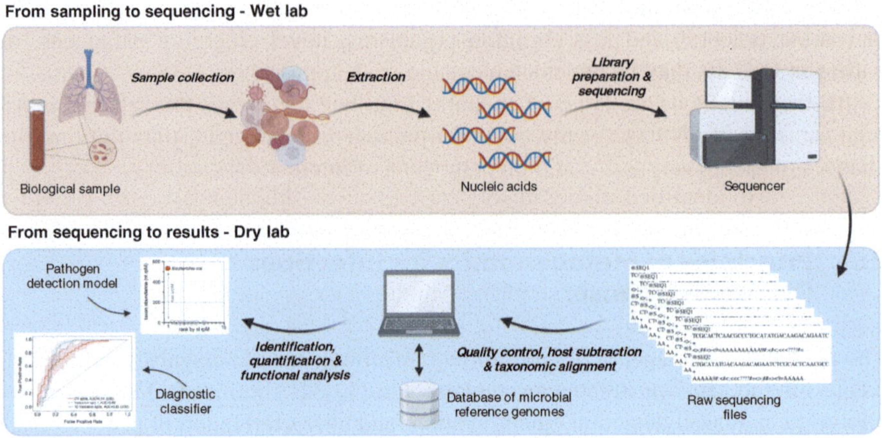


**Fig. 2.1** Simplified overview of a metagenomics workflow, which is broken down into two main steps. Sample collection, nucleic acid extraction, library preparation, and sequencing are depicted in the orange panel. Once reads are sequenced, data are fed into a bioinformatics pipeline (blue panel) for quality control, host subtraction, and taxonomic alignment, followed by identification and quantification of microbial species, and functional analysis. Two possible analyses are depicted and consist of pathogen detection and disease classification (figures adapted from Kalantar et al. [16]). Created with BioRender.com

The general metagenomics workflow (Fig. 2.1) begins with nucleic acid extraction (DNA and/or RNA) from the biological sample of interest. This step is followed by library preparation, during which nucleic acid is fragmented, and short adapter sequences are ligated onto the ends of the fragments to permit PCR amplification and binding to the sequencer flow cell. Samples are typically barcoded to enable multiplexing. Long-read (e.g., Oxford nanopore, Oxford, UK) and short-read (e.g., Illumina, San Diego, CA, USA) sequencing platforms can be used clinically, with turnaround times ranging from 6 h to several days depending on instrumentation, degree of sample multiplexing, and infrastructure [17].

Prior to analysis, raw sequencing reads must be demultiplexed based on barcodes, filtered for quality and complexity, and trimmed to remove adapters and barcodes. The resulting sequencing data contains both host and non-host (i.e., microbial) components, which vary in proportions depending on type of biological specimen, though host data often represent the vast majority. The host reads can either be discarded from further analysis or, in the case of RNA sequencing, analyzed to assess host gene expression. To identify microbial taxa present in the sample, non-host sequences are aligned to reference databases, such as the NCBI nucleotide database, containing reference pathogen genomes. In cases of novel pathogens, reference database alignment will be imperfect, but generally capable of providing insight regarding the most similarly related microbes. Alternatively, to detect species and strains that might not be present in the reference database, a *de novo* assembly and annotation approach can be taken.

Additionally, quantification can be performed to estimate the relative abundance of different taxonomic groups, and functional analysis can be carried out (Fig. 2.1). Functional analysis can involve the identification of antimicrobial resistance and/or virulence factor genes, using for example publicly available databases.

## 2.4 DNA Sequencing vs. RNA Sequencing

DNA sequencing is considered the usual method of choice for the detection of pathogens in a range of different sample types [18] because it targets all DNA present in a sample and will capture non-actively transcribed or non-functional genes as well, providing additional taxonomic and functional information. However, DNA sequencing will not allow detection of RNA viruses, as only DNA will be amplified during the sequencing process. Conversely, metatranscriptomics can be used to detect RNA as well as replicating DNA viruses and might thus allow a broader detection of pathogens. For the detection of bacterial species when performing RNA sequencing, even though more bacterial sequences will be detected, differences in bacterial transcript abundances might lead to fewer species being detected as a species might be contributing more transcripts than others [19]. To add more complexity, organisms detected via DNA sequencing might not reflect active infection, but may instead represent nonviable organisms and/or environmental deposition [20]. For researchers interested in the interplay between pathogens and the host response, RNA sequencing enables simultaneous sequencing of pathogens and host gene expression from a single sample to provide a comprehensive snapshot of interactions [21].

While each sequencing approach provides complementary and valuable information, conducting both DNA and RNA sequencing is often prohibitively expensive and/or time-consuming. In essence, the decision to sequence one or the other should be carefully considered in the early phases of the project and should be based on the questions and samples of interest.

## 2.5 Proof of Concept and Clinical Trial Data for Metagenomic Diagnostics

Metagenomic strategies have been successfully used for the diagnosis of infections in critically ill patients using a variety of sample types, such as cerebrospinal fluid (CSF) to identify meningitis and/or encephalitis [22–24], circulating blood to identify sepsis [18, 24], and respiratory samples (tracheal aspirate [25] and bronchoalveolar lavage [BAL] [23, 24]) to diagnose lower respiratory tract infections, among others.

In one of the initial demonstrations of the clinical utility of this approach, metagenomics for diagnosis of central nervous system infections in CSF samples was investigated in 204 severely ill hospitalized patients [22]; 58 infections were identified, 13 of which had not been identified via clinical testing but were solely diagnosed using metagenomics testing. In seven of these cases, the results of metagenomics testing led to clinically impactful changes in antibiotic treatment (i.e., extension, narrowing, or adjusting of spectrum) and enabled timely resolution of the infection. Notably, metagenomic testing also had a significant false negative rate, with 26/58 (45%) clinically confirmed infections not detected by metagenomic sequencing. Gu and colleagues [23] reported the results of metagenomic sequencing in 182 samples from 160 patients with acute illness, with comparison to culture and PCR testing as the gold standard for infection diagnosis. Body fluid samples included abscess aspirate, synovial fluid, pleural fluid, ascites, CSF, BAL, and others. In this dataset, the sensitivity of metagenomic sequencing for bacterial infection ranged from 75% to 79% (depending on the sequencing method), with specificity of 81–91%, with even higher sensitivity and specificity for fungal species. With the important exception of plasma, metagenomic sequencing appeared to perform well across body fluid sample types studied.

The diagnostic utility of metagenomics has also been studied in sepsis. In one cohort of 350 patients [18] a 94% concordance between blood culture and plasma-based metagenomics testing was reported. Metagenomics also permitted the identification of disease-causing organisms in more cases than culture (169 vs. 132, respectively). In another study of 193 patients with sepsis, a higher rate of pathogen detection was reported using metagenomics (85%) when compared to culture (31%) [24]. In that study, concordance for metagenomics testing and culture was 30%, and 55% of microbial species were detected solely with metagenomics. These results were consistent across several samples, including CSF, circulating blood, and BAL. Of note, in this study, metagenomics showed high detection rates for bacteria and viruses, but lower rates than culture when considering fungal species such as *Candida*.

Metagenomics has also been evaluated for the diagnosis of lower respiratory tract infections in the ICU using BAL samples. In one study of 22 hematopoietic stem cell transplant patients [25], identification of a putative pathogen was reported in 12 patients; 6 had not been detected using routine clinical diagnostic tests. Another larger study of lower respiratory tract infection in 92 patients with acute respiratory failure found that metagenomic analyses of tracheal aspirate could identify pathogens with 96% accuracy compared to culture, and also identify putative missed pathogens in over 60% of cases with clinically suspected lower respiratory tract infection but negative standard of care microbiologic testing [26]. More recently, a similar study focusing on children with lower respiratory tract infection investigated the use of metagenomics for diagnosis and pathogen identification in 397 individuals [27]. In that analysis, the disease-causing organism was identified in 92% of lower respiratory tract infection cases, and the integration of clinical testing and metagenomics enabled a diagnosis in 90% of cases vs. 67% for routinely ordered testing.

**Table 2.2** Case examples using metagenomics for the diagnosis of infectious disease and identification of disease-causing organisms

| Disease of interest | Samples | Studies [Ref] |
|---|---|---|
| CNS infection | CSF | Wilson et al. [22]<br>Gu et al. [23] |
| Sepsis | Plasma | Blauwkamp et al. [18]<br>Ren et al. [24]<br>Kalantar et al. [16] |
| Respiratory infection | BAL<br>Pleural fluid<br>Tracheal aspirate | Gu et al. [23]<br>Langelier et al. [25]<br>Langelier et al. [26]<br>Tsitsiklis et al. [27] |
| Abscess | Abscess fluid | Gu et al. [23] |
| Peritonitis | Peritoneal fluid | Gu et al. [23] |
| Urinary tract infection | Urine | Gu et al. [23] |
| Septic arthritis | Joint fluid | Gu et al. [23] |

*CNS* central nervous system, *CSF* cerebrospinal fluid, *BAL* bronchoalveolar lavage

An overview of these studies and selected additional exemplary clinical investigations of metagenomic studies is presented in Table 2.2.

## 2.6 Metagenomics for Prediction of Pathogen Antimicrobial Resistance

Antimicrobial resistance is one of the most urgent threats to human health and a major challenge for managing infections in the ICU [28, 29]. Historically, detection of antimicrobial resistant pathogens has necessitated phenotypic susceptibility testing of clinician-ordered bacterial cultures. Direct detection of antimicrobial resistance gene products through metagenomics offers an opportunity to overcome the limitations of culture by directly detecting the pathogen genes conferring antimicrobial resistance. Databases such as the Comprehensive Antibiotic Resistance Gene Database (CARD) [30] can map reads to known antimicrobial resistance genes from a diverse set of organisms [31]. Further, some bioinformatics pipelines, such as the ID-seq pipeline [32], enable integrated taxonomic and antimicrobial resistance gene identification. Metagenomics has been employed in hospital settings to study the distribution of resistant organisms [33–35], and a recent proof of concept study demonstrated utility for antimicrobial resistance prediction in critically ill patients with pneumonia [29]. Advances in machine learning algorithms may ultimately enable genotype to phenotype prediction for a broad range of organisms, although limitations in genome coverage of low abundance resistance genes in metagenomic datasets are currently an important barrier to overcome [36]. Metagenomics holds promise for expanding the functionality of existing public health surveillance systems by enabling surveillance for known and emerging antimicrobial resistant pathogens in the hospital, community, and environment [31].

## 2.7 Assessing the Host Response to Enhance Metagenomic Pathogen Detection

In most metagenomic approaches, only host or only microbial data is generated and analyzed, permitting *either* the detection of microbial species *or* the profiling of the host response. However, capturing *both* components with RNA sequencing, which can enable pathogen detection *and* profiling of the host response, can provide a more complete picture of the complex interplay between pathogens and host. In the context of infection, it can be challenging to distinguish commensals from disease-causing organisms; however, combining pathogen identification data with host response profiling can help with this distinction.

Two recent studies have reported approaches integrating microbe and host response to improve diagnosis and understand infectious diseases in lower respiratory tract infections and sepsis, respectively [25, 16]. In the study of 92 respiratory failure patients described earlier [25], a combined microbe and host signature was employed to distinguish lower respiratory tract infections from non-infectious etiologies of respiratory failure in tracheal aspirate samples. This approach also identified pathogens and recognizing pathogens from commensal organisms, because of the complimentary of the datasets, was further enhanced by integrating the host-derived data. In integrating host and microbe data, cases of infection were diagnosed with high accuracy (96%). Another recent study took a similar approach to sepsis diagnostics, integrating host and microbe data from blood metagenomic and metatranscriptomic sequencing of 221 critically ill patients for a diagnosis of sepsis and identification of pathogens in blood samples [16]. Notably, the integrated metagenomic model identified 99% of sepsis cases with positive microbiology, predicted sepsis in 74% of the suspected sepsis cases with negative conventional microbiology, and was consistent with a diagnosis of sepsis in 89% of unclear sepsis cases. Furthermore, patients without sepsis were correctly predicted as non-sepsis with a specificity of 78%, highlighting the model's potential utility as a rule-out diagnostic test. This proof-of-concept study highlighted the potential of integrating host and microbe data to diagnose sepsis and identify relevant pathogens, especially for cases without positive microbiology or more complex cases.

## 2.8 Metagenomics: Potential Hurdles and Important Considerations

In addition to choosing the sample to perform the sequencing on and the type of sequencing (DNA- vs. RNA-sequencing), there are some limitations, challenges, and important questions to consider when considering a metagenomics-based approach for the detection of pathogens in the ICU. First, metagenomics-based approaches permit the detection of not only relevant pathogens, but also all low abundance commensal and environmental contaminating organisms that may be present in a sample. Identifying commensal organisms is especially relevant in the context of non-sterile-site samples (e.g., lung and gut) that contain complex microbial backgrounds, as opposed to typically sterile samples such as CSF. Recent advances in algorithms to distinguish pathogenic microbes from commensal or contaminating organisms have been an important step to interpreting the significance of the hundreds of microbial alignments that result from analysis. One algorithm, for example, is designed to identify disproportionately abundant microbes within samples and only report those with established pathogenicity [25]. For all samples, to ensure the taxonomic alignments detected are relevant and not due to environmental contaminants, both negative (water or synthetic matrix) and positive controls must be included and processed in the same way as test samples [37].

Second, the proportion of host-derived sequences in metagenomic data can be quite high, ranging from 10% (gut) to over 95% (respiratory) of total sequences depending on the anatomical site of sampling [38]. If the goal of sequencing is to detect pathogens alone, then increasing coverage by generating more sequencing reads or using targeted enrichment methods [39] should be considered, though these approaches will increase cost and complexity. A larger proportion of host nucleotide sequences will lead to decreased sensitivity for microbial detection due to lower coverage of non-host sequences [40].

Third, metagenomics remains a costly diagnostic approach that has not yet been incorporated into standard of care in most clinical settings. Despite an increased cost with respect to culture- or PCR-based methods, clinically practical metagenomics assays have comparable costs (~2000 US dollars) to a computed tomography (CT) scan with contrast. While this cost is still a major barrier in many settings, particularly in low- and middle-income countries, sequencing costs continue to decrease each year as technology improves [41]. Historically, intensive computational requirements have also been a barrier to the broader clinical use of metagenomics assays; however, the availability of free, cloud-based bioinformatics pipelines [32] has democratized the bioinformatics steps needed to go from sequence to pathogen identification.

## 2.9 Conclusion

Despite promising results, metagenomics remains underutilized in the ICU. Several factors still limit its inclusion in routine critical care, including the lack of definitive clinical trials testing its utility, few laboratories with the infrastructure needed to afford rapid turnaround, cost in low resource settings, and the fact that few metagenomics assays have undergone the clinical validation needed to permit use in patient care. These barriers will need to be overcome before wide adoption of metagenomics into clinical practice. However, an increasing number of studies are demonstrating the potential utility of metagenomics in a range of settings relevant to critically ill patients. Moving forward, a gradual inclusion of metagenomics into current clinical diagnosis pipelines, starting from a complementary inclusion along with currently used tests in severely ill patients, may demonstrate the full potential of this technology in the ICU.

## References

1. WHO. The top 10 causes of death. Available at: https://www.who.int/news-room/fact-sheets/detail/the-top-10-causes-of-death. Accessed 28 Jun 2022.
2. Jain S, Self WH, Wunderink RG, et al. Community-acquired pneumonia requiring hospitalization among U.S. adults. N Engl J Med. 2015;373:415–27.
3. Nannan Panday RS, Lammers EMJ, Alam N, Nanayakkara PWB. An overview of positive cultures and clinical outcomes in septic patients: a sub-analysis of the Prehospital Antibiotics Against Sepsis (PHANTASi) trial. Crit Care. 2019;23:182.
4. Nannan Panday RS, Wang S, van de Ven PM, Hekker TAM, Alam N, Nanayakkara PWB. Evaluation of blood culture epidemiology and efficiency in a large European teaching hospital. PLoS One. 2019;14:e0214052.
5. Baur D, Gladstone BP, Burkert F, et al. Effect of antibiotic stewardship on the incidence of infection and colonisation with antibiotic-resistant bacteria and Clostridium difficile infection: a systematic review and meta-analysis. Lancet Infect Dis. 2017;17:990–1001.
6. Edgeworth J. Antibiotic resistance in the ICU. In: Webb A, Angus D, Finfer S, Gattinoni L, Singer M, editors. Oxford Textbook of Critical Care. 2nd ed. Oxford: Oxford Academic; 2016. p. 1378–81.
7. Lai CC, Chen SY, Ko WC, Hsueh PR. Increased antimicrobial resistance during the COVID-19 pandemic. Int J Antimicrob Agents. 2021;57:106324.
8. Lansbury LE, Rodrigo C, Leonardi-Bee J, Nguyen-Van-Tam J, Shen Lim W. Corticosteroids as adjunctive therapy in the treatment of influenza: an updated Cochrane systematic review and meta-analysis. Crit Care Med. 2020;48:e98–e106.
9. Chun K, Syndergaard C, Damas C, et al. Sepsis pathogen identification. SLAS Technol. 2015;20:539–61.
10. Beekmann SE, Diekema DJ, Chapin KC, Doern GV. Effects of rapid detection of bloodstream infections on length of hospitalization and hospital charges. J Clin Microbiol. 2003;41:3119–25.
11. Kumar A, Roberts D, Wood KE, et al. Duration of hypotension before initiation of effective antimicrobial therapy is the critical determinant of survival in human septic shock. Crit Care Med. 2006;34:1589–96.
12. Fenollar F. Raoult D Molecular diagnosis of bloodstream infections caused by non-cultivable bacteria. Int J Antimicrob Agents. 2007;30:7–15.
13. Peeling RW, Wedderburn CJ, Garcia PJ, et al. Serology testing in the COVID-19 pandemic response. Lancet Infect Dis. 2020;20:e245–9.
14. Liesenfeld O, Lehman L, Hunfeld KP, Kost G. Molecular diagnosis of sepsis: new aspects and recent developments. Eur J Microbiol Immunol. 2014;4:1–25.
15. FDA Center for Devices and Radiological Health. Nucleic acid based tests. Available at: https://www.fda.gov/medical-devices/in-vitro-diagnostics/nucleic-acid-based-tests#microbial. Accessed 28 Jun 2022.
16. Kalantar K, Neyton L, Abdelghany M, et al. Integrated host-microbe plasma metagenomics for sepsis diagnosis in a prospective cohort of critically ill adults. Nat Microbiol. 2022;7:1805–16.
17. Simner PJ, Miller S, Carroll KC. Understanding the promises and hurdles of metagenomic next-generation sequencing as a diagnostic tool for infectious diseases. Clin Infect Dis. 2018;66:778–88.
18. Blauwkamp TA, Thair S, Rosen MJ, et al. Analytical and clinical validation of a microbial cell-free DNA sequencing test for infectious disease. Nat Microbiol. 2019;4:663–74.
19. Arroyo Mühr LS, Dillner J, Ure AE, Sundström K, Hultin E. Comparison of DNA and RNA sequencing of total nucleic acids from human cervix for metagenomics. Sci Rep. 2021;11:18852.
20. Hultin E, Mühr LSA, Lagheden C, Dillner J. HPV transcription in skin tumors. PLoS One. 2019;14:e0217942.

21. Westermann AJ, Gorski SA, Vogel J. Dual RNA-seq of pathogen and host. Nat Rev Microbiol. 2012;10:618–30.
22. Wilson MR, Sample HA, Zorn KC, et al. Clinical metagenomic sequencing for diagnosis of meningitis and encephalitis. N Engl J Med. 2019;380:2327–40.
23. Gu W, Deng X, Lee M, et al. Rapid pathogen detection by metagenomic next-generation sequencing of infected body fluids. Nat Med. 2021;27:115–24.
24. Ren D, Ren C, Yao R, et al. The microbiological diagnostic performance of metagenomic next-generation sequencing in patients with sepsis. BMC Infect Dis. 2021;21:1257.
25. Langelier C, Kalantar KL, Moazed F, et al. Integrating host response and unbiased microbe detection for lower respiratory tract infection diagnosis in critically ill adults. Proc Natl Acad Sci U S A. 2018;115:E12353–62.
26. Langelier C, Zinter MS, Kalantar K, et al. Metagenomic sequencing detects respiratory pathogens in hematopoietic cellular transplant patients. Am J Respir Crit Care Med. 2018;197:524–8.
27. Tsitsiklis A, Osborne CM, Kamm J, et al. Lower respiratory tract infections in children requiring mechanical ventilation: a multicentre prospective surveillance study incorporating airway metagenomics. Lancet Microbe. 2022;3:e284–93.
28. Brusselaers N, Vogelaers D, Blot S. The rising problem of antimicrobial resistance in the intensive care unit. Ann Intensive Care. 2011;1:47.
29. Serpa PH, Deng X, Abdelghany M, et al. Metagenomic prediction of antimicrobial resistance in critically ill patients with lower respiratory tract infections. Genome Med. 2022;14:74.
30. McArthur AG, Waglechner N, Nizam F, et al. The comprehensive antibiotic resistance database. Antimicrob Agents Chemother. 2013;57:3348–57.
31. Hendriksen RS, Bortolaia V, Tate H, Tyson GH, Aarestrup FM, McDermott PF. Using genomics to track global antimicrobial resistance. Front Public Health. 2019;7:242.
32. Kalantar KL, Carvalho T, de Bourcy CFA, et al. IDseq—an open source cloud-based pipeline and analysis service for metagenomic pathogen detection and monitoring. GigaScience. 2020;9:giaa111.
33. Brooks B, Olm MR, Firek BA, et al. Strain-resolved analysis of hospital rooms and infants reveals overlap between the human and room microbiome. Nat Commun. 2017;8:1814.
34. Chng KR, Li C, Bertrand D, et al. Cartography of opportunistic pathogens and antibiotic resistance genes in a tertiary hospital environment. Nat Med. 2020;26:941–51.
35. Charalampous T, Alcolea-Medina A, Snell LB, et al. Evaluating the potential for respiratory metagenomics to improve treatment of secondary infection and detection of nosocomial transmission on expanded COVID-19 intensive care units. Genome Med. 2021;13:182.
36. Nguyen M, Long SW, McDermott PF, et al. Using machine learning to predict antimicrobial MICs and associated genomic features for nontyphoidal Salmonella. J Clin Microbiol. 2019;57:e01260–18.
37. Dickson RP, Singer BH, Newstead MW, et al. Enrichment of the lung microbiome with gut bacteria in sepsis and the acute respiratory distress syndrome. Nat Microbiol. 2016;1:1–9.
38. Lloyd-Price J, Mahurkar A, Rahnavard G, et al. Strains, functions and dynamics in the expanded Human Microbiome Project. Nature. 2017;550:61–6.
39. Quan J, Langelier C, Kuchta A, et al. FLASH: a next-generation CRISPR diagnostic for multiplexed detection of antimicrobial resistance sequences. Nucleic Acids Res. 2019;47:e83.
40. Pereira-Marques J, Hout A, Ferreira RM, et al. Impact of host DNA and sequencing depth on the taxonomic resolution of whole metagenome sequencing for microbiome analysis. Front Microbiol. 2019;10:1277.
41. National Human Genome Research Institute. The cost of sequencing a human genome. Available at: https://www.genome.gov/about-genomics/fact-sheets/Sequencing-Human-Genome-cost. Accessed 6 Sep 2022.

# Risk Stratification and Precision Medicine: Is It Feasible for Severe Infections?

3

E. J. Giamarellos-Bourboulis, M. Mouktaroudi, and M. G. Netea

## 3.1 Introduction

According to the definition provided by the USA Food and Drug Administration (FDA) "Precision medicine, sometimes known as 'personalized medicine' is an innovative approach to tailoring disease prevention and treatment that takes into account differences in people's genes, environments, and lifestyles" [1]. In other terms, although patients with a disease may appear phenotypically similar, the mechanism underlying the disease may be different and require different treatment. The main challenge is how this approach may easily be implemented in everyday clinical practice in patients with severe infections when decision-making should be fast. In this chapter, we discuss developments over the last 5 years towards application of the principles of precision medicine for severe infections. We present current knowledge on endotypes, the use of biomarkers for risk classification, the development of biomarkers informing on the mechanisms of disease, and the published trials of precision interventions guided by biomarkers. The two main severe infections that will be discussed are sepsis and severe coronavirus disease 2019 (COVID-19).

E. J. Giamarellos-Bourboulis (✉) · M. Mouktaroudi
4th Department of Internal Medicine, National and Kapodistrian University of Athens, Medical School, Athens, Greece
e-mail: egiamarel@med.uoa.gr

M. G. Netea
Department of Internal Medicine and Radboud Center for Infectious Diseases, Radboud University, Nijmegen, The Netherlands

Department of Immunology and Metabolism, Life and Medical Sciences Institute, University of Bonn, Bonn, Germany



J.-L. Vincent (ed.), *Annual Update in Intensive Care and Emergency Medicine 2023*, Annual Update in Intensive Care and Emergency Medicine,
https://doi.org/10.1007/978-3-031-23005-9_3

## 3.2 Endotypes of Severe Infections

The classification of patients with severe infection into separate groups of pathophysiology requires clustering into disease endotypes. This can be achieved only through the extensive analysis of gene expression and the definition of the main pathways that determine disease severity. In sepsis there are two published studies that have associated unfavorable outcome with endotypes. Both studies included discovery and validation cohorts. In the discovery cohorts, transcriptomic analysis was applied in whole blood samples from patients. Then, using systems biology and bioinformatics, endotypes of pathways associated with unfavorable outcome were identified. Finally, results were confirmed in the validation cohorts in which patients were clustered according to endotypes and unfavorable outcome analyzed per endotype.

The first publication was from the GAiNS (UK Genomic Advances in Sepsis) study. Enrolled patients had sepsis as a result of community-acquired pneumonia and were divided into a discovery cohort (n = 270) and a validation cohort (n = 114). Two transcriptomic sepsis-response signatures (SRS) were identified; SRS1 and SRS2. The predominant mechanisms expressed among patients with the SRS1 endotype were downregulation of the major histocompatibility complex II and human leukocyte antigen (HLA)-DR, integrins, and cell adhesion, and differentiation of the immune response. Patients with SRS1 had worse outcomes than those with SRS2 [2]. In the second study, Scicluna et al. identified four endotypes by analyzing the transcriptomic profile and clinical data from patients enrolled in the Molecular Diagnosis and Risk Stratification of Sepsis (MARS) study [3]. One discovery cohort with 306 patients, one validation cohort with 216 patients from the MARS study, and another validation cohort with 265 patients from the GAiNS study were included. Patients were classified into four endotypes, namely Mars1 to Mars 4. The Mars1 endotype was characterized by a pronounced decrease of several immune function mechanisms, including pattern recognition receptor signaling, cytokine signaling, and T-cell receptor signaling. In the discovery and both validation cohorts, patients with the Mars1 endotype had the worse outcome.

Published data from patients with severe COVID-19 involved significantly lower numbers of patients compared to publications of sepsis patients. In one study with 39 participants (7 patients with mild disease, 10 patients with moderate/severe disease, and 12 patients with critical disease), it was not possible to classify distinct endotypes as significant overlap in gene expression was found between patients with mild, moderate, and severe disease. However, critically ill patients were clearly distinct with the upregulation of *FCGR1A*, *GBP1*, *GBP2*, *IRF7*, *STAT1*, *TAP1*, and *TLR2* genes and the downregulation of *BCL2*, *CCL4*, *CN8A*, *GNLY*, and *IL7R* genes [4]. In another study of 39 patients with COVID-19, the transcriptomic profile of the granulocytes enabled classification into six endotypes, namely G1 to G6. Worse outcomes were observed for patients with endotypes G2 and G3. A total of 2289 genes were upregulated and 912 genes downregulated compared to healthy controls. In the first 10 days after onset of symptoms, patients with severe disease had 314 upregulated and 703 downregulated genes compared to patients with mild disease. However, on days 11–20 after onset of symptoms, these genes increased to

445 and 1924 respectively [5]. The authors managed to integrate this information into decision-making. Using artificial intelligence, they provided the best candidate drug for every patient according to his or her needs as defined by the gene expression profile.

## 3.3 How to Transfer Endotypes into Everyday Clinical Practice

In everyday clinical reality, endotyping cannot yet be run real-time. A full transcriptomic analysis and bioinformatics processing requires a lot of time, and the time course of severe infection is rapid. One approach would be to select single genes or a set of genes that are diagnostic of one specific endotype and develop them into one diagnostic platform. It is likely that the selected genes may be different in sepsis than in COVID-19. The data from the GAiNS and MARS studies revealed that the endotypes associated with the worse outcomes were those which provided information on sepsis-induced immunoparalysis, an entity known to infer deterioration of the host with susceptibility for secondary infections and high mortality [6]. One approach to characterize sepsis-induced immunoparalysis is measurement of copies of the interleukin (IL)-7 receptor and namely of the transcripts encoding for the membrane form of CD127 and of the soluble form of sCD127. Both these compounds are decreased in non-survivors and fewer than 0.20 transcripts of the membrane form by day 3 is independently associated with an unfavorable outcome [7]. Using the same reasoning, an immune profiling panel has been developed integrating information from 16 genes. Results in septic shock showed that the expression of *CD3D*, *CD74*, *CX3CR1* and *IFNγ* genes was decreased and the expression of *IL-10* and *S100A9* genes was increased in patients with sepsis-induced immunoparalysis [8].

Sweeny et al. followed an entirely new approach using data from three previously published cohorts. The discovery set included patients with community-acquired infections from seven different countries; the first validation set was patients with community-acquired infections from three different countries; and the second validation set was patients with hospital-acquired infections from the United States [9]. A set of 33 genes was selected, which can be informative of both the predominant mechanism of pathophysiology and of the outcome. These genes were classified into three endotypes, namely inflammopathic, adaptive, and coagulopathic. Classification into the inflammopathic endotype included the expression of five genes (*ARG1*, *LCN2*, *LTF*, *OLFM4*, *HLA-DMB*), into the adaptive endotype included the expression of 17 genes (*YKT6*, *PDE4B*, *TWISTNB*, *BTN2A2*, *ZBTB33*, *PSMB9*, *CAMK4*, *TMEM19*, *SLC12A7*, *TP53BP1*, *PLEKHO1*, *SLC25A22*, *FRS2*, *GADD45A*, *CD24*, *S100A12*, *STX1A*), and into the coagulopathic endotype included the expression of 12 genes (*KCNMB4*, *CRISP2*, *HTRA1*, *PPL*, *RHBDF2*, *ZCCHC4*, *YKT6*, *DDX6*, *SENP5*, *RAPGEF1*, *DTX2*, *RELB*). This endotyping was associated with 28-day mortality rates of 29.3%, 18.5%, and 31.1%, respectively, in sepsis [10]. However, mortality rates among patients with severe COVID-19 were different, being 29%, 42%, and 27%, for the three endotypes, respectively [11]. Finally, analysis of the G1 to G6 neutrophil specific transcripts of COVID-19 shows that patients with severe disease over-express *CD177* and *S100A12* compared to patients with mild disease [5].

## 3.4 Protein Biomarkers for Unselected Risk Classification

It is always interesting to investigate how one easily measurable protein biomarker can develop into a laboratory test to predict the likelihood of unfavorable outcome. However, this is often done in an unsophisticated manner without focusing on the association between the candidate molecule and the mechanism of the disease. More than 258 protein molecules have been suggested as biomarkers of sepsis [12]. We narrowed our search in the PubMed database to the last 5 years and used the terms "risk stratification AND sepsis". The search retrieved 164 publications. After excluding case-studies, editorials, reviews, and meta-analyses we narrowed the list to 25 publications. Among these publications, only six classified patients with sepsis using biomarkers that were informative of the underlying mechanism of disease progression. A synopsis of these publications is provided in Table 3.1 [13–18]. Studies in small cohorts showed that increases in mciroRNA-122 were associated with hepatobiliary dysfunction [13], increases in angiopoietin-2 were associated with disseminated intravascular coagulation (DIC) [14], and increases in calprotectin were associated with excess stimulation by circulating danger-associated molecular patterns (DAMPs) [15].

Two main approaches towards the classification of the underlying immune mechanism need to be cited because they are built on cohorts with large numbers of patients. The first approach is for the diagnosis of sepsis-induced immunoparalysis as described in two publications. The first study analyzed 189 patients from the REALISM study and developed the REALIST score. In this score, every patient is given one point for each of the following: 23.5% or more of immature neutrophils; serum IL-10 ≥8.5 pg/ml; and 7627 or fewer HLA-DR receptors per CD14-monocyte. The incidence of secondary infections by day 30 for patients scoring 0, 1, 2 and 3 points was 8.2%, 11.9%, 30.6%, and 46.0%, respectively [16]. The second study analyzed the change in HLA-DR/CD14-monocytes. According to the authors, fewer than 8000 receptors was the diagnostic cut-off for sepsis-induced immunnoparalysis. Patients with a significant decrease in HLA-DR/CD14-monocyte over the first 3 days had a 61% risk of developing secondary infection [17].

The second classification approach is for the diagnosis of cytokine storm or macrophage activation-like syndrome. This entity is characterized by hepatobiliary dysfunction and DIC and is associated with early death in the first 10 days. Using a test cohort of 3417 patients, a validation cohort of 1704 patients from Greece, and another small validation cohort of 109 patients from Sweden, circulating ferritin >4420 ng/ml classified macrophage activation-like syndrome with 97.1% specificity and 98.0% negative predictive value. Mortality after 28 days for patients with ferritin >4420 ng/ml was 66.0% in the test cohort, 66.7% in the Greek validation cohort, and 52.9% in the Swedish validation cohort. Macrophage activation-like

**Table 3.1** Main biomarkers informative of the mechanism of disease progression in sepsis. Analysis refers to studies published between 2017 and 2022

| Authors [Ref] | Design | Groups | Criteria for sepsis diagnosis | Biomarker studied | Risk stratification | Association with mechanism |
|---|---|---|---|---|---|---|
| Rahmel et al. [13] | Prospective | 108 pts with sepsis | Sepsis-3 | miR-122 | Sixfold increase in non-survivors | Liver damage (↑ AST, ALT, LDH) |
| Statz et al. [14] | Retrospective | 102 pts with sepsis | Sepsis-2 | Ang-2 | Increase in non-survivors | Overt DIC |
| Dubois et al. [15] | Prospective | 49 pts with septic shock | Sepsis-3 | S100A8/S100A9 and S100A12 | Predictive of 7-day mortality | Increased circulating DAMPs |
| Tremblay et al. [16] | Prospective | 189 pts with sepsis | Sepsis-3 | REALISTIC score integrating immature PMNs, IL-10 and mHLA-DR | HR 4.41 for secondary infections with score 3 | Sepsis-induced immunoparalysis |
| De Roquetaillade et al. [17] | Prospective | 592 ICU admissions | Sepsis-3 | High slope of decrease of mHLA-DR the first 3 days | HR 1.61 for secondary infection | Sepsis-induced immunoparalysis |
| Kyriazopoulou et al. [18] | Retrospective | 5121 pts from Greece; 109 pts from Sweden | Sepsis-3 | Ferritin >4420 ng/ml | 66.0% 28-day mortality | Macrophage activation-like syndrome |

*ALT* alanine aminotransferase, *Ang* angiopoietin, *AST* aspartate aminotransferase, *DAMP* danger-associated molecular patterns, *DIC* disseminated intravascular coagulation, *HR* hazard ratio, *IL* interleukin, *LDH* lactate dehydrogenase, *mHLA-DR* membrane expression of human leukocyte antigen-DR on CD14-monocytes by flow cytometry, *PMNs* polymorphonuclear neutrophils, *pts* patients syndrome was an independent entity for early mortality also when patients presented with acute respiratory distress syndrome (ARDS), shock, or acute kidney injury (AKI) [18].

Regarding risk stratification for COVID-19, we searched the PubMed database using the terms "risk stratification AND COVID-19". The search retrieved 253 results. After excluding case-studies, editorials, reviews and meta-analyses we narrowed down to five publications providing prognostic risk classification for hospitalized patients with COVID-19 [19–23]. The main risk classifiers are given in Table 3.2. However, the only biomarkers for which some mechanistic insight was

**Table 3.2** Main biomarkers associated with risk stratification in COVID-19. Analysis refers to studies published between 2017 and 2022

| Authors [Ref] | Design | Groups | Biomarker studied | Risk stratification |
|---|---|---|---|---|
| Sharifpour et al. [19] | Prospective | 268 hospitalized pts | CRP | Sensitivity 95.5% for mortality when 150 mg/l or more |
| de Guadiana-Romualdo et al. [20] | Prospective | 359 hospitalized pts | MR-proADM | AUC of ROC for 90-day mortality greater than AUC of ROC of PCT, IL-6 and lymphocyte count |
| Stefanini et al. [21] | Prospective | 397 hospitalized pts | TnI, BNP | Mortality 55.6% when TnI+/BNP+; 22.5% when TnI+/BNP-; 33.9% when TnI-/BNP+; 6.3% when TnI-/BNP- |
| Singh et al. [22] | Prospective | 276 hospitalized pts | TnT ≥17 ng/ml | OR 2.35 for in-hospital mortality, intubation or cardiac arrest |
| Laguna-Goya et al. [23] | Prospective | 276 hospitalized pts | Score by: IL-6 >86 pg/ml; NLR >6.5; LDH >424 U/l; $SpO_2$/$FiO_2$ >211 | AUC 0.94 for classification of non-survivors |
| Rovina et al. [24] | Prospective | 57 hospitalized pts | suPAR ≥6 ng/ml | OR 66.0 for SRF/death the first 14 days |
| Azam et al. [25] | Prospective | 352 hospitalized pts | suPAR tertiles (<4.60 ng/ml; 4.60–6.86 ng/ml; >6.87 ng/ml) | OR second tertile vs. first tertile 5.42 for AKI<br>OR third tertile vs. first tertile 13.25 for AKI<br>OR 2.49 of suPAR as continuous variable for SRF |
| Vasbinder et al. [26] | Prospective | 2044 hospitalized pts | suPAR ≥14.8 ng/ml | 53.8% incidence of SRF, need for renal replacement therapy or death among patients with DM2 |

– not increased, + increased, *AUC* area under the curve, *BNP* brain natriuretic peptide, *CRP* C-reactive protein, *DM2* type 2 diabetes mellitus, $FiO_2$ fraction of inspired oxygen, *IL* interleukin, *LDH* lactate dehydrogenase, *MR-proADM* pro-adrenomedullin, *NLR* neutrophil to lymphocyte ratio, *NR* not-reported, *OR* odds ratio, *ROC* receiver operating characteristics curve, *PCT* procalcitonin, *pts* patients, $SpO_2$ oxygen saturation, *SRF* severe respiratory failure, *suPAR* soluble urokinase plasminogen activator receptor, *Tn* troponin provided were MR-proADM (pro-adrenomedullin) and troponins, which are indexes of endothelial dysfunction and of myocardial dysfunction, respectively.

The only biomarker identified so far that provides evidence of an underlying mechanism for disease progression in COVID-19 is soluble urokinase plasminogen activator receptor (suPAR). In a small cohort of patients from Greece early in the pandemic, the sensitivity and the positive predictive value of suPAR ≥6 ng/ml for the prediction of progression into severe respiratory failure or death during the first 14 days after hospital admission were 85.7% [24]. The early increase in suPAR as a classifier of risk of death or of COVID-19-associated adverse events was later validated in larger cohorts [25, 26]. However, suPAR is not just a classifier of risk in COVID-19 but it is also the only biomarker, so far, which is informative of activation of the IL-1 pathway. Patients with suPAR ≥6 ng/ml have increased circulating concentrations of the DAMP, calprotectin. The injection into mice of calprotectin-enriched plasma from patients with increased suPAR concentrations, leads to organ-specific inflammation of the lung and of the colon, but sparing the liver and the kidney [27]. Administration of the drug anakinra, a recombinant form of IL-1 receptor antagonist, attenuated the inflammation of the lung and colon. When mice were treated with a calprotectin antibody, lung and colon inflammation were attenuated. These findings suggest that suPAR may be diagnostic of the stimulation of the production of IL-1β from tissue macrophages and IL-1α from the lung [27]. Activation of these pathways leads to severe respiratory failure.

## 3.5 The Use of Biomarkers to Guide Immunotherapy in Severe Infections

Biomarker-guided precision medicine for severe infection is still at the early stage. Four conditions need to be met in order for a biomarker to guide immunotherapy:

- The chosen biomarker is indicative of a specific mechanism that is fundamental for disease progression
- There is one available drug that can modulate the specific mechanism indicated by the biomarker
- The time window from biomarker measurement until start of the immunointervention should be short since the sequence of pathophysiological mechanisms in severe infections changes quickly over-time
- The efficacy and safety of the biomarker-guided immunotherapy is proven through double-blind, placebo-controlled, randomized clinical trials (RCTs)

No such high-level evidence is available for sepsis. However, there is proof-of-concept from the retrospective analysis of patients with septic shock and from case-studies of patients with sepsis-induced immunoparalysis on biomarkers that can maximize the therapeutic efficacy of hydrocortisone and of recombinant human interferon-gamma (rhIFNγ), respectively. Retrospective analysis of 83 patients with septic shock enrolled in the CORTICUS trial showed that patients randomized in the placebo arm had greater chance for survival when the baseline ratio of circulating IFNγ to IL-10 was high. However, the opposite was true for patients treated with low-dose hydrocortisone, who had a better outcome when the ratio of circulating IFNγ to IL-10 before start of treatment was low. This observation was confirmed in two independent validation cohorts [28]. In a case-series of 13 sepsis patients with <8000 HLA-DR receptors/CD14-monocyte, subcutaneous recombinant human IFNγ was administered. Treatment led to an increase to >8000 HLA-DR receptors/CD14-monocyte in nine patients and to a decrease in the sequential organ failure assessment (SOFA) score in 10 patients [29]. Retrospective analysis of data from a large-scale RCT showed that treatment with anakinra of patients with clinical signs compatible with macrophage activation syndrome was associated with a 30% decrease in 28-day mortality [30].

The above evidence should be seen as proof-of-concept that biomarker-guided immunotherapy may be promising for sepsis. However, results from a properly designed and conducted RCT are missing. The ImmunoSep RCT which was launched in August 2021 aims to provide solid proof-of-concept for this precision approach (ClinicalTrials.gov Identifier: NCT04990232). In the ImmunoSep RCT, patients with sepsis due to lung infection or primary bloodstream infection are randomized to treatment with anakinra/rhIFNγ or placebo. Study participants should meet the Sepsis-3 criteria and should have signs of macrophage activation syndrome or sepsis-induced immunoparalysis. Patients are classified as having macrophage activation syndrome if their ferritin concentration is >4420 ng/ml, and as having immunoparalysis if their ferritin concentration is ≤4420 ng/ml and they have <5000 HLA-DR receptors/CD14-monocyte. The study is double-blind and double-dummy and patients are compared according to their allocation to the personalized immunotherapy arm and to the placebo immunotherapy arm.

The SAVE-MORE (suPAR-guided Anakinra treatment for Validation of the risk and Early Management Of seveRE respiratory failure by COVID-19) trial is the only RCT of precision treatment for COVID-19 available so far [31]. The rationale behind this RCT was to use suPAR as a selection tool to enroll patients with evidence of early activation of the IL-1 cascade as described earlier. Study participants were adults with COVID-19 pneumonia in need of hospitalization, receiving oxygen delivered through mask or nasal prongs, and with plasma suPAR ≥6 ng/ml. Patients were randomized to treatment with placebo and standard-of-care (n = 189) or anakinra and standard-of-care (n = 405). The study drug was administered once daily subcutaneously for 10 days; the dose of anakinra was 100 mg. The standard-of-care included dexamethasone 6 mg once daily for 10 days. The primary endpoint was the 11-point of the World Health Organization Clinical Progression Scale (WHO-CPS) on day 28. The results showed that anakinra treatment was accompanied by a 0.36 odds (confidence intervals 0.26–0.50) for worse outcome than placebo treatment ($p < 0.0001$). Analysis of key secondary endpoints showed that anakinra treatment had a 0.62 hazard ratio compared to placebo for progression into severe respiratory failure or death during the first 14 days ($p = 0.005$). Anakinra treatment increased the odds for full COVID-19 resolution by day 28 by 64% and decreased the odds for severe disease or death by day 28 by 54% [31]. These favorable results led to the approval of anakinra treatment by the European Medicines Agency for adults with COVID-19 requiring low or high flow oxygen who are considered at risk as defined by suPAR levels ≥6 ng/ml [32]. The treatment efficacy of anakinra was significantly greater than that of any other drug studied for COVID-19 treatment. This example should be conceived as the real potential of precision treatment.

## 3.6 Conclusion

The background for future steps toward precision management of severe infection has already been set. The positive results of the SAVE-MORE RCT and the registration of anakinra guided by the suPAR biomarker provide evidence of how one precision approach may maximize clinical efficacy. We are not just in need of biomarkers that classify risk but of biomarkers that translate as indexes of the activation of specific immune pathways. Successful RCTs of treatments guided by these biomarkers are anticipated to increase efficacy (Fig. 3.1).

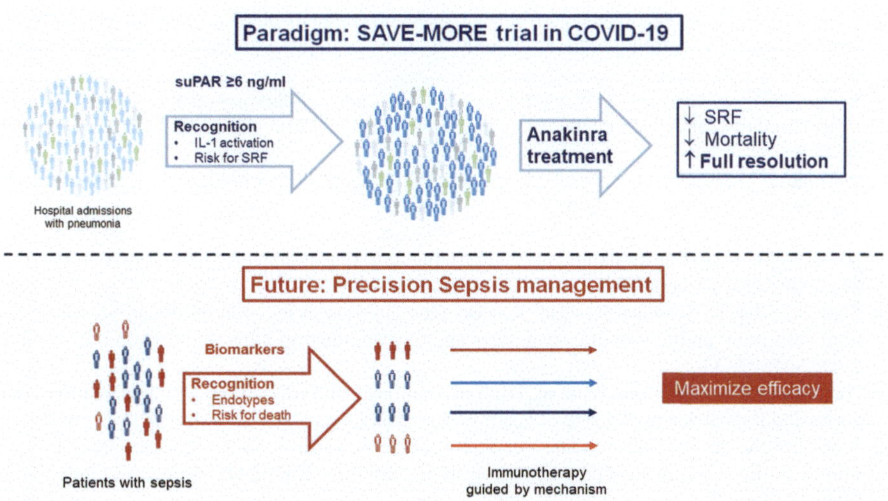


**Fig. 3.1** How the SAVE-MORE trial may guide the future of precision management of sepsis. The increase in soluble urokinase plasminogen activator receptor (suPAR) selects patients at risk or severe respiratory failure (SRF) through early interleukin (IL)-1 activation in coronavirus disease (COVID)-19 pneumonia. This selection guides treatment with anakinra. In a similar approach, patients with sepsis can be stratified into different immune endotypes, which may be recognized by specific biomarkers. This can guide specific immunotherapy aimed at modulating the precise immune mechanism. ↑ increase, ↓ decrease

## References


1. FDA. Precision medicine. Available at: https://www.fda.gov/medical-devices/in-vitro-diagnostics/precision-medicine. Accessed 5 Sep 2022.
2. Davenport EE, Burnham KL, Radhakrishnan J, et al. Genomic landscape of the individual host response and outcomes in sepsis: a prospective cohort study. Lancet Respir Med. 2016;4:259–71.
3. Scicluna BP, van Vught LA, Zwinderman AH, et al. Classification of patients with sepsis according to blood genomic endotype: a prospective cohort study. Lancet Respir Med. 2017;5:816–26.
4. Persson J, Andersson B, van Veen S, et al. Stratification of COVID-19 patients based on quantitative immune-related gene expression in whole blood. Mol Immunol. 2022;145:17–26.
5. Aschenbrenner AC, Mouktaroudi M, Krämer B, et al. Disease severity-specific neutrophil signatures in blood transcriptomes stratify COVID-19 patients. Genome Med. 2021;13:7.
6. Monneret G, Lepape A, Voirin A, et al. Persisting low monocyte human leukocyte antigen-DR expression predicts mortality in septic shock. Intensive Care Med. 2006;32:1175–83.
7. Delwarde B, Peronnet E, Venet F, et al. Low interleukin-7 receptor messenger RNA expression is independently associated with day 28 mortality in septic shock patients. Crit Care Med. 2018;46:1739–46.
8. Tawfik DM, Vachot L, Bocquet A, et al. Immune profiling panel: a proof-of-concept study of a new multiplex molecular tool to assess the immune status of critically ill patients. J Infect Dis. 2020;222(Suppl 2):S84–94.
9. Sweeney TE, Perumal TM, Henao R, et al. A community approach to mortality prediction in sepsis via gene expression analysis. Nat Commun. 2018;9:694.
10. Sweeney TE, Azad TD, Donato M, et al. Unsupervised analysis of transcriptomics in bacterial sepsis across multiple datasets reveals three robust clusters. Crit Care Med. 2018;46: 915–25.
11. Sweeney TE, Liesenfeld O, Wacker J, et al. Validation of inflammatopathic, adaptive, and coagulopathic sepsis endotypes in coronavirus disease 2019. Crit Care Med. 2021;49: e170–8.
12. Pierrakos C, Velissaris D, Bisdorff M, Marshall JC, Vincent JL. Biomarkers of sepsis: time for a reappraisal. Crit Care. 2020;24:287.
13. Rahmel T, Schäfer ST, Frey UH, Adamzik M, Peters J. Increased circulating microRNA-122 is a biomarker for discrimination and risk stratification in patients defined by sepsis-3 criteria. PLoS One. 2018;13:e0197637.
14. Statz S, Sabal G, Walborn A, et al. Angiopoietic 2 levels in the risk stratification and mortality outcome prediction of sepsis-associated coagulopathy. Clin Appl Thomb Hemost. 2018;24:1223–33.
15. Dubois C, Marcé D, Faiver V, et al. High plasma level of S100A8/S100A9 and S100A12 at admission indicates a higher risk of death in septic shock patients. Sci Rep. 2019;9:15660.
16. Tremblay JA, Peron F, Kreitmann L, et al. A stratification strategy to predict secondary infection in critical illness-induced immune dysfunction: the REALISTIC score. Ann Intensive Care. 2022;12:76.
17. De Roquetaillade C, Dupuis C, Faivre V, Lukaszewicz AC, Brumpt C, Payen D. Monitoring of circulating monocyte HLA-DR expression in a large cohort of intensive care patients: relation with secondary infections. Ann Intensive Care. 2022;12:39.
18. Kyriazopoulou K, Leventogiannis K, Norrby-Teglund A, et al. Macrophage activation-like syndrome: an immunological entity associated with rapid progression to death in sepsis. BMC Med. 2017;15:172.
19. Sharifpour M, Rangaraju S, Lu M, et al. C-reactive protein as a prognostic indicator in hospitalized patients with COVID-19. PLoS One. 2020;15:e0242400.
20. de Guadiana-Romualdo LC, Martínez Martínez M, Rodríguez MD, et al. Circulating MR-proADM levels, as an indicator of endothelial dysfunction, for early risk stratification of mid-term mortality in COVID-19 patients. Int J Infect Dis. 2021;111:211–8.

21. Stefanini GG, Chiarito M, Ferrante G, et al. Early detection of elevated cardia biomarkers to optimise risk stratification in patients with COVID-19. Heart. 2020;106:1512–8.
22. Singh N, Anchan RK, Besser SA, et al. High sensitivity troponin-T for prediction of adverse events in patients with COVID-19. Biomarkers. 2020;25:626–33.
23. Laguna-Goya R, Utero-Rico A, Talayero P, et al. IL-6-based mortality risk model for hospitalized patients with COVID-19. J Allergy Clin Immunol. 2020;146:799–807.
24. Rovina N, Akinosoglou K, Eugen-Olsen E, Hayek S, Reiser J, Giamarellos-Bourboulis EJ. Soluble urokinase plasminogen activator receptor (suPAR) as an early predictor of severe respiratory failure in patients with COVID-19 pneumonia. Crit Care. 2020;24:187.
25. Azam TU, Shadid HR, Blakely P, et al. Soluble urokinase receptor (suPAR) in COVID-19-related AKI. J Am Soc Nephrol. 2020;31:2725–35.
26. Vasbinder A, Anderson E, Shadid H, et al. Inflammation, hyperglycemia, and adverse outcomes in individuals with diabetes mellitus hospitalized for COVID-19. Diabetes Care. 2022;45:692–700.
27. Renieris G, Karakike E, Gkavogianni, et al. IL-1 mediates tissue-specific inflammation and severe respiratory failure in COVID-19. J Innate Immun. 2022;14:643–56.
28. König R, Kolte A, Ahlers O, et al. Use of IFNg/IL10 ratio for stratification of hydrocortisone therapy in patients with septic shock. Front Immunol. 2021;12:607217.
29. Payen D, Faivre V, Miatello J, et al. Multicentric experience with interferon gamma therapy in sepsis induced immunosuppression. A case series. BMC Infect Dis. 2019;19:931.
30. Shakoory B, Carcillo JA, Chatham WW, et al. Interleukin-1 receptor blockade is associated with reduced mortality in sepsis patients with features of macrophage activation syndrome: reanalysis of a prior phase III trial. Crit Care Med. 2016;44:275–81.
31. Kyriazopoulou E, Poulakou G, Milionis H, et al. Early treatment of COVID-19 with anakinra guided by soluble urokinase plasminogen activator receptor: a double-blind, randomized controlled phase 3 trial. Nat Med. 2021;27:1752–60.
32. EMA. EMA recommends approval for use of Kineret in adults with COVID-19. Available at: https://www.ema.europa.eu/en/news/ema-recommends-approval-use-kineret-adults-covid-19. Accessed 5 Sep 2022.

# 4 Interrogating the Sepsis Host Immune Response Using Cytomics

R. B. Lindell and N. J. Meyer

## 4.1 Introduction

Sepsis, the syndrome of life-threatening organ dysfunction due to infection, affects an estimated 48 million people annually around the globe and is the most common cause of death in hospitals [1, 2]. Although sepsis is defined as a dysregulated host response to infection [3], our ability to discriminate adaptive and maladaptive immune response is limited. In most serious infections, there exists a complex interplay between pathogen-induced tissue injury, pathogen-directed host inflammation, injury resulting from host immune activation, and potential secondary infections due to impaired or exhausted immune defense. Simultaneous exuberant innate immune activation and hypofunctioning adaptive immune processes are frequently detected in septic individuals [4], and we lack clinical tools to quantify the balance between hyper- and hypo-inflammation [5]. In addition, we cannot confidently

R. B. Lindell
Division of Critical Care Medicine, Department of Anesthesia and Critical Care Medicine, Children's Hospital of Philadelphia, University of Pennsylvania Perelman School of Medicine, Philadelphia, PA, USA

Institute for Immunology, University of Pennsylvania Perelman School of Medicine, Philadelphia, PA, USA

Pediatric Sepsis Program, Children's Hospital of Philadelphia, Philadelphia, PA, USA

N. J. Meyer (✉)
Institute for Immunology, University of Pennsylvania Perelman School of Medicine, Philadelphia, PA, USA

Division of Pulmonary, Allergy, and Critical Care Medicine, University of Pennsylvania Perelman School of Medicine, Philadelphia, PA, USA

Center for Translational Lung Biology and Lung Biology Institute, University of Pennsylvania Perelman School of Medicine, Philadelphia, PA, USA
e-mail: nuala.meyer@pennmedicine.upenn.edu



J.-L. Vincent (ed.), *Annual Update in Intensive Care and Emergency Medicine 2023*, Annual Update in Intensive Care and Emergency Medicine,
https://doi.org/10.1007/978-3-031-23005-9_4

ascertain which responses are necessary for microbial control and which may propagate organ injury without influencing pathogen killing. This complexity, and the demonstrated heterogeneity in patient immune response, has contributed to a major void in specific pharmacotherapy for sepsis and prompted calls for immunophenotyping that might allow more precise therapeutic targeting [6].

Circulating blood cells offer a unique window to the immune response and reflect both innate and adaptive immune programs. They are relatively easy to obtain and suitable for repeat sampling, thus their trajectories can manifest the dynamic and evolving host response to infection and inflammation. Flow cytometry is the technique of measuring single cells within a suspension by directing a laser or light source at the fluid stream and separating cells by their physical properties such as size and intracellular complexity (granularity), along with fluorescence from chemicals in the cells themselves or from fluorescent-conjugated antibodies to cellular antigens. Detectors capture the light and fluorescence emitted from cells, and the combination of light scatter and fluorescence categorizes cells with uniform size, scatter, and fluorescent features. Whereas early cytometers had only a single laser, modern cytometers combined 4, then 7, then 14 and higher numbers of lasers to facilitate characterization of more than 40 features [7]. This revolution in flow cytometry throughput in turn catalyzed an explosive growth in cellular identification, improving recognition of immune cells and tumor cells in increasing detail. A technical limitation of flow cytometry has been the spectral overlap between fluorophores, which could limit precise identification or constrain the dyes used together. In response, investigators developed mass spectrometry or cytometry by time-of-flight (CyTOF), a technique which replaces fluorescent antibodies with heavy metal isotopes that are not naturally occurring and that have unique mass spectrometry characteristics [7]. Approximately 60 heavy metal isotopes to date have sufficient purity and antibody conjugation chemistry to be studied in a single panel, greatly expanding the dimensionality of cellular characterization [7]. Although CyTOF applications in critical illness are still relatively infrequent [8], we expect applications to grow exponentially as the technology matures and costs decrease.

Peripheral blood profiling has limitations including the compartmentalization of immune reactions [9] and the inability of circulating cells to capture tissue-resident immune processes. Nonetheless, understanding which immune cells participate in the host response during sepsis may elucidate a clearer picture of regulated and dysregulated host response. In this chapter, we highlight the knowledge attained by cytometric profiling during adult and pediatric sepsis and propose key future research priorities to best harness this information.

## 4.2 Historical Focus on Immature Granulocytes in Sepsis

Long before the molecular era of medicine, hematopathologists had described the association between numeric and morphologic changes in peripheral blood leukocytes and severe infections across the age spectrum. Elevated peripheral white blood cells and a shift to more immature neutrophils or "bands" were codified as part of the systemic inflammatory response syndrome (SIRS) criteria, although with acknowledgement that SIRS could occur due to both infectious and non-infectious causes [10] and that sepsis can occur in the absence of SIRS [11]. As early as the 1970s, investigators had demonstrated that hospitalized patients with infection, both pediatric and adult, were more likely to have immature neutrophils, toxic granulation within neutrophils, and vacuolization of neutrophil cytoplasm on blood smear review [12]. Furthermore, when tested *ex vivo*, neutrophils from subjects with such morphological changes were more likely to have delayed bacterial killing and a higher proportion of neutrophils with visible intracellular bacteria [12], linking altered leukocyte morphology to impaired pathogen response. Along with the discovery of inflammatory cytokines and chemokines that were highly expressed in the circulation of septic patients, a paradigm emerged that posited that sepsis represented unrivaled and uncontrolled inflammation [13].

With the rapid advances of flow cytometric techniques, applications to the granulocyte fraction highlighted the shift to more immature neutrophil forms and significant heterogeneity among circulating leukocytes in sepsis. Neutrophils from hospitalized patients with sepsis were more likely to have reduced CD10 and CD16 expression compared to either uninfected outpatients or to patients with community-acquired infection but without SIRS, and the manual band count was correlated with $CD10^{dim}$ $CD16^{dim}$ neutrophils [14]. The antigen CD10 is not restricted to granulocytes—indeed, it is also known as acute lymphoblastic lymphoma antigen—but neutrophils express this antigen only in the latest stages of differentiation [15]. In addition, low or absent CD10 expression was shown to discriminate immature neutrophils in a study of donors treated with exogenous granulocyte colony stimulating factor (G-CSF), the growth factor most known for stimulating neutrophil production from the bone marrow. In contrast to mature $CD10^+$ neutrophils, $CD10^-$ neutrophils exhibited immunostimulatory effects on $CD4^+$ and $CD8^+$ T cells, enhancing T cell proliferation, survival, and interferon-gamma (IFNγ) production [15]. Neutrophils with $CD10^{dim}$ $CD16^{dim}$ expression persisted at 3 and 8 days after the onset of septic shock and non-survivors had a higher proportion of these cells compared to septic shock survivors [16]. In addition, neutrophils from patients with septic shock manifested altered function, with lower intracellular myeloperoxidase and lactoferrin expression, reduced chemotaxis, and impaired phagocytosis [16], suggesting that immune dysregulation in sepsis involves both immune stimulation and defective immune functions.

More recently, a class of granulocytes that has a density closer to monocytes, and thus separates with the peripheral blood mononuclear cell fraction when using density gradient separation, has been described. These 'low density neutrophils (LDN)' express markers that classically identify granulocyte origin (CD15) and suppress T cell proliferation through the elaboration of arginase which downregulates the T cell receptor zeta-chain expression [17, 18]. Given their suppressive effect on T cell effector function, these cells are known as granulocytic myeloid derived suppressor cells (gMDSC), and they seem to be especially upregulated in sepsis compared to comparably critically ill controls [18]. In addition, gMDSC express high levels of arginase-1 and neutrophil degranulation markers, many of which contribute to a transcriptomic phenotype corresponding to plasma protein hyperinflammation during acute respiratory distress syndrome (ARDS) [19]. Thus, gMDSC/LDN are a unique class of cells that may contribute to both arms of the dysregulated immune response in sepsis, innate inflammation with neutrophil degranulation, and suppression of T cell effector function.

## 4.3 Compensatory Anti-Inflammatory Response and Sepsis Immune Paresis

The past 25 years have witnessed an increasing focus on the downregulated aspects of immune function during sepsis, sometimes termed sepsis immune paresis or the compensatory anti-inflammatory response [13, 20]. Building from animal studies in which significant lymphoid apoptosis was observed in models of uncontrolled infection, investigators leveraged rapid autopsy studies to demonstrate that septic patients frequently had at least focal apoptosis in the spleen and colon [21]. Striking lymphopenia was often observed in patients with sepsis, and persistent lymphopenia beyond day 4 predicted a higher risk of death [22]. Applying flow cytometry, studies demonstrated that exogenous endotoxin, which typically stimulates an increased density of human leukocyte antigen-DR isotype (HLA-DR), a ligand for the T-cell receptor, on monocytes, failed to stimulate monocyte HLA-DR (mHLA-DR) expression in patients with sepsis or following severe trauma [23]. Elegant studies used endotoxin to stimulate *ex vivo* peripheral white blood cells collected from patients with sepsis and demonstrated that the monocytes lacking HLA-DR were also deficient in antigen-presenting capacity and in producing inflammatory cytokines, such as tumor necrosis factor alpha (TNF-α), in response to endotoxin [24]. In many ways, the monocytes from human subjects with sepsis seemed to resemble cells that had been desensitized with repeated doses of endotoxin [24], and CD14-expressing (monocytic) cells with HLA-$DR^{dim}$ expression are sometimes termed monocytic MDSC.

Monneret and colleagues profiled more than 90 subjects with septic shock and observed that whereas the proportion of low mHLA-DR cells was similar between survivors and non-survivors at admission, the persistent expression of fewer than 30% mHLA-$DR^{+}$ cells after 48 h was strongly associated with mortality [25]. Since this pivotal early work establishing mHLA-DR as a potential marker for sepsis immunosuppression, it has remained a strong candidate to identify subjects in real time with immune deficits. In an early phase 2 precision medicine sepsis trial, subjects with sepsis and confirmed low mHLA-DR were randomized to placebo or a daily dose of granulocyte-macrophage colony-stimulating factor (GM-CSF) for 8 days. Subjects randomized to GM-CSF restored their mHLA-DR expression and *in vitro/ex vivo* endotoxin-stimulated cytokine production [26]. GM-CSF-treated subjects also had improved severity of illness scores and shorter duration of mechanical ventilation, though the trial was not powered for clinical outcomes [26]. Larger trials in unselected patients with acute respiratory failure did not reproduce these findings [27], leaving many to wonder whether limiting the drug to those with low mHLA-DR might have been more effective. The expression of mHLA-DR remains a strong candidate for identifying sepsis immunosuppression in real time and newer trials may use this marker as a criterion for entry.

## 4.4 Lymphocyte Activation and Exhaustion

The past 5 years have brought more of an appreciation that rather than a compensatory anti-inflammatory response following immune hyperactivity, both hyperactivation and immunosuppression occur simultaneously, across different cell types and in different compartments [4, 9]. A focused interrogation of the B lymphocyte fraction demonstrated that this population undergoes specific depletion of memory B cells through activation-associated apoptosis pathways [28]. The significance of this finding is that in order to preferentially restore B cell function, a strategy may need to not only restore the number of B-cells but also expand or replenish the memory cell pool, which could necessitate antigen challenge [28].

A potential link between excessive activation and another aspect of lymphocyte dysregulation, exhaustion, is also observed in the T cell fraction. In a prospective study of subjects with sepsis compared to those with non-infectious critical illness, and with healthy controls, the T lymphocytes from patients with sepsis demonstrated increased markers of activation and of exhaustion [29]. Both B- and $CD4^+$ T-lymphocytes from patients with sepsis seem to overexpress the exhaustion marker programmed death 1 (PD-1) and its ligand PD-L1 [30], and T-lymphocytes also have been shown to overexpress inhibitory markers such as T-cell immunoglobulin and mucin domain-containing protein-1 (TIM-1), lymphocyte activation gene 3 (LAG-3), and cytotoxic T-lymphocyte-associated protein 4 (CTLA4) [29]. At the same time, populations of hyperactivated, proliferating T cells have been identified in adult and pediatric sepsis [31, 32].

Coronavirus disease 2019 (COVID-19) also focused attention on T cell hyperactivation as a potential marker for more severe immune dysregulation. High dimensional flow cytometric profiling of subjects highlighted considerable heterogeneity in the immune response even among hospitalized patients with COVID-19 [33]. Whereas some patients displayed almost no activation of B- or T-lymphocytes, others exhibited dramatic $CD4^+$ and $CD8^+$ T lymphocyte activation and proliferation, and the integrated immunotype characterized by this activation was associated with severity of illness, greater need for respiratory support, and higher mortality [33]. Pediatric subjects with multisystem inflammatory syndrome in children (MIS-C) also demonstrated highly activated T-lymphocytes [34], although with particular activation in the 'vascular patrolling' $CX3CR1^+$ $CD8^+$ T cell population that was not observed in hospitalized adult patients with acute COVID-19 [33]. Because the poor prognosis immunotype of acute COVID-19 was dominated by highly activated T cells but also enriched in exhaustion markers including PD-1 [33], there is strong interest in understanding better the relationship between T cell exhaustion and activation.

The mechanism by which these critically ill patients develop T cell hyperactivation is unknown, which limits our ability to deploy precision immunotherapeutics for these patients. Early in critical illness, T cell hyperactivation can occur via two distinct mechanisms: antigen-dependent activation via T cell receptor signaling [35], or a dysregulated, antigen-independent 'bystander' activation [36], as shown in Fig. 4.1. In a precision medicine paradigm for sepsis, different approaches to immune modulation could be indicated based on the antigen-specificity of the T cell

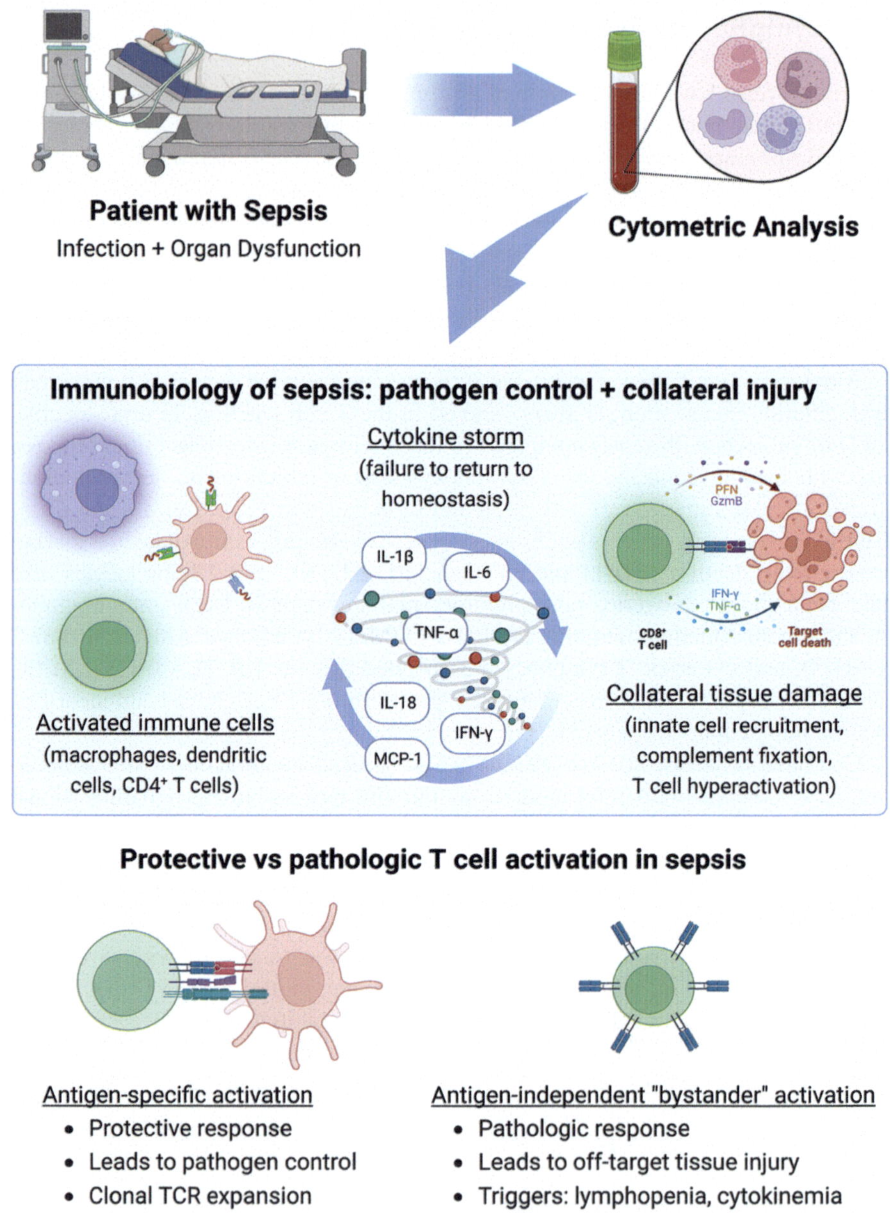


**Fig. 4.1** Potential utility of cytometric profiling to understand the sepsis immune response. Peripheral blood leukocytes from patients with sepsis can be assayed by either flow cytometry or mass cytometry (cytometry by time-of-flight [CyTOF]) to understand cell populations and, via their expression patterns, their degree of activation or exhaustion. Along with plasma protein analysis which could inform about cytokine elaboration, immune cell profiling might detect the source of inflammatory proteins and identify specific deleterious patterns. Cytotoxic T cell activation, which is associated with poor outcomes in sepsis and COVID-19 and contributes to tissue damage, may be due to antigen-driven processes that are necessary for pathogen control, or it may result from bystander activation. Discriminating between these patterns may be essential to best design strategies to intervene in pathologic activation yet preserve pathogen clearance. *TNF* tumor necrosis factor, *IL* interleukin, *IFN* interferon, *MCP* monocyte chemoattractant protein, *PFN* perforin, *GzmB* granzyme B, *TCR* T-cell receptor. Figure created with BioRender.com

response. Antigen-specific hyperactivated responses might improve pathogen clearance, and thus we might attempt to preserve this activation. In contrast, bystander activation might drive off-target tissue injury, and a precision paradigm might try to blunt such activation. If we could use cytometric profiling to distinguish these patterns of T-cell hyperactivation, more precise immunomodulation might be possible.

## 4.5 Pediatric Sepsis: Cytomics in the Developing Immune System

Since pediatric-specific criteria for sepsis were defined in 2005 [37], the burden of sepsis in children has been studied extensively [38, 39]. Although less prevalent than adult sepsis, pediatric sepsis is the leading cause of death of hospitalized children worldwide [1]. Sepsis incidence and outcomes vary dramatically by age and comorbidities, with younger children [39], immunocompromised children [40, 41], and children who develop immune dysfunction in the setting of sepsis [42] representing the highest risk clinical phenotypes.

As in adults, sepsis in children is characterized by concurrent pro- and anti-inflammatory states with dysregulation of the innate and adaptive immune responses to infection [37]. Mirroring translational investigations in adults, pediatric sepsis research has increasingly focused on defining the molecular biology of the disease. Many pediatric patients with sepsis develop innate and adaptive immune dysfunction, which is typically referred to as "immune paralysis" [43, 44] and can be identified by impaired whole blood *ex vivo* TNF-$\alpha$ and IFN$\gamma$ production capacity in response to antigen stimulation. Immune paralysis in pediatric sepsis is associated with secondary infection, persistent organ dysfunction [42], and mortality [40, 41, 45]. Mitochondrial dysfunction is a hallmark of this sepsis-associated immune suppression and has been associated with organ failure in both pediatric and adult sepsis [46].

In contrast to these functional assays, cellular and molecular approaches to immune profiling have also been applied to cohorts of pediatric sepsis patients with the goal of identifying sepsis subphenotypes that could be amenable to precision therapy. Using clinical characteristics and candidate biomarkers, investigators have identified three major inflammation subphenotypes in pediatric sepsis patients: immune paralysis (characterized by persistent antigen stimulation, decreased mHLA-DR expression, and decreased cytokine production in the setting of mitogen stimulation), sequential multiple organ failure (characterized by respiratory and liver failure, and oligogenic mutations in FAS/FAS ligand), and thrombocytopenia-associated multiple organ failure (characterized by hemolysis, thrombocytopenia, and oligogenic mutations in complement or ADAMTS13 signaling) [47]. Investigators studying the adaptive immune response in pediatric sepsis have employed unsupervised clustering of bulk transcriptomics data to identify two major subclasses of sepsis driven primarily by differences in T cell and B cell receptor signaling pathways [48]. These subclasses have been shown to have differential response to corticosteroid administration [49], and hospital mortality is substantially increased in the subgroup with downregulated signaling [48]. Finally, investigators have recently employed flow cytometry and metabolomics to demonstrate an association between T cell immunometabolic dysregulation and other markers of immune paralysis in a pilot study of pediatric sepsis patients [31].

In recognition of the association between immune dysfunction and clinical outcomes in pediatric sepsis, the most recent guidelines for monitoring organ dysfunction in pediatric critical illness specifically highlighted the need to develop capabilities for clinical monitoring of immune dysfunction in the pediatric intensive care unit (ICU) [50]. Because the pediatric immune system exhibits remarkable biologic heterogeneity driven by host characteristics, infectious exposures, and pubertal status among other factors, future research searching for a 'treatable trait' in pediatric sepsis patients with immune dysregulation will require a detailed understanding of the developing pediatric immune system in both health and disease.

## 4.6 Conclusion

Sepsis remains a critical threat to the health of adults and children worldwide. In the search for markers of dysregulated host immune reactions to infection, cytometric profiling of circulating leukocytes has yielded potential candidates to identify both hyperactive *and* hypofunctioning immune responses. If precision immunomodulatory approaches are to be successful, validated tools that reliably identify favorable and maladaptive patterns will be essential. Clinical trials are encouraged to collect peripheral blood leukocytes to enable discovery and validation of the most reliable cytometric features. Future research could focus on whether these markers, if determined prospectively, might act as enrichment tools to select patients at high risk for poor outcomes or with a differential therapeutic response.

## References

1. Rudd KE, Johnson SC, Agesa KM, et al. Global, regional, and national sepsis incidence and mortality, 1990-2017: analysis for the Global Burden of Disease Study. Lancet. 2020;395:200–11.
2. Liu V, Escobar GJ, Greene JD, et al. Hospital deaths in patients with sepsis from 2 independent cohorts. JAMA. 2014;312:90–2.
3. Singer M, Deutschman CS, Seymour C, et al. The third international consensus definitions for sepsis and septic shock (Sepsis-3). JAMA. 2016;315:801–10.
4. Delano MJ, Ward PA. Sepsis-induced immune dysfunction: can immune therapies reduce mortality? J Clin Invest. 2016;126:23–31.
5. Rubio I, Osuchowski MF, Shankar-Hari M, et al. Current gaps in sepsis immunology: new opportunities for translational research. Lancet Infect Dis. 2019;19:e422–36.
6. van Peters Ton AM, Kox M, Abdo WF, Pickkers P. Precision immunotherapy for sepsis. Front Immunol. 2018;9:1926.
7. Iyer A, Hamers AAJ, Pillai AB. CyTOF(®) for the masses. Front Immunol. 2022;13:815828.
8. Gossez M, Rimmelé T, Andrieu T, et al. Proof of concept study of mass cytometry in septic shock patients reveals novel immune alterations. Sci Rep. 2018;8:17296.

9. Conway Morris A, Rynne J, Shankar-Hari M. Compartmentalisation of immune responses in critical illness: does it matter? Intensive Care Med. 2022;48:1617–20.
10. Bone RC, Balk RA, Cerra FB, et al. American College of Chest Physicians/Society of Critical Care Medicine Consensus Conference: definitions for sepsis and organ failure and guidelines for the use of innovative therapies in sepsis. Crit Care Med. 1992;20:864–74.
11. Kaukonen KM, Bailey M, Pilcher D, Cooper DJ, Bellomo R. Systemic inflammatory response syndrome criteria in defining severe sepsis. N Engl J Med. 2015;372:1629–38.
12. Solberg CO, Hellum KB. Neutrophil granulocyte function in bacterial infections. Lancet. 1972;300:727–30.
13. Bone RC. Sir Isaac Newton, sepsis, SIRS, and CARS. Crit Care Med. 1996;24:1125–8.
14. Guérin E, Orabona M, Raquil MA, et al. Circulating immature granulocytes with T-cell killing functions predict sepsis deterioration. Crit Care Med. 2014;42:2007–18.
15. Marini O, Costa S, Bevilacqua D, et al. Mature CD10+ and immature CD10− neutrophils present in G-CSF–treated donors display opposite effects on T cells. Blood. 2017;129:1343–56.
16. Demaret J, Venet F, Friggeri A, et al. Marked alterations of neutrophil functions during sepsis-induced immunosuppression. J Leukoc Biol. 2015;98:1081–90.
17. Darcy CJ, Minigo G, Piera KA, et al. Neutrophils with myeloid derived suppressor function deplete arginine and constrain T cell function in septic shock patients. Crit Care. 2014;18:R163.
18. Uhel F, Azzaoui I, Grégoire M, et al. Early expansion of circulating granulocytic myeloid-derived suppressor cells predicts development of nosocomial infections in patients with sepsis. Am J Respir Crit Care Med. 2017;196:315–27.
19. Bos LDJ, Scicluna BP, Ong DSY, Cremer O, van der Poll T, Schultz MJ. Understanding heterogeneity in biologic phenotypes of acute respiratory distress syndrome by leukocyte expression profiles. Am J Respir Crit Care Med. 2019;200:42–50.
20. Reddy RC, Chen GH, Tekchandani PK, Standiford TJ. Sepsis-induced immunosuppression. Immunol Res. 2001;24:273–87.
21. Hotchkiss RS, Swanson PE, Freeman BD, et al. Apoptotic cell death in patients with sepsis, shock, and multiple organ dysfunction. Crit Care Med. 1999;27:1230–51.
22. Drewry AM, Samra N, Skrupky LP, Fuller BM, Compton SM, Hotchkiss RS. Persistent lymphopenia after diagnosis of sepsis predicts mortality. Shock. 2014;42:383–91.
23. Appel SH, Wellhausen SR, Montgomery R, DeWeese RC, Polk HC Jr. Experimental and clinical significance of endotoxin-dependent HLA-DR expression on monocytes. J Surg Res. 1989;47:39–44.
24. Döcke WD, Randow F, Syrbe U, et al. Monocyte deactivation in septic patients: restoration by IFN-gamma treatment. Nat Med. 1997;3:678–81.
25. Monneret G, Lepape A, Voirin N, et al. Persisting low monocyte human leukocyte antigen-DR expression predicts mortality in septic shock. Intensive Care Med. 2006;32:1175–83.
26. Meisel C, Schefold JC, Pschowski R, et al. Granulocyte-macrophage colony-stimulating factor to reverse sepsis-associated immunosuppression: a double-blind, randomized, placebo-controlled multicenter trial. Am J Respir Crit Care Med. 2009;180:640–8.
27. Paine R III, Standiford TJ, Dechert RE, et al. A randomized trial of recombinant human granulocyte-macrophage colony stimulating factor for patients with acute lung injury. Crit Care Med. 2012;40:90–7.
28. Shankar-Hari M, Fear D, Lavender P, et al. Activation-associated accelerated apoptosis of memory B cells in critically ill patients with sepsis. Crit Care Med. 2017;45:875–82.
29. Boomer JS, Shuherk-Shaffer J, Hotchkiss RS, Green JM. A prospective analysis of lymphocyte phenotype and function over the course of acute sepsis. Crit Care. 2012;16:R112.
30. Wilson JK, Zhao Y, Singer M, Spencer J, Shankar-Hari M. Lymphocyte subset expression and serum concentrations of PD-1/PD-L1 in sepsis - pilot study. Crit Care. 2018;22:95.
31. Lindell RB, Zhang D, Bush J, et al. Impaired lymphocyte responses in pediatric sepsis vary by pathogen type and are associated with features of immunometabolic dysregulation. Shock. 2022;57:191–9.

32. Zeerleder S, Hack CE, Caliezi C, et al. Activated cytotoxic T cells and NK cells in severe sepsis and septic shock and their role in multiple organ dysfunction. Clin Immunol. 2005;116:158–65.
33. Mathew D, Giles JR, Baxter AE, et al. Deep immune profiling of COVID-19 patients reveals distinct immunotypes with therapeutic implications. Science. 2020;369:eabc8511.
34. Vella LA, Giles JR, Baxter AE, et al. Deep immune profiling of MIS-C demonstrates marked but transient immune activation compared to adult and pediatric COVID-19. Sci Immunol. 2021;6:57.
35. van Heijst JW, Gerlach C, Swart E, et al. Recruitment of antigen-specific CD8+ T cells in response to infection is markedly efficient. Science. 2009;325:1265–9.
36. Tough DF, Borrow P, Sprent J. Induction of bystander T cell proliferation by viruses and type I interferon in vivo. Science. 1996;272:1947–50.
37. Goldstein B, Giroir B, Randolph A. International Consensus Conference on Pediatric Sepsis. International Pediatric Sepsis Consensus Conference: definitions for sepsis and organ dysfunction in pediatrics. Pediatr Crit Care Med. 2005;6:2–8.
38. Balamuth F, Weiss SL, Neuman MI, et al. Pediatric severe sepsis in U.S. Children's Hospitals. Pediatr Crit Care Med. 2014;15:798–805.
39. Watson RS, Carcillo JA, Linde-Zwirble WT, Clermont G, Lidicker J, Angus DC. The epidemiology of severe sepsis in children in the United States. Am J Respir Crit Care Med. 2003;167:695–701.
40. Lindell RB, Nishisaki A, Weiss SL, Traynor DM, Fitzgerald JC. Risk of mortality in immunocompromised children with severe sepsis and septic shock. Crit Care Med. 2020;48:1026–33.
41. Lindell RB, Gertz SJ, Rowan CM, et al. High levels of morbidity and mortality among pediatric hematopoietic cell transplant recipients with severe sepsis: insights from the Sepsis PRevalence, OUtcomes, and Therapies International Point Prevalence Study. Pediatr Crit Care Med. 2017;18:1114–25.
42. Muszynski JA, Nofziger R, Moore-Clingenpeel M, et al. Early immune function and duration of organ dysfunction in critically iii children with sepsis. Am J Respir Crit Care Med. 2018;198:361–9.
43. Hall MW, Knatz NL, Vetterly C, et al. Immunoparalysis and nosocomial infection in children with multiple organ dysfunction syndrome. Intensive Care Med. 2011;37:525–32.
44. Wong HR, Freishtat RJ, Monaco M, Odoms K, Shanley TP. Leukocyte subset-derived genomewide expression profiles in pediatric septic shock. Pediatr Crit Care Med. 2010;11:349–55.
45. Hall MW, Geyer SM, Guo CY, et al. Innate immune function and mortality in critically ill children with influenza: a multicenter study. Crit Care Med. 2013;41:224–36.
46. Weiss SL, Zhang D, Bush J, et al. Mitochondrial dysfunction is associated with an immune paralysis phenotype in pediatric sepsis. Shock. 2020;54:285–93.
47. Carcillo JA, Berg RA, Wessel D, et al. A Multicenter network assessment of three inflammation phenotypes in pediatric sepsis-induced multiple organ failure. Pediatr Crit Care Med. 2019;20:1137–46.
48. Wong HR, Cvijanovich NZ, Anas N, et al. Pediatric sepsis biomarker risk model-II: redefining the pediatric sepsis biomarker risk model with septic shock phenotype. Crit Care Med. 2016;44:2010–7.
49. Wong HR, Cvijanovich NZ, Allen GL, et al. Corticosteroids are associated with repression of adaptive immunity gene programs in pediatric septic shock. Am J Respir Crit Care Med. 2014;189:940–6.
50. Schlapbach LJ, Weiss SL, Bembea MM, et al. Scoring systems for organ dysfunction and multiple organ dysfunction: the PODIUM Consensus Conference. Pediatrics. 2022;149(Suppl 1):S23–31.

# 5 Precision Medicine in Septic Shock

L. Chiscano-Camón, J. C. Ruiz-Rodriguez, and R. Ferrer

## 5.1 Introduction

Septic shock needs appropriate, protocolized care, as recommended most recently in the latest version of the Surviving Sepsis Campaign (SSC) guidelines published in 2021 [1]. The implementation of the SSC recommendations and bundles is associated with a substantial mortality reduction [2]. However, mortality from sepsis remains inappropriately high [3].

Specific subgroups of patients who do not respond to conventional therapy may benefit from other therapies, which can be considered as rescue strategies. The current consensus definition of sepsis—"life-threatening organ dysfunction caused by a dysregulated host response to infection"—is broad, reflecting the intrinsic heterogeneity of the disease [4]. The source of this heterogeneity is multifaceted: infection etiologies vary, individual host comorbidities and genetics are unique, and the timeliness of diagnosis and treatment differ from patient to patient. These factors not only impact the evolution of sepsis at the individual patient level but also their responses to a therapeutic intervention.

L. Chiscano-Camón · J. C. Ruiz-Rodriguez
Intensive Care Department, Vall d'Hebron University Hospital, Barcelona, Spain

Shock, Organ Dysfunction and Resuscitation Research Group, Vall d'Hebron Institut de Recerca (VHIR), Vall d'Hebron University Hospital, Barcelona, Spain

Departament de Medicina, Universitat Autònoma de Barcelona, Barcelona, Spain

R. Ferrer (✉)
Intensive Care Department, Vall d'Hebron University Hospital, Barcelona, Spain

Shock, Organ Dysfunction and Resuscitation Research Group, Vall d'Hebron Institut de Recerca (VHIR), Vall d'Hebron University Hospital, Barcelona, Spain

Departament de Medicina, Universitat Autònoma de Barcelona, Barcelona, Spain

Ciber Enfermedades Respiratorias (Ciberes), Instituto de Salud Carlos III, Madrid, Spain
e-mail: ricard.ferrer@vallhebron.cat



J.-L. Vincent (ed.), *Annual Update in Intensive Care and Emergency Medicine 2023*, Annual Update in Intensive Care and Emergency Medicine,
https://doi.org/10.1007/978-3-031-23005-9_5

Seymour et al., using a large database, described four sepsis phenotypes with different demographics, laboratory values, and patterns of organ dysfunction that were shown to correlate with biomarker concentrations and mortality [5]. Patients with a high risk of clinical deterioration could also profit from more specific or individualized therapies [6]. This raises the need for so-called precision medicine. Precision medicine permits healthcare interventions to be tailored to groups of patients based on their disease susceptibility, diagnostic or prognostic, as well as their treatment response. The use of omics technology is a key element to identify these subgroups of patients.

We propose a translation of precision medicine to sepsis to try to personalize the management of patients with septic shock and identify different endotypes or subgroups of patients, based on biological differences that will make them more homogeneous in terms of evolution, symptoms, and response to specific treatments (Table 5.1).

**Table 5.1** Clinical applicability of precision medicine strategies in refractory septic shock based on detection of subgroups of patients, either early by gene expression to identify mediators on which to act (omics therapy), or later once the patient is moving toward a situation of being refractory to conventional measures and rescue treatment can be applied (hemoadsorption, metabolic resuscitation, other vasopressors)

| Precision medicine strategies | | Target (s) | Clinical application |
|---|---|---|---|
| Omics technologies | Genomics and epigenomics | Genetic variants | Prognosis, severity |
| | | Genotypes | Susceptibility to sepsis |
| | Transcriptomics | Gene expression, activity and regulation | Susceptibility to sepsis |
| | | Sepsis response signatures | Severity, prognosis |
| | Metabolomics | Small molecules produced by cells | Prognosis |
| | | Metabolomic profile | Response to treatment |
| | Proteomics | Proteins expressed by the genome under certain conditions | Diagnosis, prognosis |
| | | Biomarkers | Diagnosis, prognosis |
| Immunoglobulins | | Immunoglobulin levels | Sepsis-associated hypogammaglobulinemia |
| Hemoadsorption | High endotoxemia | Endotoxemia | Rescue therapy |
| | Severe hypercytokinemia | Cytokine levels | Rescue therapy |
| | Sequential hemoadsorption | Endotoxin and cytokine hemoadsorption | Rescue therapy |
| Non-catecholaminergic vasopressors | | Vasopressin<br>Selepressin<br>Terlipressin<br>Methylene blue<br>Angiotensin II | Catecholamine sparing agent<br>Rescue therapy |
| Metabolic resuscitation | | HAT therapy (hydrocortisone, ascorbic acid, thiamine)<br>Hydroxocobalamin | Restoring mitochondrial damage<br>Rescue therapy |

## 5.2 Omics Technologies

High-throughput omics technologies may revolutionize medical practice by aiding implementation of precision and personalized medicine approaches to tailor diagnostic, therapeutic, and monitoring strategies for individual patients based on their genetic and molecular signatures. Understanding the molecular sepsis signature of a patient will likely be crucial to improving the treatment of sepsis. These technologies have been used in recent years to identify various evolutionary patterns in reaction to different therapies in septic shock. They include omic platforms and novel bioinformatics techniques, notably genomics and epigenomics (study of genes and their roles), transcriptomics (study of the transcriptome of a specific cell or tissue in a certain circumstance, centered on the analysis of gene expression profiles), metabolomics (pattern analysis of molecules created by cells), and proteomics (set of all proteins expressed by the genome of a cell, tissue, or organism at a specific time and under particular conditions). These technologies can identify different endotypes or phenotypes indistinguishable clinically at the bedside but which may react differently to specific treatments [7]. These technologies can also be used to detect molecules at which therapies can be targeted in patients refractory to conventional therapy.

Most studies in this context have been directed toward patients in early stages of infection without sepsis; however, some describe a septic shock setting. For example, using transcriptomics, Wong et al. [8] performed genome-wide expression profiling using whole blood-derived RNA from 98 children with septic shock and found three subclasses of patients: A, B, and C. Patients in subclass A were characterized by suppression of genes corresponding to adaptive immunity and glucocorticoid receptor signaling. Subclass A patients had higher disease severity and mortality ratio than patients in subclasses B and C. Using metabolomics, Ferrario et al. analyzed the variations in lipid homeostasis that arise during sepsis progression [9]. Plasma samples from 20 patients with septic shock were analyzed on days 1 and 7 of sepsis progression. The authors identified 137 metabolites, several of which were distinct between survivors and non-survivors. Lysophosphatidylcholine (LPC) and phosphatidylcholine were present in smaller concentrations in non-survivors than in survivors on days 1 and day 7. Using regression models, the lowest levels of LPC on day 7 were the best prognosticator of mortality. Using proteomics, Punyadeera et al. [10] studied 16 critically ill patients and observed that a mixture of various proteins (interleukin-1 alpha [IL-1$\alpha$], interferon gamma-induced protein 10 [IP-10], soluble tumor necrosis factor receptor 2 [sTNF-R2], and soluble cell death receptor [sFAS]) were associated with the progression of sepsis to septic shock [10]. Bauzá-Martínez et al. [11] reported a larger number of circulating peptides in patients with septic shock than in sepsis patients or non-hospitalized healthy subjects. The peptide count in patients with septic shock was higher in non-survivors than in survivors, suggesting an association between the magnitude of proteolysis and outcome [11].

## 5.3 Treatments for Specific Endotypes of Patients with Septic Shock

Currently, we can identify different sepsis endotypes, with a distinct functional or pathobiological mechanism, as candidates for a precision medicine approach.

### 5.3.1 Hypogammaglobulinemia

The pathogenesis of septic shock is linked with dysregulation of the innate and adaptive immune systems. The altered mechanism in the adaptive immune system is the function of antibodies and immunoglobulins [12]. As hypogammaglobulinemia is associated with greater mortality in sepsis, it has been considered as a marker for a potential subgroup of patients for immunoglobulin treatment [13].

Although the definition of hypogammaglobulinemia is not established, low concentrations of gammaglobulins (IgG) can be defined as values less than 500 mg/dl in individuals older than 5 years or 2 standard deviations below reference values for age [14]. Hypo-IgG, especially on the day of diagnosis and the subsequent 48 h, is linked with an augmented hazard of severe illness, a greater risk of acute respiratory distress syndrome (ARDS), and a longer duration of shock [15, 16]. In addition, a synergistic role of IgG, IgM, and IgA has been reported in sepsis and septic shock [17]. The shared existence of low concentrations of endogenous IgG, IgM, and IgA in plasma is related to reduced survival in patients with septic shock [18].

Polyvalent intravenous immunoglobulins embody a rational approach to modulate pro-and anti-inflammatory responses [19]. In adults with sepsis, the use of IgM/A-enriched intravenous immunoglobulin was associated with positive results [20]. A recent meta-analysis of 19 trials and >1500 patients showed a marked decrease in mortality when using IgM- and IgA-enriched intravenous immunoglobulin compared to human albumin solution or no treatment [21]. Although, the eligibility criteria for treatment with polyvalent intravenous immunoglobulin and the best treatment strategy need to be better defined, administration of a single dose of polyclonal IgG of 1 or 2 g/kg has been recommended (level of evidence 2C) [22].

Standard administration of intravenous immunoglobulin in patients with sepsis is not recommended, as stated in the 2021 SSC guidelines [1]. Patients with hypogammaglobulinemia respond better to treatment [23] and may profit. More studies are desirable, especially in those with hypogammaglobulinemia.

### 5.3.2 Endotoxemia

Endotoxin is a lipopolysaccharide (LPS) present in the outer membrane of Gram-negative bacteria and is one of the best samples of pathogen-associated molecular patterns (PAMPs). Its presence results in an increase in pro-inflammatory and anti-inflammatory cytokines [24], enhancing the immune response and facilitating sepsis.

Endotoxin activity has been found to be a useful marker of disease severity as the lipid-A domain of endotoxin is responsible for most of the toxicity associated with LPS, typified by fever, diarrhea, hemodynamic instability, multiple organ failure, and death [25]. An early study emphasized the clinical significance of circulating levels of LPS, showing a substantial correlation between plasma endotoxin concentrations and severity of septic shock, organ dysfunction, and mortality [26]. The occurrence of endotoxemia in patients with septic shock was elevated, and up to 82% of patients had medium or high endotoxin activity [27] showing much higher lactate concentrations and inotropic score values.

In human disease, the measurement of endotoxin is extremely difficult. Since 2004, measurement of endotoxemia in humans has been made using the Endotoxin Activity Assay (EAA), a chemiluminescent rapid 30 min assay described by Romaschin in 1998 [28]. Results are expressed in EAA units, with values $\leq 0.39$ considered low, 0.40–0.59 intermediate, and $\geq 0.60$ high.

Endotoxin has been considered as one of the therapeutic objectives for sepsis and septic shock. Removing endotoxin through blood purification techniques and, specifically, by hemoadsorption has been suggested. Adsorption with a fiber column immobilized with polymyxin B (PMX; Toraymyxin®; Toray, Tokyo, Japan), is one of the best-known endotoxin removal therapies; another is the oXiris® hemofilter (Baxter, Meyzieu, France). Four clinical trials have assessed the usefulness of endotoxin hemoadsorption in septic shock. In a multicenter, open-label, pilot, randomized controlled trial (RCT) performed in Europe, 36 postsurgical patients with severe sepsis or septic shock secondary to intra-abdominal infection were randomized to receive PMX treatment for 2 h (n = 17) or standard therapy (n = 19) [29]. There were no statistically differences in endotoxin levels from baseline to 6, 8, or 24 h after treatment in the two groups. Five of 18 (28%) patients in the control group and 5 of 17 (29%) in the PMX group died during the study period; the survival analysis showed no statistical significance between the groups. There was no statistically significant difference in the mean duration of intensive care unit (ICU) stay or the number of ICU-free days between the groups. However, patients treated with PMX had substantial increases in cardiac index and oxygen delivery index, and the need for continuous renal replacement therapy (CRRT) after study entrance was decreased. PMX was well tolerated and demonstrated no significant adverse effects. This study demonstrated that the PMX cartridge is safe and may alleviate cardiac and renal dysfunction due to sepsis or septic shock. The Early Use of Polymyxin B Hemoperfusion in Abdominal Septic shock (EUPHAS) trial [30] assessed hemoperfusion with PMX compared to conventional therapy in a small sample of 64 patients with intra-abdominal infection-related severe sepsis and septic shock. The study was oriented to assess hemodynamic recovery. The improvement in mean arterial pressure (MAP) permitted the reduction of doses of vasoactive drugs in the PMX group. Sequential organ failure assessment (SOFA) scores improved in the PMX group. Additionally, a significant decrease in 28-day mortality was noted in the intervention group (32%) compared to the standard treatment group (53%). The ABDOMIX trial [31] studied 243 patients with septic shock within 12 h after emergency surgical treatment for secondary peritonitis due to organ perforation. Patients receiving hemoperfusion with PMX (119 patients) received conventional therapy plus two sessions of PMX hemoperfusion. There were no significant differences in the SOFA score or the 28-day mortality rate between the PMX and control groups (27.7% vs. 19.5%). The severity of disease and mortality rates were low in the study population. Among the 220 sessions performed, early interruption was observed in 25 cases (11%), mostly during the first session and mainly due to circuit coagulation. The two PMX hemoperfusion sessions were achieved in only 81 of 119 patients (69.8%). Of note, plasma EAA levels were not measured in any of the RCTs previously discussed.

A recent review [32] analyzing a Japanese database of patients with septic shock who received PMX hemoperfusion demonstrated a survival benefit of this treatment, as well as an increased number of ventilator-, CRRT-, and vasoactive drug-free days following early improvements in organ dysfunction.

The Euphrates trial [33] is one of the RCTs with the greatest sample of patients. This trial analyzed 450 critically ill patients with septic shock and an EAA level of ≥0.6. The intervention involved two PMX hemoperfusion treatments (90–120 min) plus standard therapy, completed within 24 h of enrollment (n = 224 patients) or sham hemoperfusion as well as standard therapy (n = 226 patients). PMX hemoperfusion was not associated with a significant difference in 28-day mortality. However, Klein et al. completed a *post hoc* study of 194 of the patients with EAA values between 0.6 and 0.89 and observed an improvement in survival in patients who received therapy with PMX [34]. Monti et al. [35] published the first study describing the use of PMX hemoperfusion as rescue therapy in 52 patients with refractory septic shock not responding to standard therapy. The SOFA score was 10 (8–14) and serum lactate was 5.89 ± 4.04 mmol/l. All patients were receiving mechanical ventilation and 90% were receiving corticosteroids. Quick reversal of circulatory dysfunction and other organ failure was achieved. The 30-day mortality was lower (29%) than projected by the SAPS II score (47%). Recently, Shoji et al. [32], in a review of recent studies, demonstrated a survival benefit of PMX hemoperfusion; an increase in the number of ventilator-free days, renal replacement-free days, and norepinephrine-free days was observed in patients treated with PMX hemoperfusion. These studies provide important insight into the patient population likely to benefit from PMX hemoperfusion, i.e., those with higher levels of endotoxemia.

It seems reasonable to consider patients with refractory septic shock and severe multi-organ dysfunction, who have had adequate control of the infectious focus and have an EAA of 0.6–0.9 as potential candidates for endotoxin hemoadsorption. The ongoing TIGRIS study [36] is enrolling patients with EAA levels between 0.60 and 0.89 and randomizing them to PMX hemoperfusion or standard medical care. The results of this study will provide more data on the possible benefits of endotoxin hemoadsorption in patients with septic shock and multi-organ dysfunction.

### 5.3.3 Hypercytokinemia

Sepsis occurs when the initially appropriate host response to infection becomes amplified and subsequently dysregulated, leading to an imbalance of pro-inflammatory and anti-inflammatory responses [37]. An overabundance of pro-inflammatory cytokines can lead to endothelial injury and systemic inflammatory response syndrome.

A tightly regulated equilibrium of the cytokine web is vital for eliminating invasive pathogens on the one hand and restricting tissue-damaging inflammation on the other. Various studies have suggested an association of IL-6 hypercytokinemia with organ dysfunction, response to treatment, and prognosis in sepsis. Kellum et al. found that 82% of patients with community-acquired pneumonia had a systemic increase in cytokine levels [38]. Moreover, patients with greater levels of IL-6 and IL-10 had associated severe organ dysfunction and higher mortality [39]. Patients who survive sepsis show a rapid decline in IL-6 levels, in comparison to the slow and gradual decrease in non-survivors [40]. Thus, the decrease in IL-6 concentrations is associated with a better prognosis [41], and IL-10 overproduction is the most important predictor of severity and mortality [42, 43].

Extracorporeal blood purification therapies have been suggested as an approach to improve the outcome of septic patients, lessening the systemic expression of pro-inflammatory and anti-inflammatory mediators and rebuilding immune homeostasis [39]. Presently, there are several methods available for cytokine adsorption: Cytosorb, oXiris, Alteco LPS Adsorber (Alteco Medical, Lund, Sweden), and HA 330 and 380 (Jafron, Zhuhai City, China). The most commonly used cartridge and the one for which most data are available is CytoSorb® (CytoSorbents Corporation, Monmouth Junction, NJ, USA).

Several observational studies have suggested the clinical advantages of using Cytosorb® in septic shock to reduce vasopressor support and even mortality. Friesecke et al. studied 20 consecutive patients with refractory septic shock and hypercytokinemia after 6 h of basic treatment. Refractory septic shock was defined as progressive shock despite full-standard therapy, lactate concentrations ≥2.9 mmol/l (or increased compared to baseline), and high norepinephrine requirements (>0.3 μg/kg/min). The average IL-6 levels were 25,523 ng/ml (1052–491,260 ng/ml). In this study, Cytosorb® use was associated with a substantial decrease in norepinephrine requirements and an increase in lactate clearance, which resulted in shock resolution in 13 patients [44]. In a case series of 45 patients with septic shock treated with hemadsorption, Paul et al. defined a significant vasopressor dose decrease (norepinephrine 51.4%, epinephrine 69.4%, and vasopressin 13.9%) [45]. Likewise, a reduction in IL-6 levels (52.3%) and lactate levels (39.4%) was detected in the survivors. A survival rate of 75% was reported in patients who received treatment within 24 h of admission to the ICU. Patients who had treatment within 24–48 h after ICU admission had a survival rate of 68%. In a retrospective study performed by Brouwer et al., Cytosorb® was associated with decreased 28-day all-cause mortality in patients with septic shock [46].

Scientific data on the clinical advantages of cytokine elimination obtained from RCTs are limited. Hawchar et al. performed a proof-of-concept, prospective, randomized pilot trial of use of Cytosorb® in 20 patients with early onset septic shock. A major reduction in the need for vasopressor support was observed. In the control group, this difference was not achieved with standard therapy [47]. Rugg et al. compared patients with septic shock who received CytoSorb® in addition to CRRT ($n = 42$) versus matched controls ($n = 42$). Median catecholamine requirements approximately halved within 24 h after the initiation of Cytosorb®. In-hospital mortality was significantly lower in the CytoSorb® group (35.7% vs. 61.9%; $p = 0.015$) [48]. Neither of the above studies reported plasma cytokine levels prior to the initiation of the hemoadsorptive technique.

Cytokine hemadsorption may have a position as a rescue therapy in a particular subgroup of patients with refractory septic shock, hyperlactatemia, multi-organ failure, and very high hypercytokinemia. Well-designed RCTs should be performed in patients with this clinical picture to validate its advantages.

### 5.3.4 Sequential Hemadsorption

Current practice has demonstrated that hemadsorption helps recovery of immune homeostasis. However, in particular patients, endotoxin-only adsorption may be insufficient [49]. Endotoxemia and the overproduction of inflammatory mediators, in the form of a cytokine storm, are associated with the severity of sepsis and septic shock and determine prognosis [50]. Sequential hemadsorption (endotoxin hemadsorption with PMX, Toraymyxin®, and subsequent cytokine hemadsorption with Cytosorb®) has been applied in highly selected patients [51]. Precision medicine has allowed for a better selection of individuals according to their phenotypic and genetic profile to identify patients who could benefit from sequential hemadsorption (cytokine and endotoxin hemadsorption). Sequential hemadsorption is intended to remove the primary stimulus that induces the dysregulated inflammatory response. The candidates for sequential hemadsorption are patients with refractory septic shock, multi-organ dysfunction, high endotoxemia, and hypercytokinemia (extremely high levels of IL-6). Realtime monitoring of plasma cytokines (IL-6, IL-10) can guide clinicians to withhold therapy [52].

Hybrid therapies, such as the mixed use of endotoxin hemadsorption and coupled plasma filtration in a single circuit [53], have been examined in a specific group of post-cardiac surgery patients with sepsis and EAA levels $\geq 0.6$. However, some investigators did not include patients with high vasopressor requirements and acute severity scores in their analyses. The presence of adequate source control and the severity profile of patients should be studied before using hybrid hemadsorption as adjunctive therapy.

In addition to sequential techniques, novel advances have shown the scientific community that complementary hemadsorption strategies are plausible to achieve homeostasis, and are safe with no adverse effects.

## 5.4 Non-catecholaminergic Vasopressors

There are situations in which, despite the initiation of high-dose catecholaminergic vasoactive therapy, it is not possible to achieve a MAP ≥65 mmHg. In hemodynamic terms, this tends to be called refractory septic shock, and although there is not a universally established definition, a dose of norepinephrine >0.5 μg/kg/min is generally considered the cut-off value; these patients have a mortality rate between 50 and 94% [54]. There are, however, so-called non-catecholaminergic agents, which act as sparing vasoactive agents. Here we present some of them currently in use.

### 5.4.1 Vasopressin

Arginine vasopressin is a non-catecholaminergic vasopressor hormone released by the posterior pituitary in response to hypotension and hypernatremia. It acts through a family of receptors: V1a, V1b, V2, oxytocin (vasodilator), and purinergic receptors (of limited importance in sepsis). Vasopressin induces synthesis of nitric oxide (NO), which paradoxically can limit vasoconstriction, while preserving kidney perfusion; it can also induce some degree of cardiac depression. Activation of the V1a receptor occurs at the level of vascular smooth muscle and is independent of the action of catecholamines, which explains why vasopressin complements norepinephrine in refractory shock situations. On the other hand, in certain septic shock situations, vasopressin deficiency has been observed in relation to a depletion of hormone stores and inadequate synthesis and release at the level of the hypothalamic-pituitary axis [55]. In several RCTs, infusion of low doses of vasopressin (0.01–0.04 U/min), increased MAP and decreased the need for norepinephrine [56, 57]. In the VASST [58] study, 778 patients with septic shock and receiving at least 5 g/min of norepinephrine were randomized to receive vasopressin (0.01–0.03 U/min) or increasing doses of norepinephrine. In general, no differences were observed in mortality at 28 or 90 days. The rate of adverse events was also similar. But in the subgroup of patients with less severe septic shock (those receiving norepinephrine doses <15 g/min), longer survival was seen in the vasopressin arm. More recently, the VANISH study [59] compared the effects of vasopressin vs. norepinephrine ± hydrocortisone in 409 patients with septic shock. Although there were no significant mortality differences between the groups, use of vasopressin reduced the need for renal replacement therapy (RRT). Both these studies showed a sparing effect on catecholamines; therefore, the early use of vasopressin in combination with norepinephrine can help reduce the adrenergic load associated with traditional vasoactive agents. In a recent meta-analysis of four RCTs [60] comparing vasopressin with other vasopressors, vasopressin reduced the requirement for RRT. There are still controversies involving vasopressin use, specially directed to practical considerations (when to start, which dosage, and when to discontinue), which are elegantly cited by Der-Nigoghossian et al. [61]. Vasopressin was approved in 2021 by the

European Medicines Agency for use in adult septic shock refractory to catecholamines. The latest SSC recommendations suggest adding vasopressin instead of scaling norepinephrine above 0.25–0.5 g/kg/min when it is not possible to reach a MAP ≥ 65 mmHg (weak recommendation, moderate quality of evidence) [1]. It should be considered that it is not only the dose of norepinephrine that is a trigger to start vasopressin, but also the trend to increasing doses of catecholaminergic drugs [62].

### 5.4.2 Selepressin

Selepressin is a selective vasopressin type 1A (V1A) receptor agonist and may be a valid option in the field of refractoriness to conventional catecholaminergic drugs, but few clinical data support its administration in this setting. Antonucci et al. [63] reviewed 17 articles, only two of which were in humans, and concluded that there may be some beneficial findings, specifically in patients with associated renal dysfunction. Regarding those human studies, a phase 2a randomized, double-blinded, placebo-controlled multicenter trial investigated the efficacy of selepressin in patients with early septic shock and concluded that doses of 2.5 ng/kg/min were effective as a norepinephrine sparing agent and associated with a lower rate of cumulative net fluid balance [64]. A phase 2b/3, multicenter, double-blinded, randomized clinical trial investigated the efficacy and safety of selepressin at different dosages in vasopressor-dependent septic shock; despite achieving a catecholaminergic-sparing effect during the first hours without increasing adverse events, the primary and secondary outcomes were not achieved [65].

### 5.4.3 Terlipressin

Terlipressin is a synthetic analog of vasopressin with greater selectivity for the V1-receptor. The most recent research has been in the form of a meta-analysis of RCTs [66]; 10 studies with 928 patients were included. Despite a shorter duration of mechanical ventilation and reduced norepinephrine requirements, use of terlipressin did not reduce the mortality rate. Lactate clearance, length of stay in ICU or hospital, and total adverse events were also similar between the studied groups (although there was a tendency showing that digital ischemia was more common in the terlipressin group). This is an extensive field to study with considerable patient heterogeneity and the optimal terlipressin-dosing regimen might be variable.

### 5.4.4 Methylene Blue

Methylene blue is a cGMP blocker, which inhibits guanylate cyclase and thus relaxation of smooth muscle mediated by NO. It may decrease pulmonary vascular leak, increase MAP, and decrease norepinephrine needs in refractory shock after extracorporeal circulation and in septic shock. Most of the available studies are observational and with small sample sizes in which treatment was started late in the course of the shock. In the most recent one, conducted in 20 refractory septic shock patients, there was limited hemodynamic responsiveness to methylene blue administration; however, those who responded had significantly improved survival as non-responders were in a more profound state of tissue hypoxia [67]. Recently, Sari-Yavuz et al. [68] performed a retrospective cohort study of 262 patients in shock treated with methylene blue. Shock was defined as a norepinephrine dose >0.1 μg/kg/min and serum lactate level > 2 mmol/l at the start of methylene blue administration. Three different dosing strategies were identified: bolus injection followed by continuous infusion, bolus injection only, or continuous infusion only (bolus 2 mg/kg; continuous infusion with 0.25 mg/kg/min). In all groups, vasoactive-inotropic scores decreased over time. The main finding was that the bolus injection followed by a continuous infusion decreased 28-day mortality. There are no randomized clinical trials using this drug, which limits its use in septic shock [69].

### 5.4.5 Angiotensin II

Angiotensin II (ATII) is a natural hormone with endocrine properties, autocrine and paracrine effects recently approved by the USA Food and Drug Administration (FDA) for the treatment of distributive shock. It has vasoconstrictor effects at both arterial and venous levels. In the ATHOS-3 trial [70] 344 patients refractory to catecholamine treatment with norepinephrine (0.2 g/kg/min or equivalent) were randomized to receive ATII or placebo. The main objective of the study was to achieve an increase in baseline MAP ≥ 10 mmHg or raise arterial pressure > 75 mmHg; this was achieved in 69.9% of ATII patients and in 23.4% of the placebo group without significant differences in side effects. Recently, Bellomo et al. [71] observed that renin levels are markedly elevated in vasodilatory shock and could identify patients in whom treatment with ATII may be more beneficial. Currently, ATII should not be considered as a first-line agent, but having demonstrated its safety and physiological efficacy, it may have a future role as a vasopressor adjuvant.

## 5.5 Metabolic Resuscitation

During septic shock, progression of tissue damage occurs, with mitochondrial damage being the main actor in this process. This mitochondrial dysfunction causes altered energy production and decoupling of oxidative phosphorylation leading to what is known as oxidative stress. This oxidative stress is shown with an increase in reactive oxygen (ROS) and nitrogen (RNS) species, which cause damage to the cell membrane, intercellular junctions, and endothelial barrier with damage to the glycocalyx [72], altered vascular tone, and increased capillary permeability, with a certain degree of refractoriness to the action of catecholamines [73]. Because of their intracellular biological effects, use of corticosteroids, ascorbic acid, and thiamine has been proposed as part of the complementary treatment of sepsis, in the so-called "metabolic resuscitation".

### 5.5.1 Vitamin C (Ascorbic Acid)

The clinical significance of high-dose vitamin C given as a "sepsis cocktail" with hydrocortisone and thiamine was popularized by Marik et al. [74] who showed significantly reduced hospital mortality, duration of vasopressor dependence, and organ injury.

Several RCTs assessing the effects of intravenous vitamin C were therefore performed in critically ill patients followed by several systematic reviews and meta-analyses, demonstrating benefits including reduced organ dysfunction and reduced duration on vasopressor support in patients receiving high-dose vitamin C [75], but an effect on reducing mortality is still not clear. A meta-analysis [76] that deserves to be highlighted for its review not exclusively of corticosteroids, but of the so-called "metabolic resuscitation cocktail" (hydrocortisone, vitamin C and thiamine), did not show statistical significance regarding mortality. However, it did show that the combination of these three compounds improved organ failure (measured by ΔSOFA in the first 72 h of treatment), as well as the need for vasoactive amines.

However, recently, Lamontagne et al. [77] showed that vitamin C administration in sepsis was harmful with an increase in morbidity and 28-day mortality. This was a very elegant study that resolves the open question about the use of vitamin C in patients with sepsis. Nevertheless, the subpopulation of patients with refractory septic shock is a matter of concern because they have high mortality and were not well represented in this study: fewer than 60% of the study population met septic shock criteria. In fact, the administration of vitamin C in the subgroup of the most severe patients showed neutral results. In addition, hydrocortisone, vitamin C and thiamine therapy was not evaluated, despite this having the most pathophysiological basis [78]. Information about markers of oxidative stress may help to understand the results. Imbalances in baseline characteristics may also have contributed to the observed differences. Patients in the intervention group had 10% higher lactate levels, were more often in shock, and more often receiving mechanical ventilation already at baseline.

These three elements of metabolic resuscitation separately or in combinations that do not include the three substances have not yet shown the expected results, but further thoughts should be considered in the interpretation of recent trials and for future studies: was the dose of vitamin C adequate? Should vitamin C administration be triggered by plasma vitamin C levels? What is the optimal timing for vitamin C administration, and the optimal duration? Is there a biomarker relevant to vitamin C use? What outcome should be measured? Which critically ill patients may benefit the most? [79]. The future direction may be to evaluate combined hydrocortisone, vitamin C, and thiamine therapy in refractory septic shock.

### 5.5.2 Hydroxocobalamin

Hydroxocobalamin has an FDA indication for treatment of confirmed or suspected cyanide poisoning. It is also used off-label for postoperative vasoplegia, which can develop after stopping cardiopulmonary bypass (CPB). Hydroxocobalamin increases vascular tone by acting as a sink for circulating NO and hydrogen sulfide ($H_2S$). Mechanistically, NO oxidizes the cobalt atom of hydroxocobalamin forming a Co-NO complex that can subsequently transfer NO to hemoglobin or glutathione. $H_2S$ is produced by bacteria during septic shock resulting in vasodilation and hydroxocobalamin has been shown to bind and reduce the circulating volume of $H_2S$ [80]. Data from two case series provide the rationale for its use in this context. The first demonstrated that 24 of 33 patients with vasoplegia secondary to CPB had at least a 33% reduction in vasopressor dose 30 min after hydroxocobalamin administration [81]. The second demonstrated a 14 mmHg increase in MAP 30 min after hydroxocobalamin administration [82]. However, in the largest case series to date, Ritter et al. [83] studied 35 patients in septic shock who received a single bolus of hydroxocobalamin; the analysis included 3992 hemodynamic data points. They found that there was no difference in MAP 24 h after hydroxocobalamin administration. This study was different from previous studies by incorporating hourly hemodynamic measurements into the analysis, but there was still a small number of patients so that subgroup analyses could not be performed.

In this context, an ongoing phase 2 RCT is investigating a single dose of hydroxocobalamin versus placebo on vasopressor use at 3, 24 and 48 h (ClinicalTrials.gov Identifier: NCT03783091) in a septic shock setting.

## 5.6 New Molecules for Adjuvant Treatment of Sepsis

Translational scientific research has contributed to the study of several molecules in phase 2–3 clinical trials. The concept of enrichment—including both prognostic and predictive enrichment—is fundamental to enabling precision medicine. These recent trials in sepsis have used enrichment strategies based on different endotypes and biomarkers.

### 5.6.1 Nangibotide

Human triggering receptor expressed on myeloid cells (TREM)-1 is a 30-kDa glycoprotein of the immunoglobulin superfamily. TREM-1 is expressed at late stages of myeloid cell differentiation [84], and it associates with DNAX activation protein (DAP)12 for signaling and function [85], inducing the secretion of pro-inflammatory chemokines and cytokines in response to bacterial and fungal infections. Blockade of TREM-1 reduces inflammation and increases survival in animal models of bacterial sepsis. Nangibotide is a 12 amino-acid peptidic fragment derived from TREM-like transcript-1 (TELT-1), a receptor protein of the TREM-1 family. Nangibotide can bind to TREM-1 ligand and modulate the amplification of the immune response caused by the activation of TREM-1 in sepsis. In preclinical animal studies of peritonitis with septic shock, analogs of nangibotide reduced inflammatory response and improved organ function, cardiovascular status, and survival [86, 87]. In a recent phase 2a clinical trial that investigated the safety and tolerability of three doses of nangibotide in septic shock, nangibotide-treated patients had improved organ function biomarkers [88]. This effect was larger in the subgroup of patients with high circulating soluble TREM-1 (sTREM-1) levels. A phase 2b clinical trial, ASTONISH, is currently being conducted to evaluate its efficacy, safety, and tolerability in patients with septic shock, specially focused on the high sTREM-1 subgroup (ClinicalTrials.gov Identifier: NCT04055909) [89].

### 5.6.2 Recombinant Alkaline Phosphatase

Alkaline phosphatase is an endogenous homodimeric enzyme present in many cells and organs (e.g., intestines, placenta, liver, bone, kidney, and granulocytes) that exerts detoxifying effects through dephosphorylation of endotoxins and other pro-inflammatory compounds, including extracellular ATP by hydrolysis [90, 91]. Alkaline phosphatase may also attenuate the innate immune response induced by endotoxin release, as dephosphorylation of endotoxin abolishes its biological activity and the dephosphorylated LPS acts as a Toll-like receptor (TLR)4 antagonist [92]. In animal models of sepsis, alkaline phosphatase administration attenuated the inflammatory response and reduced mortality [93]. There are some clinical trials evaluating the effects of alkaline phosphatase in sepsis. The STOP-AKI trial was a double-blind, placebo-controlled, dose-finding adaptive phase 2a/2b trial that enrolled 301 adults with sepsis-associated acute kidney injury (AKI). The optimal therapeutic dose of recombinant alkaline phosphatase was 1.6 mg/kg. The 3-day treatment did not improve kidney function in the first week of treatment, but all-cause mortality at day 28 was lower in the recombinant alkaline phosphatase group than in placebo-treated patients. This effect persisted to day 90 [94]. A clinical phase 3 study, the REVIVAL trial (ClinicalTrials.gov Identifier: NCT04411472), to investigate the effect of recombinant alkaline phosphatase on 28-day mortality in patients with sepsis-associated AKI is underway.

### 5.6.3 Adrecizumab

Adrenomedullin (ADM), a 52-amino acid peptide belonging to the calcitonin gene-related peptide family [95], plays an important role in sepsis. ADM has immunomodulatory and endothelial barrier-stabilizing properties, maintaining vascular integrity [96]. Its tropism for the vascular endothelium, interstitium, and smooth muscle, and its vasodilatory properties, may contribute to sepsis-associated hypotension and increased vascular permeability. At high concentrations, ADM leads to excessive vasodilation, and increased plasma levels of ADM are associated with high vasopressor requirements, multiorgan dysfunction, and mortality [97, 98]. By binding to ADM, adrecizumab (HAM8101) does not entirely block ADM function, though it reduces its capacity to elicit a second messenger response. Under normal conditions, the concentration of ADM is higher in the interstitium than in the circulating blood. The net effect is an increase in adrecizumab-bound ADM in the circulation, removed from the interstitium, and only partial functional inhibition of ADM. Because of this redistribution, the ADM concentration in the interstitium decreases, and ADM cannot act on smooth muscle cells to exert its vasodilatory activity. Thus, adrecizumab can reduce vasodilation by reducing excessive levels of interstitially located ADM. The increased net activity of ADM in the circulation could promote stabilization of endothelial permeability [99]. Preclinical studies performed in a porcine model of sepsis showed that administration of adrecizumab reduced the progression to septic shock, renal granulocyte extravasation, and inflammatory response [100]. The AdrenOSS-2 study, a phase 2a double-blind, randomized, placebo-controlled, biomarker-guided trial, addressed the safety and tolerability of adrecizumab in patients with septic shock and elevated plasma concentrations of circulating biologically active ADM (>70 pg/ml) [101]. Although it was not the primary objective of the study, an improvement in multi-organ dysfunction was observed. A subsequent phase 2b/3 clinical trial, the ENCOURAGE study, will assess adrecizumab (4 mg/kg) in septic shock patients immediately after initiation of vasopressors.

### 5.6.4 Apoptotic Cells

Allocetra-OTS is a cell-based therapeutic composed of donor apoptotic cells. The product contains allogeneic mononuclear enriched cells in a liquid suspension with at least 40% early apoptotic cells. Apoptotic cells contribute to the maintenance of peripheral immune homeostasis. Allocetra-OTS was shown to have a beneficial effect on cytokine storm, with downregulation of anti- and pro-inflammatory cytokines. Experimental animal models have demonstrated that apoptotic cell infusion in mice is associated with a reduction in circulating pro-inflammatory cytokines, suppression of polymorphonuclear neutrophil infiltration in target organs, decreased serum LPS levels, and decreased mortality [102]. Van Heerden et al. performed a phase 1b clinical trial with Allocetra-OTS in 10 patients with sepsis and SOFA scores ranging from 2 to 6 [103]. All 10 patients survived, while matched historical controls had a mortality rate of 27%. The authors concluded that infusion of apoptotic cells to patients with mild-to-moderate sepsis was safe and had a significant immunomodulating effect, leading to early resolution of the cytokine storm. A phase 2 study evaluating the efficacy, safety, and tolerability of different doses and regimens of Allocetra-OTS to treat organ failure in sepsis patients (ClinicalTrials.gov Identifier: NCT04612413) is currently underway.

## 5.7 Conclusion

The heterogeneity of septic shock is a complex and engaging feature of the disease that demands novel strategies for improved classification of patients. Precision medicine identifies subgroups of septic shock patients with a high risk of adverse outcomes who may benefit from specific treatments or rescue therapies according to their particular characteristics. Although some clinical tools are still being evaluated in early stages of research, precision medicine is becoming a reality that improves our clinical approach.

## References

1. Evans L, Rhodes A, Alhazzani W, et al. Surviving sepsis campaign: international guidelines for management of sepsis and septic shock 2021. Intensive Care Med. 2021;47:1181–247.
2. Levy MM, Rhodes A, Phillips GS, et al. Surviving sepsis campaign: association between performance metrics and outcomes in a 7.5-year study. Crit Care Med. 2015;43:3–12.
3. Yébenes JC, Ruiz-Rodriguez JC, Ferrer R, et al. Epidemiology of sepsis in Catalonia: analysis of incidence and outcomes in a European setting. Ann Intensive Care. 2017;7:19.
4. Singer M, Deutschman CS, Seymour CW, et al. The third international consensus definitions for sepsis and septic shock (Sepsis-3). JAMA. 2016;315:801–10.
5. Seymour CW, Kennedy JN, Wang S, et al. Derivation, validation, and potential treatment implications of novel clinical phenotypes for sepsis. JAMA. 2019;321:2003–17.
6. Ruiz-Rodriguez JC, Plata-Menchaca EP, Chiscano-Camón L, et al. Precision medicine in sepsis and septic shock: from omics to clinical tools. World J Crit Care Med. 2022;11:1–21.
7. Leligdowicz A, Matthay MA. Heterogeneity in sepsis: new biological evidence with clinical applications. Crit Care. 2019;23:80.
8. Wong HR, Cvijanovich NZ, Allen GL, et al. Validation of a gene expression-based subclassification strategy for pediatric septic shock. Crit Care Med. 2011;39:2511–7.
9. Ferrario M, Cambiaghi A, Brunelli L, et al. Mortality prediction in patients with severe septic shock: a pilot study using a target metabolomics approach. Sci Rep. 2016;6:20391.
10. Punyadeera C, Schneider EM, Schaffer D, et al. A biomarker panel to discriminate between systemic inflammatory response syndrome and sepsis and sepsis severity. J Emerg Trauma Shock. 2010;3:26–35.
11. Bauzá-Martinez J, Aletti F, Pinto BB, et al. Proteolysis in septic shock patients: plasma peptidomic patterns are associated with mortality. Br J Anaesth. 2018;121:1065–74.
12. Angus DC, van der Poll T. Severe sepsis and septic shock. N Engl J Med. 2013;369:840–51.
13. Alejandria MM, Lansang MA, Dans LF, Mantaring JB III. Intravenous immunoglobulin for treating sepsis, severe sepsis and septic shock. Cochrane Database Syst Rev. 2013;2013:Cd001090.
14. Bermejo-Martín JF, Rodriguez-Fernandez A, Herrán-Monge R, et al. Immunoglobulins IgG1, IgM and IgA: a synergistic team influencing survival in sepsis. J Intern Med. 2014;276:404–12.
15. Taccone FS, Stordeur P, De Backer D, Creteur J, Vincent JL. Gamma-globulin levels in patients with community-acquired septic shock. Shock. 2009;32:379–85.
16. Andaluz-Ojeda D, Iglesias V, Bobillo F, et al. Early natural killer cell counts in blood predict mortality in severe sepsis. Crit Care. 2011;15:R243.
17. Tian L, Zhu J, Jin J, et al. Prognostic value of circulating lymphocyte B and plasma immunoglobulin M on septic shock and sepsis: a systematic review and meta-analysis. Am J Transl Res. 2019;11:7223–32.

18. Krautz C, Maier SL, Brunner M, et al. Reduced circulating B cells and plasma IgM levels are associated with decreased survival in sepsis - a meta-analysis. J Crit Care. 2018;45:71–5.
19. Busani S, Damiani E, Cavazzuti I, Donati A, Girardis M. Intravenous immunoglobulin in septic shock: review of the mechanisms of action and meta-analysis of the clinical effectiveness. Minerva Anestesiol. 2016;82:559–72.
20. Nierhaus A, Berlot G, Kindgen-Milles D, Müller E, Girardis M. Best-practice IgM- and IgA-enriched immunoglobulin use in patients with sepsis. Ann Intensive Care. 2020;10:132.
21. Cui J, Wei X, Lv H, et al. The clinical efficacy of intravenous IgM-enriched immunoglobulin (pentaglobin) in sepsis or septic shock: a meta-analysis with trial sequential analysis. Ann Intensive Care. 2019;9:27.
22. Olivares MM, Olmos CE, Álvarez MI, et al. Colombian guidelines of clinical practice for the use of immunoglobulins in the treatment of replacement and immunomodulation. Rev Alerg Mex. 2017;64(Suppl 2):s5–s65.
23. Welte T, Dellinger RP, Ebelt H, et al. Efficacy and safety of trimodulin, a novel polyclonal antibody preparation, in patients with severe community acquired pneumonia: a randomized, placebo-controlled, double-blind, multicenter, phase II trial (CIGMA study). Intensive Care Med. 2018;44:438–48.
24. Ankawi G, Neri M, Zhang J, Breglia A, Ricci Z, Ronco C. Extracorporeal techniques for the treatment of critically ill patients with sepsis beyond conventional blood purification therapy: the promises and the pitfalls. Crit Care. 2018;22:262.
25. Ronco C. Endotoxin removal: history of a mission. Blood Purif. 2014;37(Suppl 1):5–8.
26. Marshall JC, Foster D, Vincent JL, et al. Diagnostic and prognostic implications of endotoxemia in critical illness: results of the MEDIC study. J Infect Dis. 2004;190:527–34.
27. Bottiroli M, Monti G, Pinciroli R, et al. Prevalence and clinical significance of early high endotoxin activity in septic shock: an observational study. J Crit Care. 2017;41:124–9.
28. Romaschin AD, Harris DM, Ribeiro MB, Paice J, Foster DM, Walker PM, Marshall JC. A rapid assay of endotoxin in whole blood using autologous neutrophil dependent chemiluminescence. J Immunol Methods. 1998;212:169–85.
29. Vincent JL, Laterre PF, Cohen J, et al. A pilot-controlled study of a polymyxin B-immobilized hemoperfusion cartridge in patients with severe sepsis secondary to intra-abdominal infection. Shock. 2005;23:400–5.
30. Cruz DN, Antonelli M, Fumagalli R, et al. Early use of polymyxin B hemoperfusion in abdominal septic shock: the EUPHAS randomized controlled trial. JAMA. 2009;301:2445–52.
31. Payen DM, Guilhot J, Launey Y, et al. Early use of polymyxin B hemoperfusion in patients with septic shock due to peritonitis: a multicenter randomized control trial. Intensive Care Med. 2015;41:975–84.
32. Shoji H, Ferrer R. Potential survival benefit and early recovery from organ dysfunction with polymyxin B hemoperfusion: perspectives from a real-world big data analysis and the supporting mechanisms of action. J Anesth Analg Crit Care. 2022;2:27.
33. Dellinger RP, Bagshaw SM, Antonelli M, et al. Effect of targeted polymyxin B hemoperfusion on 28-day mortality in patients with septic shock and elevated endotoxin level: the EUPHRATES randomized clinical trial. JAMA. 2018;320(14):1455–63.
34. Klein DJ, Foster D, Walker PM, Bagshaw SM, Mekonnen H, Antonelli M. Polymyxin B hemoperfusion in endotoxemic septic shock patients without extreme endotoxemia: a post hoc analysis of the EUPHRATES trial. Intensive Care Med. 2018;44:2205–12.
35. Monti G, Terzi V, Calini A, et al. Rescue therapy with polymyxin B hemoperfusion in high-dose vasopressor therapy refractory septic shock. Minerva Anestesiol. 2015;81:516–25.
36. Iba T, Klein DJ. The wind changed direction and the big river still flows: from EUPHRATES to TIGRIS. J Intensive Care. 2019;7:31.
37. Cohen J. The immunopathogenesis of sepsis. Nature. 2002;420:885–91.
38. Kellum JA, Kong L, Fink MP, et al. Understanding the inflammatory cytokine response in pneumonia and sepsis: results of the Genetic and Inflammatory Markers of Sepsis (GenIMS) study. Arch Intern Med. 2007;167:1655–63.

39. Bozza FA, Salluh JI, Japiassu AM, et al. Cytokine profiles as markers of disease severity in sepsis: a multiplex analysis. Crit Care. 2007;11:R49.
40. Jekarl DW, Lee SY, Lee J, et al. Procalcitonin as a diagnostic marker and IL-6 as a prognostic marker for sepsis. Diagn Microbiol Infect Dis. 2013;75:342–7.
41. Kumar AT, Sudhir U, Punith K, Kumar R, Ravi Kumar VN, Rao MY. Cytokine profile in elderly patients with sepsis. Indian J Crit Care Med. 2009;13:74–8.
42. Gogos CA, Drosou E, Bassaris HP, Skoutelis A. Pro- versus anti-inflammatory cytokine profile in patients with severe sepsis: a marker for prognosis and future therapeutic options. J Infect Dis. 2000;181:176–80.
43. Chaudhry H, Zhou J, Zhong Y, et al. Role of cytokines as a double-edged sword in sepsis. In Vivo. 2013;27:669–84.
44. Friesecke S, Stecher SS, Gross S, Felix SB, Nierhaus A. Extracorporeal cytokine elimination as rescue therapy in refractory septic shock: a prospective single-center study. J Artif Organs. 2017;20:252–9.
45. Paul R, Sathe P, Kumar S, Prasad S, Aleem M, Sakhalvalkar P. Multicentered prospective investigator initiated study to evaluate the clinical outcomes with extracorporeal cytokine adsorption device (CytoSorb(®)) in patients with sepsis and septic shock. World J Crit Care Med. 2021;10:22–34.
46. Brouwer WP, Duran S, Kuijper M, Ince C. Hemoadsorption with CytoSorb shows a decreased observed versus expected 28-day all-cause mortality in ICU patients with septic shock: a propensity-score-weighted retrospective study. Crit Care. 2019;23:317.
47. Hawchar F, László I, Öveges N, Trásy D, Ondrik Z, Molnar Z. Extracorporeal cytokine adsorption in septic shock: a proof of concept randomized, controlled pilot study. J Crit Care. 2019;49:172–8.
48. Rugg C, Klose R, Hornung R, et al. Hemoadsorption with CytoSorb in septic shock reduces catecholamine requirements and in-hospital mortality: a single-center retrospective 'genetic' matched analysis. Biomedicine. 2020;8:539.
49. Malard B, Lambert C, Kellum JA. In vitro comparison of the adsorption of inflammatory mediators by blood purification devices. Intensive Care Med Exp. 2018;6:12.
50. Chousterman BG, Swirski FK, Weber GF. Cytokine storm and sepsis disease pathogenesis. Semin Immunopathol. 2017;39:517–28.
51. Ruiz-Rodríguez JC, Chiscano-Camón L, Palmada C, et al. Endotoxin and cytokine sequential hemoadsorption in septic shock and multi-organ failure. Blood Purif. 2022;51:630–3.
52. Ruiz-Rodríguez JC, Chiscano-Camón L, Ruiz-Sanmartin A, et al. Cytokine hemoadsorption as rescue therapy for critically ill patients with SARS-CoV-2 pneumonia with severe respiratory failure and hypercytokinemia. Front Med (Lausanne). 2022;8:779038.
53. Yaroustovsky M, Abramyan M, Krotenko N, Popov D, Plyushch M, Rogalskaya E. A pilot study of selective lipopolysaccharide adsorption and coupled plasma filtration and adsorption in adult patients with severe sepsis. Blood Purif. 2015;39:210–7.
54. Nandhabalan P, Ioannou N, Meadows C, Wyncoll D. Refractory septic shock: our pragmatic approach. Crit Care. 2018;22:215.
55. Landry DW, Levin HR, Gallant EM, et al. Vasopressin deficiency contributes to the vasodilation of septic shock. Circulation. 1997;95:1122–5.
56. Patel BM, Chittock DR, Russell JA, Walley KR. Beneficial effects of short-term vasopressin infusion during severe septic shock. Anesthesiology. 2002;96:576–82.
57. Holmes CL, Walley KR, Chittock DR, Lehman T, Russell JA. The effects of vasopressin on hemodynamics and renal function in severe septic shock: a case series. Intensive Care Med. 2001;27:1416–21.
58. Russell JA, Walley KR, Singer J, et al. Vasopressin versus norepinephrine infusion in patients with septic shock. N Engl J Med. 2008;358:877–87.
59. Gordon AC, Mason AJ, Thirunavukkarasu N, et al. Effect of early vasopressin vs norepinephrine on kidney failure in patients with septic shock: the VANISH randomized clinical trial. JAMA. 2016;316:509–18.

60. Nagendran M, Russell JA, Walley KR, et al. Vasopressin in septic shock: an individual patient data meta-analysis of randomised controlled trials. Intensive Care Med. 2019;45:844–55.
61. Der-Nigoghossian C, Hammond DA, Ammar MA. Narrative review of controversies involving vasopressin use in septic shock and practical considerations. Ann Pharmacother. 2020;54:706–14.
62. Guerci P, Belveyre T, Mongardon N, Novy E. When to start vasopressin in septic shock: the strategy we propose. Crit Care. 2022;26:125.
63. Antonucci E, Giovini M, Agosta S, Sakr Y, Leone M. Selepressin in septic shock. Shock. 2022;57:172–9.
64. Russell JA, Vincent JL, Kjølbye AL, et al. Selepressin, a novel selective vasopressin V1A agonist, is an effective substitute for norepinephrine in a phase IIa randomized, placebo-controlled trial in septic shock patients. Crit Care. 2017;21:213.
65. Laterre PF, Berry SM, Blemings A, et al. Effect of selepressin vs placebo on ventilator- and vasopressor-free days in patients with septic shock: the SEPSIS-ACT randomized clinical trial. JAMA. 2019;322:1476–85.
66. Zhu Y, Huang H, Xi X, Du B. Terlipressin for septic shock patients: a meta-analysis of randomized controlled study. J Intensive Care. 2019;7:16.
67. Porizka M, Kopecky P, Dvorakova H, et al. Methylene blue administration in patients with refractory distributive shock – a retrospective study. Sci Rep. 2020;10:1828.
68. Sari-Yavuz S, Heck-Swain K, Keller M, et al. Methylene blue dosing strategies in critically ill adults with shock – a retrospective cohort study. Res Square. 2022. https://doi.org/10.21203/rs.3.rs-1752415/v1.
69. Paciullo CA, McMahon Horner D, Hatton KW, Flynn JD. Methylene blue for the treatment of septic shock. Pharmacotherapy. 2010;30:702–15.
70. Khanna A, English SW, Wang XS, et al. Angiotensin II for the treatment of vasodilatory shock. N Engl J Med. 2017;377:419–30.
71. Bellomo R, Forni LG, Busse LW, et al. Renin and survival in patients given angiotensin ii for catecholamine-resistant vasodilatory shock. A clinical trial. Am J Respir Crit Care Med. 2020;202:1253–61.
72. Burke-Gaffney A, Evans TW. Lest we forget the endothelial glycocalyx in sepsis. Crit Care. 2012;16:121.
73. Bedard K, Krause KH. The NOX family of ROS-generating NADPH oxidases: physiology and pathophysiology. Physiol Rev. 2007;87:245–313.
74. Marik PE, Khangoora V, Rivera R, Hooper MH, Catravas J. Hydrocortisone, vitamin c, and thiamine for the treatment of severe sepsis and septic shock: a retrospective before-after study. Chest. 2017;151:1229–38.
75. Stoppe C, Lee ZY, Ortiz L, Heyland DK, Patel JJ. The potential role of intravenous vitamin C monotherapy in critical illness. JPEN J Parenter Enteral Nutr. 2022;46:972–6.
76. Assouline B, Faivre A, Verissimo T, et al. Thiamine, ascorbic acid, and hydrocortisone as a metabolic resuscitation cocktail in sepsis: a meta-analysis of randomized controlled trials with trial sequential analysis. Crit Care Med. 2021;49:2112–20.
77. Lamontagne F, Masse MH, Menard J, et al; LOVIT Investigators and the Canadian Critical Care Trials Group. Intravenous vitamin C in adults with sepsis in the intensive care unit. N Engl J Med. 2022;386:2387–98.
78. Marik PE. Hydrocortisone, ascorbic acid and thiamine (HAT therapy) for the treatment of sepsis. Focus on ascorbic acid. Nutrients. 2018;10:1762.
79. Stoppe C, Preiser JC, de Backer D, Elke G. Intravenous vitamin C in adults with sepsis in the intensive care unit: still LOV'IT? Crit Care. 2022;26:230.
80. Brouwer M, Chamulitrat W, Ferruzzi G, Sauls DL, Weinberg JB. Nitric oxide interactions with cobalamins: biochemical and functional consequences. Blood. 1996;88:1857–64.
81. Shah PR, Reynolds PS, Pal N, Tang D, McCarthy H, Spiess BD. Hydroxocobalamin for the treatment of cardiac surgery-associated vasoplegia: a case series. Can J Anaesth. 2018;65:560–8.

82. Armour S, Armour TK, Joppa WR, Maltais S, Nelson JA, Wittwer E. Use of hydroxocobalamin (vitamin B12a) in patients with vasopressor refractory hypotension after cardiopulmonary bypass: a case series. Anesth Analg. 2019;129:e1–4.
83. Ritter LA, Maldarelli M, McCurdy MT, et al. Effects of a single bolus of hydroxocobalamin on hemodynamics in vasodilatory shock. J Crit Care. 2022;67:66–71.
84. Bouchon A, Dietrich J, Colonna M. Cutting edge: inflammatory responses can be triggered by TREM-1, a novel receptor expressed on neutrophils and monocytes. J Immunol. 2000;164:4991–5.
85. Lanier LL, Bakker AB. The ITAM-bearing transmembrane adaptor DAP12 in lymphoid and myeloid cell function. Immunol Today. 2000;21:611–4.
86. Derive M, Boufenzer A, Bouazza Y, et al. Effects of a TREM-like transcript 1-derived peptide during hypodynamic septic shock in pigs. Shock. 2013;39:176–82.
87. Derive M, Bouazza Y, Sennoun N, et al. Soluble TREM-like transcript-1 regulates leukocyte activation and controls microbial sepsis. J Immunol. 2012;188:5585–92.
88. François B, Wittebole X, Ferrer R, et al. Nangibotide in patients with septic shock: a phase 2a randomized controlled clinical trial. Intensive Care Med. 2022;46:1425–37.
89. Francois B, Lambden S, Gibot S, et al. Rationale and protocol for the efficacy, safety and tolerability of nangibotide in patients with septic shock (ASTONISH) phase IIb randomised controlled trial. BMJ Open. 2021;11:e042921.
90. Koyama I, Matsunaga T, Harada T, Hokari S, Komoda T. Alkaline phosphatases reduce toxicity of lipopolysaccharides in vivo and in vitro through dephosphorylation. Clin Biochem. 2002;35:455–61.
91. Bentala H, Verweij WR, Huizinga-Van der Vlag A, van Loenen-Weemaes AM, Meijer DK, Poelstra K. Removal of phosphate from lipid A as a strategy to detoxify lipopolysaccharide. Shock. 2002;18:561–6.
92. Wy CA, Goto M, Young RI, Myers TF, Muraskas J. Prophylactic treatment of endotoxic shock with monophosphoryl lipid A in newborn rats. Biol Neonate. 2000;77:191–5.
93. Su F, Brands R, Wang Z, et al. Beneficial effects of alkaline phosphatase in septic shock. Crit Care Med. 2006;34:2182–7.
94. Pickkers P, Mehta RL, Murray PT, et al. Effect of human recombinant alkaline phosphatase on 7-day creatinine clearance in patients with sepsis-associated acute kidney injury: a randomized clinical trial. JAMA. 2018;320:1998–2009.
95. Poyner DR, Sexton PM, Marshall I, et al. International Union of Pharmacology. XXXII. The mammalian calcitonin gene-related peptides, adrenomedullin, amylin, and calcitonin receptors. Pharmacol Rev. 2002;54:233–46.
96. Geven C, Kox M, Pickkers P. Adrenomedullin and adrenomedullin-targeted therapy as treatment strategies relevant for sepsis. Front Immunol. 2018;9:292.
97. Marino R, Struck J, Maisel AS, et al. Plasma adrenomedullin is associated with short-term mortality and vasopressor requirement in patients admitted with sepsis. Crit Care. 2014;18:R34.
98. Caironi P, Latini R, Struck J, et al. Circulating biologically active adrenomedullin (bio-ADM) predicts hemodynamic support requirement and mortality during sepsis. Chest. 2017;152:312–20.
99. Geven C, Pickkers P. The mechanism of action of the adrenomedullin-binding antibody adrecizumab. Crit Care. 2018;22:159.
100. Thiele C, Simon TP, Szymanski J, et al. Effects of the non-neutralizing humanized monoclonal anti-adrenomedullin antibody adrecizumab on hemodynamic and renal injury in a porcine two-hit model. Shock. 2020;54:810–8.
101. Laterre PF, Pickkers P, Marx G, et al. Safety and tolerability of non-neutralizing adrenomedullin antibody adrecizumab (HAM8101) in septic shock patients: the AdrenOSS-2 phase 2a biomarker-guided trial. Intensive Care Med. 2021;47:1284–94.
102. Ren Y, Xie Y, Jiang G, Fan J, Yeung J, Li W, Tam PK, Savill J. Apoptotic cells protect mice against lipopolysaccharide-induced shock. J Immunol. 2008;180:4978–85.
103. van Heerden PV, Abutbul A, Sviri S, et al. Apoptotic cells for therapeutic use in cytokine storm associated with sepsis- a phase Ib clinical trial. Front Immunol. 2021;12:718191.

# Part II

# Sepsis Biomarkers and Organ Dysfunction Scores

# Host Response Biomarkers for Sepsis in the Emergency Room

6

O. Turgman, M. Schinkel, and W. J. Wiersinga

## 6.1 Introduction

Sepsis is a medical emergency currently defined as life-threatening organ dysfunction caused by a dysregulated host response to infection [1]. With a recent estimate of 11 million sepsis-related deaths out of 48.9 million yearly sepsis cases, it is a global health priority [2]. Current sepsis treatment guidelines recommend general measures, such as antibiotic treatment, source control, and resuscitation [3]. The heterogeneity of the sepsis syndrome however makes early and consistent diagnosis difficult [4] and has resulted in a lack of sepsis-specific treatments [5, 6]. An essential factor limiting our ability to detect sepsis is the lack of clinically relevant biomarkers for the early phases of the syndrome.

The benefits of early diagnosis and treatment have been well-studied and protocolized in specialties such as trauma medicine, cardiology (e.g., myocardial infarction and cardiac arrest) and neurology (e.g., stroke management), but less so in the field of sepsis [7]. This can potentially lead to longer time-to-antibiotics and higher mortality [8]. Sepsis patients often undergo their first extensive evaluation in the emergency room (ER). Decisions made at this stage, such as choice of antibiotic treatment and discharge destination, are likely to highly impact the rest of the

O. Turgman
Center for Experimental and Molecular Medicine, Amsterdam Institute for Infection and Immunity, Amsterdam UMC, Location Academic Medical Center, University of Amsterdam, Amsterdam, The Netherlands

M. Schinkel · W. J. Wiersinga (✉)
Center for Experimental and Molecular Medicine, Amsterdam Institute for Infection and Immunity, Amsterdam UMC, Location Academic Medical Center, University of Amsterdam, Amsterdam, The Netherlands

Division of Infectious Diseases, Department of Medicine, Amsterdam UMC, Location Academic Medical Center, University of Amsterdam, Amsterdam, The Netherlands
e-mail: w.j.wiersinga@amsterdamumc.nl



J.-L. Vincent (ed.), *Annual Update in Intensive Care and Emergency Medicine 2023*, Annual Update in Intensive Care and Emergency Medicine,
https://doi.org/10.1007/978-3-031-23005-9_6

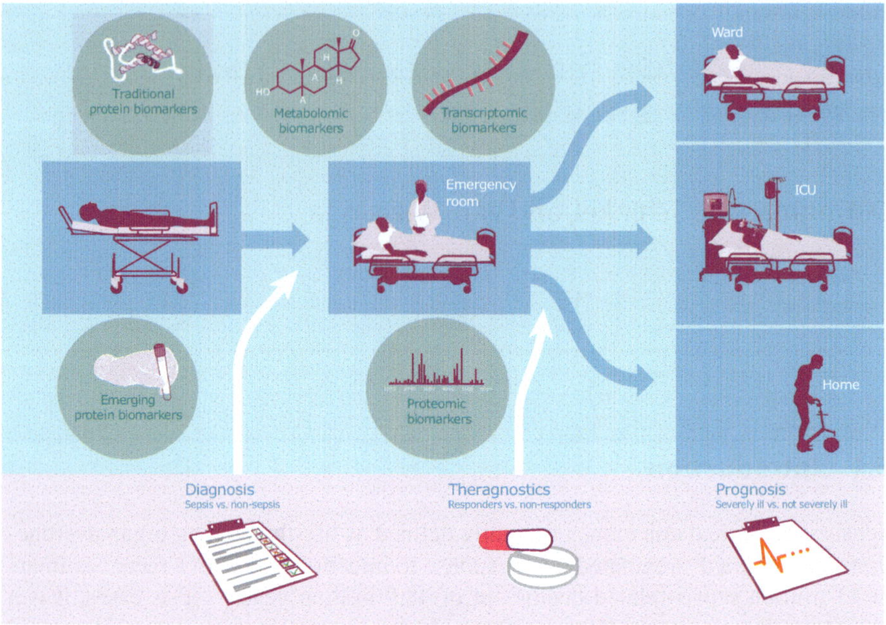


**Fig. 6.1** Host response biomarkers for sepsis in the emergency room (ER). A visualization of the patient flow through the ER and of the different types of sepsis biomarkers and their respective roles in this process

hospital stay. Biomarkers are able to reduce the heterogeneity among sepsis patients in the ER and could improve their care.

This review aims to provide a high-level overview of sepsis biomarkers that are relevant for the ER setting. It focuses on markers found in the systemic compartment and includes traditional and emerging protein biomarkers, but also those arising from the fields of transcriptomics, proteomics, and metabolomics (Fig. 6.1).

## 6.2 Biomarkers in the Context of Sepsis

Biomarkers can be defined as any objective, reproducible characteristics by which (patho)physiologic processes can be identified and measured [9]. Within the field of sepsis, one can differentiate between diagnostic, prognostic, and therapeutic biomarkers [10, 11]. Diagnostic biomarkers differentiate between infectious and non-infectious disease or help identify specific pathogens. Prognostic biomarkers are useful for assessing the risk of poor outcomes in septic patients and can help us stratify patients by their risk profiles. Lastly, therapeutic biomarkers are used to assess the effectiveness of a treatment. In recent years, biomarkers have been used for a fourth category: theragnostics. Theragnostics describes an approach in which patients are stratified based on specific biomarkers or pathways that might be more susceptible to specific intervention [5, 12]. Also termed predictive enrichment, this approach stands in contrast to prognostic enrichment wherein patients with a higher likelihood of having a certain outcome are identified. Prognostic enrichment in trials can improve power and reduce the number of patients needed [12]. This is underscored by recent studies in patients with severe coronavirus disease 2019 (COVID-19) in which C-reactive protein (CRP) and soluble urokinase plasminogen receptor (suPAR) plasma levels were successfully used to guide treatment with respectively anti-interleukin (IL)-6 and anti-IL-1 [13, 14]. In the later study, allocation of patients to treatment groups was guided by suPAR, a biomarker that predicts progression to severe respiratory failure or death in COVID-19 patients. The study only included patients with suPAR levels >6 ng/ml, and randomized them to receive either IL-1 receptor antagonist or placebo in addition to the standard-of-care treatment. The sepsis field is moving from traditional ways of diagnosis and treatment towards a precision medicine approach, in which more homogeneous patient groups with shared pathophysiologic pathways are identified that are amenable to a specific treatment [15]. Biomarkers will be essential to expedite this transition.

### 6.2.1 Traditional Biomarkers: CRP and Procalcitonin (PCT)

From the hundreds of biomarkers evaluated for diagnosing infection and sepsis, only a handful are used by clinicians on a large scale. Although non-specific for the diagnosis of sepsis, CRP and procalcitonin (PCT) are often used to detect inflammation because of their high sensitivity [16]. CRP is an acute-phase reactant protein synthesized by the liver, primarily induced by IL-6 [17], whereas PCT is a precursor for the calcitonin hormone, normally made in the thyroid gland. When compared to CRP, PCT levels increase faster after stimulation, reach their peak faster, and also decline faster after resolution of infection [18]. These are desirable characteristics for a biomarker, especially in the ER, as they describe the current state of a patient more accurately. A systematic review, which assessed the accuracy and clinical value of PCT for diagnosis of sepsis in intensive care unit (ICU) and ER patients, reported an area under the curve (AUC) value of 0.85 (95% confidence interval (CI) 0.81–0.88) for diagnosis of sepsis [19]. One of the included studies, among ER patients with suspected infection, reported an AUC value for PCT of 0.79 for diagnosis of sepsis, which was better than that of IL-6 (AUC 0.70) or CRP (AUC 0.67) [20]. This finding was confirmed in a recent systematic review that specifically addressed the role of PCT in the ER setting [21]; according to most included studies, PCT performed better than CRP or lactate as a diagnostic biomarker for sepsis. As a predictor of adverse outcomes, the data on PCT are more inconsistent. In some studies PCT was superior to CRP and lactate, but in others it was not [21]. There is, however, solid evidence that PCT can be of added value for effectively and safely reducing the duration of antibiotic therapy in critically ill patients. This is underlined by a recent meta-analysis that included 21 studies in patients with sepsis and/or respiratory infection, demonstrating that duration of antibiotic treatment was significantly reduced in both groups when PCT was used as a guiding biomarker compared with clinical evaluation alone [18]; as a secondary outcome, in-hospital mortality was also significantly lower among these patients [18]. Currently, the Surviving Sepsis Campaign (SSC) guidelines advise against using PCT to aid the decision of when to start antimicrobials and suggest clinical evaluation alone [3]. However, PCT use is suggested to help decide when to discontinue antimicrobials among adult patients with sepsis where the optimal duration of therapy is unclear [3].

### 6.2.2 Emerging Biomarkers

Over 250 biomarkers for sepsis have been evaluated in clinical and experimental studies [10]. Examples of emerging biomarkers that have been studied in the ER setting for either diagnostic or prognostic value include presepsin, IL-6, lipopolysaccharide-binding protein (LBP), pancreatic stone protein (PSP), bactericidal/permeability-increasing protein (BPI), group II phospholipase A2 (PLA2GIIA), brain natriuretic peptide (BNP), soluble triggering receptor expressed on myeloid cells-1 (sTREM-1), suPAR, pro-adrenomedullin (MR-proADM), macrophage migration inhibitory factor (MIF), heparin-binding protein, D-dimer, soluble IL-2 receptor alpha chain (sCD25), and cell-free DNA [10]. Many more potential sepsis biomarkers have been studied in non-ER patient groups, but these are outside the scope of this review. Those discussed herein were selected based on the presence of recent literature, the number of included patients in the relevant studies, and the setting in which the biomarker was tested (i.e., in the ER). A full overview of sepsis biomarkers can be found elsewhere [10, 11].

#### 6.2.2.1 Presepsin

Presepsin, first described as soluble CD14 subtype in 2005 [22], is a soluble fragment of CD14, a broad-spectrum affinity component of the innate immune system. Serum presepsin levels start to rise 2 h after infection and already reach their peak after 3 h, making it a potentially valuable early biomarker for sepsis in the ER [23, 24]. A 2013 study from China in 859 ER patients with at least two diagnostic criteria for systemic inflammatory response syndrome (SIRS), showed superior performance characteristics of presepsin compared to PCT for sepsis diagnosis (AUC of 0.820 vs. 0.724 for PCT) as well as prediction of severe sepsis (AUC 0.840 vs. 0.741) [25]. A more recent meta-analysis from 2017 concluded that presepsin had a pooled sensitivity of 0.84 (95% CI 0.80–0.87) and specificity of 0.76 (95% CI 0.67–0.84) for diagnosing sepsis among critically ill patients (admitted to the ER, ICU or cardiac care unit) [23]. Interestingly, when subgroups were analyzed, presepsin had better specificity in ER patients when compared to ICU patients (0.82, 95% CI 0.69–0.91 vs. 0.64, 95% CI 0.51–0.76) with an AUC indicative of higher accuracy in the ER group (0.91 vs. 0.85) [23]. However, when compared to CRP or PCT in ER patients, presepsin did not perform better in terms of diagnosing sepsis in this meta-analysis [23]. Finally, in a recent South Korean prospective observational study among 420 ER patients, presepsin performed better than CRP in terms of differentiating between non-infectious organ failure, sepsis, and septic shock, defined according to Sepsis-3 criteria [24]. However, presepsin was described as having equal performance compared to PCT [24]. In this study, patients with high serum presepsin levels (≥ 821 pg/ml) had a higher mortality rate compared to patients with lower levels (33.3% vs. 18.4% respectively) [24]. These results indicate that presepsin has value as a diagnostic and prognostic biomarker for sepsis in the ER, but whether it outperforms PCT or CRP has not been conclusively shown.

#### 6.2.2.2 sTREM-1

TREM-1 is a member of the immunoglobulin superfamily expressed on neutrophils and monocytes [26]. During bacterial and fungal infections, TREM-1 is upregulated, which causes release of sTREM-1. In a 2021 meta-analysis, sTREM-1 was described as having a sensitivity of 0.85 (95% CI 0.76–0.91) and a specificity of 0.79 (95% CI 0.70–0.86) for differentiating sepsis from SIRS among critically ill patients from various countries worldwide [27]. sTREM-1 was also able to predict 28-day mortality with a sensitivity of 0.80 (95% CI 0.66–0.89) and a specificity of 0.75 95% (CI 0.70–0.86) [27]. Looking at the ER specifically, a recent Taiwanese study investigated the prognostic value of sTREM-1 in 155 ER patients with sepsis [28]. Significantly higher and sustained levels of sTREM-1 were found among nonsurvivors on days 1, 4, and 7 after admission. sTREM-1 and sequential organ failure assessment (SOFA) scores were the only factors independently associated with sepsis-related death, with AUC values of 0.726 (95% CI 0.613–0.838; $p = 0.028$) and 0.705 (95% CI 0.602–0.808; $p = 0.042$), respectively [28]. Taken together, sTREM-1 has been shown to have diagnostic and prognostic value as a biomarker for sepsis in critically ill patients. However, studies that evaluate the added value of sTREM-1 on meaningful patient-related outcome parameters in comparison to other biomarkers specifically in the ER are lacking.

#### 6.2.2.3 Proadrenomedullin

MR-proADM, derived from adrenomedullin (ADM), has been shown to play a role in preserving the integrity and stability of the endothelium after severe infection [29]. ADM acts directly on the sympathetic nervous system, causing arterial and venous vasodilation, natriuresis, bronchodilation, and positive inotropy. MR-proADM as a compound is more stable than ADM and accurately reflects ADM levels [30]. A recent systematic review that investigated MR-proADM as an early biomarker for sepsis, included 11 studies with 1176 sepsis patients and 823 controls [30]. ER, ICU, and ward patients were included. Diagnostic criteria for sepsis varied between studies. Pooled data concerning the ability of MR-proADM to diagnose sepsis showed a sensitivity of 0.83% (95% CI 0.79–0.87%) and specificity of 0.90% (95% CI 0.83–0.94%). Less is known about MR-proADM as a prognostic biomarker of sepsis. MR-proADM levels measured within 24 h of ICU admission have been shown to be positively correlated with organ failure in patients with sepsis [30]. Among ER patients, MR-proADM was the only biomarker associated with blood culture status, i.e., low levels were correlated with a negative blood culture, when compared to CRP, PCT, lactate, soluble PLA2GIIA, sTREM-1, presepsin, and sCD25 [31]. An English study among ER patients with COVID-19, found that MR-proADM could predict 30-day mortality more accurately than CRP, PCT, white blood cell count, and lymphocyte or neutrophil count. Elevated MR-proADM levels were also associated with critical care admission and non-invasive ventilation among these patients [29]. Taken together, MR-proADM can assist in the diagnosis of sepsis as well as prediction of severe disease among patients with suspected infection in the ER. However, there are no studies addressing its true potential for improving the outcome of patients in the ER with (suspected) sepsis.

## 6.3 Transcriptomics

Recent advances in omic technologies have shifted the focus from traditional protein biomarkers to the fields of genomics, transcriptomics, proteomics, and metabolomics [32]. Transcriptomics and proteomics have been studied the most in the context of sepsis biomarkers. By analyzing relevant data on a molecular level, it has become possible to identify sepsis and stratify patients according to information pertaining to cellular proteins, metabolites, genes, and their expression. This allows for more homogenous cohorts of patients that share biological similarities, which might open the door for effective treatment strategies, designed to address a certain pathophysiological pathway.

A recent study aimed to identify novel transcriptional diagnostic and risk stratification biomarkers among ER and ICU patients from various countries worldwide with suspected infection and at least two SIRS/Sepsis-1 criteria [33]. Using unsupervised machine learning, several immune-related processes were found to differ among severely ill patients (24-h SOFA score >5) compared to patients who were less sick. For example, neutrophil degranulation was the most enriched pathway among severely ill patients, indicating that sepsis severity in the early stages is strongly associated with neutrophil activity. Interferon-gamma (IFNγ) was notably downregulated among non-survivors. Using RNAseq data, a 40-gene classification set was identified that was able to categorize patients into one of five mechanistic endotypes with an accuracy of 96% [33]. Different endotypes were found to have different enriched pathways and severity of disease. For example, neutrophilic-suppressive (NPS) and inflammatory (INF) endotypes were associated with more severe disease based on organ failure probability, SOFA scores, length of hospital stay, requirement for oxygen supplementation, and positive blood culture tests. The NPS endotype was found to include the most immunosuppressed patients with severe disease, with downregulation of IFN signaling, CD28 co-stimulation, and programmed-death (PD)-1 signaling. Conversely, the INF endotype, which also included the most severely ill patients, was found to have upregulation of multiple inflammatory pathways, such as IFNγ and TNF-α signaling [33].

In a different study from the USA, using 29 preselected mRNA inputs inflammatix-bacterial-viral-non-infected-version 1 (IMX-BVN-1) was created, a neural network classifier trained to differentiate between bacterial, viral, and non-infectious disease among ICU patients [34]. When infection adjudications were unanimous, IMX-BVN-1 was shown to have AUC values of 0.86 (bacterial-vs.-other), 0.85 (viral-vs.-other), and 0.82 (non-infected-vs.-other). In a later validation study among 312 ER patients with suspected acute infections and at least one abnormal vital sign, IMX-BVN-2 (an updated version of IMX-BVN-1) was described to have AUC values of 0.82–0.90 for differentiating between bacterial infection and no infection [35]. This was superior to PCT (AUC 0.80–0.89), CRP (0.79–0.84), and white blood cell count (0.69–0.77). AUC values ranged due to varying degrees of certainty in the retrospective adjudication of infection status. When differentiating between viral infections and no infection, IMX-BVN-2 showed an AUC value of 0.82–0.83, whereas PCT, CRP, and white blood cell count could not differentiate between these groups (AUC <0.4). Most recently, IMX-SEV-2, a variant of IMX-BVN-2 developed for predicting disease severity in patients with sepsis, was described to have an AUC value of 0.84 (95% CI 0.76–0.93) for predicting in-hospital mortality [36]. This was superior to lactate (AUC 0.76; 95% CI 0.64–0.87), qSOFA (0.68; 95% CI 0.57–0.79), and the National Early Warning Score 2 (0.75; 95% CI 0.65–0.85) ($p = 0.015$, 0.001, and 0.013, respectively).

Other tools that use transcriptomic data and have been developed as biomarkers for sepsis are SeptiCyte Lab [37], the sepsis mortality score (SMS) for prediction of death in septic patients [38], and the FAIM3:PLAC8 ratio, originally derived to identify community-acquired pneumonia in ICU patients but later studied as a biomarker for sepsis [39]. These promising tools await validation in an ER setting where clinical sepsis is not always overt.

## 6.4 Proteomics and Metabolomics

The proteome is defined as the entire set of proteins that can be expressed by a genome while the metabolome is defined as all the small molecules in cells that are a product of the genome and of genome-environment interactions [40]. These novel analytes have been used to diagnose sepsis, reveal profiles of patients that relate to clinical outcomes, and identify future targets for intervention. Techniques such as chromatography and mass-spectrometry have enabled us to study very small particles that provide information of underlying biological processes. A novel technique, Raman spectroscopy, uses light scattering to non-destructively provide a structural fingerprint by which particles can be identified and has been used for identifying pathogens and metabolites, such as IL-6 [41, 42]. In a cohort of 63 critically ill patients with sepsis and 43 controls, Chen et al. used a combined proteomics and metabolomics approach to identify specific profiles in amino acid metabolism that could differentiate between patients with sepsis and healthy controls, with AUC values ranging from 0.81 to 0.96 [43]. In a validation group, the AUC value ranged from 0.62 to 1.00. Among the most discriminative metabolites were fatty acids and glycerophospholipids, which have roles in energy production and lipid signal transduction, respectively. Pathways and proteins involved in the acute inflammatory response, Toll-like receptor (TLR) signaling, defense response, and activation of myeloid cells were correlated with sepsis and sepsis-associated kidney injury.

Multi-omics analysis has also been used to develop tools for triage of pediatric sepsis. A study published in 2015 used metabolomic and proteomic profiling data to assess the accuracy of these profiles in retrospectively differentiating between pediatric patients with sepsis who were admitted to the pediatric ICU (PICU) (n = 94) and those who presented to the ER but were not admitted to the PICU (n = 81). Reported AUC values ranged from 0.88–0.96 [44]. Multi-omic-based profiles that can be used to predict severity of disease and necessity for certain treatments are valuable, especially when certain expertise is not available. In a more recent study, van Houten et al. investigated whether a host-protein-based assay could differentiate between bacterial and viral infection among preschool children [45]. The assay integrates concentrations of three biomarkers: TNF-related apoptosis-inducing ligand (TRAIL), IFNγ induced protein-10 (IP10), and CRP. Patients (n = 577) were aged 2–60 months and were included from four hospitals in the Netherlands and two hospitals in Israel. Patients were either diagnosed with lower respiratory tract infection or had a clinical presentation with fever with unknown source. Reference diagnoses were adjudicated by a panel of three experienced pediatricians, based on all clinical information including follow-up at 28 days. AUC values for differentiating between viral and bacterial infection ranged from 0.90–0.92, depending on the degree of certainty of the adjudicating panelists [45].

A metabolomics approach has also been used to diagnose bacteremic sepsis among 114 Swedish adult ER patients [46]. Of these patients, 65 had laboratory-confirmed bacteremia and fulfilled the 1992 criteria for sepsis (i.e., SIRS criteria plus infection). The remaining 45 patients were initially also suspected of bacteremic sepsis, but were found to have negative blood cultures and laboratory-confirmed alternative diagnoses. After analysis, six metabolites were integrated into a diagnostic tool, which was tested in a subgroup of the cohort and was found to be able to predict bacteremic sepsis with an accuracy of 88.1% [46]. Metabolomics has also brought possibilities for personalizing drug treatment as was exemplified in a study in the USA in 21 patients with vasopressor-dependent septic shock treated with l-carnitine [47]. Responders to l-carnitine had significant changes in their metabolomic signatures. Taken together, these data show that metabolic signatures can be used for the diagnosis of sepsis, for the stratification of patients towards a specific treatment, and as a marker of disease severity.

## 6.5 Conclusion

Biomarkers for sepsis in the ER can be of diagnostic, prognostic, and therapeutic value. Theragnostics entails the use of biomarkers for predictive or prognostic enrichment [11]. A large number of sepsis markers has been identified and studied recently, but only a few are being used widely in everyday clinical practice [10]. Ideally, a biomarker can diagnose sepsis, predict its severity, and help to ascertain appropriate treatment. It should be able to stratify patients according to their disease severity or susceptibility to a specific treatment. Unfortunately, biomarkers that can achieve these goals consistently in the heterogeneous population found in the ER setting have not yet been identified. Widely known and used are CRP and PCT, which can have important roles in the ER but do not meet the aforementioned criteria for the ideal biomarker. Emerging protein biomarkers, such as presepsin and MR-proADM, have shown promise in several specific homogeneous populations but validation in large and diverse cohorts is lacking. From the field of omics, several promising new techniques have emerged, enabling health care providers to integrate high-dimensional data, which can increase power and efficiency for identifying clinically relevant biomarkers for sepsis in the ER setting [32]. However, further validation of these biomarkers should be done first. Furthermore, their effect on clinically meaningful patient-related outcome measures, let alone their cost-effectiveness, is often ill-defined and should be the subject of further studies. It is very unlikely that a single biomarker will provide us with the answers to all our needs. Panels of biomarkers have been shown to be more effective in many aspects than single ones [48]. The field of biomarkers for sepsis in the ER is developing rapidly. In the near future, management of sepsis in the ER is likely to be guided by repeated measurements of biomarker arrays, which utilize point-of-care tests. These tests limit hands-on time and reflect abnormalities in host response pathways that are amenable to targeted therapeutics.

**Acknowledgments** This work is supported by a H2020 Eurostars grant (ESTAR22116, SEP-RAID) from the European Union. WJW is supported by the Netherlands Organization for Scientific Research (NWO Vidi grant no. 91716475). We would like to thank Maartje Kunen for help in the preparation of the figure.

## References

1. Singer M, Deutschman CS, Seymour CW, et al. The Third International Consensus Definitions for Sepsis and Septic Shock (Sepsis-3). JAMA. 2016;315:801–10.
2. Rudd KE, Johnson SC, Agesa KM, et al. Global, regional, and national sepsis incidence and mortality, 1990-2017: analysis for the Global Burden of Disease Study. Lancet. 2020;395:200–11.
3. Evans L, Rhodes A, Alhazzani W, et al. Surviving sepsis campaign: international guidelines for management of sepsis and septic shock 2021. Intensive Care Med. 2021;47:1181–247.
4. Peltan ID, McLean SR, Murnin E, et al. Prevalence, characteristics, and outcomes of emergency department discharge among patients with sepsis. JAMA Netw Open. 2022;5:e2147882.
5. van der Poll T, Shankar-Hari M, Wiersinga WJ. The immunology of sepsis. Immunity. 2021;54:2450–64.
6. Maslove DM, Tang B, Shankar-Hari M, et al. Redefining critical illness. Nat Med. 2022;28:1141–8.
7. Seymour CW, Band RA, Cooke CR, et al. Out-of-hospital characteristics and care of patients with severe sepsis: a cohort study. J Crit Care. 2010;25:553–62.
8. Filbin MR, Lynch J, Gillingham TD, et al. Presenting symptoms independently predict mortality in septic shock: importance of a previously unmeasured confounder. Crit Care Med. 2018;46:1592–9.
9. Biomarkers Definitions Working G. Biomarkers and surrogate endpoints: preferred definitions and conceptual framework. Clin Pharmacol Ther. 2001;69:89–95.
10. Pierrakos C, Velissaris D, Bisdorff M, Marshall JC, Vincent JL. Biomarkers of sepsis: time for a reappraisal. Crit Care. 2020;24:287.

11. van Engelen TSR, Wiersinga WJ, Scicluna BP, van der Poll T. Biomarkers in Sepsis. Crit Care Clin. 2018;34:139–52.
12. Stanski NL, Wong HR. Prognostic and predictive enrichment in sepsis. Nat Rev Nephrol. 2020;16:20–31.
13. Kyriazopoulou E, Poulakou G, Milionis H, et al. Early treatment of COVID-19 with anakinra guided by soluble urokinase plasminogen receptor plasma levels: a double-blind, randomized controlled phase 3 trial. Nat Med. 2021;27:1752–60.
14. Group RC. Tocilizumab in patients admitted to hospital with COVID-19 (RECOVERY): a randomised, controlled, open-label, platform trial. Lancet. 2021;397:1637–45.
15. van der Poll T, van de Veerdonk FL, Scicluna BP, Netea MG. The immunopathology of sepsis and potential therapeutic targets. Nat Rev Immunol. 2017;17:407–20.
16. Simon L, Gauvin F, Amre DK, Saint-Louis P, Lacroix J. Serum procalcitonin and C-reactive protein levels as markers of bacterial infection: a systematic review and meta-analysis. Clin Infect Dis. 2004;39:206–17.
17. Nehring SM, Goyal A, Patel BC. C reactive protein. In: StatPearls [Internet]. Treasure Island, FL: StatPearls; 2022.
18. Elnajdy D, El-Dahiyat F. Antibiotics duration guided by biomarkers in hospitalized adult patients; a systematic review and meta-analysis. Infect Dis (Lond). 2022;54:387–402.
19. Wacker C, Prkno A, Brunkhorst FM, Schlattmann P. Procalcitonin as a diagnostic marker for sepsis: a systematic review and meta-analysis. Lancet Infect Dis. 2013;13:426–35.
20. Tsalik EL, Jaggers LB, Glickman SW, et al. Discriminative value of inflammatory biomarkers for suspected sepsis. J Emerg Med. 2012;43:97–106.
21. Velissaris D, Zareifopoulos N, Lagadinou M, et al. Procalcitonin and sepsis in the Emergency Department: an update. Eur Rev Med Pharmacol Sci. 2021;25:466–79.
22. Yaegashi Y, Shirakawa K, Sato N, et al. Evaluation of a newly identified soluble CD14 subtype as a marker for sepsis. J Infect Chemother. 2005;11:234–8.
23. Wu CC, Lan HM, Han ST, et al. Comparison of diagnostic accuracy in sepsis between presepsin, procalcitonin, and C-reactive protein: a systematic review and meta-analysis. Ann Intensive Care. 2017;7:91.
24. Lee S, Song J, Park DW, et al. Diagnostic and prognostic value of presepsin and procalcitonin in non-infectious organ failure, sepsis, and septic shock: a prospective observational study according to the Sepsis-3 definitions. BMC Infect Dis. 2022;22:8.
25. Liu B, Chen YX, Yin Q, Zhao YZ, Li CS. Diagnostic value and prognostic evaluation of Presepsin for sepsis in an emergency department. Crit Care. 2013;17:R244.
26. Lemarie J, Gibot S. Soluble triggering receptor expressed on myeloid cells-1: diagnosis or prognosis? Crit Care Clin. 2020;36:41–54.
27. Qin Q, Liang L, Xia Y. Diagnostic and prognostic predictive values of circulating sTREM-1 in sepsis: a meta-analysis. Infect Genet Evol. 2021;96:105074.
28. Kung CT, Su CM, Hsiao SY, et al. The prognostic value of serum soluble TREM-1 on outcome in adult patients with sepsis. Diagnostics (Basel). 2021;11:1979.
29. Moore N, Williams R, Mori M, et al. Mid-regional proadrenomedullin (MR-proADM), C-reactive protein (CRP) and other biomarkers in the early identification of disease progression in patients with COVID-19 in the acute NHS setting. J Clin Pathol. 2022. (published online ahead of print). https://doi.org/10.1136/jclinpath-2021-207750.
30. Li P, Wang C, Pang S. The diagnostic accuracy of mid-regional pro-adrenomedullin for sepsis: a systematic review and meta-analysis. Minerva Anestesiol. 2021;87:1117–27.
31. Mearelli F, Barbati G, Spagnol F, et al. The role of mid-regional proadrenomedullin in the differential diagnosis between culture-negative and culture-positive sepsis at emergency department admission. Biomedicine. 2022;10:357.
32. Schuurman AR, Reijnders TDY, Kullberg RFJ, Butler JM, van der Poll T, Wiersinga WJ. Sepsis: deriving biological meaning and clinical applications from high-dimensional data. Intensive Care Med Exp. 2021;9:27.
33. Baghela A, Pena OM, Lee AH, et al. Predicting sepsis severity at first clinical presentation: the role of endotypes and mechanistic signatures. EBioMedicine. 2022;75:103776.

34. Mayhew MB, Buturovic L, Luethy R, et al. A generalizable 29-mRNA neural-network classifier for acute bacterial and viral infections. Nat Commun. 2020;11:1177.
35. Bauer W, Kappert K, Galtung N, et al. A novel 29-messenger RNA host-response assay from whole blood accurately identifies bacterial and viral infections in patients presenting to the emergency department with suspected infections: a prospective observational study. Crit Care Med. 2021;49:1664–73.
36. Galtung N, Diehl-Wiesenecker E, Lehmann D, et al. Prospective validation of a transcriptomic severity classifier among patients with suspected acute infection and sepsis in the emergency department. Eur J Emerg Med. 2022;29:357–65.
37. McHugh L, Seldon TA, Brandon RA, et al. A molecular host response assay to discriminate between sepsis and infection-negative systemic inflammation in critically ill patients: discovery and validation in independent cohorts. PLoS Med. 2015;12:e1001916.
38. Shukeri W, Ralib AM, Abdulah NZ, Mat-Nor MB. Sepsis mortality score for the prediction of mortality in septic patients. J Crit Care. 2018;43:163–8.
39. Maslove DM, Shapira T, Tyryshkin K, Veldhoen RA, Marshall JC, Muscedere J. Validation of diagnostic gene sets to identify critically ill patients with sepsis. J Crit Care. 2019;49: 92–8.
40. Karczewski KJ, Snyder MP. Integrative omics for health and disease. Nat Rev Genet. 2018;19:299–310.
41. Lima C, Ahmed S, Xu Y, et al. Simultaneous Raman and infrared spectroscopy: a novel combination for studying bacterial infections at the single cell level. Chem Sci. 2022;13:8171–9.
42. Crapnell RD, Jesadabundit W, Garcia-Miranda Ferrari A, et al. Toward the rapid diagnosis of sepsis: detecting interleukin-6 in blood plasma using functionalized screen-printed electrodes with a thermal detection methodology. Anal Chem. 2021;93:5931–8.
43. Chen Q, Liang X, Wu T, et al. Integrative analysis of metabolomics and proteomics reveals amino acid metabolism disorder in sepsis. J Transl Med. 2022;20:123.
44. Mickiewicz B, Thompson GC, Blackwood J, et al. Development of metabolic and inflammatory mediator biomarker phenotyping for early diagnosis and triage of pediatric sepsis. Crit Care. 2015;19:320.
45. van Houten CB, de Groot JAH, Klein A, et al. A host-protein based assay to differentiate between bacterial and viral infections in preschool children (OPPORTUNITY): a double-blind, multicentre, validation study. Lancet Infect Dis. 2017;17:431–40.
46. Kauppi AM, Edin A, Ziegler I, et al. Metabolites in blood for prediction of bacteremic sepsis in the emergency room. PLoS One. 2016;11:e0147670.
47. Evans CR, Karnovsky A, Puskarich MA, Michailidis G, Jones AE, Stringer KA. Untargeted metabolomics differentiates l-carnitine treated septic shock 1-year survivors and nonsurvivors. J Proteome Res. 2019;18:2004–11.
48. Villar J, Herran-Monge R, Gonzalez-Higueras E, et al. Clinical and biological markers for predicting ARDS and outcome in septic patients. Sci Rep. 2021;11:22702.

# Repetitive Assessment of Biomarker Combinations as a New Paradigm to Detect Sepsis Early

7

P. Eggimann, Y. -A. Que, and F. Ventura

## 7.1 Introduction

Sepsis is defined as a dysregulated host response to an infection [1]. Septic shock – a subset of sepsis with severe organ failure and cellular/metabolic dysfunction – is associated with a higher risk of mortality [1]. Rapid identification and initiation of treatment remains the major challenge in sepsis management, as any delay in the initiation of effective anti-infective therapy, rapid source control, and, if required, organ failure support, is associated with incremental mortality [2]. Accordingly, the overarching goal of all sepsis definitions/guidelines that have been proposed over the last decades has been to improve accurate and early diagnosis of sepsis, with the goal to initiate prompt management [2].

Unfortunately, the lack of specificity of this clinical-based approach resulted in increased prescriptions of empirical broad-spectrum antibiotics in patients that might not have sepsis. Indeed, only 30 to 40% of patients receiving empirical therapy for presumed sepsis at the initiation of treatment are eventually shown to have definite infection [3]. While this approach might save lives, it largely contributes to antimicrobial resistance. The burden of bacterial antimicrobial resistance for the

P. Eggimann (✉)
Department of Locomotor Apparatus, Lausanne University Hospital (CHUV), University of Lausanne, Lausanne, Switzerland
e-mail: philippe.eggimann@chuv.ch

Y.-A. Que
Department of Intensive Care Medicine, Inselspital—Bern University Hospital, University of Bern, Bern, Switzerland

F. Ventura
Intensive Care Unit, Hirslanden Clinique des Grangettes, Chêne-Bougeries, Switzerland

Division of Anesthesiology, University Hospitals of Geneva, Geneva, Switzerland



J.-L. Vincent (ed.), *Annual Update in Intensive Care and Emergency Medicine 2023*,
Annual Update in Intensive Care and Emergency Medicine,
https://doi.org/10.1007/978-3-031-23005-9_7

year 2019 reached close to five million associated deaths of which 1.27 million were directly attributable [4]. The May 2022 G7 Health Summit thus urged for solutions that would allow better-targeted administration of antibiotics [5].

## 7.2 Limited Usefulness of Routinely Used Biomarkers of Sepsis

In this context, many biomarkers potentially of use to improve the diagnostic accuracy of sepsis have been investigated, but only a few are widely used at the bedside [6]. C-reactive protein (CRP) and procalcitonin (PCT) displayed limited performance for the diagnosis of infection and as such are not integrated within guidelines [2]. A meta-analysis of 30 studies including 3244 patients reported a sensitivity of 77% and specificity of 79% for PCT to detect infection [7]. Another meta-analysis including three randomized controlled trials (RCTs) failed to demonstrate a difference in short-term mortality when antibiotic administration was started according to PCT levels compared to clinical suspicion of infection [8]. In contrast, PCT, and to a lesser extent CRP, has repeatedly been shown to be useful to guide antibiotic de-escalation and has been integrated into antibiotic stewardship programs targeting a reduction of antibiotic use [2].

## 7.3 Time for a Paradigm Change in the Use of Sepsis Biomarkers

In a Swiss survey performed in 2020, 92.3% (37 out of 40) of physicians certified in critical care or anesthesiology declared that they measured CRP concentrations when they suspected sepsis, 84.6% PCT, and 89.7% leukocytes; all said they measured lactate concentrations [9]. There is thus a need for biomarkers that would help physicians in their difficult task of detecting and managing sepsis at the bedside.

So far sepsis biomarkers have been evaluated almost exclusively for their ability to diagnose/confirm infection and/or sepsis with high sensitivity and positive predictive value (PPV) as the main criteria [6, 10]. However, being able to exclude sepsis by using biomarkers with high specificity and negative predictive value (NPV) might help reduce the overconsumption of unnecessary antibiotics and decrease the burden of antimicrobial resistance. In other contexts, for example, in the diagnostic workup of acute coronary syndromes, repetitive measurements of biomarkers are part of routine assessment. Such an approach for sepsis deserves further attention. Indeed, reliable biomarkers that could easily be used at the bedside to quickly diagnose or rule out sepsis are eagerly awaited.

## 7.4 Pancreatic Stone Protein, A Novel Sepsis Biomarker That Is Released Early

Pancreatic stone protein (PSP) is a 16 kDa C-type lectin protein mostly produced by the pancreas and the intestine [11]. Its first described function was the inhibition of the growth and nucleation of calcium carbonate crystals in the pancreatic juice [11]. As such, PSP is elevated in acute pancreatitis even in the absence of infection and should not be used to diagnose infection/sepsis in this setting [12] (Fig. 7.1). A seminal study from the group of Rolf Graf in Zurich identified PSP as a potential biomarker of infection and sepsis in a cohort of trauma patients [11]. PSP concentrations increased early in trauma patients who subsequently developed either infection or sepsis. Later, several studies confirmed that PSP can be used to differentiate infection and sepsis from other non-infectious severe inflammatory states in critically ill patients [13, 14], in patients with ventilator-associated pneumonia (VAP) [15], after cardiac surgery [14, 16], after severe burn trauma [17], after inhalation injury [18], and in neonates [19] (Table 7.1). In addition, PSP was shown to predict outcome in some of these studies (reviewed in 2019 [20] and in 2022 [21]) (Table 7.2).

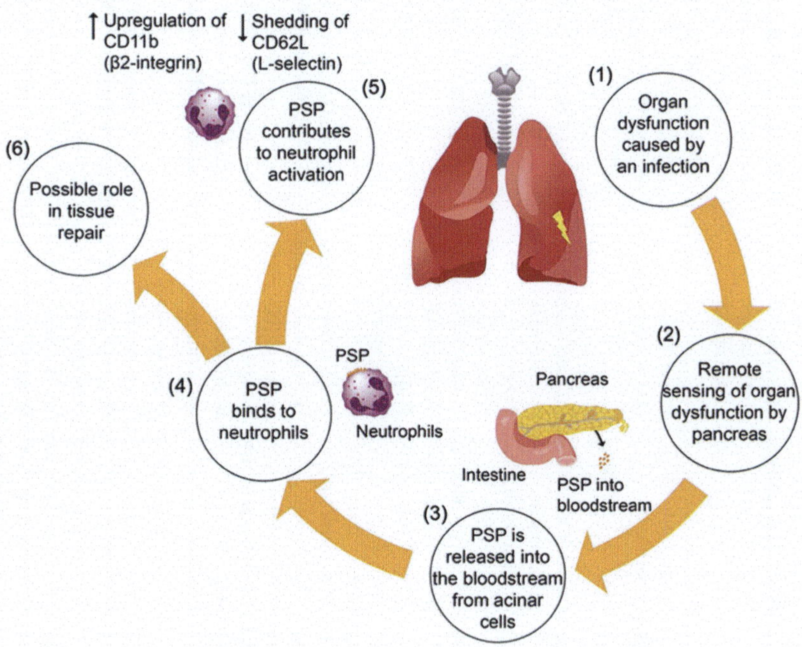


**Fig. 7.1** Hypothetical model of pancreatic stone protein (PSP) physiopathology. The pancreas remotely senses infection and/or organ dysfunction (2) and releases PSP, a C-type lectin protein family member from acinar cells, into the blood stream (3) [34]. PSP has been shown to promote the shedding of CD62L and to upregulate the expression of CD11b on the cell surface of neutrophils (4) [13]. Neutrophils with an increased CD11b expression interact with ligands on damaged endothelial cells, resulting in high affinity adhesion to the vascular endothelium, extravasation, and migration to the site of tissue damage (5) [35, 36]. PSP might play a role in tissue regeneration, the relevance of which remains to be demonstrated in sepsis (6). (Adapted from [13, 34])

**Table 7.1** Performance of pancreatic stone protein (PSP) for diagnosis of infection and/or sepsis

| Study | Type of patients | Type of study | Infection/sepsis prediction | Comparison with other biomarkers |
|---|---|---|---|---|
| **Keel et al.** [13] | **83 ICU adult trauma patients** | **Retrospective, single-center, observational** | **PSP increased from 22.8 ng/ml in patients without infection to 111.4 ng/ml in patients developing infection and 146.4 ng/ml in patients developing sepsis** | **PSP > PCT > CRP > IL-6** |
| García de Guadiana-Romualdo et al. [25] | 83 unselected adult patients Emergency department | Prospective, single-center observational | Infection: AUC 0.84 (0.77–0.90), cut-off 41.5 ng/ml<br>Sepsis: AUC 0.87 (0.81–0.94), cut-off 96.6 ng/ml | PSP = PCT = sCD25 |
| Llewelyn et al. [26] | 219 unselected adult ICU or intermediate care patients | Prospective, multicenter, observational | Sepsis: AUC 0.93 (0.89–0.97) cut-off 30 ng/ml | PSP = sCD25<br>PSP > PCT = IL-6 > HBP |
| Klein et al. 2015 [16] | 120 adult ICU patients after elective cardiac surgery | Prospective, single-center, observational | Infection: AUC 0.77 (0.62–0.89) cut-off of 41.5 ng/ml | PSP > CRP<br>PSP > WBC |
| Parlato et al. [27] | 279 adult ICU patients admitted with SIRS (CAPITAIN study) | Prospective, multicenter, observational | Sepsis: AUC 0.63 (0.54–0.71) | CRP < PSP < CD74 < IL-6 < PCT < IL-8 |
| García de Guadiana-Romualdo et al. [28] | 114 cases of febrile neutropenia in 105 adult patients in emergency room | Prospective, single-center, observational | Infection: AUC 0.75 (0.66–0.84) cut-off 29.0 ng/ml | PCT > PSP<br>PSP > sCD25 |
| **Klein et al.** [17] | **90 adult ICU patients with burns >15% total body surface area** | **Prospective, single-center, observational** | **Sepsis: Day 7 post-op PSP AUC 0.89 (0.81–0.96) cut-off 60.12 ng/ml** | **PSP > PCT > CRP > WBC** |
| **Pugin et al.** [23] | **243 adult ICU patients at risk for nosocomial infection** | **Prospective, multicenter, observational** | **Sepsis: AUC 0.75 (0.67–0.82) cut-off: 290.5 ng/ml; cut-off CRP 167.2 mg/l, cut-off PCT 0.94 ng/ml** | **PSP = PCT = CPR**<br>**[a]PSP + CRP > PSP** |

Studies highlighted in bold: Pre-symptomatic diagnosis of infection/sepsis

Cut-off for PSP: in most studies, PSP has been measured using a standardized ELISA technique developed in 1999, not available for real-time use [29]. Nanofluidic technology developed by Abionic translated into a CE-IVDR 2022 certified PSP-abioKIT® on the *in vitro* diagnostic platform abioSCOPE® (CE marked) that has been used recently and is commercially available (Abionic, Epalinges, Switzerland). Compared to the previous ELISA technique on which most data were generated, PSP baseline levels are higher using this novel point-of-care technology. Both technologies correlate and the abioSCOPE® PSP level in ng/ml equals approximately to 4.6 × previous ELISA ng/ml (95% CI 0.39–0.59) [30]. As such, the 44 ng/ml PSP cut-off for the diagnosis of infection according to the meta-analysis [22] would translate to 203.3 ng/ml using the abioSCOPE® technology.

*IL* interleukin, *CRP* C-reactive protein, *PCT* procalcitonin, *WBC* white blood cell count, *AUC* area under the receiver operating characteristic curve, *HPB* heparin binding protein

[a]Combined biomarkers improved prediction

**Table 7.2** Performance of pancreatic stone protein (PSP) to predict outcome in patients with sepsis

| Study | Type of patients | Type of study | Outcome prediction | Comparison with other biomarkers |
|---|---|---|---|---|
| Boeck et al. [15] | 101 adult ICU patients with VAP | Multicenter, retrospective, observational | AUC survival day 1: 0.69 (0.57–0.80) cut-off 24 ng/ml<br>AUC death day 7: 0.76 (0.62–0.91) cut-off 177 ng/ml | No |
| Que et al. [31] | 107 adult ICU patients with sepsis | Single center, prospective, observational | AUC 0.65 (0.51–0.80) | PSP > IL-8 > IL-6 > PCT > CRP |
| García de Guadiana-Romualdo et al. [28] | 122 adult ICU patients with sepsis | Single center, prospective, observational | Baseline PSP plus lactate: AUC 0.796<br>Baseline SOFA: AUC 0.826<br>On day 2 PSP: AUC 0.844; SOFA AUC-ROC 0.923 | PSP > PCT |
| Gukasjan et al. [32] | 91 adult ICU patients with secondary peritonitis | Two centers, prospective, observational | PSP: AUC 0.775 cut-off 130 ng/ml | PSP > IL-6 > PCT > WBC > CRP |
| Que et al. [37] | 249 (158 + 91) adult ICU patients with sepsis | Two centers, prospective, observational | PSP + SAPS II AUC 0.659 (0.563–0.755)<br>PSP + APACHE II AUC 0.679 (0.584–0.772)<br>PSP + PCT + SAPS II AUC 0.721 (0.632–0.812) | [a]PSP > PCT > CRP |
| Van Singer et al. [33] | 173 PCR-confirmed SARS-CoV-2 patients in emergency room | Single center, prospective, observational | PSP: AUC 0.83: (0.74–0.92)<br>PSP + CRP: AUC 0.90 (0.84–0.97)<br>PSP + severity score CRB-65: AUC 0.95 (0.91–0.98) | CRP > PSP<br>[a]PSP + CRP > PSP |

Cut-off for PSP: in most studies, PSP has been measured using a standardized ELISA technique developed in 1999, not available for real-time use [29]. Nanofluidic technology developed by Abionic translated into a CE-IVDR 2022 certified PSP-abioKIT® on the *in vitro* diagnostic platform abioSCOPE® (CE marked) that has been used recently and is commercially available (Abionic, Epalinges, Switzerland). Compared to the previous ELISA technique on which most data were generated, PSP baseline levels are higher using this novel point-of-care technology. Both technologies correlate and the abioSCOPE® PSP level in ng/ml equals approximately to 4.6 × previous ELISA ng/ml (95% CI 0.39–0.59) [30]. As such, the 44 ng/ml PSP cut-off for the diagnosis of infection according to the meta-analysis [22] would translate to 203.3 ng/ml using the abioSCOPE® technology

*IL* interleukin, *CRP* C-reactive protein, *PCT* procalcitonin, *WBC* white blood cell count, *AUC* area under the receiver operating characteristic curve

[a]Combined biomarkers improved prediction

**Table 7.3** Performance of combined biomarkers to predict infection

| | AUC (95% CI) | Sensitivity (95% CI) | Specificity (95% CI) | PPV (95% CI) | NPV (95% CI) | PLR (95% CI) | NLR (95% CI) |
|---|---|---|---|---|---|---|---|
| PSP + CRP | 0.90 [0.87, 0.92] | 0.82 [0.78, 0.86] | 0.85 [0.79, 0.90] | 0.91 [0.88, 0.94] | 0.70 [0.64, 0.76] | 5.30 [3.74, 7.53] | 0.21 [0.17, 0.27] |
| PSP + PCT | 0.83 [0.80, 0.87] | 0.72 [0.68, 0.78] | 0.84 [0.78, 0.89] | 0.90 [0.86, 0.93] | 0.59 [0.54, 0.67] | 4.41 [3.14, 6.18] | 0.32 [0.27, 0.39] |
| CRP + PCT | 0.87 [0.84, 0.90] | 0.73 [0.69, 0.78] | 0.85 [0.80, 0.90] | 0.91 [0.88, 0.94] | 0.61 [0.55, 0.67] | 4.93 [3.44, 7.07] | 0.31 [0.26, 0.38] |
| PSP + CRP + PCT | 0.90 [0.87, 0.92] | 0.82 [0.78, 0.86] | 0.84 [0.79, 0.90] | 0.92 [0.88, 0.94] | 0.69 [0.63, 0.75] | 5.27 [3.71, 7.48] | 0.22 [0.18, 0.28] |

Data from [22]

*AUC* area under the receiver operating characteristic curve, *PPV* positive predictive value, *NPV* negative predictive value, *PLR* positive likelihood ratio, *NLR* negative likelihood ratio, *CI* confidence interval, *PSP* pancreatic stone protein, *CRP* C-reactive protein, *PCT* procalcitonin

A meta-analysis [22] showed that PSP performed better (area under the receiver operating curve [AUC] 0.81, 95% CI 0.78–0.85, SE 0.017) than CRP (AUC 0.77, 95% CI 0.73–0.80, SE 0.019) or PCT (AUC 0.78, 95% CI 0.74–0.82, SE 0.022) for the diagnosis of infection. The combination of CRP with PSP further enhanced accuracy (AUC 0.90, 95% CI 0.87–0.92), with higher sensitivity (0.82 (0.78–0.86)) and specificity (0.85 (0.79–0.90)) for discriminating infectious from non-infectious states (Table 7.3).

A recent prospective multicenter study confirmed that repeated PSP measurements were able to detect nosocomial sepsis in critically ill patients requiring intensive care unit (ICU) admission before the occurrence of clinical signs/symptoms [23]. The diagnostic accuracy of PSP (AUC 0.75, 95% CI 0.67–0.82) was similar to that of CRP (AUC 0.77, 95% CI 0.69–0.84) and PCT (AUC 0.75, 95% CI 0.68–0.82), but its combination with CRP further increased accuracy (AUC 0.79, 95% CI 0.72–0.86), confirming the usefulness of this combination in that context. Of note, PSP levels increased early, i.e., 48–72 h before the occurrence of symptoms or clinical signs, paving the way for the detection of nosocomial sepsis before the symptomatic phase. These data were further confirmed in a cohort of patients after severe burn trauma, in whom PSP showed a 3.3 to 5.5-fold increase within the 72 h preceding the occurrence of signs and symptoms of nosocomial sepsis. In contrast, CRP, PCT, and leukocyte levels did not vary significantly [17].

## 7.5 Role of Repetitive Serial Assessments of CRP and PSP in the Diagnostic Workup of Sepsis

As CRP and PSP have consistently demonstrated high performance in various patient populations when assessed together in the context of sepsis, we propose to include their repetitive assessment in the diagnostic process to exclude/confirm the

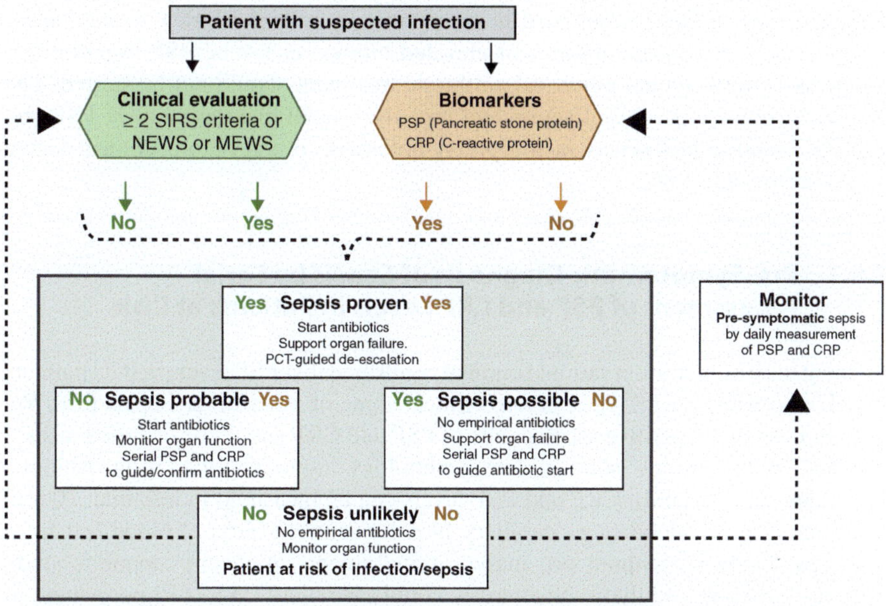


**Fig. 7.2** Serial C-reactive protein (CRP) and pancreatic stone protein (PSP) measurement in patients suspected of having infection and/or at risk of sepsis. *SIRS* systemic inflammatory response syndrome, *NEWS* National Early Warning Score, *MEWS* Modified Early Warning Score

presence of infection and/or sepsis (Fig. 7.2). Depending on the presence/absence of a dysregulated host response, organ failure and the levels of biomarkers, we suggest the following scenarios:

1. In the presence of a clear dysregulated host response (as suggested by the computation of clinical measures, such as systemic inflammatory response syndrome (SIRS) criteria, the National Early Warning Score (NEWS) and the Modified Early Warning Score (MEWS) [2]), elevated biomarker levels may confirm the diagnosis of sepsis and the need for urgent and aggressive management (antibiotics, infection source control, organ failure support).
2. When the dysregulated host response is limited or doubtful (clinical scores below threshold), elevated biomarker levels might suggest the presence of an infection and sepsis is therefore probable, which might validate the start of antibiotic therapy and justify intensive monitoring of organ function and the search for a possible source of infection.
3. In the presence of a clear dysregulated host response (clinical scores above threshold), but in the absence of elevated biomarker levels, especially those of PSP, sepsis is possible and empirical antibiotic treatment could be delayed according to the clinical context until infection has been proven. In this situation, repetitive serial measurements of CRP and PSP should further contribute to refine the management strategy according to their evolution.

4. Finally, when the dysregulated host response is limited (clinical scores below threshold), and in the absence of elevated biomarker levels, PSP in particular, sepsis is unlikely and empirical antibiotic treatment should not be started. The patient remains at risk of sepsis and repetitive serial measurement of PSP and CRP could detect sepsis in the pre-symptomatic phase before clinical signs/symptoms develop.

### 7.5.1 Pre-Symptomatic Diagnosis of Sepsis by Serial Assessment of PSP and CRP Levels in Patients at Risk

A recent multicenter observational clinical confirmed that PSP levels in ICU patients at risk of sepsis rose 48–72 h before clinical signs of nosocomial sepsis [23]. We thus propose that repetitive assessments of PSP and CRP should be included in such patients. With current point-of-care technology (abioSCOPE® from Abionic, Epalinges, Switzerland), CRP and PSP levels can be measured in less than 10 min from one drop of blood (e.g., capillary blood, venous or arterial blood left from blood gas analysis) without pre-analytic requirements. A recent economic study from the USA showed that such an assay could save up to US$ 1688 per patient in the emergency room, and US$ 3315 for those in intensive care (potential nationwide savings of US$ 7 billion per year) [24].

## 7.6 Conclusion

Sepsis is a major public health problem, and its early diagnosis currently mostly relies on a thorough clinical evaluation. The lack of a demonstrated added value of biomarkers, even those with good sensitivity, precludes their generalized use at the bedside to guide the initiation of antibiotic therapies. PSP has recently emerged as a promising biomarker of sepsis. PSP performed better than CRP and PCT at detecting sepsis in various critically ill populations. PSP levels increase 48 to 72 h before clinical signs and symptoms of sepsis. PSP can be measured within less than 10 min using point-of-care testing on one drop of whole blood without a pre-analytical phase. Given the reported performance of CPR and PSP, we propose to include combined assessment of their blood levels to confirm or rule out sepsis in patients with a suspicion of infection. In addition, as PSP levels increase 48–72 h before the development of clinically overt sepsis, we also propose to integrate repetitive CRP and PSP measurement in the routine assessment of critically ill patients at risk of sepsis.

## References

1. Singer M, Deutschman CS, Seymour CW, et al. The Third International Consensus Definitions for Sepsis and Septic Shock (Sepsis-3). JAMA. 2016;315:801.

2. Evans L, Rhodes A, Alhazzani W, et al. Surviving Sepsis Campaign: International Guidelines for Management of Sepsis and Septic Shock 2021. Crit Care Med. 2021;49:e1063.
3. Klein Klouwenberg PMC, Cremer OL, van Vught LA, et al. Likelihood of infection in patients with presumed sepsis at the time of intensive care unit admission: a cohort study. Crit Care. 2015;19:319.
4. Murray CJ, Ikuta KS, Sharara F, et al. Global burden of bacterial antimicrobial resistance in 2019: a systematic analysis. Lancet. 2022;399:629–55.
5. G7 Health Ministers' Communiqué. Available at: https://www.g7germany.de/resource/blob/974430/2042058/5651daa321517b089cdccfaffd1e37a1/2022-05-20-g7-health-ministers-communique-data.pdf?download=1. Accessed 6 Nov 22.
6. Barichello T, Generoso JS, Singer M, Dal-Pizzol F. Biomarkers for sepsis: more than just fever and leukocytosis—a narrative review. Crit Care. 2022;26:14.
7. Wacker C, Prkno A, Brunkhorst FM, Schlattmann P. Procalcitonin as a diagnostic marker for sepsis: a systematic review and meta-analysis. Lancet Infect Dis. 2013;13:426–35.
8. Lam SW, Bauer SR, Fowler R, Duggal A. Systematic review and meta-analysis of procalcitonin-guidance versus usual care for antimicrobial management in critically ill patients: focus on subgroups based on antibiotic initiation, cessation, or mixed strategies. Crit Care Med. 2018;46:684–90.
9. Ventura F. Diagnosis of sepsis. Presented at Area Critica, Bologna, 2 Dec 2021.
10. Pierrakos C, Velissaris D, Bisdorff M, Marshall JC, Vincent JL. Biomarkers of sepsis: time for a reappraisal. Crit Care. 2020;24:287.
11. Graf R. Pancreatic stone protein—sepsis and the riddles of the exocrine pancreas. Pancreatology. 2020;20:301–4.
12. Rodríguez Rojas C, García de Guadiana-Romualdo L, Morán Sánchez S, et al. Role of pancreatic stone protein as an early biomarker for risk stratification of acute pancreatitis. Dig Dis Sci. 2022;67:3275–83.
13. Keel M, Härter L, Reding T, et al. Pancreatic stone protein is highly increased during posttraumatic sepsis and activates neutrophil granulocytes. Crit Care Med. 2009;37:1642–8.
14. Klein HJ, Buehler PK, Niggemann P, et al. Expression of pancreatic stone protein is unaffected by trauma and subsequent surgery in burn patients. World J Surg. 2020;44:3000–9.
15. Boeck L, Graf R, Eggimann P, et al. Pancreatic stone protein: a marker of organ failure and outcome in ventilator-associated pneumonia. Chest. 2011;140:925–32.
16. Klein HJ, Csordas A, Falk V, et al. Pancreatic stone protein predicts postoperative infection in cardiac surgery patients irrespective of cardiopulmonary bypass or surgical technique. PLoS One. 2015;10:e0120276.
17. Klein HJ, Niggemann P, Buehler PK, et al. Pancreatic stone protein predicts sepsis in severely burned patients irrespective of trauma severity: a monocentric observational study. Ann Surg. 2021;274:e1179–86.
18. Klein HJ, Rittirsch D, Buehler PK, et al. Response of routine inflammatory biomarkers and novel pancreatic stone protein to inhalation injury and its interference with sepsis detection in severely burned patients. Burns. 2021;47:338–48.
19. Schlapbach LJ, Graf R, Woerner A, et al. Pancreatic stone protein as a novel marker for neonatal sepsis. Intensive Care Med. 2013;39:754–63.
20. Eggimann P, Que Y-A, Rebeaud F. Measurement of pancreatic stone protein in the identification and management of sepsis. Biomark Med. 2019;13:135–45.
21. Fidalgo P, Nora D, Coelho L, Povoa P. Pancreatic stone protein: review of a new biomarker in sepsis. J Clin Med. 2022;11:1085.
22. Prazak J, Irincheeva I, Llewelyn MJ, et al. Accuracy of pancreatic stone protein for the diagnosis of infection in hospitalized adults: a systematic review and individual patient level meta-analysis. Crit Care. 2021;25:182.
23. Pugin J, Daix T, Pagani JL, et al. Serial measurement of pancreatic stone protein for the early detection of sepsis in intensive care unit patients: a prospective multicentric study. Crit Care. 2021;25:151.

24. Schneider JE, Dick K, Cooper JT, Chami N. Pancreatic stone protein point-of-care testing can reduce healthcare expenditure in sepsis. Health Econ Rev. 2022;12:39.
25. García de Guadiana-Romualdo L, Berger M, Jiménez-Santos E, et al. Pancreatic stone protein and soluble CD25 for infection and sepsis in an emergency department. Eur J Clin Investig. 2017;47:297–304.
26. Llewelyn MJ, Berger M, Gregory M, et al. Sepsis biomarkers in unselected patients on admission to intensive or high-dependency care. Crit Care. 2013;17:R60.
27. Parlato M, Philippart F, Rouquette A, et al. Circulating biomarkers may be unable to detect infection at the early phase of sepsis in ICU patients: the CAPTAIN prospective multicenter cohort study. Intensive Care Med. 2018;44:1061–70.
28. García de Guadiana-Romualdo L, Jiménez-Santos E, Cerezuela-Fuentes P, et al. Analyzing the capability of PSP, PCT and sCD25 to support the diagnosis of infection in cancer patients with febrile neutropenia. Clin Chem Lab Med. 2019;57:540–8.
29. Bimmler D, Angst E, Valeri F, et al. Regulation of PSP/reg in rat pancreas: immediate and steady-state adaptation to different diets. Pancreas. 1999;19:255–67.
30. Benninga R, Haquette G, Ventura F, Cateau C, Maerki I. Nanofluidic technology enables rapid quantification of pancreatic stone protein as an early biomarker of sepsis: method comparison of the abioSCOPE in-vitro diagnostic device. J Appl Lab Med. 2022. 28th AACC International CPOCT Symposium (abst).
31. Que YA, Delodder F, Guessous I, et al. Pancreatic stone protein as an early biomarker predicting mortality in a prospective cohort of patients with sepsis requiring ICU management. Crit Care. 2012;16:R114.
32. Gukasjan R, Raptis DA, Schulz H-U, Halangk W, Graf R. Pancreatic stone protein predicts outcome in patients with peritonitis in the ICU. Crit Care Med. 2013;41:1027–36.
33. Van Singer M, Brahier T, Brochu Vez MJ, Gerhard Donnet H, Hugli O, Boillat-Blanco N. Pancreatic stone protein for early mortality prediction in COVID-19 patients. Crit Care. 2021;25:267.
34. Reding T, Palmiere C, Pazhepurackel C, et al. The pancreas responds to remote damage and systemic stress by secretion of the pancreatic secretory proteins PSP/regI and PAP/regIII. Oncotarget. 2017;8:30162.
35. Lerman YV, Kim M. Neutrophil migration under normal and sepsis conditions. Cardiovasc Hematol Disord Drug Targets. 2015;15:19–28.
36. Kovach MA, Standiford TJ. The function of neutrophils in sepsis. Curr Opin Infect Dis. 2012;25:321–7.
37. Que YA, Guessous I, Dupuis-Lozeron E, et al. Prognostication of mortality in critically ill patients with severe infections. Chest. 2015;148:674–82.

# Organ Dysfunction Scores in the Adult ICU

# 8

A. Reintam Blaser, K. F. Bachmann, and Y. M. Arabi

## 8.1 Introduction

Multiple organ dysfunction, historically first recognized as a consequence of sepsis [1], is the main cause of morbidity and mortality in the intensive care unit (ICU) [2]. In the 1990s, the rationale of assessing organ systems concomitantly was raised [3, 4] and, shortly thereafter, the need to quantify each of these organ dysfunctions was realized. Three similar scoring systems (the multiple organ dysfunction score (MODS), the logistic organ dysfunction score (LODS), and the sequential organ failure assessment (SOFA)), all of them including six organ systems, were proposed [5–7]. The organ systems assessed were the respiratory, cardiovascular, hematological, liver, renal and neurological systems. All the scores have shown comparable performance in predicting ICU mortality [8].

A literature search in PubMed for each of these scores in adult patients (search formulas (respective score[Title/Abstract]) AND (adult[MeSH Terms])) resulted in 13 titles for LODS, 50 for MODS, and 1957 for the SOFA score. Clearly, the SOFA score is the most established, studied, and widely used multiple organ dysfunction score within the critical care community. Therefore, we use the SOFA score as a reference for assessment of multiple organ dysfunction in the ICU. The SOFA score has been used for multiple purposes (Fig. 8.1).

A. Reintam Blaser (✉) · K. F. Bachmann
Department of Anaesthesiology and Intensive Care, University of Tartu, Tartu, Estonia

Department of Intensive Care Medicine, Lucerne Cantonal Hospital, Lucerne, Switzerland
e-mail: annika.reintam.blaser@ut.ee

Y. M. Arabi
Intensive Care Department, Ministry of National Guard Health Affairs, King Abdullah International Medical Research Center, King Saud bin Abdulaziz University for Health Sciences, Riyadh, Saudi Arabia



J.-L. Vincent (ed.), *Annual Update in Intensive Care and Emergency Medicine 2023*, Annual Update in Intensive Care and Emergency Medicine,
https://doi.org/10.1007/978-3-031-23005-9_8

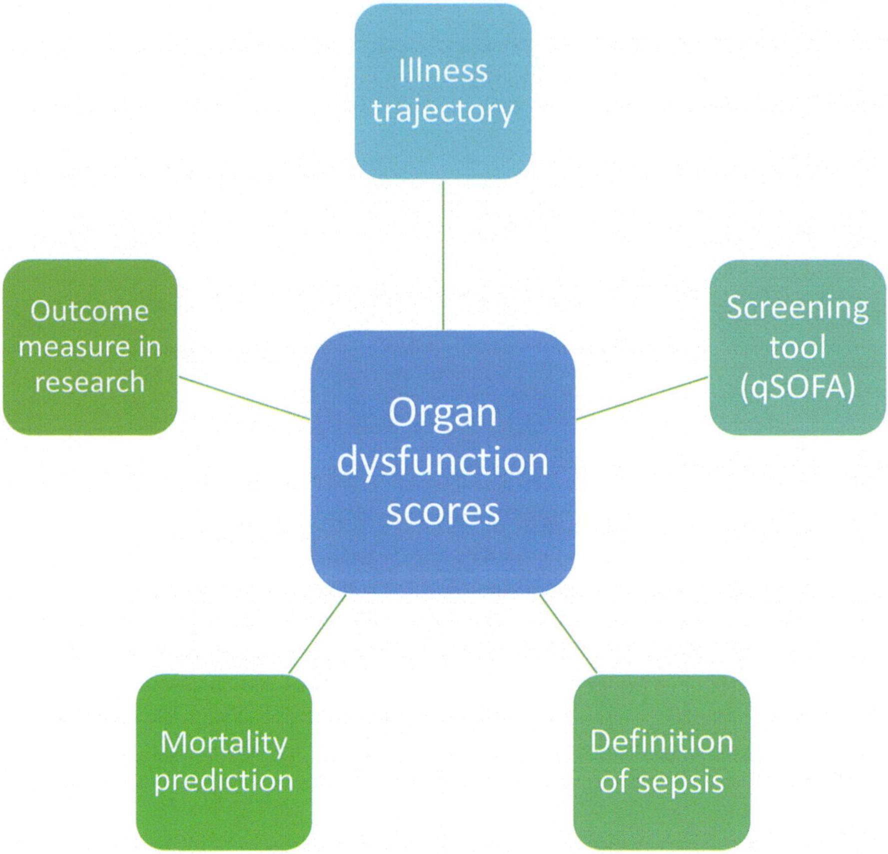


**Fig. 8.1** Organ dysfunction scores and their clinical use. *qSOFA* quick sequential organ failure assessment score

After its original development, the name of the SOFA score was modified from "sepsis-related" to "sequential" illustrating further broadening of the concept and recognizing the importance of multiple organ dysfunction also in patients without severe infection [9]. The goal of the SOFA score, published by Vincent and colleagues, was "to describe quantitatively and as objectively as possible the degree of organ dysfunction/failure over time" [7]. The time factor seems particularly important, as most ICU prediction scores such as the APACHE II, SAPS II and others, are based on admission day values and do not enable assessment of the patient's trajectory over time [10].

Over the three decades since SOFA was introduced, several aspects of critical care practice have evolved, and may have implications for the assessment of organ dysfunction. The aim of this chapter is to revisit the concept and definitions of organ dysfunction and failure as well as the concepts involved in establishing an organ dysfunction scoring system for the adult ICU population. We review the evolution of assessment of organ dysfunction in- and outside of the ICU, summarize possible variables reflecting organ dysfunction, and discuss their current use in organ dysfunction scoring systems. We point out the strengths and weaknesses of organ dysfunction assessment today, elaborate on the quantification of organ failure as a system for mortality prediction and study endpoints, and propose future perspectives.

## 8.2 Definition and Rationale for Assessment of Organ Dysfunction

Septic shock is the main reason for organ dysfunction and failure in the ICU [11]. Macro- and microvascular dysfunction caused by excessive humoral mediators lead to the development of organ dysfunction and failure [12]. The process of organ dysfunction is continuous and may progress to organ failure or to full recovery, highlighting the importance of assessing trends over multiple time points. Dysfunctions of different organs have different time courses; cardiovascular dysfunction commonly presents early in the course of critical illness, whereas thrombocytopenia and hyperbilirubinemia (defining hematologic and hepatic dysfunction) often develop later in the course (Fig. 8.2) [9, 13]. Although organ dysfunction is common and may serve as an early warning system, organ failure is usually a life-threatening condition that requires immediate recognition and treatment. Assessing patients with potential organ dysfunction on a daily basis therefore seems to be a valid strategy to prevent catastrophic events [14]. Organ dysfunction scores were created in the 1990s to quantify organ dysfunction and to follow the dynamics of the disease process and not for mortality prediction. However, they were all validated for their ability to predict mortality and are nowadays commonly used to predict mortality and poor prognosis. A recent study assessing the SOFA score, systematic inflammatory response syndrome (SIRS) criteria, and quick SOFA (qSOFA) score in 184,875 patients with an infection-related primary admission diagnosis showed that the SOFA score had a significantly higher predictive power for in-hospital mortality [15]. This was further confirmed in 2350 sepsis patients with SOFA outperforming qSOFA and the SIRS criteria [16]. This finding may not be generalizable to more selected patient populations. In the recent coronavirus disease 2019 (COVID-19) pandemic, SOFA did not accurately predict short-term hospital mortality in a retrospective analysis of 15,122 patients with COVID, with a low area under the receiver operating characteristic curve (AUC) of 0.66 (0.65–0.67) [17].

The SOFA score has also become an important study endpoint in large trials [18]. A recent systematic review and meta-regression analysis by de Grooth and colleagues demonstrated that treatment effects on delta SOFA appear to be steadily linked to mortality in randomized controlled trials (RCTs) [19]. In contrast, results from 87 RCTs suggested that fixed-day SOFA scores were not significantly linked to mortality [19]. This further emphasizes the importance of following trends rather than assessing single time points. A recent publication by Xu and colleagues identified four subphenotypes using categories of worsening and improving 72 h SOFA

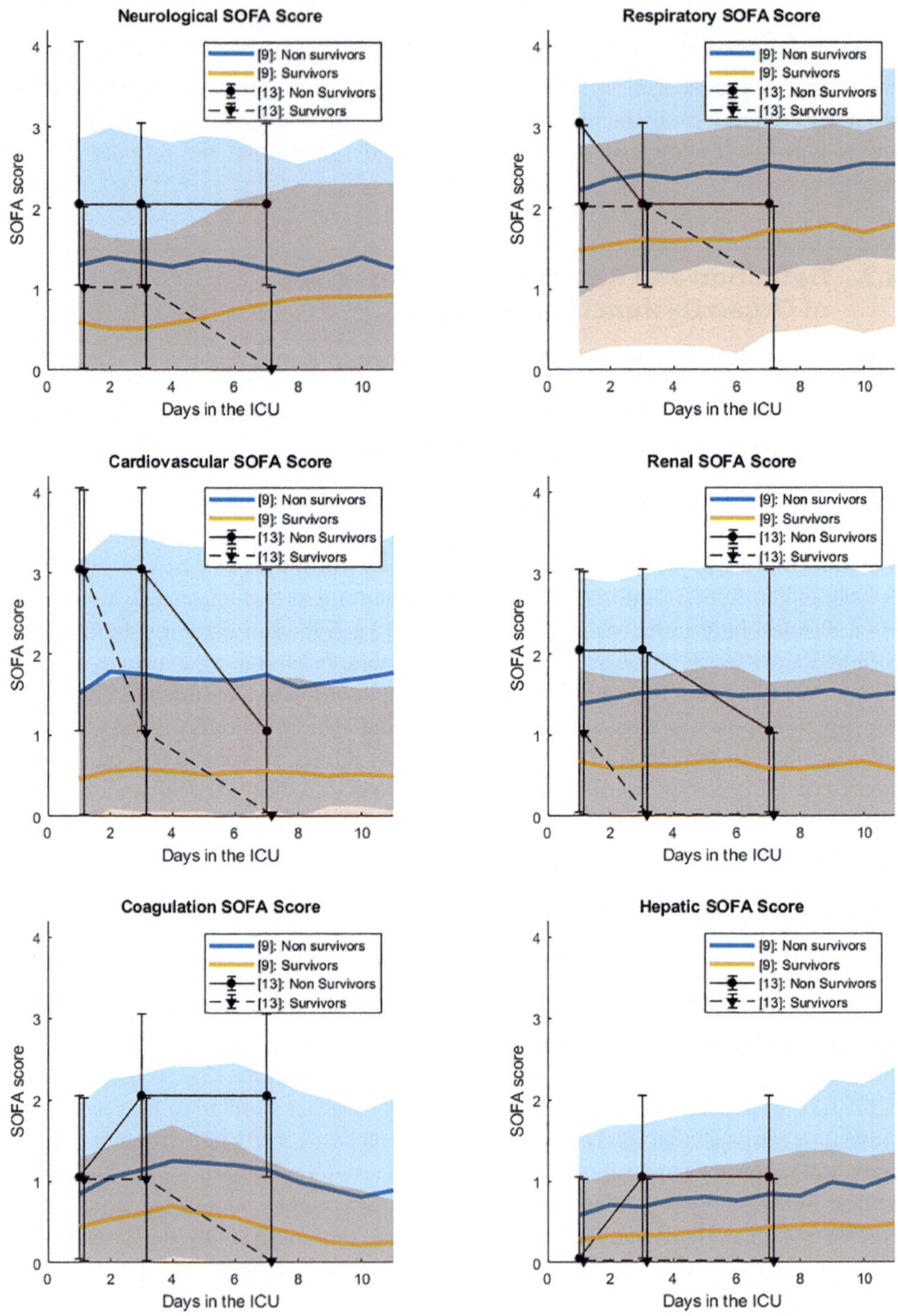


**Fig. 8.2** Development of individual organ sequential organ failure assessment (SOFA) scores in critically ill patients over time. Data are taken from Vincent and colleagues [9], published in 1998 including 1449 patients (presented as mean with standard deviation, blue and orange plots) and Nakashima and colleagues [13] published in 2020 including 2732 patients (presented as median with IQR, black plots)

trajectories and subdividing the trajectories into rapid and delayed changes. The authors found that this phenotyping enabled identification of patients with the highest mortality risk and highest rates of mechanical ventilation [20]. Machine learning models further incorporate organ dysfunction scores in order to boost mortality prediction [21].

## 8.3 Variables Representing Organ Dysfunction and Their Implementation into Scoring Systems

For the purpose of this chapter, different variables that may reflect organ dysfunction and failure are divided into four categories. First, clinical signs that can be assessed at the bedside, such as heart rate, respiratory rate or blood pressure. This category may also include point-of-care sonography, which has become increasingly used at the bedside in the last decade and may complement clinical examination [22]. Second, laboratory findings, e.g., creatinine for the assessment of renal dysfunction and failure. Third, measurements and tests that are not rapidly available at the bedside and may require patient transport, e.g., computed tomography (CT) or magnetic resonance imaging (MRI). Fourth, organ system support, including medications and devices. Although organ support may differ significantly between different regions and institutions, the level of support still corresponds to the degree of organ dysfunction. Furthermore, variables that are obtainable only in the ICU should be distinguished from variables that may be obtainable in the ward or emergency room. Laboratory markers are obtainable in the emergency room as well as on the general ward, but repetitive measurements may be cumbersome in these settings. Additional tests, such as advanced measurements (e.g., CT scan) may not be readily available and daily assessment is not applicable.

Table 8.1 gives a list of important variables for each organ system in the four abovementioned categories.

The main characteristics of ideal variables to be used in the organ dysfunction scores are [10]:

- Simple, inexpensive, and routinely available in ICUs
- Reliable (intra- and inter-observer) and objective (independent of observer)
- Organ specific and independent of therapy
- Sequentially available, including on admission and at fixed time points during the ICU course
- Reflect acute dysfunction of the organ in question but not chronic dysfunction
- Reproducible in large, heterogeneous groups of ICU patients, as well as in several types of ICU in different regions

**Table 8.1** Relevant variables for organ dysfunction classification divided into four categories and presented by organ system

| Organ system | Bedside signs and measurements | Laboratory variables | Advanced tests and measurements | Organ support |
|---|---|---|---|---|
| Neurological | **GCS**, **RASS**, **CAM(-ICU)** | NSE | EEG, CT, MRI, ICP, tissue oxygenation, transcranial Doppler, opticus sheath assessment | Delirium medication (e.g., dexmedetomidine or haloperidol), deep sedation? temperature control? |
| Cardiovascular | **Heart rate**, **blood pressure**, **mottling, capillary refill** | **Troponin**, **NT-proBNP**, **lactate** | **Cardiac output**, pulmonary artery and filling pressures, $SvO_2$, **echocardiography** | Vasopressors and inotropes, devices |
| Respiratory | **Respiratory rate, $SpO_2$**, PEEP, Plateau pressure | **$SpO_2/FiO_2$**, $PaO_2/FiO_2$, deadspace indices (e.g. $PaCO_2/etCO_2$) | Esophageal balloon, CT, electrical impedance tomography | Oxygen supplementation, high flow nasal oxygen, NIV, mechanical ventilation, neuromuscular blockade, VV-ECMO |
| Renal | **Urine output, POC US** | **Creatinine**, cystatin C, albumin/creatinine quotient, urine sediment, non-anion gap acidosis | Doppler, biopsy | Dialysis |
| Liver | **Ascites, hepatic encephalopathy**, **icterus, jaundice**, variceal bleeding | **Bilirubin**, **transaminases**, **INR**, **glucose, ammonia, gamma-GT, alkaline phosphatase, coagulation factors** | CT, MRI, Doppler, ICG-PDR | **Glucose**, **lactulose/lactitol, rifaximin,** liver support (e.g. MARS; plasmapheresis) |
| Hematological/coagulation | **Bleeding**, **petechiae** | **Thrombocytes, aPTT, anti-factor Xa activity, fibrinogen, neutrophil-to-lymphocyte ratio, neutropenia, mean platelet volume** | Biopsy | Neutrophil stimulation |

| | | | | |
|---|---|---|---|---|
| Abdomen/GI | Gastric residual volumes, **stool passage, bowel sounds, diarrhea, abdominal distension, GI bleeding**, IAP, POC US | **Lactate**, citrulline, I-FABP | CT, MRI, absorption tests (3-O-methyl-D-glucose, paracetamol) | Prokinetic use, laxatives, open abdomen |
| Metabolism/ electrolytes | | **Electrolytes** | | Electrolyte correction |
| Physical/muscle function | MRC | ? | CT, myography, biopsy, US | Level of assistance needed |

Variables given in bold can most likely be acquired on the general ward or emergency room (ER), whereas acquisition of the remaining variables is more intensive care unit (ICU) specific

*GCS* Glasgow coma scale, *RASS* Richmond agitation-sedation scale, *CAM-ICU* confusion assessment method for the ICU, *NSE* neuron specific enolase, *EEG* electroencephalogram, *CT* computed tomography, *NIV* non-invasive ventilation, *MRI* magnetic resonance image, *ICP* intracranial pressure, $SvO_2$ mixed venous saturation, $SpO_2$ pulse oximetry, $FiO_2$ fraction of inspired oxygen, $PaCO_2$ arterial carbon dioxide partial pressure, $etCO_2$ end-tidal carbon dioxide partial pressure, *VV-ECMO* veno-venous extracorporeal membrane oxygenation, *POC US* point of care ultrasonography, *INR* international normalized ratio, *ICG-PDR* indocyanine green plasma disappearance rate, *aPTT* activated partial thromboplastin time, *MARS* molecular adsorbent recirculating system, *IAP* intra-abdominal pressure, *MRC* Medical Research Council scale, *US* ultrasonography

Table 8.2 provides a list of these criteria and indicates whether the proposed four categories (clinical signs, laboratory findings, additional tests not available at the bedside, and the level of organ support) adhere to these criteria. Real world variables will most likely never fulfill all of the proposed criteria and a consensus on what aspects of the list should be prioritized, e.g., simplicity and low cost versus organ specificity and independence of therapy, has to be found. The Glasgow Coma Scale (GCS) score may illustrate this point, as the variable is simple and inexpensive but highly therapy dependent when the use of sedation in the ICU is taken into account.

**Table 8.2** The four proposed categories of available variables for organ dysfunction assessment rated by the list of criteria for ideal descriptors of organ dysfunction [10]

| | Bedside signs and measurements | Laboratory findings | Advanced tests and measurements | Organ support |
|---|---|---|---|---|
| Simple and inexpensive | ++ | + | −− | −− |
| Routinely available in all ICUs | ++ | ++ | −− | −− |
| Reliable (intra- and inter-observer independent) | − | ++ | + | + |
| Objective (observer independent) | − | ++ | + | + |
| Specific to the function of the organ in question | +/− | + | ++ | ++ |
| Therapy independent | +/− | +/− | + | −− |
| Sequential (available at ICU admission or shortly thereafter and then at fixed periods of time) | ++ | ++ | −− | ++ |
| Not affected by transient, reversible abnormalities associated with therapeutic or practical interventions | + | + | ++ | −− |
| Reflect acute dysfunction of the organ in question but not chronic dysfunction | + | +/− | +/− | −− |
| Reproducible in large, heterogeneous groups of ICU patients | − | ++ | − | −− |
| Reproducible in several types of ICU from different regions of the globe | + | ++ | −− | −− |
| Abnormal in one direction only | + | +/− | − | ++ |
| Use continuous rather than dichotomous variables | −− | ++ | +/− | − |

(−−) does not apply, (−) rather does not apply, (+/−) unclear or different for specific variables in this category, (+) partially applies, (++) fully applies

## 8.4 Organ Systems Included in the Organ Dysfunction Scores in the ICU

The original SOFA score includes some of the listed variables in Table 8.1, namely the arterial oxygen partial pressure to fraction of inspired oxygen ($PaO_2/FiO_2$) ratio, bilirubin, thrombocyte count, vasopressor use, blood pressure, creatinine, urine output, and GCS. There have been many proposed adaptations to the original SOFA score for single organ systems and some additional variables presented in Table 8.1 have been assessed:

### 8.4.1 Neurological Component

The neurological system component of the SOFA score is based on the GCS, which is easily available and shows good mortality prediction. One issue with the GCS, however, is that it is unclear whether to use the actual GCS score or the presumed GCS score, as the GCS score may be reduced due to sedation without an underlying neurological condition. This issue was already discussed in the original SOFA publication [7]. In order to expand the neurological SOFA component, inclusion of the Richmond Agitation-Sedation Scale (RASS) when GCS data are not available has shown adequate performance [23].

### 8.4.2 Cardiovascular Component

The cardiovascular component of the SOFA score has been discussed extensively [24, 25], and recently the need for an update has been raised [26, 27]. The main reason for this suggestion is that the use of dopamine, which was the most used vasoactive drug in the 1990s, has disappeared almost completely from many ICUs. Accordingly, the score lost its linearity in prediction of mortality [26, 27]. The original MODS score used a product of heart rate and blood pressure as the cardiovascular component of the score [5]. A modified cardiovascular SOFA score consisting of lactate, shock index, and vasoactive agents has been proposed [24]. Additionally, norepinephrine equivalents have been suggested as an alternative strategy to quantify cardiovascular organ dysfunction [28, 29]. Lactate and capillary refill time are surrogates frequently used in resuscitation [30] and troponin has been associated with adverse cardiovascular outcome in sepsis patients [31]. These are variables that might be considered to describe the cardiovascular component of multiple organ dysfunction. Over recent decades, there have been major developments in devices to support the heart [32], which are currently not considered in organ dysfunction scores. However, a patient in cardiogenic shock receiving extracorporeal membrane oxygenation (ECMO) or left ventricular support (Impella) should be categorized higher on the organ dysfunction scale independent of additional need for vasopressors or inotropes.

### 8.4.3 Respiratory Component

The respiratory system in the current SOFA score is assessed using oxygenation parameters but somewhat neglects ventilation parameters, such as dead space indices, low compliance, or the use of continuous neuromuscular blockade, all of which are linked to mortality [33, 34]. Also newer devices, such as non-invasive ventilation and high flow nasal oxygen, are not included in the score. Chronic respiratory dysfunction currently cannot be distinguished from acute.

### 8.4.4 Hematological Component

The current main hematological component—the platelet count (used additionally to the white blood cell count in MODS and as the only variable in others)—appears to be strongly linked with mortality [35]. However, some other markers, such as the neutrophil-to-lymphocyte ratio [36] or the mean platelet volume [37], also appear to be good independent predictors of mortality. When assessing coagulation in clinical practice, variables other than platelet count (e.g., International Normalized Ratio [INR]) are regularly considered. On the other hand, a low platelet count may reflect hemopoietic as well as coagulation disorder. While a very low platelet count is usually an acute event, a milder decrease in platelet count can be chronic. Anti-platelet drugs influencing function and not the platelet count are currently not considered.

### 8.4.5 Renal Component

The renal component relies on creatinine levels, urine output, and renal replacement therapy (RRT), except when the latter is used for non-renal reasons (intoxication, metabolic disorders, rhabdomyolysis, aggressive fluid removal). In terms of mortality and compared to several other organ systems, such as cardiovascular and respiratory, it should be considered that renal function can be well supported also outside of the ICU. Moreover, patients with chronic renal dysfunction of different degree are common among critically ill patients. Scores that exclude the renal system component for patients on chronic RRT have been proposed in pediatric patients, but this approach has not been validated in the adult population [38].

### 8.4.6 Hepatic Component

Hepatic dysfunction relies on bilirubin solely, which does not cover the manifold functions of the liver. A modified SOFA score for patients with end-stage liver disease (CLIF-SOFA), using INR and encephalopathy as new variables outperformed specific liver dysfunction/cirrhosis scores as well as the SOFA score in these patients [39].

### 8.4.7 Abdominal Component

The abdominal component beyond the hepatic system was neglected in the original SOFA score, based on the reason that "attempting to include dysfunction/failure of the gut was felt to be very important, but also too complex and therefore abandoned" [7]. More recently it has been concluded that the challenges of measuring gastrointestinal dysfunction prevent inclusion of the gut system into organ dysfunction scores [40]. A European Society of Intensive Care Medicine (ESICM)-endorsed study recently addressed this problem and developed the GastroIntestinal Dysfunction Score (GIDS), which improved overall performance of the SOFA score in prediction of mortality [41]. Unfortunately, the two tested biomarkers (citrulline and intestinal fatty-acid binding protein [I-FABP]) did not improve the performance of the score, leaving the score based on subjective variables. Intra-abdominal hypertension was included in the GIDS score as a variable reflecting the abdominal compartment, interacting with enteral nutrition and gastrointestinal dysfunction [42] and being a cause of morbidity and mortality [43]. Multiple studies have shown the importance of the abdominal/gastrointestinal component in the multiple organ dysfunction syndrome, justifying attempts to include it in future scores [41, 44].

### 8.4.8 Metabolic Component

Metabolic dysfunction with acid-base/electrolyte disturbances as well as physical/muscle function has not been considered in organ dysfunction scores so far. Multiple electrolyte disorders, including refeeding syndrome, have been linked to mortality, but knowledge on the interplay of electrolytes is scarce [45], and interactions with other organ dysfunctions poorly studied.

### 8.4.9 Physical Component

Physical function is a mainstay of recovery far beyond the ICU and ICU-acquired weakness could be considered to be the organ dysfunction with the longest duration, also associated with long-term mortality.

## 8.5 Modified SOFA Scores

The strength of the original SOFA score is that most variables can be assessed at the bedside and it relies on laboratory measurements that are broadly available and part of daily measurements on the ICU. Grissom and colleagues proposed a modified SOFA score in order to perform an assessment with fewer resources, e.g., in an emergency room during a mass influx of patients [46]. In particular, the modified score used the pulse oximetry oxygen saturation ($SpO_2$) to $FiO_2$ ratio rather than the $PaO_2/FiO_2$ ratio, did not score the coagulation system, and relied on clinical signs, such as icterus or jaundice, for the liver system. The other systems were left unchanged. The score performed similarly to the original SOFA score in a cohort of 1770 patients [46]. Vacheron and colleagues developed a simplified sa-SOFA score in 2020, in which they reduced each dimension to a 3 point ordinal scale (0 to 2 points) rather than the original 5 point ordinal scale (0 to 4 points) [47]. The score does not rely on creatinine or blood pressure values and considers total catecholamine use rather than only norepinephrine and epinephrine. The score outperformed the original SOFA score in a cohort of 1436 patients [47]. Whether these modified scores continue to be accurate should be assessed in larger cohorts.

Mortality in critically ill patients stems from multiorgan failure. The risk of developing multiorgan failure may be mediated by preexisting conditions, which are not assessed by the SOFA score. Lee and colleagues proposed a complemented SOFA score by adding comorbidity parameters and age to the SOFA score [48]. Adding these parameters improved mortality prediction compared to the original SOFA score in a cohort of 1049 consecutive patients [48]. However, assessing acute organ dysfunction should be possible independent of preexisting conditions. Moreover, age and comorbidities will remain fixed over time, possibly distorting the dynamic/delta scores.

In order to detect states of multiple organ failure, organ systems have to be assessed simultaneously. One single organ system will not provide sufficient prognostic information. Adding several different organ systems complements the score. One possible exception to this may be the neurological SOFA score (based on GCS), which has been shown to dominate the association between admission score and 30-day mortality [49].

## 8.6 The Future of Organ Dysfunction Scores

Although many aspects of assessing organ dysfunction are still valid, changes in clinical practice may have impacted the performance of organ dysfunction scores and newer practices may no longer be reflected within the original scoring system [26, 27]. Table 8.3 lists some examples of new practices that are currently not assessed within the current SOFA score. Indeed, each component of existing organ dysfunction scores can be criticized as being not comprehensive for the particular organ function. However, the advantage of these scores from the 1990s is their simplicity and assessment of components simultaneously. Additionally, the SOFA score has been the most used scoring system for organ dysfunction and failure in the critically ill population. It has gained widespread interest as a marker of morbidity and mortality beyond sepsis patients and has become an international standard in research reporting and outcome measurement [5, 14]. This has enabled comparison of patients and research results within an established system. Such a consensus has yet to be found within the pediatric critical care community [50]. An established scoring system, such as the SOFA score, should therefore not be jeopardized lightly

**Table 8.3** Current approaches to quantified assessment of organ dysfunction in- and outside the intensive care unit (ICU)

| Organ system | Current approach in the ICU as part of an organ dysfunction score | Current approach outside of the ICU as single organ dysfunction | (Newer) practices not reflected in scores |
|---|---|---|---|
| Neurology | GCS | GCS | Sedation |
| Cardiovascular | cvSOFA | NYHA | VA-ECMO, Impella, LVAD, vasoactive and inotropic agents such as vasopressin, angiotensin II, milrinone, levosimendan |
| Respiratory | $PO_2/FiO_2$, mechanical ventilation | GOLD, FEV1 | High flow nasal oxygen, NIV, VV-ECMO, $ECCO_2R$ |
| Renal | Creatinine, urine output | KDIGO | CVVHD, CVVHF, IHD |
| Coagulation | Platelet count | INR, bleeding events | Coagulation factors, use of anticoagulants and/or anti-platelet agents |
| Liver | Bilirubin | MELD, Child-Pugh | MARS |
| Additional organ dysfunctions to be considered in an organ dysfunction score | | | |
| | Current approach in the ICU | Current approach outside of the ICU | Possible future approach |
| Abdomen/GI | GI symptoms, AGI, IAP | Weight loss, chronic diarrhea or constipation | GIDS, assessment of motility (US, pressure waves) and malabsorption (biomarkers) |
| Electrolytes | Measurement and correction of single electrolytes | Measurement and correction of single electrolytes | Assessment of all electrolytes, management considering interactions |
| Muscle | MRC | Physical performance tests, myography | US, myography, physical performance tests? |

*GCS* Glasgow coma scale, *cvSOFA* cardiovascular SOFA, *NYHA* New York Heart Association functional classification, *VA-ECMO* veno-arterial extracorporeal membrane oxygenation, *LVAD* left-ventricular assist device, $pO_2$ arterial oxygen partial pressure, $FiO_2$ fraction of inspired oxygen, *GOLD* global initiative for chronic lung disease classification system, *FEV1* expired volume at the end of first second of forced expiration, *NIV* non-invasive ventilation, *VV-ECMO* veno-venous extracorporeal membrane oxygenation, $ECCO_2R$ extracorporeal $CO_2$ removal, *KDIGO* Kidney Disease Improving Global Outcomes, *CVVHD* continuous veno-venous hemodialysis, *CVVHF* continuous veno-venous hemofiltration, *IHD* intermittent hemodialysis, *MELD* Model for end-stage liver disease, *MARS* molecular adsorbent recirculating system, *GI* gastrointestinal, *AGI* acute gastrointestinal injury grading, *IAP* intra-abdominal pressure, *GIDS* gastrointestinal dysfunction score, *MRC* Medical Research Council scale, *US* ultrasonography

by new adaptations. However, since its original publication in 1996, practices within the critical care community have clearly changed which may be reflected in the dynamics of SOFA subscores (Fig. 8.2). Thus, discussion about the need and possible options to update the score is probably justified. At the same time, development of many alternative scores may be futile and confusing. Therefore, if undertaken, this process of update should be well coordinated and based on a broad consensus in the ICU community.

## 8.7 Conclusion

The introduction of organ dysfunction scoring systems was a major development in critical care. Over the last three decades, several aspects of clinical practice have evolved. As such, revisiting some of the components and underlying concepts of organ dysfunction scores may be warranted. Such a revision would need to be guided by data. Independent of discussions about an update, the application of organ dysfunction scores as dynamic tools assisting in treatment decisions, rather than as prediction tools, needs to be further developed. Studies assessing the time course and interactions of different organ dysfunctions are therefore warranted.

## References


1. Bone RC, Balk RA, Cerra FB, et al. Definitions for sepsis and organ failure and guidelines for the use of innovative therapies in sepsis. Chest. 1992;101:1644–55.
2. Evans L, Rhodes A, Alhazzani W, et al. Surviving sepsis campaign: International guidelines for management of sepsis and septic shock 2021. Crit Care Med. 2021;49:e1063–143.
3. Goris RJA. Mediators of multiple organ failure. Intensive Care Med. 1990;16:S192–6.
4. Tran DD, Groeneveld AB, van der Meulen J, Nauta JJ, Strack van Schijndel RJ, Thijs LG. Age, chronic disease, sepsis, organ system failure, and mortality in a medical intensive care unit. Crit Care Med. 1990;18:474–9.
5. Marshall JC, Cook DJ, Christou NV, Bernard GR, Sprung CL, Sibbald WJ. Multiple organ dysfunction score: a reliable descriptor of a complex clinical outcome. Crit Care Med. 1995;23:1638–52.
6. Le Gall JR, Klar J, Lemeshow S, et al. The Logistic Organ Dysfunction system. A new way to assess organ dysfunction in the intensive care unit. ICU Scoring Group. JAMA. 1996;276:802–10.
7. Vincent JL, Moreno R, Takala J, et al. The SOFA (Sepsis-related Organ Failure Assessment) score to describe organ dysfunction/failure. Intensive Care Med. 1996;22:707–10.
8. Khwannimit B. A comparison of three organ dysfunction scores: MODS, SOFA and LOD for predicting ICU mortality in critically ill patients. J Med Assoc Thai. 2007;90:1074–81.
9. Vincent JL, de Mendonça A, Cantraine F, et al. Use of the SOFA score to assess the incidence of organ dysfunction/failure in intensive care units: results of a multicenter, prospective study. Working group on "sepsis-related problems" of the European Society of Intensive Care Medicine. Crit Care Med. 1998;26:1793–800.
10. Vincent JL, Moreno R. Clinical review: scoring systems in the critically ill. Crit Care. 2010;14:207.
11. Blanco J, Muriel-Bombín A, Sagredo V, et al. Incidence, organ dysfunction and mortality in severe sepsis: a Spanish Multicentre Study. Crit Care. 2008;12:R158.
12. Chierego M, Verdant C, De Backer D. Microcirculatory alterations in critically ill patients. Minerva Anestesiol. 2006;72:199–205.
13. Nakashima T, Miyamoto K, Shimokawa T, Kato S, Hayakawa M. The association between sequential organ failure assessment scores and mortality in patients with sepsis during the first week: the JSEPTIC DIC Study. J Intensive Care Med. 2020;35:656–62.
14. Soo A, Zuege DJ, Fick GH, et al. Describing organ dysfunction in the intensive care unit: a cohort study of 20,000 patients. Crit Care. 2019;23:186.
15. Raith EP, Udy AA, Bailey M, et al. Prognostic accuracy of the SOFA score, SIRS Criteria, and qSOFA score for in-hospital mortality among adults with suspected infection admitted to the intensive care unit. JAMA. 2017;317:290–300.

16. Khwannimit B, Bhurayanontachai R, Vattanavanit V. Comparison of the performance of SOFA, qSOFA, and SIRS for predicting mortality and organ failure among sepsis patients admitted to the intensive care unit in a middle-income country. J Crit Care. 2018;44:156–60.
17. Keller MB, Wang J, Nason M, Warner S, Follmann D, Kadri SS. Preintubation sequential organ failure assessment score for predicting COVID-19 mortality: external validation using electronic health record from 86 U.S. healthcare systems to appraise current ventilator triage algorithms. Crit Care Med. 2022;50:1051–62.
18. Gelissen H, de Grooth HJ, Smulders Y, et al. Effect of low-normal vs high-normal oxygenation targets on organ dysfunction in critically ill patients: a randomized clinical trial. JAMA. 2021;326:940–8.
19. de Grooth HJ, Geenen IL, Girbes AR, Vincent JL, Parienti JJ, Oudemans-van Straaten HM. SOFA and mortality endpoints in randomized controlled trials: a systematic review and meta-regression analysis. Crit Care. 2017;21:38.
20. Xu Z, Mao C, Su C, et al. Sepsis subphenotyping based on organ dysfunction trajectory. Crit Care. 2022;26:197.
21. Liu Y, Gao K, Deng H, et al. A time-incorporated SOFA score-based machine learning model for predicting mortality in critically ill patients: a multicenter, real-world study. Int J Med Inform. 2022;163:104776.
22. Zieleskiewicz L, Muller L, Lakhal K, et al. Point-of-care ultrasound in intensive care units: assessment of 1073 procedures in a multicentric, prospective, observational study. Intensive Care Med. 2015;41:1638–47.
23. Vasilevskis EE, Pandharipande PP, Graves AJ, et al. Validity of a modified sequential organ failure assessment score using the Richmond Agitation-Sedation Scale. Crit Care Med. 2016;44:138–46.
24. Yadav H, Harrison AM, Hanson AC, Gajic O, Kor DJ, Cartin-Ceba R. Improving the accuracy of cardiovascular component of the sequential organ failure assessment score. Crit Care Med. 2015;43:1449–57.
25. Szczeklik W, Fronczek J. Should we revise the SOFA score? Yes. Acta Anaesthesiol Scand. 2022;66:658–9.
26. Bachmann KF, Arabi YM, Regli A, Starkopf J, Reintam BA. Cardiovascular SOFA score may not reflect current practice. Intensive Care Med. 2022;48:119–20.
27. Pölkki A, Pekkarinen PT, Takala J, Selander T, Reinikainen M. Association of Sequential Organ Failure Assessment (SOFA) components with mortality. Acta Anaesthesiol Scand. 2022;66:731–41.
28. Bosch NA, Teja B, Wunsch H, Walkey AJ. Characterization and validation of a novel measure of septic shock severity. Intensive Care Med. 2020;46:135–7.
29. Vallabhajosyula S, Jentzer JC, Kotecha AA, et al. Development and performance of a novel vasopressor-driven mortality prediction model in septic shock. Ann Intensive Care. 2018;8:112.
30. Hernández G, Ospina-Tascón GA, Damiani LP, et al. Effect of a resuscitation strategy targeting peripheral perfusion status vs serum lactate levels on 28-day mortality among patients with septic shock. JAMA. 2019;321:654.
31. Garcia MA, Rucci JM, Thai KK, et al. Association between troponin i levels during sepsis and postsepsis cardiovascular complications. Am J Respir Crit Care Med. 2021;204:557–65.
32. Attinger-Toller A, Bossard M, Cioffi GM, et al. Ventricular unloading using the Impella(TM) device in cardiogenic shock. Front Cardiovasc Med. 2022;9:856870.
33. Lee BY, Lee S-I, Baek MS, et al. Lower driving pressure and neuromuscular blocker use are associated with decreased mortality in patients with COVID-19 ARDS. Respir Care. 2022;67:216–26.
34. Lecompte-Osorio P, Pearson SD, Pieroni CH, et al. Bedside estimates of dead space using end-tidal CO2 are independently associated with mortality in ARDS. Crit Care. 2021;25:333.
35. Akca S, Haji-Michael P, de Mendonça A, Suter P, Levi M, Vincent JL. Time course of platelet counts in critically ill patients. Crit Care Med. 2002;30:753–6.

36. Liang P, Yu F. Value of CRP, PCT, and NLR in prediction of severity and prognosis of patients with bloodstream infections and sepsis. Front Surg. 2022;9:857218.
37. Tajarernmuang P, Phrommintikul A, Limsukon A, Pothirat C, Chittawatanarat K. The role of mean platelet volume as a predictor of mortality in critically ill patients: a systematic review and meta-analysis. Crit Care Res Prac. 2016;2016:1–8.
38. Jhang WK, Kim YA, Ha EJ, et al. Extrarenal sequential organ failure assessment score as an outcome predictor of critically ill children on continuous renal replacement therapy. Pediatr Nephrol. 2014;29:1089–95.
39. Pan HC, Jenq CC, Tsai MH, et al. Scoring systems for 6-month mortality in critically ill cirrhotic patients: a prospective analysis of chronic liver failure—sequential organ failure assessment score (CLIF-SOFA). Aliment Pharmacol Ther. 2014;40:1056–65.
40. Marshall JC. Measuring organ dysfunction. Med Klin Intensivmed Notfmed. 2020;115(Suppl 1):15–20.
41. Reintam Blaser A, Padar M, Mändul M, et al. Development of the Gastrointestinal Dysfunction Score (GIDS) for critically ill patients—a prospective multicenter observational study (iSOFA study). Clin Nutr. 2021;40:4932–40.
42. Reintam Blaser A, Regli A, De Keulenaer B, et al. Incidence, risk factors, and outcomes of intra-abdominal hypertension in critically ill patients—a prospective multicenter study (IROI Study). Crit Care Med. 2019;47:535–42.
43. Regli A, Reintam Blaser A, De Keulenaer B, et al. Intra-abdominal hypertension and hypoxic respiratory failure together predict adverse outcome—a sub-analysis of a prospective cohort. J Crit Care. 2021;64:165–72.
44. Aperstein Y, Cohen L, Bendavid I, et al. Improved ICU mortality prediction based on SOFA scores and gastrointestinal parameters. PLoS One. 2019;14:e0222599.
45. Reintam Blaser A, van Zanten ARH, de Man AME. Electrolytes in the ICU. In: Vincent JL, editor. Annual Update in Intensive Care and Emergency Medicine 2022. Heidelberg: Springer; 2022. p. 183–200.
46. Grissom CK, Brown SM, Kuttler KG, et al. A modified sequential organ failure assessment score for critical care triage. Disaster Med Public Health Prep. 2010;4:277–84.
47. Vacheron CH, Friggeri A, Iwaz J, et al. A new simplified and accurate sa-SOFA score. J Crit Care. 2020;57:240–5.
48. Lee KS, Sheen SS, Jung YJ, et al. Consideration of additional factors in Sequential Organ Failure Assessment score. J Crit Care. 2014;29:185.e189–185.e12.
49. Knox DB, Lanspa MJ, Pratt CM, Kuttler KG, Jones JP, Brown SM. Glasgow Coma Scale score dominates the association between admission Sequential Organ Failure Assessment score and 30-day mortality in a mixed intensive care unit population. J Crit Care. 2014;29:780–5.
50. Kawasaki T, Shime N, Straney L, et al. Paediatric sequential organ failure assessment score (pSOFA): a plea for the world-wide collaboration for consensus. Intensive Care Med. 2018;44:995–7.

# Part III

# ARDS

# *Ex Vivo* Lung Perfusion Models to Explore the Pathobiology of ARDS

9

A. Abdalla, K. Dhaliwal, and M. Shankar-Hari

## 9.1 Introduction

Acute respiratory distress syndrome (ARDS) is an acute diffuse, inflammatory lung injury that occurs in response to a variety of insults, such as trauma, pneumonia, sepsis, and pancreatitis. At the bedside, ARDS is defined as respiratory failure within 1 week of a known insult, non-cardiogenic or volume-related etiology, bilateral presence of pulmonary infiltrates, and acute onset of hypoxemia that is graded based on the required fraction of inspiratory oxygen [1].

ARDS is a common cause of mortality and long-term morbidity. An international, multicenter, prospective cohort study in a convenience sample of patients in 459 intensive care units (ICUs) from 50 countries across five continents undergoing invasive mechanical (IMV) or non-invasive (NIV) ventilation reported a period prevalence of 10.4% of ICU admissions [2]. This equates to an estimated potential global burden of 11.5–55 × $10^5$ ARDS cases per year [3]. ARDS affects all age groups; has a high mortality in excess of 40%; and causes a long-term reduction in quality of life for survivors. ARDS survivors have exercise limitations,

A. Abdalla · K. Dhaliwal
Centre for Inflammation Research, Queen's Medical Research Institute, University of Edinburgh, Edinburgh, UK

Translational Healthcare Technologies Group, Centre for Inflammation Research, Queen's Medical Research Institute, University of Edinburgh, Edinburgh, UK

M. Shankar-Hari (✉)
Centre for Inflammation Research, Queen's Medical Research Institute, University of Edinburgh, Edinburgh, UK

Translational Healthcare Technologies Group, Centre for Inflammation Research, Queen's Medical Research Institute, University of Edinburgh, Edinburgh, UK

Intensive Care Unit, Royal Infirmary of Edinburgh, Edinburgh, UK
e-mail: manu.shankar-hari@ed.ac.uk



J.-L. Vincent (ed.), *Annual Update in Intensive Care and Emergency Medicine 2023*, Annual Update in Intensive Care and Emergency Medicine,
https://doi.org/10.1007/978-3-031-23005-9_9

psychological sequelae, decreased physical quality of life, increased costs, and high use of health care services for up to 5 years after they recover from their acute illness [4].

Recently, a systematic review of randomized controlled trials (RCTs) in ARDS highlighted the lack of any pharmacological success in clinical effectiveness trials [5]. An important explanation for lack of RCT success in ARDS could be inability of drug targets identified in pre-clinical models to favorably alter the complex immune changes within the lung in patients with ARDS. This prompted us to explore the utility of human *ex vivo* lung perfusion (EVLP) models to inform ARDS pathobiology to facilitate accelerated translation of preclinical research to patient care.

EVLP is a technique to maintain lung viability outside the body for several hours to allow assessment and reconditioning, traditionally used in the context of lung transplantation. Our rationale was that human EVLP models may enhance our understanding of ARDS pathobiology beyond animal models and *in silico* co-culture models. Because EVLP models maintain lung tissue viability, they would enable us to generate the spatial landscape of early ARDS pathobiology with delineation of the cell-cell interactions among the alveolar epithelium, alveolar endothelium, and lung resident immune cells occurring following different insults to the human lung. These changes could be studied at the cell phenotype, cell function, and molecular levels (transcript/proteins).

## 9.2 ARDS Pathobiology Overview

In health, the alveolar-capillary membrane consists of a continuous layer of squamous epithelial cells (type 1) interspersed with type 2 alveolar epithelial cells and a basement membrane that separates them from underlying capillaries with non-fenestrated endothelial cells. These cells are tightly bound to each other in their respective compartments by intercellular tight junctions expressing epithelial cadherin (E-cadherin) and vascular endothelial cadherin (VE-cadherin), respectively on their plasma membranes. The function of the alveolar-capillary membrane is to maintain barrier integrity, permit efficient gaseous diffusion, and regulate the movement of fluid, cells, and ions between the two compartments [6]. Resident immune cells that respond to pathogens and environmental insults to this barrier include alveolar macrophages, marginated neutrophils, as well as resident lymphocytes in the interstitial spaces.

Broadly, insults to the alveolar-capillary membrane are categorized into direct (epithelial) or indirect (endothelial) injury, based on the compartment where the injury starts, or perhaps is dominant (Fig. 9.1). Direct and indirect injuries have distinct histological features [7]. One in five patients with ARDS has features of direct and indirect injury or mixed etiologies of lung injury. With direct injuries, the discontinuous hyaline membranes formed are thicker when compared with indirect injuries, often with greater fibrin and collagen deposition. Of note, an early cardinal feature of indirect injuries is VE-cadherin destabilization resulting in loss of tight junctions between endothelial cells. The final common pathway in direct and indirect injuries is increased alveolar-capillary membrane permeability, alveolar

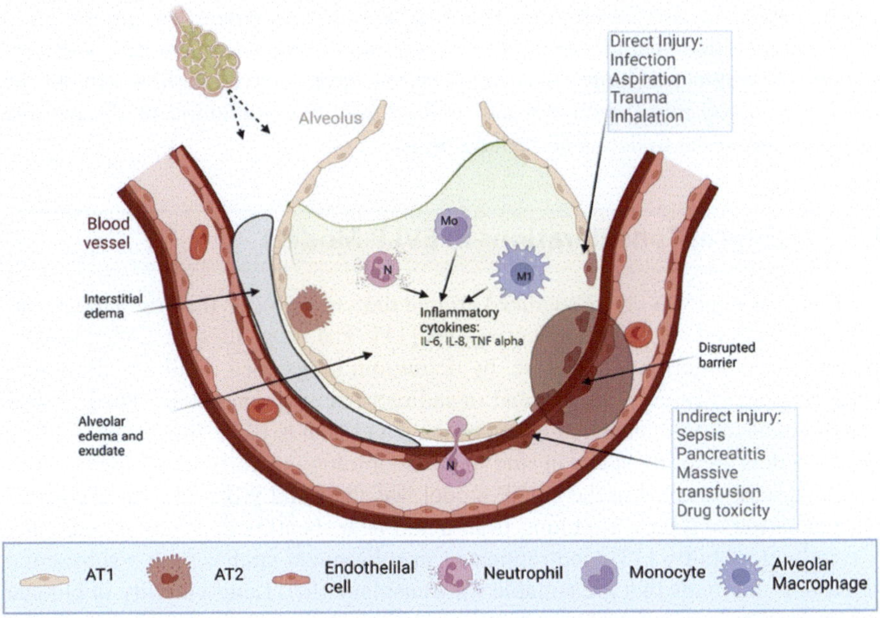


**Fig. 9.1** Alveolar capillary membrane injury. *IL* interleukin, *TNF* tumor necrosis factor, *AT1* alveolar type 1 cells, *AT2* alveolar type 2 cells. Created with Biorender.com

congestion, loss of functional lung architecture and decrease in the volume of aerated lung tissue [8].

## 9.3 Different Approaches to Inducing and Attenuating Lung Injury in EVLP Models: Lipopolysaccharide Challenge as an Example

Insult can be administered via the airway or via the perfusate. Airway insults resemble direct and perfusate insults indirect injuries causing ARDS. Lipopolysaccharide (LPS), a Toll-like receptor 4 (TLR4) agonist, has been used in other experimental models of lung injury both for direct and indirect insults. Two studies have evaluated it using the EVLP model, each using a different mode of injury. Lee et al. instilled LPS into the right middle lobe of a single lung EVLP to simulate direct lung injury [9]. Weathington et al. used EVLP to model indirect lung injury by infusing LPS through the pulmonary artery [10]. In the study by Lee et al., the primary endpoint measured was alveolar fluid clearance, as a surrogate of alveolar flooding and alveolar-capillary membrane dysfunction, whereas in the study by Weathington et al., the endpoints were lung function, cytokine induction, and transcriptional profiles. The histological pattern observed in the two studies correlated with the type of injury: endobronchially delivered LPS causing an increase in cellularity with mainly neutrophilic and alveolar edema, while indirect injury caused an increase in septal thickness. These two experiments [9, 10] show the utility of

EVLP in studying two different mechanisms of action to induce lung injury; however, they also demonstrate variability in how this experimental model is set up. Namely, the number of lungs used, the perfusate solution used with or without the addition of blood into the circuit and its flow rate, the ventilation mode, and the endpoints measured to define acute lung injury.

## 9.4 Technical Considerations in EVLP Models

The EVLP system was conceptualized around the same time as the original descriptions of ARDS by Asbaugh and colleagues [11]. The lungs used in EVLP models are sourced postmortem. Therefore, by definition, lungs used in all EVLP models will have some degree of direct, and or indirect insult, prior to harvesting. EVLP models enable experiments that last between 4 and 12 h to be performed [12]. Thus, EVLP models are of most use in studying pathobiology of early lung injury.

A landmark advance in the EVLP model was the Lund protocol, which enabled transplantation of a harvested lung from a non-heart-beating donor by maintaining *ex vivo* lung viability [13], and replicated in subsequent studies with a substantial increase in the lungs that are suitable for transplant [14]. Lung viability in clinical transplantation is based on functional assessment encompassing lung airway pressures, compliance, and gas exchange throughout EVLP (Box 9.1). EVLP models have also been used to study the physiological as well as the histological and molecular phenotype of pulmonary arterial hypertension, idiopathic pulmonary fibrosis, and emphysema [15]. Many of these assessments have similarities with unanswered questions around early ARDS pathobiology, which could be addressed with EVLP models. For example, EVLP models have been used to induce lung injury directly or indirectly with a variety of pathogenic organisms and LPS [9, 10, 16, 17], and then to test therapies ranging from mesenchymal stem cells to small molecules, which are currently being tested in early phase clinical trials [18–20].

**Box 9.1 Acceptance criteria after EVLP**

- The ratio of arterial oxygen partial pressure ($PaO_2$ in mmHg) to fraction of inspired oxygen ≥350 mmHg
- Stable or improving pulmonary artery pressure
- Stable or improving airway pressures
- Stable or improving pulmonary compliance

The basic technique for EVLP is very similar across protocols; the circuit is illustrated in Fig. 9.2. A pump drives perfusate around the circuit through a gas membrane attached to a heater-cooler, then through a leukocyte filter. The perfusate then enters the pulmonary artery and drains from the left atrium to a reservoir or cannula back into the circuit. Transducers, thermometers, and flow meters are placed within the circuit for monitoring purposes. The differences in the protocols lie in whether the left atrium is left open or closed, the targeted perfusate flow rate, the ventilation strategy, and whether red cell concentrate is added or not to the perfusate (Table 9.1).

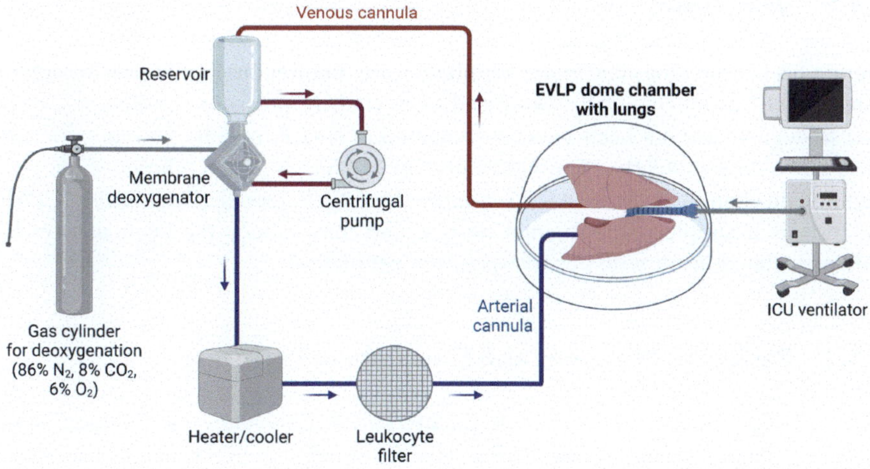


**Fig. 9.2** *Ex vivo* lung perfusion (EVLP) circuit. Created with Biorender.com

**Table 9.1** Variables to consider in *ex vivo* lung perfusion models

| Parameter | Options | Description | Advantages | Disadvantages |
|---|---|---|---|---|
| Lungs | Single | Single lung used | Increases number of experiments | Less physiological |
| | En-bloc | Both lungs used | More physiological | Lack of internal control |
| Ventilation | Continuous positive airway pressure | | Easier set-up | Less physiological |
| | Positive pressure ventilation | | More physiological | Ventilator-associated lung injury |
| Perfusion flow rate | 100% cardiac output | | More physiological | May reduce experimental time by endothelial damage |
| | 40% cardiac output | | More physiological | Ideally requires a left atrium for cannulation |
| | 0.2–0.5 l/min | | Prolonged period under experimental conditions | Less physiological |
| Perfusate | Cellular | Addition of either red cell concentrate or whole blood to perfusion fluid | Increased oxygen carrying capacity, more physiological, whole blood provides peripheral leukocytes to study injury | More complex set-up |
| | Acellular | No cellular additions to the perfusion fluid | Easier set-up, can study resident cells in isolation | Less physiological |

### 9.4.1 Ventilation

During EVLP, the lungs can either be inflated with continuous positive airway pressure (CPAP) or mechanically ventilated with positive-pressure ventilation. These two strategies have not been directly compared in EVLP models. We can only surmise that a lung protective ventilation strategy is more likely to reproduce the pulmonary mechanics seen in ARDS within the EVLP model. In contrast, CPAP inflation is a simpler experimental design, and may reduce the cyclical stretch-collapse related insult with positive-pressure ventilation.

### 9.4.2 Perfusion Pressures and Flow Rate of Perfusate

The pulmonary vascular resistance is usually raised. Depending on the duration of hypoxic time, the extent of endothelial injury will differ between lungs. Therefore, studies thus far using EVLP models have used varying flow rates, ranging from 40% to 100%, with flow rates ranging from 0.2–0.5 l/min [9, 10, 15–17]. The inspired fraction of oxygen delivered can also be adjusted to ensure normoxemia of the perfusate.

The choice of perfusion strategy should therefore be guided by the underlying hypothesis being tested. For example, if a physiological response is sought, clinical EVLP perfusate flows are appropriate; however for a more mechanistic study at the cellular network level with length of time in the system important, a more conservative flow strategy should be adopted.

### 9.4.3 Controls for Experiments

Due to the heterogeneity of lung harvesting and of individual donors, the EVLP model provides an excellent opportunity for internal control. Thus, lungs can be perfused in a single lung preparation, using direct injury models, with an uninjured lobe acting as the control [9, 19], or using indirect injury with the contralateral lung acting as the control [21]. En-bloc preparations have also been used [10, 15], and again the choice is determined by the underlying experimental question.

### 9.4.4 Cellular or Acellular Perfusion?

A major difference between the three commonly used clinical protocols for EVLP (Table 9.1) is whether red cell concentrate is used as part of the perfusate. When red cell concentrate is used, it is termed cellular, and acellular when not (e.g., the 'Toronto' protocol is acellular). When red cell concentrate is used, the target hematocrit is usually 10–15%. Two main indications for using a cellular perfusate in the clinical setting are to better mimic physiological flow through the pulmonary vasculature and to allow for more accurate oxygen blood gas analysis [22]. In the context of experimental studies of lung injury, cellular perfusion usually entails the addition of whole blood into the circuit to provide peripheral leukocytes to respond to the injury. In these studies, authors have found that alveolar fluid clearance, a measure of lung injury, was only impacted once whole blood was added to the system [16, 23]. The advantage of using an acellular perfusate is the ability to study the resident lung cell population in isolation, thus simplifying experimental design and logistics [10, 18, 24]. Blood gas analyses of acellular perfusates are unreliable. Therefore other physiologic parameters of lung injury, such as markers of reduction in lung compliance, should be monitored [22].

## 9.5 Defining ARDS in EVLP Models

Guidance from the American Thoracic Society for animal models of ARDS recommends at least three of four key features: (1) histologic evidence of tissue injury; (2) alteration of the alveolar-capillary barrier; (3) presence of an acute inflammatory response; and (4) evidence of physiologic dysfunction [25]. These criteria are easily adapted for EVLP models, as shown in Table 9.2, into the experimental design in Fig. 9.3.

**Table 9.2** Assessment of presence of lung injury in *ex vivo* lung perfusion (EVLP) models

| Feature | EVLP information |
|---|---|
| Alteration of the alveolar-capillary barrier/ evidence of physiologic dysfunction | Physiological parameters—pulmonary arterial pressure, lung compliance, alveolar fluid clearance<br>Alveolar-capillary barrier function—lung wet-to-dry ratio, BAL albumin, protein or Evan's blue dye accumulation in lung homogenates |
| Histologic evidence of tissue injury | Light and electron microscopy |
| Presence of an acute inflammatory response | Tissue imaging for markers<br>Flow cytometry<br>Activation markers on leukocytes<br>Chemokine or cytokine measurement in BAL fluid or lung tissue |

*BAL* bronchoalveolar lavage

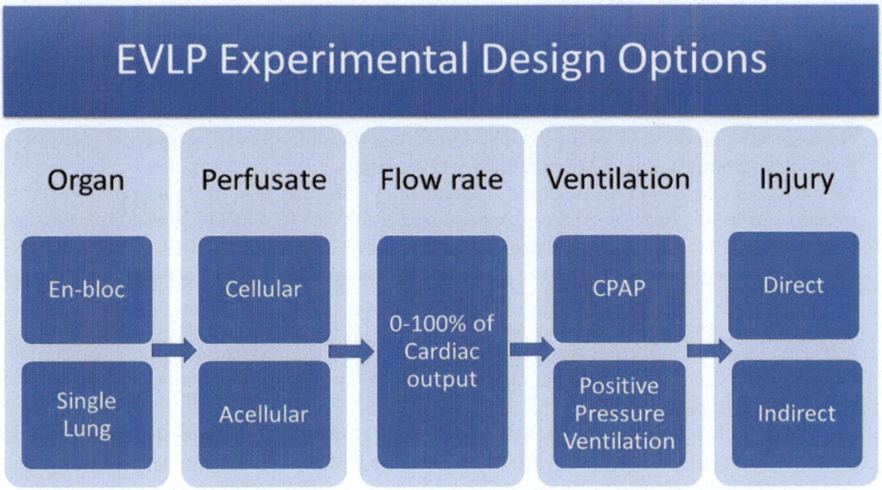


**Fig. 9.3** *Ex vivo* lung perfusion (EVLP) experimental options. *CPAP* continuous positive airway pressure

## 9.6 EVLP Challenges

The lung environment in experimental EVLP models tends to be 'primed' by the illness of the deceased, the harvesting, and the cold ischemic time. For example, in the case of brain-dead donors, the immune system is activated [26, 27], and the warm ischemic time after cardiac arrest also results in immune activation along with cell death [28, 29]. Placement of harvested lung, and rewarding during EVLP also triggers an inflammatory response with increases in cytokines, such as interleukin (IL)-6, IL-8, IL-1β, and monocyte chemoattractant protein (MCP)-1 [15, 30], and an altered transcriptional state characterized by altered tumor necrosis factor (TNF)-α signaling, apoptosis, and vascular pathways [15, 31]. Thus, when interpreting experimental results in lung injury models, these factors must be considered However, it is possible to draw mechanistic insight by separating the baseline changes from post-injury changes using appropriate controls.

## 9.7 Conclusion

EVLP models offer a translatable insult-injury-testing platform for functional and molecular characterization of acute lung injury. The platform could become an essential step in the translational pipeline for ARDS management.

**Acknowledgement** MS-H is funded by a clinician scientist fellowship from the National Institute for Health Research [CS-2016-16-011].

## References

1. Force ADT, Ranieri VM, Rubenfeld GD, et al. Acute respiratory distress syndrome: the Berlin definition. JAMA. 2012;307:2526–33.
2. Bellani G, Laffey JG, Pham T, et al. Epidemiology, patterns of care, and mortality for patients with acute respiratory distress syndrome in intensive care units in 50 countries. JAMA. 2016;315:788–800.
3. Adhikari NK, Fowler RA, Bhagwanjee S, Rubenfeld GD. Critical care and the global burden of critical illness in adults. Lancet. 2010;376:1339–46.
4. Herridge MS, Tansey CM, Matte A, et al. Functional disability 5 years after acute respiratory distress syndrome. N Engl J Med. 2011;364:1293–304.
5. Saha R, Assouline B, Mason G, Douiri A, Summers C, Shankar-Hari M. Impact of differences in acute respiratory distress syndrome randomised controlled trial inclusion and exclusion criteria: systematic review and meta-analysis. Br J Anaesth. 2021;127:85–101.
6. Matthay MA, Folkesson HG, Clerici C. Lung epithelial fluid transport and the resolution of pulmonary edema. Physiol Rev. 2002;82:569–600.
7. Capelozzi VL. What have anatomic and pathologic studies taught us about acute lung injury and acute respiratory distress syndrome? Curr Opin Crit Care. 2008;14:56–63.
8. Matthay MA, Zemans RL, Zimmerman GA, et al. Acute respiratory distress syndrome. Nat Rev Dis Primers. 2019;5:18.
9. Lee JW, Krasnodembskaya A, McKenna DH, Song Y, Abbott J, Matthay MA. Therapeutic effects of human mesenchymal stem cells in ex vivo human lungs injured with live bacteria. Am J Respir Crit Care Med. 2013;187:751–60.

10. Weathington NM, Alvarez D, Sembrat J, et al. Ex vivo lung perfusion as a human platform for preclinical small molecule testing. JCI Insight. 2018;3:e95515.
11. Ashbaugh DG, Bigelow DB, Petty TL, Levine BE. Acute respiratory distress in adults. Lancet. 1967;2:319–23.
12. Cypel M, Yeung JC, Hirayama S, et al. Technique for prolonged normothermic ex vivo lung perfusion. J Heart Lung Transplant. 2008;27:1319–25.
13. Steen S, Sjöberg T, Pierre L, Liao Q, Eriksson L, Algotsson L. Transplantation of lungs from a non-heart-beating donor. Lancet. 2001;357:825–9.
14. Luo Q, Zhu L, Wang Y, Wang L, Lv W, Hu J. The conversional efficacy of ex vivo lung perfusion and clinical outcomes in patients undergoing transplantation of donor lungs by ex vivo lung perfusion: a meta-analysis. Ann Transplant. 2019;24:647–60.
15. Cardenes N, Sembrat J, Noda K, et al. Human ex vivo lung perfusion: a novel model to study human lung diseases. Sci Rep. 2021;11:490.
16. Lee JW, Fang X, Gupta N, Serikov V, Matthay MA. Allogeneic human mesenchymal stem cells for treatment of E. coli endotoxin-induced acute lung injury in the ex vivo perfused human lung. Proc Natl Acad Sci U S A. 2009;106:16357–62.
17. Ross JT, Nesseler N, Leligdowicz A, et al. The ex vivo perfused human lung is resistant to injury by high-dose S. pneumoniae bacteremia. Am J Physiol Lung Cell Mol Physiol. 2020;319:L218–27.
18. Gennai S, Monsel A, Hao Q, Park J, Matthay MA, Lee JW. Microvesicles derived from human mesenchymal stem cells restore alveolar fluid clearance in human lungs rejected for transplantation. Am J Transplant. 2015;15:2404–12.
19. Park J, Kim S, Lim H, et al. Therapeutic effects of human mesenchymal stem cell microvesicles in an ex vivo perfused human lung injured with severe E. coli pneumonia. Thorax. 2019;74:43–50.
20. McAuley DF, Cross LM, Hamid U, et al. Keratinocyte growth factor for the treatment of the acute respiratory distress syndrome (KARE): a randomised, double-blind, placebo-controlled phase 2 trial. Lancet Respir Med. 2017;5:484–91.
21. Cypel M, Feld JJ, Galasso M, et al. Prevention of viral transmission during lung transplantation with hepatitis C-viraemic donors: an open-label, single-Centre, pilot trial. Lancet Respir Med. 2020;8:192 201.
22. Yeung JC, Cypel M, Machuca TN, et al. Physiologic assessment of the ex vivo donor lung for transplantation. J Heart Lung Transplant. 2012;31:1120–6.
23. Shaver CM, Wickersham N, McNeil JB, et al. Cell-free hemoglobin promotes primary graft dysfunction through oxidative lung endothelial injury. JCI Insight. 2018;3:e98546.
24. Snyder ME, Sembrat J, Noda K, et al. Human lung-resident macrophages colocalize with and provide costimulation to PD1(hi) tissue-resident memory T cells. Am J Respir Crit Care Med. 2021;203:1230–44.
25. Kulkarni HS, Lee JS, Bastarache JA, et al. Update on the features and measurements of experimental acute lung injury in animals: an official American Thoracic Society workshop report. Am J Respir Cell Mol Biol. 2022;66:e1–e14.
26. Korovesi I, Papadomichelakis E, Orfanos SE, et al. Exhaled breath condensate in mechanically ventilated brain-injured patients with no lung injury or sepsis. Anesthesiology. 2011;114:1118–29.
27. Takada M, Nadeau KC, Hancock WW, et al. Effects of explosive brain death on cytokine activation of peripheral organs in the rat. Transplantation. 1998;65:1533–42.
28. Gori F, Fumagalli J, Lonati C, et al. Lung biomolecular profile and function of grafts from donors after cardiocirculatory death with prolonged donor warm ischemia time. J Clin Med. 2022;11:3066.
29. Wong A, Liu M. Inflammatory responses in lungs from donation after brain death: mechanisms and potential therapeutic targets. J Heart Lung Transplant. 2021;40:890–6.
30. Sadaria MR, Smith PD, Fullerton DA, et al. Cytokine expression profile in human lungs undergoing normothermic ex-vivo lung perfusion. Ann Thorac Surg. 2011;92:478–84.
31. Wong A, Zamel R, Yeung J, et al. Potential therapeutic targets for lung repair during human ex vivo lung perfusion. Eur Respir J. 2020;55:902222.

# Interpretation of Lung Perfusion in ARDS

10

L. Ball, F. Marchese, and P. Pelosi

## 10.1 Introduction

Supportive treatments in patients with acute respiratory distress syndrome (ARDS) are mainly aimed at ensuring gas exchange, which is determined by the matching of lung ventilation and perfusion [1]. Clinical practice is typically more focused on manipulating ventilation through changes of ventilator settings, rather than balancing ventilation and perfusion, although these two components are equally important in determining the adequacy of oxygenation and carbon dioxide ($CO_2$) removal. The body of evidence shaping the current clinical management of ARDS [2] is built based on the randomized trials conducted in the last three decades, most of which were centered on ventilatory management targeting oxygenation and/or respiratory mechanics [3]. Nonetheless, lung perfusion is indirectly affected by several factors characterizing the care of patients with ARDS admitted to the intensive care unit (ICU), including hemodynamic management and mechanical ventilation itself [4]. Therefore, understanding the mechanisms of lung perfusion and ventilation matching seems crucial for optimizing the clinical management of patients with ARDS

L. Ball (✉) · P. Pelosi
Department of Surgical Sciences and Integrated Diagnostics (DISC), University of Genoa, Genoa, Italy

Department of Anesthesia and Intensive Care, Ospedale Policlinico San Martino, IRCCS per l'Oncologia e le Neuroscienze, Genoa, Italy
e-mail: lorenzo.ball@unige.it

F. Marchese
Department of Surgical Sciences and Integrated Diagnostics (DISC), University of Genoa, Genoa, Italy



J.-L. Vincent (ed.), *Annual Update in Intensive Care and Emergency Medicine 2023*, Annual Update in Intensive Care and Emergency Medicine, https://doi.org/10.1007/978-3-031-23005-9_10

[5]. Despite the availability of several techniques to assess lung perfusion in the clinical setting, the basic concepts of the modeling of ventilation-perfusion matching are derived from earlier studies conducted on healthy subjects, subsequently translated to ARDS. The inhomogeneity of ARDS lungs [6] substantially complicates the interpretation of ventilation-perfusion matching and imbalances between ventilation and perfusion are rarely taken into account when treating patients with ARDS [7]. The aim of this chapter is to provide a critical approach to the interpretation of lung perfusion in ARDS, from pathophysiology to clinical practice.

## 10.2 Determinants of Gas Exchange

Blood gas exchange represents the core task of the respiratory system and depends on three components: ventilation (), diffusion, and perfusion ( $\dot{Q}$ ). All these mechanisms can be impaired in ARDS, with a major role of the matching between $\dot{V}$ and $\dot{Q}$ [8].

### 10.2.1 Ventilation

Ventilation includes alveolar and physiological dead space ventilation, with anatomic dead space accounting for 2–3 ml/kg of body weight in healthy subjects during spontaneous breathing and alveolar dead space caused by unperfused respiratory units [9]. In normal conditions, convective movements drive gas through the airways, while diffusive movements drive gas through the respiratory zone [10]. Once ventilation has reached the alveolus, diffusion occurs according to Fick's law [1]. At constant dead space, the elimination of $CO_2$ $(\dot{V}CO_2)$ is proportional to alveolar ventilation $(\dot{V}_A)$, i.e., $\dot{V}CO_2 = k \cdot \dot{V}_A \cdot PaCO_2$, thus the $PaCO_2$ is inversely proportional to $\dot{V}_A$ [11]. Ventilation can be impaired by several mechanisms including alveolar flooding, loss of aeration, atelectasis, hyperinflation, and pneumolysis (Fig. 10.1, left panel). All these alterations can coexist in ARDS from different etiologies [12, 13].

### 10.2.2 Perfusion

When considering the lung as a whole organ, lung perfusion ($\dot{Q}$) equals the cardiac output, while at the regional level it is represented by the alveolar capillary blood flow. The cardiac output streams through the lungs with low pressures as compared to the systemic circulation, and its regional distribution depends on several mechanisms including hypoxic vasoconstriction and is affected by ventilation itself. Certain capillaries are not perfused in resting conditions, but can be reopened at higher right heart pressures or lung volumes in a process known as vascular recruitment [14]. Perfusion can be altered in ARDS through several mechanisms including aberrant regulation of vasal tone, endothelial swelling, embolism or thrombosis, and vascular lysis [15], as illustrated in Fig. 10.1, right panel.

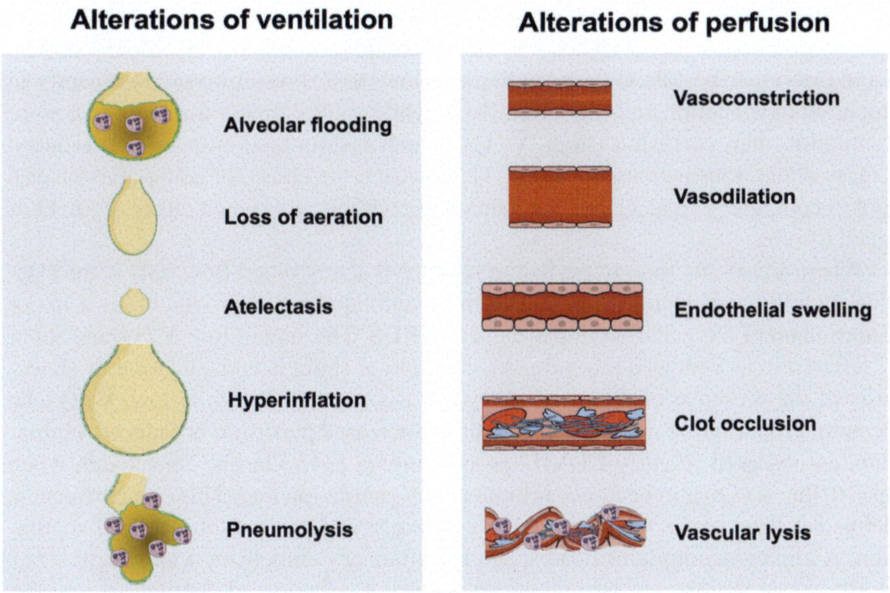


**Fig. 10.1** Left panel, main pathological alterations of ventilation. Right panel, main pathological alterations of perfusion

The distribution of regional perfusion in the supine position has been traditionally described as gravity-dependent, with dorsal regions receiving more perfusion than ventral ones [16]. However, in inhomogeneous ARDS lungs where weight distribution is massively skewed towards the dorsal regions [17], the increase of perfusion in the dependent regions could only derive from the backward dislocation of most of the lung tissue and vasculature. To compensate for this, perfusion in ARDS lungs should be related to the amount of lung tissue. The few studies that have investigated the distribution of perfusion accounting for the amount of lung tissue observed different patterns—an anti-gravitational distribution in coronavirus disease 2019 (COVID-19) [18] and a bell-shaped, linear or gravitational ventral-to-dorsal distribution in conventional ARDS [19]—depending on the level of applied positive end-expiratory pressure (PEEP) [20] and the position [21].

## 10.3 The Ventilation:Perfusion Ratio: Definition and Pitfalls

In healthy lungs, ventilation and perfusion are balanced not only from a conceptual point of view, but also numerically. In fact, when minute ventilation (corresponding to $\dot{V}$) and cardiac output (corresponding to $\dot{Q}$) are measured at rest, they are both in the order of magnitude of 5 l/min. While this absolute value may vary, the approximation $\dot{V} \approx \dot{Q}$ remains valid in uninjured lungs of several animal species [16]. Mismatching between $\dot{V}$ and $\dot{Q}$ is responsible for most of the pathophysiological and clinical conditions where gas exchange is impaired [22], including ARDS [23].

Earlier studies on ventilation and perfusion matching investigated their ratio, namely dividing $\dot{V}$ by $\dot{Q}$: when these are equal their ratio is 1 [11]. Values less than 1 indicate more perfusion than ventilation (low $\dot{V}/\dot{Q}$) resulting predominantly in impaired oxygenation and decreased $PaO_2$, while values greater than 1 denote more ventilation than perfusion (high $\dot{V}/\dot{Q}$), which results predominantly in reduced $CO_2$ washout, thus increased $PaCO_2$ [1]. However, the choice of using division as a tool to compare $\dot{V}$ and $\dot{Q}$ has mathematical consequences when either $\dot{V}$ or $\dot{Q}$ is equal to zero.

When $\dot{V} = 0$, its ratio to perfusion remains 0 at any blood flow: this is the classical definition of shunt, or perfused, non-ventilated regions, which are a major determinant of oxygenation impairment in ARDS. The sum of low $\dot{V}/\dot{Q}$ and shunt is referred to as venous admixture. An example of shunt is consolidation or atelectasis in the presence of impaired hypoxic vasoconstriction, while low $\dot{V}/\dot{Q}$ can occur in ground-glass opacities due to either increased perfusion or reduced ventilation, as observed in early COVID-19 pneumonia [24]. On the other hand, when $\dot{Q} = 0$ the $\dot{V}/\dot{Q}$ ratio becomes infinite at any ventilation rate. This compartment is defined as dead space, which, together with high $\dot{V}/\dot{Q}$, constitutes wasted ventilation. A clinical example of dead space is pulmonary embolism, while high $\dot{V}/\dot{Q}$ may occur in regions receiving reduced perfusion or increased ventilation, e.g., for the application of high PEEP and consequent mechanical compression of pulmonary vasculature or excessive spontaneous ventilation at higher lung volumes. A last and underexplored anomaly of $\dot{V}/\dot{Q}$ is when both $\dot{V}$ and $\dot{Q}$ equal zero, corresponding to lung regions that are simultaneously non-ventilated and non-perfused. While from a mathematical standpoint 0/0 is an indefinite form (i.e., it cannot be computed and is neglected in the classical model describing $\dot{V}/\dot{Q}$ matching), from a pathophysiological point of view this corresponds to clear clinical entities in ARDS, such as consolidation or atelectasis in the presence of hypoxic vasoconstriction or pulmonary vascular thrombosis occurring in an injured, non-ventilated lung region. This non-ventilated, non-perfused compartment can only be explored regionally with a few imaging techniques and has been very rarely addressed by traditional studies of lung perfusion. Nonetheless, in a study in COVID-19-related ARDS, the size of this compartment ranged from 0% to 30% of the total lung mass, with a median value of 7% in endotracheally intubated patients [18].

Figure 10.2 shows all possible combinations of ventilation and perfusion. When interpreting lung perfusion at the regional level, $\dot{V}/\dot{Q} = 1$ represents an ideal condition (the white diagonal area) derived from any combination of proportionally matched ventilation and perfusion, including non-physiological regions with low ventilation and low perfusion or high ventilation and high perfusion. An example of the latter case is represented by a septic patient with increased ventilation demands due to a hypermetabolic state, compensated by an increased cardiac output, with a paradoxical matching of ventilation and perfusion in the presence of pathological changes on both sides. The blue and red boxes in Fig. 10.2 represent shunt and dead space, which are considered homogeneous in the classical interpretation of $\dot{V}/\dot{Q}$, being respectively $\dot{V}/\dot{Q} = 0$ and $\dot{V}/\dot{Q} = \infty$. However, their contribution to gas

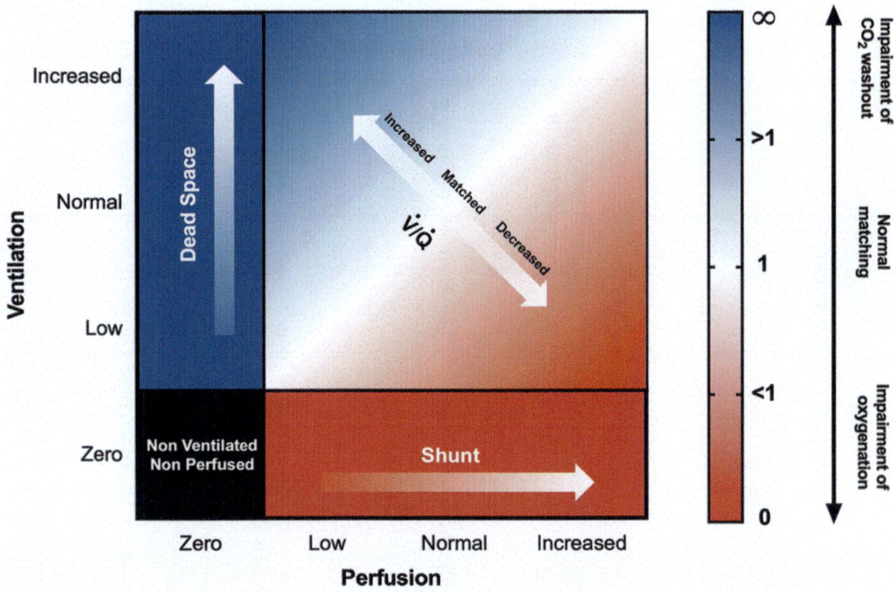


**Fig. 10.2** Relationship between ventilation (y axis) and perfusion (x axis)

exchange impairment in ARDS is different at the regional level, considering that dead space areas could receive low to high fractions of the minute ventilation, and shunt regions could be perfused by low to high proportions of the cardiac output.

Overall, while the interpretation of $\dot{V}/\dot{Q}$ matching at the whole-lung level is well established, caution should be posed when translating these concepts at a granular regional scale especially in ARDS. These considerations might only appear theoretical. However, we should strive to bring them to the bedside when caring for patients with ARDS, considering the cardiopulmonary system as targeting continuously matching of ventilation and perfusion while ensuring metabolic needs.

## 10.4 Static and Dynamic Assessment of Ventilation and Perfusion

Ventilation and perfusion are difficult to assess, especially at the bedside, with the contemporary reference technique for evaluating their regional matching being single photon emission computed tomography (SPECT) [25]. Several diagnostic tools are in fact unable to actually measure ventilation and perfusion, but rather provide a snapshot of the distribution of gases and blood in the lungs (see Table 10.1) [26]. As illustrated in Fig. 10.3, ventilation can be defined at the regional level as the change in volume from

**Table 10.1** Tools to assess lung perfusion

| Target | Technique | Principle of functioning | Radiation burden | Available at the bedside | Advantages | Pitfalls |
|---|---|---|---|---|---|---|
| Whole lung | Multiple inert gas elimination technique (MIGET) | Intravenous administration of several inert gases and measurement of their removal through exhaled gases | None | Yes, but requires complex post-processing of blood and exhaled gas samples | • Reference measurement of $\dot{V}/\dot{Q}$ mismatch at the whole lung level | • Very complex<br>• Requires sophisticated equipment<br>• Cannot explore non-aerated non-perfused regions |
| | Automatic lung parameter estimator (ALPE) | Changes in $FiO_2$ and measurement of consequent changes in oxygenation | None | Yes | • Does not require sophisticated analyzers | • Requires lowering the $FiO_2$<br>• Limited applicability in ARDS<br>• Cannot explore non-aerated non-perfused regions |
| Regional perfusion | Scintigraphy (planar perfusion scan) | Intravenous administration of radiolabeled contrast medium | High | No | • Historical reference method for assessment of lung perfusion<br>• Can be combined with inhaled radiolabeled contrast medium to measure ventilation and ventilation-perfusion matching | • Radiation exposure<br>• Bidimensional coronal view<br>• Low spatial resolution<br>• Unavailable at the bedside<br>• Cannot normalize perfusion to lung tissue mass |
| | Single photon emission CT (SPECT) | Intravenous administration of radiolabeled contrast medium | High | No | • Provides three-dimensional, whole lung regional distribution of perfusion<br>• Can be combined with inhaled radiolabeled contrast medium to measure ventilation and ventilation-perfusion matching<br>• Can be combined with conventional CT to allow morphological assessment of lung aeration<br>• Can normalize perfusion to lung tissue mass | • Radiation exposure<br>• Long execution time<br>• Unavailable at the bedside |

| | | | | | | |
|---|---|---|---|---|---|---|
| | Positron emission tomography (PET) | Intravenous administration of contrast medium with positron-emitting isotopes | High | No | • Provides three-dimensional, regional distribution of perfusion<br>• Can be combined with conventional CT to allow morphological assessment of lung aeration<br>• Can normalize perfusion to lung tissue mass | • High radiation exposure<br>• Long execution time<br>• Limited to research in ARDS |
| | Perfusion CT | Continuous acquisition of CT images during intravenous administration of iodinated contrast medium | High | No | • Provides three-dimensional, regional distribution of pulmonary blood flow<br>• Post-processing can extract information on lung ventilation<br>• Widely available<br>• Can normalize perfusion to lung tissue mass | • High radiation exposure<br>• Exposure to iodinated contrast medium<br>• Requires image post-processing<br>• Cannot acquire the whole lungs but only a portion of the chest |
| | Dual-energy CT (DECT) | Simultaneous acquisition of two CT scans with different energy after injection of iodinated contrast medium. Pulmonary blood volume is computed comparing the attenuation in the two scans | Intermediate | No | • Morphological evaluation<br>• Single, fast, acquisition of the whole lung<br>• Can measure non-aerated, non-perfused regions<br>• Not available on all CT scanners<br>• Can normalize perfusion to lung tissue mass | • Radiation exposure<br>• Exposure to iodinated contrast medium<br>• Does not measure ventilation and perfusion but their surrogates (aeration and pulmonary blood distribution) |
| | Lung subtraction CT angiography | Sequential acquisition of two CT scans before and after injection of iodinated contrast medium. Pulmonary blood volume is computed comparing the attenuation in the two scans after co-registration of the two CT scans. | Intermediate | No | • Morphological evaluation<br>• Single, fast, acquisition of the whole lung<br>• Can measure non-aerated, non-perfused regions<br>• Can potentially be implemented in all CT scanners<br>• Can normalize perfusion to lung tissue mass | • Requires image post-processing<br>• Not yet widely validated<br>• Not yet readily available<br>• Does not measure ventilation and perfusion but aeration and pulmonary blood distribution |

(continued)

**Table 10.1** (continued)

| Target | Technique | Principle of functioning | Radiation burden | Available at the bedside | Advantages | Pitfalls |
|---|---|---|---|---|---|---|
| | Magnetic resonance imaging (MRI) | Lung ventilation and perfusion specific MRI sequences | None | No | • Radiation free<br>• Recently proposed sequences do not imply use of contrast medium | • Not yet widely validated<br>• Not yet readily available<br>• No data in ARDS |
| | Electric impedance tomography (EIT) | Measurement of chest impedance changes with an electrode belt following injection of hypertonic saline | None | Yes | • Radiation free<br>• Available at the bedside<br>• Allows measurement of ventilation<br>• High temporal resolution<br>• Repeatable | • Limited spatial resolution<br>• Can explore a single axial slice of lungs<br>• Cannot explore non-aerated non-perfused regions<br>• Requires injection of hypertonic saline<br>• Cannot normalize perfusion to lung tissue mass |

*CT* computed tomography, *$FiO_2$* inspired oxygen fraction

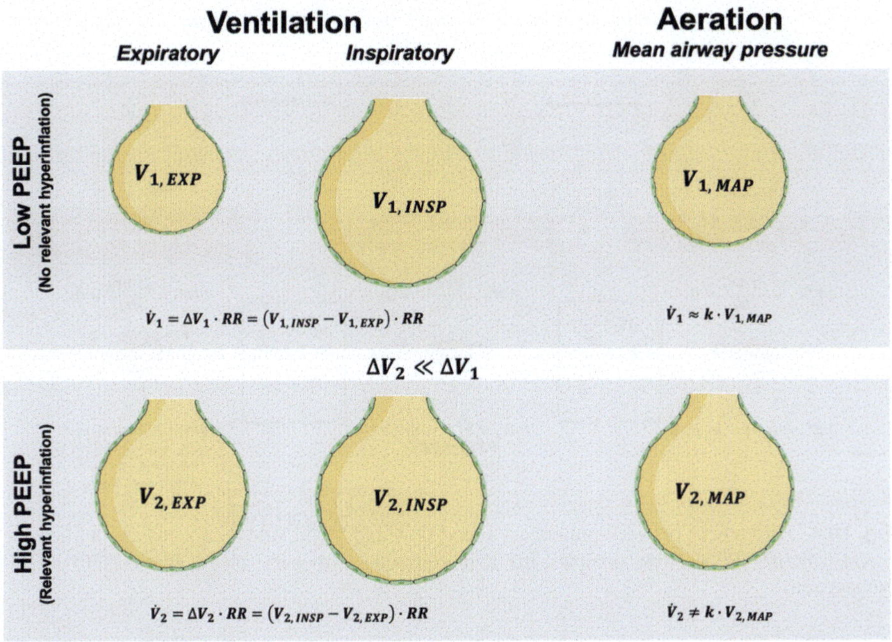


**Fig. 10.3** Differences between ventilation and aeration in case of no relevant hyperinflation (upper panel) and static hyperinflation due to high positive end-expiratory pressure (PEEP) (lower panel). $V_{exp}$ end-expiration alveolar volume, $V_{insp}$ end-inspiration alveolar volume, *MAP* mean airway pressure, *RR* respiratory rate

expiration to inspiration. The gold standard for measuring lung aeration is computed tomography (CT), and may provide a reasonable surrogate for ventilation in the absence of relevant hyperinflation [27]. However, especially when higher levels of PEEP are used, resulting in static hyperinflation at end-expiration, highly aerated lung regions may not receive ventilation, acting as dead space (Fig. 10.3, bottom panel). Estimating ventilation with non-dynamic CT would require acquiring two scans at end-expiration and end-inspiration, an approach largely confined to research purposes. The only clinically available tool capable of capturing ventilation in real time is electrical impedance tomography (EIT) [28], which will be discussed in detail later.

Similarly, assessment of perfusion would require monitoring of blood flow over time. The interaction between pulmonary blood flow, pulmonary blood volume, and size of pulmonary capillaries is illustrated in Fig. 10.4. Flow is the quantity of blood that passes through a capillary section per unit of time, while volume is the static amount of blood inside a capillary. At a given pulmonary blood volume and capillary size, different blood flows might be present. On the other hand, the same blood flow will result in different pulmonary blood volumes if passing through capillaries of different sizes. However, studies in models of ARDS showed an acceptable correlation between blood flow and blood volume, suggesting that the latter could act as a reasonable surrogate of lung perfusion [29]. EIT also offers the possibility of assessing perfusion, analyzing changes in chest impedance after injection of hypertonic saline [28].

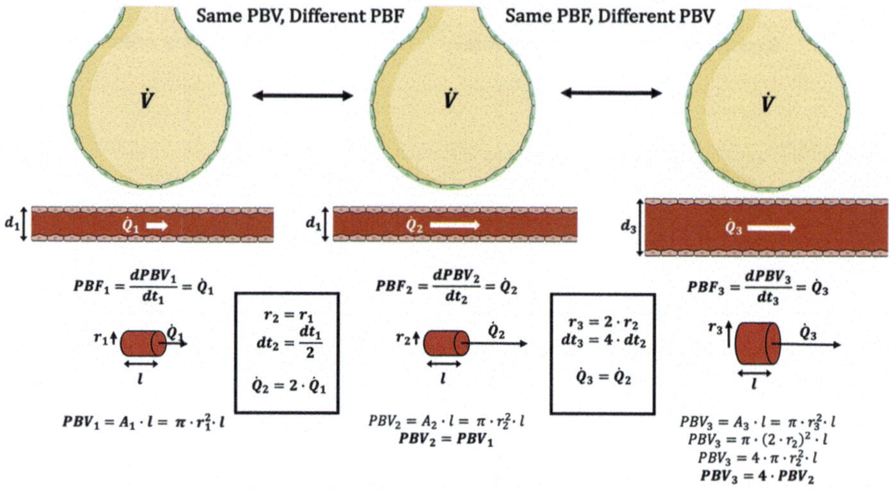


**Fig. 10.4** Differences between pulmonary blood flow and blood volume at constant pulmonary blood volume (PBV) (left comparison) and constant pulmonary blood flow (PBF) (right comparison)

## 10.5 Alveolar Perfusion Pressure

Gas exchange occurs at the interface between the alveolar and capillary surfaces, where blood flow is driven by the differential pressure between arterial and venous districts. Pulmonary capillary pressure cannot be easily measured at the bedside, being defined as $P_{cap} = LAP + PC_{RF} \cdot (PAP - LAP)$, where $PC_{RF}$ is post-capillary resistance fraction, and PAP and LAP are the mean pulmonary artery and left atrial pressures, respectively [30]. Lung capillaries are also subject to alveolar pressure ($P_{ALV}$) and pleural pressure ($P_{pl}$), thus creating a transmural pressure gradient between the epithelium and endothelium. Interestingly, the pressure in the interstitium during spontaneous breathing is more negative than is the pressure in the pleura. During inspiration, the changes in $P_{pl}$ underestimate changes in the interstitial pressure ($P_{int}$) [31, 32]: in fact, the size of capillaries, affecting perfusion, depends on the application of tensile or compressive forces, respectively seen during spontaneous breathing and positive pressure ventilation [13]. Recent data suggest that tensile stress may lead to less lung injury than compressive stress, likely depending on how the direction of applied forces acts on regional transmural pressures. Overall, the hydrostatic perfusion pressure ($P_{perf} = P_{int} - P_{cap}$) is influenced by other components, such as lymphatic drainage [13] and could increase the migration of inflammatory cells from the blood to the alveolus. The $P_{int}$ is directly proportional to $P_{ALV}$ and inversely to $P_{pl}$, thus being different in spontaneous breathing versus positive pressure ventilation. Moreover, higher hydrostatic perfusion alone does not necessarily imply higher $P_{perf}$, as $P_{perf}$ is also proportional to capillary resistance.

### 10.5.1 Perfusion as Determinant of Lung Injury

Pulmonary blood flow and pulmonary capillary pressure have both been related to the development of ventilator-induced lung injury (VILI) in an experimental model [33]. Under high capillary pressure conditions, endothelial cells are subject to mechanical stretch due to increased capillary wall tension, while high flow results in the application of shear stress forces and endothelial cell deformation [34]. These mechanisms may explain how targeting supranormal cardiac output, and thus pulmonary blood flow, may even worsen the clinical outcome in critically ill patients [35]. In the management of ARDS, conservative ventilatory strategies aimed at achieving lung rest rather than aggressive recruitment have been proposed [36]; ideally, this approach could also benefit from integration with conservative hemodynamic management.

## 10.6 How to Assess Lung Perfusion

Over the years, different diagnostic techniques have been applied to the study of pulmonary perfusion and ventilation. The study of lung perfusion is meaningful, especially if coupled with the assessment of ventilation.

### 10.6.1 Assessment of Global Lung Perfusion

At the whole-lung level, the reference method is the multiple inert gas elimination technique (MIGET) [7, 37]. This method is based on the analysis of exhaled versus pulmonary blood concentrations of six different inert gases and enables the distribution of $\dot{V}$ and $\dot{Q}$ to be plotted as a function of the $\dot{V}/\dot{Q}$ ratio. This is an extremely complex technique, never applied in clinical practice; however, it contributed enormously to the understanding of $\dot{V}/\dot{Q}$ mismatch and MIGET plots are a core part of physiology handbooks and scholarly literature [1, 8, 22]. MIGET plots have a bell-shaped distribution in healthy subjects, where $\dot{V}$ and $\dot{Q}$ are well matched, but can have a bimodal or asymmetrical distribution in ARDS [8] (Fig. 10.5, top panels).

In MIGET plots, the distributions of $\dot{V}$ and $\dot{Q}$ are plotted against their ratio in a logarithmic scale, whereas shunt and dead space, corresponding to $\dot{V}/\dot{Q}$ values of 0 and ∞, are reported as dots at the boundaries of the horizontal axis. The dead space fraction, comprising airway and anatomical dead space, is typically off scale. The MIGET method is intrinsically blind to the extent of non-ventilated, non-perfused regions. To increase clinical feasibility, a simplified MIGET-derived alternative method based on changes of the inspired oxygen fraction ($FiO_2$) has been proposed [38]; however, this method requires the $FiO_2$ to be lowered drastically, which makes it unsafe in ARDS patients [7].

More recently, especially for illustrative purposes, a histogram of $\dot{V}/\dot{Q}$ frequency distribution has also been proposed [1], showing the amount of lung tissue or volume characterized by a specific $\dot{V}/\dot{Q}$ ratio. Since these plots (Fig. 10.5,

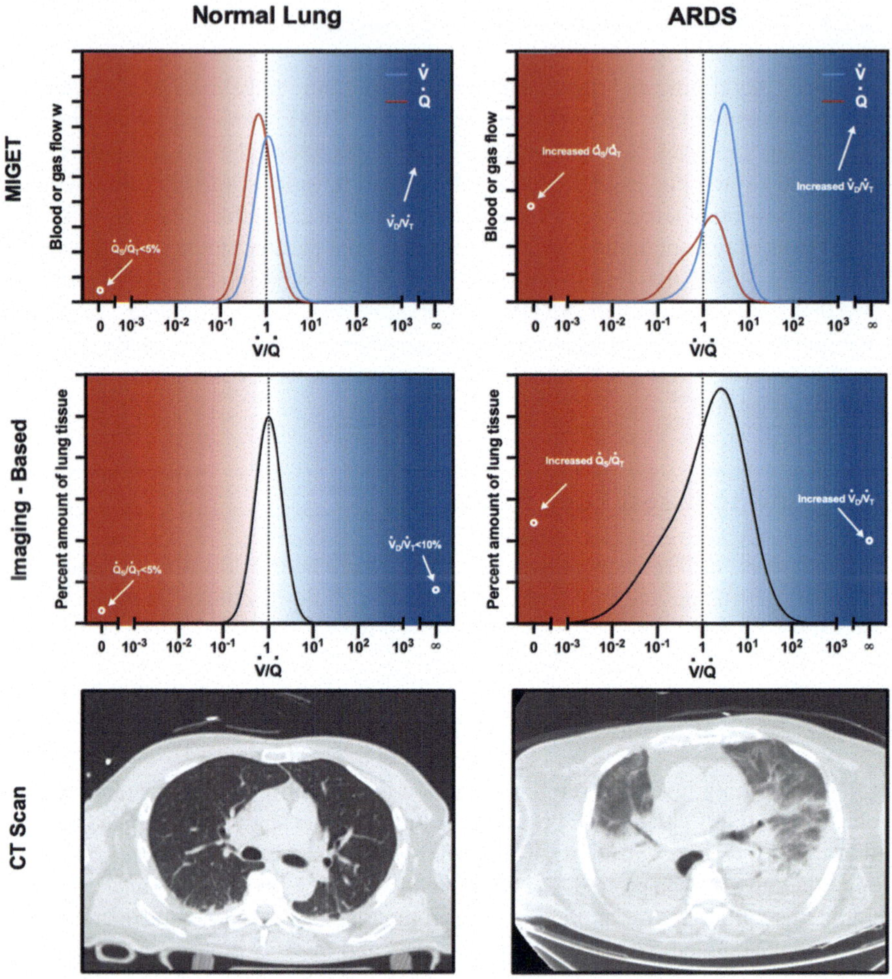


**Fig. 10.5** Example of multiple inert gas elimination technique (MIGET) plots (upper panels) in a mechanically ventilated patient with non-injured lungs (left) and one with acute respiratory distress syndrome (ARDS) (right); distribution of ventilation/perfusion ( $\dot{V}/\dot{Q}$) as a percentage of lung tissue (middle panels); corresponding computed tomography (CT) scan (bottom panels)

middle panels) resemble MIGET plots, they carry a substantial risk of misinterpretation. The MIGET plots report the amount of blood and gas flow received by portions of lung with a certain $\dot{V}/\dot{Q}$ ratio and refer to the whole lung. Conversely, $\dot{V}/\dot{Q}$ frequency distribution histograms show the amount of lung volume or tissue with a given $\dot{V}/\dot{Q}$ ratio and can be used to plot the overall distribution of regional lung $\dot{V}/\dot{Q}$ imaging techniques [18]. In the example in Fig. 10.5, $\dot{V}/\dot{Q}$ is expressed as a fraction of the total lung weight: the dead space being typically located in aerated regions, its weight is relatively low; therefore, the corresponding dot is no longer out of the Y axis scale as in the MIGET plot.

### 10.6.2 Assessment of Regional Perfusion

The assessment of regional perfusion in ARDS relies on the use of imaging techniques. Compared to the MIGET method, these approaches enable identification of the regional distribution of perfusion or its surrogates [26]. Lung perfusion imaging techniques can be classified into those requiring the administration of radionuclides, those exposing the patient to ionizing radiations, and those that are radiation-free. Unfortunately, most imaging methods require moving the patient to the radiology facility, thus strongly limiting their use in clinical practice at the bedside in critically ill patients. Table 10.1 provides an overview of available techniques, highlighting their advantages and pitfalls. This paragraph describes in more detail the most relevant techniques currently available. The reference method for assessing regional $\dot{V}/\dot{Q}$ matching is SPECT, and it is typically combined with CT acquisition (SPECT/CT) to enabling simultaneous assessment of ventilation, perfusion, and lung morphology. However, this technique requires the administration of a radiolabeled inhaled gas, such as $^{81m}$Kr or inhaled aerosolized $^{9m}$Tc-labeled particulate for the ventilation side and $^{9m}$Tc-macroaggregated albumin for perfusion [25]. The main historical indication for SPECT is pulmonary embolism in non-injured lungs, and it has been used in ARDS only for research purposes. Among radiological techniques, the reference is perfusion CT [29]. This technique requires the continuous irradiation of a thick chest slab during injection of a contrast medium; blood flow is inferred from iodine-induced changes in CT attenuation. It is associated with high radiation exposure, and cannot examine the whole lung but rather a limited axial section. As an alternative, dual-energy CT (DECT) has been introduced in some CT scanners. In a single scan, DECT can acquire the entire lung, providing a map of distribution of lung aeration and blood volume. Its application in ARDS is recent, and a study in COVID-19 introduced its quantitative analysis, proposing the use of the gas to blood ratio as a surrogate for the regional $\dot{V}/\dot{Q}$ [18]. Since DECT is available only with two CT scanner vendors, alternatives are under investigation. In particular, the possibility of deriving pulmonary blood volume maps that co-register non-contrast and contrast-enhanced conventional CT scans seems promising [39]. CT-based techniques all share the potential to explore the size of the non-aerated, non-perfused compartment.

Among radiation-free techniques, magnetic resonance imaging (MRI) has been recently validated as a tool to estimate lung aeration [40] and a lung-specific sequence, such as the perfusion mapping with phase-resolved functional lung (PREFUL) MRI, has been developed to implement $\dot{V}/\dot{Q}$ assessment on a conventional MRI scanner [41]. The applicability and clinical role of MRI in ARDS has yet to be determined.

The only available bedside, radiation-free technique is EIT. As discussed above, EIT enables measurement of both $\dot{V}$ and $\dot{Q}$ and is the only technique gaining attention as a clinical tool to guide decision-making in ARDS [26], albeit mainly limited to large teaching hospitals. The main limitations of EIT are the low spatial resolution, the ability to investigate only a single axial slice of lung, the need for further validation of the algorithms measuring perfusion, and the intrinsic inability to explore non-aerated, non-perfused areas. Despite these limitations, the extension of $\dot{V}/\dot{Q}$ mismatch assessed with EIT has been associated with mortality in ARDS [42].

## 10.7 How to Manipulate Lung Perfusion

Several pharmacological and non-pharmacological treatments commonly used in the care of patients with ARDS may influence lung perfusion. Some of these are used intentionally to manipulate perfusion; others affect it indirectly, sometimes with unwanted drawbacks.

### 10.7.1 Drugs

Several drugs commonly used in critically ill patients induce pulmonary perfusion modifications, and while some are used with this purpose, others can bring such alteration unintentionally. Traditionally used and well-known vasodilators are nitric oxide (NO) donors (inhaled NO, sodium nitroprusside, and nitroglycerin). Inhaled NO has the potential of improving $\dot{V}/\dot{Q}$ matching through selective vasodilation in ventilated regions, but its impact on mortality in patients with ARDS remains unproven [43]. Other drugs with unselective pulmonary vasodilating effects include prostacyclin, phosphodiesterase inhibitors, and endothelin antagonists [44]. Intravenous almitrine may also improve $\dot{V}/\dot{Q}$ matching, boosting hypoxic vasoconstriction in injured lung regions [44].

Other agents, less known for their effects on pulmonary perfusion, especially during hypoxic vasoconstriction, which is key in limiting hypoxemia in ARDS [8], are frequently administered with diverse purpose, and include angiotensin converting enzyme (ACE)-inhibitors [45], calcium-channel blockers [46], corticosteroids, acetazolamide, and catecholamines. The effects on pulmonary vasculature are poorly described in ARDS, and the clinical relevance of their effects on $\dot{V}/\dot{Q}$ matching is unclear.

### 10.7.2 Ventilation

Ventilation itself, in particular the choice of PEEP level, can modify perfusion considerably. In low $\dot{V}/\dot{Q}$ compartments, higher PEEP levels may produce mechanical capillary compression [1, 47] due to reduction of the alveolar perfusion pressure, possibly resulting in improved $\dot{V}/\dot{Q}$ matching and oxygenation, provided that the blood flow is not diverted towards non-aerated regions. In normal $\dot{V}/\dot{Q}$ regions, high PEEP levels may alter $\dot{V}/\dot{Q}$ matching, resulting in high $\dot{V}/\dot{Q}$ compartments, whereas in hyperinflated regions the mismatch might be further worsened with increase in dead space [13]. This phenomenon has important clinical implications, since improvement or derangements of oxygenation may be due to redistribution of regional perfusion and not to structural changes of the pulmonary parenchyma.

### 10.7.3 Positioning

Body positioning also has relevant implications, though with debated differences between healthy lungs and ARDS. Gravity draws blood towards dependent regions of the lungs [16]. Prone positioning reduces mortality in severe ARDS [48], but the main mechanism underlying oxygenation improvement in the prone position seems to be more attributable to redistribution of ventilation rather than redistribution of perfusion [21]. However, since lung loss of aeration is predominantly located in dorsal regions in ARDS, redistribution of ventilation alone will result in improvement of $\dot{V}/\dot{Q}$ even if perfusion remains substantially unchanged. Lateral positioning could also have a role in improving oxygenation in unilateral pneumonia or in ARDS with predominance of injury in one side [49]. However, lateral positioning has unclear effects on mortality and carries the risk of migration of inflammatory mediators and bacteria from the injured lung to the dependent one. For these reasons, lateral position in ARDS should be considered only in selected cases [50].

## 10.8 A Six-Compartment Model to Describe Regional V/Q Matching

A six-compartment model can be proposed to explain gas exchange impairment in ARDS, considering the $\dot{V}/\dot{Q}$ ratio to describe the relationship between ventilation and perfusion. These six, mutually exclusive compartments are illustrated in Fig. 10.6 and are here described: (1) Functional exclusion, accounting for regions with no perfusion and no ventilation. In these regions the abolition of ventilation (i.e., collapse or consolidation) is matched with the abolition of perfusion (i.e., effective hypoxic vasoconstriction or mechanical compression of blood vessels). (2) Shunt, or complete loss of ventilation with preserved perfusion, the impact of which on the impairment of oxygenation is dependent on the amount of perfusion of such regions. Shunt is not responsive to increase in $FiO_2$ but may respond, through recruitment, to higher PEEP levels. (3) Low $\dot{V}/\dot{Q}$ regions, corresponding to poorly ventilated regions with normal perfusion or normally ventilated regions with increased perfusion. This compartment contributes to oxygenation impairment, and may respond to increase in $FiO_2$ and possibly to PEEP, through reduction of perfusion by mechanical vasoconstriction. (4) Regions with matched $\dot{V}/\dot{Q}$, corresponding to lung areas with any proportional matching of ventilation and perfusion. (5) High $\dot{V}/\dot{Q}$ regions, thus normally ventilated regions with decreased perfusion or increased ventilation in normally perfused regions. (6) Dead space, corresponding

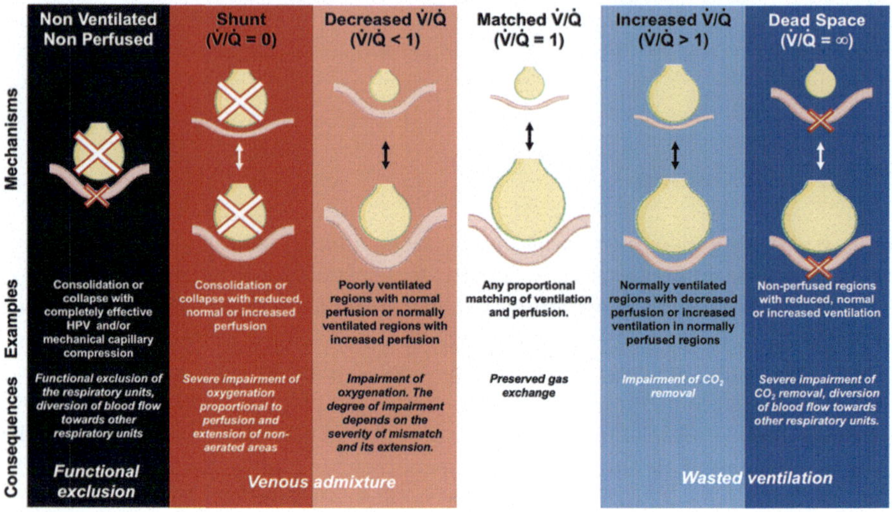


**Fig. 10.6** A six-compartment model to describe regional ventilation-perfusion ($\dot{V}/\dot{Q}$) matching. *HPV* hypoxic pulmonary vasoconstriction

to non-perfused regions with reduced, normal, or increased ventilation. The impact on $CO_2$ removal of this compartment may be worsened by the application of higher PEEP levels.

These six compartments should be thought of as a system of communicating vessels: any manipulation of ventilation or hemodynamics ideally targeting one of the compartments will necessarily affect the others, as part of the ventilation or perfusion will be diverted from one to another.

## 10.9 Conclusion

Regional lung perfusion and its abnormalities are important determinants for gas-exchange in ARDS, representing a current and future challenge for the intensivist to optimize ventilatory settings. When confronting ARDS with this mind, if we only think about ventilation, we might realize that we are missing 'the dark side of the moon'. However, the assessment of regional perfusion is not easy at the bedside and new techniques should be developed and validated in the near future.

## References

1. Petersson J, Glenny RW. Gas exchange and ventilation–perfusion relationships in the lung. Eur Respir J. 2014;44:1023–41.
2. Fan E, Del Sorbo L, Goligher EC, et al. An Official American Thoracic Society/European Society of Intensive Care Medicine/Society of Critical Care Medicine Clinical Practice Guideline: Mechanical Ventilation in Adult Patients with Acute Respiratory Distress Syndrome. Am J Respir Crit Care Med. 2017;195:1253–63.

3. Ball L, Serpa Neto A, Trifiletti V, et al. Effects of higher PEEP and recruitment manoeuvres on mortality in patients with ARDS: a systematic review, meta-analysis, meta-regression and trial sequential analysis of randomized controlled trials. Intensive Care Med Exp. 2020;8:39.
4. Vieillard-Baron A, Matthay M, Teboul JL, et al. Experts' opinion on management of hemodynamics in ARDS patients: focus on the effects of mechanical ventilation. Intensive Care Med. 2016;42:739–49.
5. Pelosi P, Ball L, Barbas CSV, et al. Personalized mechanical ventilation in acute respiratory distress syndrome. Crit Care. 2021;25:250.
6. Cressoni M, Cadringher P, Chiurazzi C, et al. Lung inhomogeneity in patients with acute respiratory distress syndrome. Am J Respir Crit Care Med. 2014;189:149–58.
7. Baumgardner JE, Hedenstierna G. Ventilation/perfusion distributions revisited. Curr Opin Anaesthesiol. 2016;29:2–7.
8. Radermacher P, Maggiore SM, Mercat A. Fifty years of research in ARDS. gas exchange in acute respiratory distress syndrome. Am J Respir Crit Care Med. 2017;196:964–84.
9. Hedenstierna G, Sandhagen B. Assessing dead space. A meaningful variable? Minerva Anestesiol. 2006;72:521–8.
10. Horsfield K, Cumming G. Functional consequences of airway morphology. J Appl Physiol. 1968;24:384–90.
11. Riley RL, Cournand A. Ideal alveolar air and the analysis of ventilation-perfusion relationships in the lungs. J Appl Physiol. 1949;1:825–47.
12. Huppert LA, Matthay MA, Ware LB. Pathogenesis of acute respiratory distress syndrome. Semin Respir Crit Care Med. 2019;40:31–9.
13. Silva PL, Ball L, Rocco PRM, Pelosi P. Physiological and pathophysiological consequences of mechanical ventilation. Semin Respir Crit Care Med. 2022;43:321–34.
14. Johnson RL, Hsia CC. Functional recruitment of pulmonary capillaries. J Appl Physiol. 1985;1994(76):1405–7.
15. Gattinoni L, Busana M, Giosa L, Macrì MM, Quintel M. Prone positioning in acute respiratory distress syndrome. Semin Respir Crit Care Med. 2019;40:94–100.
16. Clark AR, Burrowes KS, Tawhai MH. Ventilation/perfusion matching: of myths, mice, and men. Physiology. 2019;34:419–29.
17. Gattinoni L, Caironi P, Cressoni M, et al. Lung recruitment in patients with the acute respiratory distress syndrome. N Engl J Med. 2006;354:1775–86.
18. Ball L, Robba C, Herrmann J, et al. Lung distribution of gas and blood volume in critically ill COVID-19 patients: a quantitative dual-energy computed tomography study. Crit Care. 2021;25:214.
19. Gama de Abreu M, Spieth PM, et al. Noisy pressure support ventilation: a pilot study on a new assisted ventilation mode in experimental lung injury. Crit Care Med. 2008;36:818–27.
20. Güldner A, Braune A, Ball L, et al. Comparative effects of volutrauma and atelectrauma on lung inflammation in experimental acute respiratory distress syndrome. Crit Care Med. 2016;44:e854–65.
21. Scaramuzzo G, Ball L, Pino F, et al. Influence of positive end-expiratory pressure titration on the effects of pronation in acute respiratory distress syndrome: a comprehensive experimental study. Front Physiol. 2020;11:179.
22. West JB, Luks A. West's Respiratory Physiology: The Essentials. 11th ed. Philadelphia: Wolters Kluwer; 2021.
23. Karbing DS, Panigada M, Bottino N, et al. Changes in shunt, ventilation/perfusion mismatch, and lung aeration with PEEP in patients with ARDS: a prospective single-arm interventional study. Crit Care. 2020;24:111.
24. Robba C, Battaglini D, Ball L, et al. Distinct phenotypes require distinct respiratory management strategies in severe COVID-19. Respir Physiol Neurobiol. 2020;279:103455.
25. Bailey DL, Roach PJ. A brief history of lung ventilation and perfusion imaging over the 50-year tenure of the editors of seminars in nuclear medicine. Semin Nucl Med. 2020;50:75–86.
26. Ball L, Scaramuzzo G, Herrmann J, Cereda M. Lung aeration, ventilation, and perfusion imaging. Curr Opin Crit Care. 2022;28:302–7.

27. Gattinoni L, Caironi P, Pelosi P, Goodman LR. What has computed tomography taught us about the acute respiratory distress syndrome? Am J Respir Crit Care Med. 2001;164:1701–11.
28. Hentze B, Muders T, Luepschen H, et al. Regional lung ventilation and perfusion by electrical impedance tomography compared to single-photon emission computed tomography. Physiol Meas. 2018;39:065004.
29. Fuld MK, Halaweish AF, Haynes SE, Divekar AA, Guo J, Hoffman EA. Pulmonary perfused blood volume with dual-energy CT as surrogate for pulmonary perfusion assessed with dynamic multidetector CT. Radiology. 2013;267:747–56.
30. Gaar KA, Taylor AE, Owens LJ, Guyton AC. Pulmonary capillary pressure and filtration coefficient in the isolated perfused lung. Am J Physiol. 1967;213:910–4.
31. Pelosi P, Rocco PR. Effects of mechanical ventilation on the extracellular matrix. Intensive Care Med. 2008;34:631–9.
32. Battaglini D, Robba C, Ball L, et al. Noninvasive respiratory support and patient self-inflicted lung injury in COVID-19: a narrative review. Br J Anaesth. 2021;127:353–64.
33. López-Aguilar J, Piacentini E, Villagrá A, et al. Contributions of vascular flow and pulmonary capillary pressure to ventilator-induced lung injury. Crit Care Med. 2006;34:1106–12.
34. Ballermann BJ. Endothelial cell activation. Kidney Int. 1998;53:1810–26.
35. Hayes MA, Timmins AC, Yau EH, Palazzo M, Hinds CJ, Watson D. Elevation of systemic oxygen delivery in the treatment of critically ill patients. N Engl J Med. 1994;330:1717–22.
36. Pelosi P, Rocco PRM, Gama de Abreu M. Close down the lungs and keep them resting to minimize ventilator-induced lung injury. Crit Care. 2018;22:72.
37. Wagner PD. The multiple inert gas elimination technique (MIGET). Intensive Care Med. 2008;34:994–1001.
38. Weinreich UM, Thomsen LP, Rees SE, Rasmussen BS. The effects of oxygen induced pulmonary vasoconstriction on bedside measurement of pulmonary gas exchange. J Clin Monit Comput. 2016;30:207–14.
39. Grob D, Oostveen LJ, Prokop M, Schaefer-Prokop CM, Sechopoulos I, Brink M. Imaging of pulmonary perfusion using subtraction CT angiography is feasible in clinical practice. Eur Radiol. 2019;29:1408–14.
40. Ball L, Braune A, Spieth P, et al. Magnetic resonance imaging for quantitative assessment of lung aeration: a pilot translational study. Front Physiol. 2018;9:1120.
41. Voskrebenzev A, Gutberlet M, Klimeš F, et al. Feasibility of quantitative regional ventilation and perfusion mapping with phase-resolved functional lung (PREFUL) MRI in healthy volunteers and COPD, CTEPH, and CF patients. Magn Reson Med. 2018;79:2306–14.
42. Spinelli E, Kircher M, Stender B, et al. Unmatched ventilation and perfusion measured by electrical impedance tomography predicts the outcome of ARDS. Crit Care. 2021;25:192.
43. Lewis SR, Pritchard MW, Thomas CM, Smith AF. Pharmacological agents for adults with acute respiratory distress syndrome. Cochrane Database Syst Rev. 2019;7:CD004477.
44. Lumb AB, Slinger P. Hypoxic pulmonary vasoconstriction: physiology and anesthetic implications. Anesthesiology. 2015;122:932–46.
45. Kiely DG, Cargill RI, Lipworth BJ. Acute hypoxic pulmonary vasoconstriction in man is attenuated by type I angiotensin II receptor blockade. Cardiovasc Res. 1995;30:875–80.
46. Kennedy T, Summer W. Inhibition of hypoxic pulmonary vasoconstriction by nifedipine. Am J Cardiol. 1982;50:864–8.
47. Pesenti A, Riboni A, Marcolin R, Gattinoni L. Venous admixture (Qva/Q) and true shunt (Qs/Qt) in ARF patients: effects of PEEP at constant FIO2. Intensive Care Med. 1983;9:307–11.
48. Guérin C, Reignier J, Richard JC, et al. Prone positioning in severe acute respiratory distress syndrome. N Engl J Med. 2013;368:2159–68.
49. Tongyoo S, Vilaichone W, Ratanarat R, Permpikul C. The effect of lateral position on oxygenation in ARDS patients: a pilot study. J Med Assoc Thail Chotmaihet Thangphaet. 2006;89(Suppl 5):S55–61.
50. Bastia L, Rozé H, Brochard LJ. Asymmetrical lung injury: management and outcome. Semin Respir Crit Care Med. 2022;43:369–78.

# A Structured Diagnostic Algorithm for Patients with ARDS

# 11

L. D. J. Bos, H. -J. de Grooth, and P. R. Tuinman

## 11.1 Introduction

Patients admitted to the intensive care unit (ICU) with acute respiratory failure frequently fulfil the criteria for acute respiratory distress syndrome (ARDS) [1]. The diagnosis is based on radiological, physiological, and clinical criteria described in the 'Berlin definition' (Table 11.1) [2]. Yet establishing the diagnosis of ARDS has limited treatment consequences in and of itself, as the available evidence-based interventions are mainly related to minimizing iatrogenic damage (e.g., ventilator-induced lung injury [VILI] and fluid overload) rather than the use of specific treatments. Whereas the intervention options for the syndrome itself are limited, adequate and timely treatment of the causal underlying condition has a major impact on the improvement of outcomes for patients with ARDS [3].

The classical description of ARDS relies on the histological finding of diffuse alveolar damage secondary to another condition (one of the clinical risk factors described in Table 11.1) [4]. Diffuse alveolar damage is an untreatable finding and must be distinguished from a large number of diseases that also meet the ARDS syndrome definition but are treatable [5]. Table 11.2 provides an overview of the differential diagnoses that must be taken into account in patients suspected of having ARDS.

It should be possible to establish a definitive causal diagnosis within 7 days after onset in the vast majority of patients with ARDS. Yet, the often chaotic nature of clinical reality can lead to a delayed and haphazard search for underlying causes, especially in patients with multiple important problems.

L. D. J. Bos (✉)
Department of Intensive Care, Amsterdam UMC, Location AMC, University of Amsterdam, Amsterdam, The Netherlands
e-mail: l.d.bos@amsterdamumc.nl

H.-J. de Grooth · P. R. Tuinman
Department of Intensive Care, Amsterdam UMC, Location VUMC, Vrije Universiteit Amsterdam, Amsterdam, The Netherlands

 
J.-L. Vincent (ed.), *Annual Update in Intensive Care and Emergency Medicine 2023*, Annual Update in Intensive Care and Emergency Medicine,
https://doi.org/10.1007/978-3-031-23005-9_11

**Table 11.1** Berlin definition of acute respiratory distress syndrome (ARDS) [2]

| | | |
|---|---|---|
| Timing | | Within 1 week of risk factor[a] *or* new/increase in respiratory symptoms |
| Imaging | | Bilateral abnormalities not explained by pleural effusion, collapse or 'nodules' |
| Origin of pulmonary edema | | Insufficiently explained by cardiac failure or overload (if there is not a risk factor for ARDS, an echocardiogram should be performed) |
| Oxygenation | Mild | $200 < PaO_2/FiO_2 < 300$ mmHg ($26 < PaO_2/FiO_2 < 40$ kPa) + PEEP ≥5 cm $H_2O$ |
| | Moderate | $100 < PaO_2/FiO_2 < 200$ mmHg ($13 < PaO_2/FiO_2 < 26$ kPa) + PEEP ≥5cm$H_2O$ |
| | Severe | $PaO_2/FiO_2 < 100$ mmHg ($PaO_2/FiO_2 < 13$ kPa) + PEEP ≥5 cm $H_2O$ |

*PEEP* positive end-expiratory pressure
[a]Clinical risk factors: Pneumonia, aspiration, smoke inhalation, near drowning, sepsis, pancreatitis, trauma, major surgery, blood transfusion (this is referred to as transfusion-related lung injury; TRALI)

**Table 11.2** Differential diagnoses to consider in patients with ARDS

| | |
|---|---|
| Diffuse alveolar damage | Idiopathic; acute interstitial pneumonia |
| | First presentation of ILD |
| | Acceleration of known ILD |
| Cardiogenic pulmonary edema | |
| Infection | Bacterial pneumonia |
| | Viral pneumonia |
| | Fungal infection |
| | PJP pneumonia |
| | HSV/CMV reactivation |
| Interstitial lung diseases and vasculitis | Vasculitis (e.g., GPA, EGPA, and Goodpasture) |
| | Autoimmune disease (e.g., RA, SLE, SSc, Sjögren, antisynthetase syndrome, amyopathic (dermato) myositis and overlap syndromes) |
| | Medication-related: amiodarone/tyrosine kinase inhibitor/ chemotherapy / many others (www.pneumotox.com) |
| | Radiotherapy-associated |
| Malignancies | Lymphangitis carcinomatosa |
| | Intrapulmonary lymphoma |

*ILD* interstitial lung disease, *PJP Pneumocystis jirovecii*, *HSV Herpes simplex* virus, *CMV* cytomegalo virus, *GPA* granulomatosis with polyangiitis, *EGPA* eosinophilic granulomatosis with polyangiitis, *RA* rheumatoid artritis, *SLE* systemic lupus erythematosus, *SSc* systemic sclerosis

This narrative review aims to provide a structured approach to the diagnosis of underlying conditions in patients who fulfil the ARDS criteria according to the Berlin definition, in order to enable underlying causes to be rapidly and adequately treated. The diagnostic steps are described point by point in three phases and are summarized in a flowchart (Fig. 11.1). We also provide a summary of the most important uncertainties relevant to clinicians managing patients with ARDS.

With the steps and timeframe described here, we have intended to strike a balance between early and vigorous diagnostic investigations where needed and a more parsimonious approach where appropriate. Nevertheless, the authors' experience is one rooted in academic medicine in a resource-rich environment. The details of our

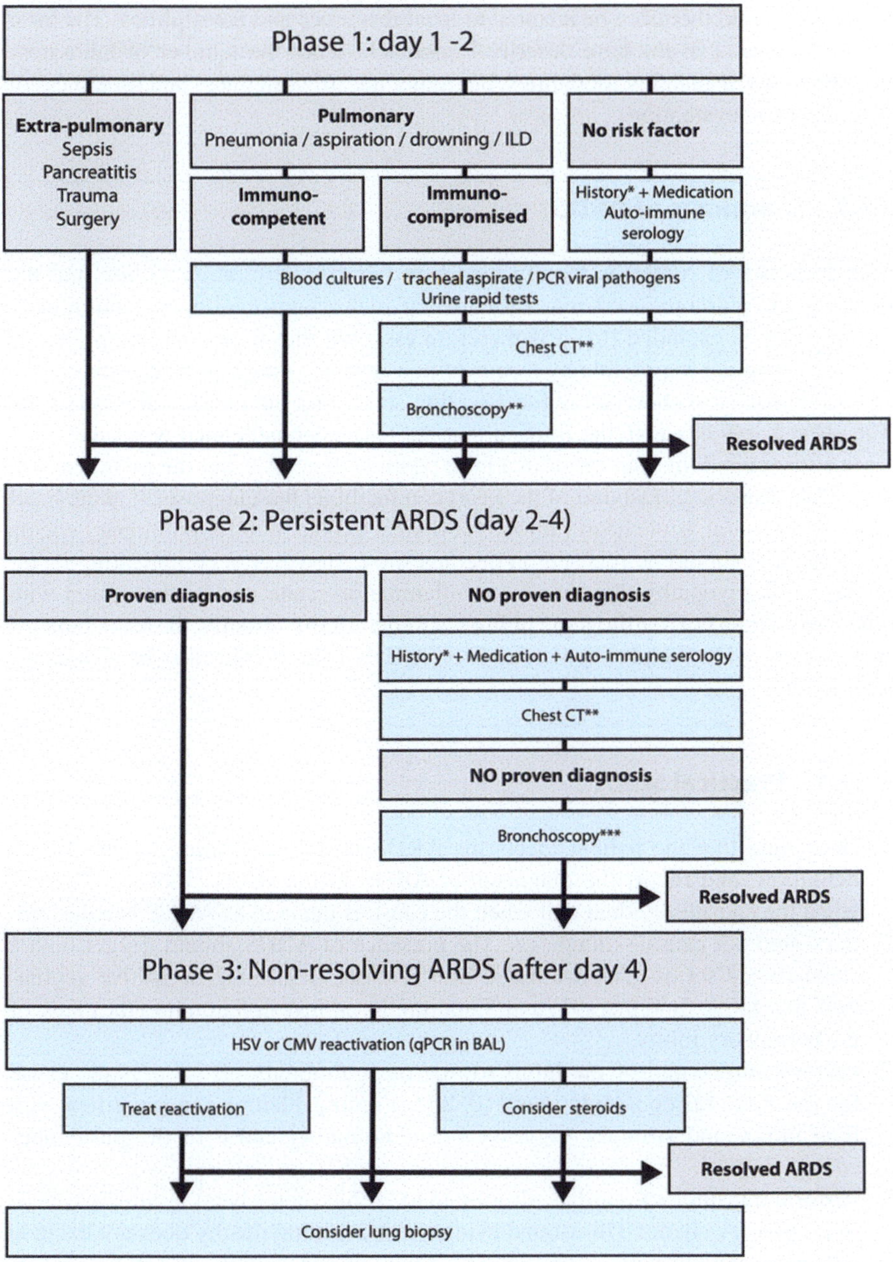


**Fig. 11.1** Flowchart for diagnostic steps in patient with ARDS. *Including exposure to drugs, animals, toxic fumes, vaping. **Chest computed tomography (CT) with high resolution (HR) images, preferably with an inspiratory hold. ***Send for tests described under point 6 in phase 1 in the text. *qPCR* quantitative polymerase chain reaction, *CMV* cytomegalovirus, *BAL* bronchoalveolar lavage, *ILD* interstitial lung disease

approach should therefore be adapted to local resources and possibilities. The most important aspect of the here described approach is not the number of laboratory investigations or imaging modalities, but rather the structuredness and timeliness of the diagnostic evaluation.

## 11.2 Diagnosis of ARDS

The diagnosis of ARDS is largely based on hypoxic respiratory failure and the detection of pulmonary edema, from which hydrostatic cardiogenic pulmonary edema must be excluded [6]. It is therefore essential that false positive results are excluded as much as possible by means of non-invasive imaging. Ultrasound of the lungs is superior to chest X-ray for detecting and ruling out pleural effusion [7, 8]. The chest X-ray can give the illusion that the lung is consolidated when there is a large effusion and this can result in a false positive diagnosis, but the treatment differs. Transthoracic ultrasound of the heart can facilitate the diagnosis of acute heart failure. In general, acute heart failure is sufficient explanation for pulmonary edema and treatment should be focused on decongestion. However, a complicating factor is that cardiomyopathy due to a hyperinflammatory state can be associated with ARDS (and thus non-cardiogenic pulmonary edema) [9]. Usually, these are patients with sepsis, with a high *a priori* risk of ARDS who should also be diagnosed with ARDS.

### 11.2.1 Practical Steps

1. Determine that the patient meets the ARDS criteria according to the 'Berlin definition' and report the diagnosis of ARDS in the status (Table 11.1), both when the cause is evident and when the cause is unclear, as ARDS is a descriptive—and not causal—diagnosis. The presence of ARDS should trigger both a standardized set of evidence-based interventions (e.g., lung protective ventilation, restrictive fluid therapy) and, importantly, an investigation into the cause of the pulmonary injury.
2. Perform ultrasound of the lungs to rule out pulmonary effusion as the cause for the bilateral consolidations [10, 11]. Finding pleural abnormalities with lung ultrasound strongly suggests an inflammatory cause of the pulmonary edema [12].
3. Perform transthoracic cardiac ultrasound to exclude acute heart failure as a cause of pulmonary edema. Ultrasound evidence of cardiomyopathy does not exclude ARDS in an underlying condition with a high pre-probability of ARDS (such as sepsis) and in this case ARDS should be diagnosed despite the contribution of acute heart failure to the onset of pulmonary edema.

### 11.2.2 Uncertainties

- Patients treated with high-flow nasal oxygenation do not meet the Berlin definition of ARDS [13], and there is considerable uncertainty about optimal lung-protective strategies in these patients. Yet the structured investigation into the cause of lung injury (outlined below) should not be delayed merely because the formal definition has not been met.
- Lung ultrasound may be used for the diagnosis of bilateral opacities and might be used to diagnose non-cardiogenic pulmonary edema [14]. There is uncertainty about the best algorithmic approach to ARDS diagnosis based on lung ultrasound and the diagnostic test characteristics.
- Cardiac ultrasound can provide diagnostic evidence in favor of heart failure, but it is unclear what cutoffs truly exclude ARDS as cause.

## 11.3 First Phase of Evaluation (Days 1 and 2)

Extra-pulmonary and pulmonary risk factors for ARDS need to be identified as soon as possible. When an evident extra-pulmonary cause for ARDS, such as septic shock, is present, timely treatment of the underlying cause determines the patient's prognosis [15]. Patients with community-acquired pneumonia *and* ARDS are indistinguishable from patients in the ICU with community-acquired pneumonia without ARDS in terms of epidemiological data, microbiological results, and outcome, and likely require the same treatment [16]. As opportunistic infections can present with specific radiological patterns that cannot be appreciated on chest X-ray, a chest computed tomography (CT) scan should be performed in patients with increased *a priori* risk for such infections (see practical steps) [17]. If no risk factor can be identified, there is an increased probability of an underlying systemic disease or drug related cause [5]. Further information for this should be obtained through history, physical examination, autoimmune serology and chest CT. The most important serological tests are: extractable nuclear antigens (ENA), anti-nuclear antibodies (ANA), anti-neutrophil cytoplasmic antibodies (ANCA), myositis blot, anti-cyclic citrulline peptide antibody (aCCP) and rheumatoid factor (RF). When hemoptysis and/or acute renal insufficiency with (microscopic) hematuria are present, anti-glomerular basal membrane (aGBM) levels should also be obtained [18].

### 11.3.1 Practical Steps

1. Determine whether there is an extra-pulmonary or a pulmonary cause for ARDS.
2. If an extra-pulmonary cause seems very likely, no search for an underlying pulmonary disease is required in the first phase. The underlying condition must be treated.

3. In case of pneumonia in a patient with a normal immune system, no invasive diagnostic tests need to be performed in the first 48 h. Required diagnostics are sputum culture, respiratory mutiplex polymerase chain reaction (PCR), antigen tests, and blood cultures.
4. An immunocompromised patient can be defined by one or more of the following criteria:
    (a) Severe neutropenia (absolute neutrophil count <500/μl) or prolonged lymphopenia (absolute lymphocyte count <1000/μl for >7 days)
    (b) Hematological malignancy
    (c) Long-term steroid exposure (≥20 mg/day prednisone equivalent for more than 2 weeks)
    (d) Status after organ transplantation
    (e) Monoclonal antibodies or other anti-inflammation immunosuppressive medications (e.g., azathioprine, mycophenolate mofetil, methotrexate)
    (f) Known immunodeficiency such as human immunodeficiency virus (HIV) with CD4+ cell count of less than 200/mm$^3$.
5. In an immunocompromised patient with suspected pneumonia, a chest CT should be performed to evaluate the radiological pattern of lung involvement.
6. In an immunocompromised patient with suspected pneumonia, bronchoscopy should be performed with bronchoalveolar lavage (BAL) for bacterial and fungal culture, galactomannan and targeted PCRs for respiratory pathogens, including but not limited to respiratory viruses, *Aspergillus*, *Pneumocystis jirovecii* (PJP), cytomegalovirus (CMV) and Herpes simplex virus (HSV)—depending on the pattern on chest CT.
    (a) For specific radiological images, additional microbiological investigation should be considered, for example *Nocardia* or *Cryptococcus* in the context of nodular abnormalities.
    (b) One fraction should be sent for cytology, especially if eosinophilic pneumonia or malignancy is in the differential diagnosis.
    (c) If diffuse alveolar hemorrhage is considered, gradual rinsing with saline should be performed.
7. If no risk factors for ARDS are present an alternative diagnosis should be investigated through a complete re-evaluation of history and complete physical examination.
    (a) Pay attention specifically to systemic diseases (Table 11.2).
    (b) If clinical signs and/or symptoms consistent with a systemic disease are found, low-threshold autoimmune serology should be used. Also determine the creatinine kinase and urine sediment on dysmorphic erythrocytes. If indicated, additional scleroderma immunoassay, complement, lupus anticoagulant test, anti-cardiolipins and B2 glycoprotein1.
    (c) If diffuse alveolar hemorrhage is considered, in the context of vasculitis or not, the anti-GBM must also be determined.
8. The medication list should be systematically reviewed to identify and discontinue potentially pulmonary toxic medications (see www.pneumotox.com)
9. A chest CT should be considered based on the diagnostic information obtained in the previous steps or if the patient deteriorates within 48 h.

### 11.3.2 Uncertainties

- Immunosuppressed patients are frequently grouped together in critical care research and it is largely unclear how different types of immunosuppression (e.g., predominant granulocyte function, T-cell or B-cell immunity) influence the risks for opportunistic infections in critically ill patients [19].
- The microbial diagnosis of opportunistic infections has shifted from traditional diagnostic techniques to PCR-based technology. There is considerable uncertainty surrounding the best cut-offs for these diagnostic tests. For example, CMV and HSV pneumonitis are nowadays frequently diagnosed using PCR, but little evidence on optimal cut-offs exists, which could result in over-diagnosis and over-treatment [20–22].
- With the increase in polypharmacy and increased use of novel drugs, there is more risk for drug-related pulmonary toxicity. Although pulmonary toxicity has been described for many of the frequently used drugs, it is very difficult to reach a definitive diagnosis as no diagnostic tests are available [23, 24].

## 11.4 Second Phase of Evaluation (Days 3–5)

A considerable proportion of patients will improve during the first phase of evaluation and in other patients it will be possible to establish a definitive causal diagnosis [25]. If after 2 days no causative agent of pneumonia has been demonstrated, and if the clinical condition of the patient does not improve, it is important to reconsider the diagnosis. To not miss any mimicking conditions, the same approach is followed as in patients without a risk factor at presentation including but not limited to a detailed history, physical examination, and autoimmune serology.

Performing a chest CT scan can help distinguish between opportunistic infections and interstitial lung diseases [17, 18, 26]. A bronchoscopy with lavage is a reliable method to take microbiological cultures from the lower respiratory tract [18], especially if PCR analyses are performed for viruses and opportunistic pathogens such as *Pneumocystis* and *Aspergillus*. Bronchoscopy can result in loss of pressure from the ventilation system and thus to collapse of previously opened parts of the lung. However, multiple studies suggest that bronchoscopy with lavage is safe in intubated patients with ARDS provided that it follows the prevailing guidelines [27–29].

### 11.4.1 Practical Steps

1. Determine whether the risk factor for ARDS has been proven, for example because a pathogen was detected in the context of an infection.
2. If the risk factor for ARDS has been proven, treatment should be continued and possibly optimized. In this case, there is no need to look further for alternative diagnoses, unless there are clear diagnostic clues pointing towards a second cause for lung injury.

3. If there was a suspected cause, but it remains unproven after day 2, a complete re-evaluation of autoimmune disorders, toxic medications, and chest CT should be performed in patients in whom this was not performed at an earlier stage (see sections 6–8 of phase 1).
4. The chest CT findings should prompt consideration of bronchoscopy with lavage (see section 6 of phase 1).

## 11.5 Third Phase of Evaluation (Days 6–7)

If ARDS persists for more than 5 days after diagnosis it is considered as 'non-resolving' and the risk of fibrosis formation is considerable if the cause for ARDS remains untreated [3, 30]. There are several studies that show that reactivation of HSV and CMV is frequent in non-resolving ARDS [31–33]. No randomized trials have been conducted on whether or not to treat HSV reactivations, but observational studies suggest independent excess mortality in the HSV and CMV group. Due to the lack of other treatable conditions in this patient group, it is therefore advisable to treat reactivation [18].

There is conflicting evidence from several randomized trials of corticosteroid treatment for non-resolving ARDS. There appears to be a positive effect on ventilation duration and possibly on mortality if treatment is started early in the non-resolving phase, e.g., before day 14 [34–36]. Apart from hyperglycemias, relatively few adverse reactions have been described [37].

In patients in whom ARDS persists and in whom the underlying cause has not been confirmed despite all the above steps, a lung biopsy should be considered. The risks of an open lung biopsy (<10% serious complications, <1% lethal complications [38]) must be weighed against the substantial burden of ongoing ICU treatment without a clear diagnosis. Open lung biopsy provided a specific diagnosis in about 75% of cases and led to an adjustment in medication in about one in three patients [38]. In addition, findings other than diffuse alveolar damage are associated with change in therapy and better outcome [32, 39–42]. Prolonged ventilation in the context of non-resolving ARDS without a diagnosis has a very poor prognosis and can result in unnecessarily prolonged ICU treatment with all the adverse consequences that this entails. All in all, this results in the recommendation to consider an open lung biopsy in all patients with non-resolving ARDS without a proven risk factor [18]. Traditionally, a surgical open lung biopsy is obtained by thoracoscopy, but there are new developments in the field of bronchoscopically obtained cryobiopsies that can be considered as an alternative [43].

### 11.5.1 Practical Steps

1. Consider HSV or CMV reactivation as a contributing factor for lung inflammation in non-resolving ARDS. A bronchoscopy with BAL should then be performed for quantitative PCR of these viruses.

**Table 11.3** Diagnostic patterns to consider for open lung biopsy in non-resolving ARDS

| |
|---|
| Infection |
| Connective tissue disease |
| Drug reaction |
| Eosinophilic pneumonia |
| Blood suggestive of vasculitis |
| Foreign material (inhaled, aspirated, injected) |
| Scarring |
| Hypersensitivity pneumonitis |

2. Consider high dose corticosteroid treatment in patients with non-resolving ARDS. Treatment early in the non-resolving phase, before day 14, is associated with a better outcome and is therefore recommended.
3. If ARDS persists on days 5–7 and the diagnosis is not confirmed despite all the above steps, it is recommended to discuss performing a lung biopsy in a multidisciplinary meeting. It is of utmost importance to provide the pathologists with all available clinical information to come to the best possible diagnosis (Table 11.3).

### 11.5.2 Uncertainties

- HSV and CMV reactivation could be a marker of severity of disease or an etiological factor hampering the resolution of ARDS. Currently, it remains unclear whether treatment of HSV or CMV reactivation actually improves clinical outcomes [22].
- There is considerable variation in the use of high dose steroids for the treatment of non-resolving ARDS. One randomized controlled trial showed steroid use was associated with shortened duration of invasive mechanical ventilation, but had no effect on mortality [44]. Furthermore, the dosage and duration of treatment is open for debate, although some guidance based on pharmacological principles is available [45].
- The available literature on the diagnostic and therapeutic consequences of open lung biopsy is largely based on data acquired before the widespread implementation of molecular testing for pathogens. Current diagnostic test characteristics are therefore uncertain.

## 11.6 Conclusion

Establishing the underlying cause of ARDS is of great importance as adequate treatment of this cause improves outcome. The proposed structured diagnostic algorithm helps clinicians to systematically evaluate patients with ARDS and to decrease time to diagnosis and thereby start of adequate treatment.

## References


1. Bellani G, Laffey JG, Pham T, et al. Epidemiology, patterns of care, and mortality for patients with acute respiratory distress syndrome in intensive care units in 50 countries. JAMA. 2016;315:788–800.
2. Ranieri VM, Rubenfeld GD, Thompson BT, et al. Acute respiratory distress syndrome: the Berlin definition. JAMA. 2012;307:2526–33.
3. Thompson BT, Chambers RCR, Liu KKD, et al. Acute respiratory distress syndrome. N Engl J Med. 2017;377:562–72.
4. Ashbaugh DG, Bigelow DB, Petty TL, Levine BE. Acute respiratory distress in adults. Lancet. 1967;2:319–23.
5. Gibelin A, Parrot A, Maitre B, et al. Acute respiratory distress syndrome mimickers lacking common risk factors of the Berlin definition. Intensive Care Med. 2016;42:164–72.
6. Ware LB, Matthay MA. Clinical practice. Acute pulmonary edema. N Engl J Med. 2005;353:2788–96.
7. Hew M, Tay TR. The efficacy of bedside chest ultrasound: from accuracy to outcomes. Eur Respir Rev. 2016;25:230–46.
8. Chiumello D, Sferrazza Papa GF, Artigas A, et al. ERS statement on chest imaging in acute respiratory failure. Eur Respir J. 2019;54:1900435.
9. Sato R, Nasu M. A review of sepsis-induced cardiomyopathy. J Intensive Care. 2015;3:1–7.
10. Walden AP, Jones QC, Matsa R, Wise MP. Pleural effusions on the intensive care unit; hidden morbidity with therapeutic potential. Respirology. 2013;18:246–54.
11. Xirouchaki N, Magkanas E, Vaporidi K, et al. Lung ultrasound in critically ill patients: comparison with bedside chest radiography. Intensive Care Med. 2011;37:1488–93.
12. Heldeweg MLA, Smit MR, Kramer-Elliott SR, et al. Lung ultrasound signs to diagnose and discriminate interstitial syndromes in ICU patients: a diagnostic accuracy study in two cohorts. Crit Care Med. 2022;50:1607–17.
13. Matthay MA, Thompson BT, Ware LB. The Berlin definition of acute respiratory distress syndrome: should patients receiving high-flow nasal oxygen be included? Lancet Respir Med. 2021;9:933–6.
14. Vercesi V, Pisani L, van Tongeren PSII, et al. External confirmation and exploration of the Kigali modification for diagnosing moderate or severe ARDS. Intensive Care Med. 2018;44:523–4.
15. Rhodes A, Evans LE, Alhazzani W, et al. Surviving sepsis campaign: international guidelines for management of sepsis and septic shock: 2016. Intensive Care Med. 2017;43:304–77.
16. Cilloniz C, Ferrer M, Liapikou A, et al. Acute respiratory distress syndrome in mechanically-ventilated patients with community-acquired pneumonia. Eur Respir J. 2018;51:1702215.
17. Zheng X, Zhang G. Imaging pulmonary infectious diseases in immunocompromised patients. Radiol Infect Dis. 2014;1:37–41.
18. Papazian L, Calfee CS, Chiumello D, et al. Diagnostic workup for ARDS patients. Intensive Care Med. 2016;42:674–85.
19. Azoulay E, Mokart D, Kouatchet A, Demoule A, Lemiale V. Acute respiratory failure in immunocompromised adults. Lancet Respir Med. 2018;7:173–86.
20. Lee HY, Rhee CK, Choi JY, Lee HY, Lee JW, Lee DG. Diagnosis of cytomegalovirus pneumonia by quantitative polymerase chain reaction using bronchial washing fluid from patients with hematologic malignancies. Oncotarget. 2017;8:39736–45.
21. Papazian L, Hraiech S, Lehingue S, et al. Cytomegalovirus reactivation in ICU patients. Intensive Care Med. 2016;42:28–37.
22. Simoons-Smit AM, Kraan EM, Beishuizen A, Strack van Schijndel RJ, Vandenbroucke-Grauls CM. Herpes simplex virus type 1 and respiratory disease in critically-ill patients: real pathogen or innocent bystander? Clin Microbiol Infect. 2006;12:1050–9.
23. Johkoh T, Lee KS, Nishino M, et al. Chest CT diagnosis and clinical management of drug-related pneumonitis in patients receiving molecular targeting agents and immune checkpoint inhibitors: a position paper from the Fleischner society. Radiology. 2021;159:550–66.

24. Skeoch S, Weatherley N, Swift AJ, et al. Drug-induced interstitial lung disease: a systematic review. J Clin Med. 2018;7:356.
25. Schenck EJ, Oromendia C, Torres LK, Berlin DA, Choi AMK, Siempos II. Rapidly improving ARDS in therapeutic randomized controlled trials. Chest. 2019;155:474–82.
26. Bajaj SK, Tombach B. Respiratory infections in immunocompromised patients: lung findings using chest computed tomography. Radiol Infect Dis. 2017;4:29–37.
27. Kalchiem-Dekel O, Shanholtz CB, Jeudy J, Sachdeva A, Pickering EM. Feasibility, safety, and utility of bronchoscopy in patients with ARDS while in the prone position. Crit Care. 2018;22:54.
28. Prebil SEW. Safety of research bronchoscopy in critically ill patients. J Crit Care. 2014;29:961–4.
29. Lisle A, Medford MA. Safety of broncho-alveolar lavage in ventilated patients with acute respiratory distress syndrome sticking to life: closure of a bronchopleural fistula with fibrin glue in a patient with recurrent pneumothoraces. J Bronchol. 2007;14:2007.
30. Cabrera-Benitez NE, Laffey JG, Parotto M, et al. Mechanical ventilation-associated lung fibrosis in acute respiratory distress syndrome: a significant contributor to poor outcome. Anesthesiology. 2014;121:189–98.
31. Tuxen DV, Cade JF, McDonald MI, Buchanan MRC, Clark RJ, Pain MCF. Herpes simplex virus from the lower respiratory tract in adult respiratory distress syndrome. Am Rev Respir Dis. 1982;126:416–9.
32. Papazian L, Doddoli C, Chetaille B, et al. A contributive result of open-lung biopsy improves survival in acute respiratory distress syndrome patients. Crit Care Med. 2007;35:755–62.
33. Ong DSY, Spitoni C, Klein Klouwenberg PMC, et al. Cytomegalovirus reactivation and mortality in patients with acute respiratory distress syndrome. Intensive Care Med. 2016;42:333–41.
34. Peter JV, John P, Graham PL, Moran JL, George IA, Bersten A. Corticosteroids in the prevention and treatment of acute respiratory distress syndrome (ARDS) in adults: meta-analysis. BMJ. 2008;336:1006–9.
35. Bihari S, Bailey M, Bersten AD. Steroids in ARDS: to be or not to be. Intensive Care Med. 2016;42:931–3.
36. Ruan SY, Lin HH, Huang CT, Kuo PH, Wu HD, Yu CJ. Exploring the heterogeneity of effects of corticosteroids on acute respiratory distress syndrome: a systematic review and meta-analysis. Crit Care. 2014;18:R63.
37. Chaudhuri D, Sasaki K, Karkar A, et al. Corticosteroids in COVID-19 and non-COVID-19 ARDS: a systematic review and meta-analysis. Intensive Care Med. 2021;47:521–37.
38. Libby LJ, Gelbman BD, Altorki NK, Christos PJ, Libby DM. Surgical lung biopsy in adult respiratory distress syndrome: a meta-analysis. Ann Thorac Surg. 2014;98:1254–60.
39. Kao KC, Hu HC, Chang CH, et al. Diffuse alveolar damage associated mortality in selected acute respiratory distress syndrome patients with open lung biopsy. Crit Care. 2015;19:228.
40. Cardinal-Fernández P, Bajwa EK, Dominguez-Calvo A, Menéndez JM, Papazian L, Thompson BT. The presence of diffuse alveolar damage on open lung biopsy is associated with mortality in patients with acute respiratory distress syndrome. Chest. 2016;149:1155–64.
41. Lorente JA, Cardinal-Fernández P, Muñoz D, et al. Acute respiratory distress syndrome in patients with and without diffuse alveolar damage: an autopsy study. Intensive Care Med. 2015;41:1921–30.
42. Guerin C, Bayle F, Leray V, et al. Open lung biopsy in nonresolving ARDS frequently identifies diffuse alveolar damage regardless of the severity stage and may have implications for patient management. Intensive Care Med. 2014;41:222–30.
43. Zhou G, Feng Y, Wang S, et al. Transbronchial lung cryobiopsy may be of value for nonresolving acute respiratory distress syndrome: case series and systematic literature review. BMC Pulm Med. 2020;20:183.
44. Steinberg KP, Hudson LD, Goodman RB, et al. Efficacy and safety of corticosteroids for persistent acute respiratory distress syndrome. N Engl J Med. 2006;354:1045–57.
45. Meduri GU, Annane D, Confalonieri M, et al. Pharmacological principles guiding prolonged glucocorticoid treatment in ARDS. Intensive Care Med. 2020;46:2284–96.

# Hemodynamic Implications of Prone Positioning in Patients with ARDS

# 12

C. Lai, X. Monnet, and J. -L. Teboul

## 12.1 Introduction

Prone positioning is recommended in patients with moderate to severe acute respiratory distress syndrome (ARDS) when the ratio of arterial oxygen partial pressure ($PaO_2$) to inspired oxygen fraction ($FiO_2$) is <150 mmHg despite optimized mechanical ventilation or use of neuromuscular blockade [1, 2]. Indeed, prone position may improve arterial oxygenation [3, 4] and sessions lasting more than 16 h are associated with reduced mortality [5]. The use of prone positioning has spread considerably in recent years. Whereas in a large observational study in 2014 only 16% of patients with severe ARDS underwent prone positioning [6], more than two thirds of patients with moderate-to-severe ARDS had several sessions of prone positioning during the first wave of the coronavirus disease 2019 (COVID-19) pandemic in 2020 [7, 8].

Prone positioning improves oxygenation through improvement of the ventilation-to-perfusion ratio since aeration and ventilation increase in the most dorsal parts of the lung, whereas pulmonary blood flow remains predominant in these parts [9]. Lung recruitment also permits a decrease in atelectrauma, reduction in the transpulmonary driving pressure, and increase in lung compliance [10]. Hence, prone positioning may limit the mechanical power [11] and might thus prevent ventilator-induced lung injury (VILI).

In addition to the effects on oxygenation and respiratory mechanics, prone positioning induces some hemodynamic effects, which may also be beneficial [12, 13]. In this article, we review how prone positioning can exert those favorable

C. Lai (✉) · X. Monnet · J.-L. Teboul
Université Paris-Saclay, AP-HP, Service de médecine intensive-réanimation, Hôpital de Bicêtre, DMU CORREVE, Inserm UMR S_999, FHU SEPSIS, Groupe de recherche clinique CARMAS, Le Kremlin-Bicêtre, France
e-mail: christopher.lai@aphp.fr

 
J.-L. Vincent (ed.), *Annual Update in Intensive Care and Emergency Medicine 2023*, Annual Update in Intensive Care and Emergency Medicine,
https://doi.org/10.1007/978-3-031-23005-9_12

cardiovascular effects. Moreover, prone position sessions are at least 16 h long [1], and even sometimes extended up to 39 h [14]. During such a long time period, the question of administering fluid therapy may arise. Thus, we will explore how preload responsiveness could be detected to guide fluid therapy in patients in the prone position.

## 12.2 Hemodynamic Effects of Prone Positioning

### 12.2.1 Prone Positioning Affects Venous Return Determinants and May Increase Right Ventricular Preload

Venous return is the blood flow from the systemic venous network towards the right heart [15]. According to Guyton's model, venous return is equal to the venous return pressure gradient divided by the resistance to venous return [16]. The pressure gradient of venous return is defined as the difference between the mean systemic pressure (Pms) and the right atrial pressure [16]. Prone positioning increases the intra-abdominal pressure (IAP) [12, 17] (Fig. 12.1). This may cause two distinct effects on venous return. On the one hand, prone positioning increases Pms and central venous pressure (CVP) to a lesser extent, resulting in an increase in the pressure gradient of venous return [17] (Fig. 12.1). These effects are due: (1) to lowering the trunk from the semi-recumbent position to the strict supine horizontal position,

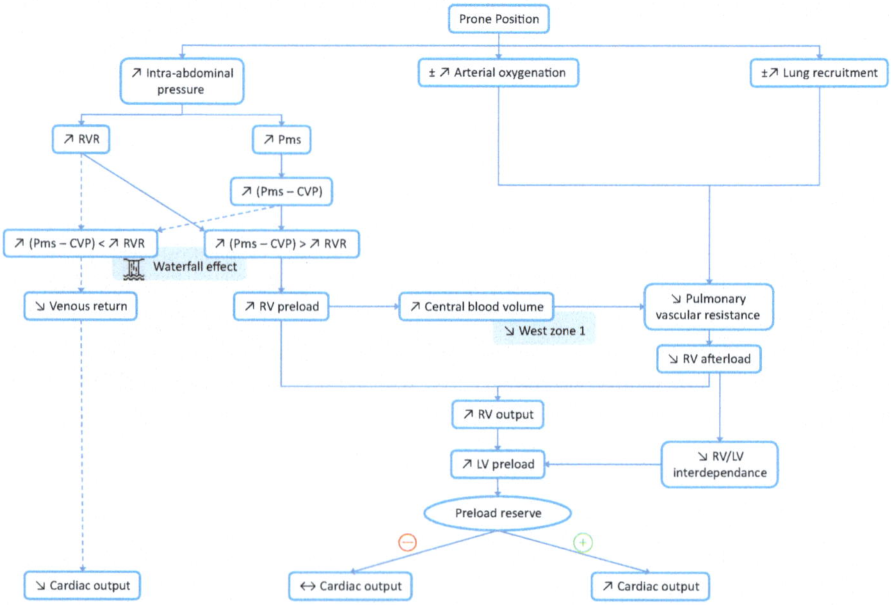


**Fig. 12.1** Hemodynamic effects of prone positioning. *CVP* central venous pressure, *LV* left ventricular, *Pms* mean systemic pressure, *RV* right ventricular, *RVR* resistance to venous return

secondary to a passive shift of blood from the splanchnic compartment to the heart, as occurs during passive leg raising [18]; and (2) to transferring the patient from the strict supine to the prone position, an effect that is predominant [17]. On the other hand, the increase in IAP induced by prone positioning also increases the resistance to venous return [17] (Fig. 12.1). An increase in venous return can be observed when the increase in its pressure gradient is not countered by the increase in its resistance [17] (Fig. 12.1). This increase in venous return results in an increase in right ventricular (RV) preload, as assessed by the increase in CVP [11, 12, 17]. The increase in CVP may be related to the simple transmission of IAP to the thorax, but this is unlikely as the esophageal pressure increases to a lesser extent than does CVP when patients are transferred from supine to prone position [11, 19].

### 12.2.2 Prone Positioning May Decrease Pulmonary Vascular Resistance and Right Ventricular Afterload

In patients with ARDS, RV dysfunction is not rare, its prevalence ranging from 10% to 30% in large observational studies [20–23]. Severe RV dysfunction was shown to be associated with increased mortality [20]. The main cause of RV dysfunction in ARDS is the increase in RV afterload secondary to the increase in pulmonary vascular resistance (PVR). The latter may be due to hypoxic pulmonary vasoconstriction [24], to inflammatory mediators [25], to microthrombi formation [26], and/or to the hemodynamic effects of mechanical ventilation [27, 28]. Regarding the latter mechanism, tidal volume at each insufflation and application of positive end-expiratory pressure (PEEP) over the entire ventilator cycle increase the lung volume. This may increase PVR by compressing the intra-alveolar vessels and, thus, increase the proportion of lung West zones 2, where the alveolar pressure is higher than the pulmonary venous pressure [29] (Fig. 12.2).

Prone positioning may reverse some of the mechanisms responsible for RV dysfunction during ARDS. First, by improving arterial oxygenation, prone position should decrease hypoxic vasoconstriction [3, 5, 12, 30]. Second, prone positioning allows the recruitment of the vertebral parts of the lungs, resulting in a more homogeneous alveoli aeration [31, 32]. This recruitment of non-aerated alveoli increases the diameter of the extra-alveolar vessels in these regions (Fig. 12.2). Prone positioning also dampens the overdistension present in hyperinflated lung areas. In this way, it should decrease the compression of intra-alveolar vessels in these zones and decrease the transpulmonary driving pressure, according to principles described by Whittenberger et al. [33] (Fig. 12.2). Moreover, by recruiting lung units, prone positioning can prevent the application of too high PEEP levels. Finally, prone positioning can increase venous return and central blood volume [17] which, in turn, increases pulmonary venous pressure, releases the compression of some previously compressed pulmonary microvessels, and shifts these vessels from West zone 2 to West zone 3 conditions. The combination of all these effects should result in a decrease in PVR and RV afterload [12, 13] (Fig. 12.1). It remains to be determined whether the effect of prone

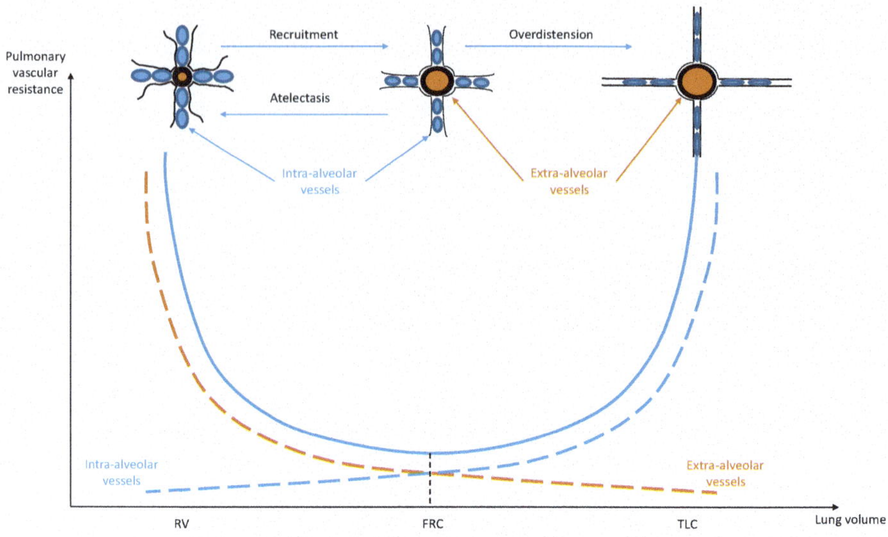


**Fig. 12.2** Relationship between lung volume and pulmonary vascular resistance. *FRC* functional residual capacity, *RV* residual volume, *TLC* total lung capacity

positioning on hemodynamics in general and on RV function in particular contributes to its beneficial effect on outcome. In this regard, we have already learned that prone positioning could be beneficial in responders as well as in non-responders defined by changes in blood gas variables (increase in $PaO_2/FiO_2$ or decrease in the arterial carbon dioxide partial pressure ($PaCO_2$)) [5, 34].

### 12.2.3 Prone Positioning May Increase Left Ventricular Preload

Left ventricular (LV) preload can increase secondary to the improvement in RV preload and afterload with prone positioning, as illustrated by the increase in the pulmonary artery occlusion pressure (PAOP) reported in previous studies [12, 35, 36]. Moreover, in patients with RV enlargement prior to prone positioning, reduction in RV afterload dampens the RV/LV interdependence, as illustrated by the decrease in the RV end-diastolic area/LV end-diastolic area ratio measured by echocardiography. This should also increase LV end-diastolic volume and thus LV preload [12, 13].

### 12.2.4 Overall Effects of Prone Positioning on Cardiac Output

Several studies have evaluated the effects of prone positioning on cardiac output with variable results. Some have found that prone positioning has little or no effect [37–39], whereas others have described an increase in cardiac output [13, 40, 41]. In a recent study evaluating 197 prone position sessions in 107 patients, Ruste et al.

found that cardiac output decreased ≥15% in 23% of the sessions, increased ≥15% in 25% of the sessions, and remained stable in 52% of the sessions [42]. The changes in cardiac output with prone positioning likely depend on the volume status and the degree of preload responsiveness prior to prone positioning. Indeed, cardiac output increases only in patients with LV preload reserve [12, 17] (Fig. 12.1). However, cardiac output may decrease in both preload responsive and unresponsive patients if IAP increases to a very large extent with prone positioning, irrespective of the IAP value in the supine position [17]. It is noteworthy that prone positioning can increase venous return, and thus cardiac output, only if the IAP is lower than the intramural pressure of the inferior vena cava (i.e., when the vena cava is in a Takata zone 3) [43, 44]. When profound hypovolemia is present and/or when the IAP under prone position is high, the venous return should be reduced, due to the extension of Takata zone non-3 conditions and to the occurrence of vascular waterfall phenomena [17, 43, 44].

Thus, a major goal when using prone positioning in patients with ARDS should be to minimize the increase in IAP, because a large increase in IAP, independent of its baseline value, may exert some detrimental effects on the circulation [17]. In this regard, in a crossover study, Michelet et al. found that using an air-cushioned mattress was associated with a limited increase in IAP (+4 mmHg) compared to a conventional foam mattress (+8 mmHg) [36]. Also, the use of thoraco-pelvic supports allows free abdominal movement and may decrease IAP. In a randomized study in 11 patients comparing prone position with or without thoraco-pelvic supports, Chiumello et al. demonstrated that application of thoraco-pelvic supports decreased chest wall compliance, increased pleural pressure, and slightly worsened hemodynamics without any advantage on gas exchange [45]. Moreover, prolonged contact with the supports could induce pressure sores. Finally, the increase in IAP with prone positioning could impair the perfusion of intra-abdominal organs. However, in studies measuring IAP during prone positioning, the increase in IAP was limited and, as long as cardiac output was preserved, hepato-splanchnic perfusion [39], liver function [40], gastric intramucosal energy balance [39, 40], and renal function [41] were not impaired. Therefore, the increase in IAP with prone positioning is rather limited. The use of thoraco-pelvic support should be avoided and limited to patients with a high increase in IAP with prone positioning [46].

## 12.3 Detecting Preload Responsiveness in Patients in the Prone Position

Acute circulatory failure is common in patients with ARDS [8, 47] whether it is secondary to sepsis, vasoplegia induced by sedative drugs, or the side-effects of mechanical ventilation. In the context of ARDS, the optimization of hemodynamics and cardiac output is important since insufficient cardiac output may worsen hypoxemia due to intrapulmonary shunt (low mixed venous oxygen tension effect). Fluid therapy is often considered as the first-line therapy to improve cardiac output and microvasculatory blood flow. However, only one half of patients would effectively benefit from fluid administration in terms of increase in cardiac output, which defines preload responsiveness [48]. Moreover, the pathophysiology of ARDS is marked by increased pulmonary microvascular permeability, with the risk of worsening lung edema when fluids are given. It is also now well demonstrated that the cumulative fluid balance is independently associated with mortality in patients with ARDS [49, 50]. The benefit/risk ratio of fluid therapy should thus be carefully evaluated before any fluid administration, and it is therefore essential to assess preload responsiveness. In this regard, several dynamic indices or tests can be performed [51]. We will review those which have been evaluated and can be used in the prone position during ARDS.

### 12.3.1 Trendelenburg Maneuver

The passive leg raising (PLR) test, consisting of transferring a patient from a semi-recumbent position to a position where the trunk is horizontal and the lower limbs are elevated at 30–45° [52], enables the prediction of fluid responsiveness with good reliability [53, 54]. Unfortunately, this postural maneuver is not applicable in the prone position. A Trendelenburg maneuver has been proposed as an alternative, as it mobilizes the blood from the splanchnic venous reservoir and the lower limbs to the intrathoracic compartment, increasing cardiac preload in patients in prone position [55] and receiving extracorporeal membrane oxygenation (ECMO) [56]. In a study of 33 patients with ARDS in the prone position, Yonis et al. found that the area under the receiver operating characteristic curve (AUC) of cardiac output changes during the Trendelenburg maneuver was 0.90 (95% CI 0.80–1.00). An increase in cardiac output ≥8% during the Trendelenburg maneuver enabled the diagnosis of fluid responsiveness with a sensitivity of 87% (95% CI 67–100), and specificity of 89% (95% CI 72–100) [55].

### 12.3.2 End-Expiratory Occlusion Test

The end-expiratory occlusion test (EEOT) is based on heart-lung interactions. A 15-s expiratory hold transitorily decreases the intrathoracic pressure and thus increases cardiac preload. This increases cardiac output in case of preload responsiveness [57]. An increase in cardiac output ≥5% during an EEOT has been shown to reliably predict fluid responsiveness in patients in the supine position [57, 58]. In the surgical setting, Messina et al. evaluated the performance of an EEOT at 6 and 8 ml/kg to predict fluid responsiveness in 40 patients having spinal surgery in the prone position [59]. They found that an EEOT at either tidal volume value did not reliably predict fluid responsiveness. However, it is important to note that the ventilator interruption during expiration lasted only 15 s, whereas the cardiac output monitor used in that study averaged hemodynamic data over a 30-s period, with a probable dampening of the changes in cardiac output potentially produced by the

EEOT [59]. In patients with ARDS, the study by Yonis et al. also found that an EEOT performed with a tidal volume of 6 ml/kg did not predict fluid responsiveness [55]. This may be due to attenuated effects of expiratory hold on venous return increase, since the IAP increase with prone positioning may promote Takata zone 2 conditions in some patients. It must be noted that cardiac arrhythmias were present in 42% of patients in this study [55]. In another study evaluating 84 prone position sessions in patients with severe ARDS with no cardiac arrhythmias, an EEOT at 6 ml/kg was reliable to predict fluid responsiveness with an AUC of 0.93 ± 0.06 (0.87–0.98) but with a low cut-off percent cardiac output increase (3.2%) [60]. Such a low cut-off, which has been reported by other studies [61], requires the use of precise cardiac output monitoring.

### 12.3.3 Pulse Pressure Variation

In the absence of cardiac output monitoring, other hemodynamic variables could be used to predict fluid responsiveness. Changes in arterial pulse pressure during mechanical ventilation—also called pulse pressure variation (PPV)—which are secondary to the changes in stroke volume occurring during the respiratory cycle [62], predict fluid responsiveness in patients receiving a tidal volume of at least 8 ml/kg provided they are perfectly adapted to their ventilator and they have no cardiac arrhythmia [63, 64]. Studies evaluating PPV in the operating room setting showed that PPV could predict fluid responsiveness in the prone position [65–67]. Nevertheless, tidal volume was ≥8 ml/kg and lung compliance was not impaired in these patients [65–67]. Such results cannot be extrapolated to patients with ARDS, who have low lung compliance and are generally ventilated with low tidal volumes, two conditions that alter the ability of PPV to predict fluid responsiveness [68–70]. In a study evaluating the predictive performance of PPV during prone positioning in patients with ARDS ventilated with a tidal volume of 6 ml/kg, Shi et al. found that PPV ≥ 6.5% enabled preload responsiveness to be assessed with an AUC of 0.85 ± 0.05 (0.77–0.92), a sensitivity of 74% (57%–95%), and a specificity of 79% (56%–96%). However, the gray zone of PPV (between 5% and 8%) included 40% of the cases [60].

### 12.3.4 Tidal Volume Challenge

To overcome the limitations of PPV interpretation in case of low tidal volume ventilation, Myatra et al. described a tidal volume challenge (TVC) that consists of a 1-min increase in tidal volume from 6 to 8 ml/kg of predicted body weight [71]. An absolute increase in PPV ≥3.5% during a TVC predicted fluid responsiveness in critically ill patients in the supine position [71]. In patients with ARDS undergoing prone positioning, Shi et al. showed that an absolute change in PPV ≥3.5% during a TVC assessed preload responsiveness with an AUC of 0.94 ± 0.03 (sensitivity: 98%, specificity: 86%) [60]. The ability of a TVC to predict preload responsiveness was better than that of baseline PPV, but comparable with an EEOT performed at 6 ml/kg [60]. In the study by Yonis et al., the Trendelenburg maneuver performed better than the TVC, but the assessment was performed in only 19 patients, since patients with arrhythmia were excluded [55]. In summary, the TVC, which has been repeatedly found to be reliable in supine patients seems also to be reliable during prone positioning [59, 60]. It has the advantage of assessing preload responsiveness without the need for cardiac output measurements and could be easily used in low and middle-resource settings.

### 12.3.5 Mini-Fluid Challenge

The mini-fluid challenge consists of administering a bolus of a small fluid volume (100–150 ml in 1 min) and measuring the changes in hemodynamic variables. The increase in cardiac output after the mini-fluid challenge can predict the increase in cardiac output when administering 400 ml of fluids, for a total of 500 ml fluid administration [72]. This test was shown to be reliable to predict fluid responsiveness in supine conditions [58, 69]. The change in PPV with a mini-fluid challenge could also predict fluid responsiveness [73]. Although it has not yet been evaluated in patients in the prone position, there is no reason why it could not be applicable to these patients. However, in contrast to other above-mentioned tests, the mini-fluid challenge is not reversible as it requires fluid administration.

## 12.4 Conclusion

Placing a patient with ARDS in the prone position has important implications for both venous return and RV function. While an increase in IAP tends to raise the upstream pressure for venous return, an increase in venous return may be observed only in the absence of a simultaneous rise in the resistance to venous return. Prone positioning can decrease RV afterload, an effect which is beneficial in patients with prior RV dysfunction. On the other hand, prone positioning could reduce cardiac output and organ perfusion in some conditions. Therefore, hemodynamic assessment, including echocardiography and cardiac output monitoring, is important when placing a patient in the prone position. Hemodynamic assessment can also guide fluid management using dynamic tests of preload responsiveness, such as the Trendelenburg maneuver, an EEOT, or a TVC.

## References

1. Papazian L, Aubron C, Brochard L, et al. Formal guidelines: management of acute respiratory distress syndrome. Ann Intensive Care. 2019;9:69.
2. Hajjar LA, Costa IBSDS, Rizk SI, et al. Intensive care management of patients with COVID-19: a practical approach. Ann Intensive Care. 2021;11:36.

3. Gattinoni L, Mascheroni D, Fumagalli R. Effect of prone positioning on the survival of patients with acute respiratory failure. N Engl J Med. 2001;345:568–73.
4. Guérin C, Constantin JM, Bellani G, et al. A prospective international observational prevalence study on prone positioning of ARDS patients: the APRONET (ARDS Prone Position Network) study. Intensive Care Med. 2018;44:22–37.
5. Guérin C, Reignier J, Richard JC, et al. Prone positioning in severe acute respiratory distress syndrome. N Engl J Med. 2013;368:2159–68.
6. Bellani G, Laffey JG, Pham T, et al. Epidemiology, patterns of care, and mortality for patients with acute respiratory distress syndrome in intensive care units in 50 countries. JAMA. 2016;315:788.
7. COVID-ICU Group on behalf of the REVA Network and the COVID-ICU Investigators. Clinical characteristics and day-90 outcomes of 4244 critically ill adults with COVID-19: a prospective cohort study. Intensive Care Med. 2021;47:60–73.
8. Greco M, De Corte T, Ercole A, et al. Clinical and organizational factors associated with mortality during the peak of first COVID-19 wave: the global UNITE-COVID study. Intensive Care Med. 2022;48:690–705.
9. Richter T, Bellani G, Harris RS, et al. Effect of prone position on regional shunt, aeration, and perfusion in experimental acute lung injury. Am J Respir Crit Care Med. 2005;172:480–7.
10. Guérin C, Albert RK, Beitler J, et al. Prone position in ARDS patients: why, when, how and for whom. Intensive Care Med. 2020;46:2385–96.
11. Boesing C, Graf PT, Schmitt F, et al. Effects of different positive end-expiratory pressure titration strategies during prone positioning in patients with acute respiratory distress syndrome: a prospective interventional study. Crit Care. 2022;26:82.
12. Jozwiak M, Teboul JL, Anguel N, et al. Beneficial hemodynamic effects of prone positioning in patients with acute respiratory distress syndrome. Am J Respir Crit Care Med. 2013;188:1428–33.
13. Vieillard-Baron A, Charron C, Caille V, Belliard G, Page B, Jardin F. Prone positioning unloads the right ventricle in severe ARDS. Chest. 2007;132:1440–6.
14. Walter T, Zucman N, Mullaert J, et al. Extended prone positioning duration for COVID-19-related ARDS: benefits and detriments. Crit Care. 2022;26:208.
15. Persichini R, Lai C, Teboul JL, Adda I, Guérin L, Monnet X. Venous return and mean systemic filling pressure: physiology and clinical applications. Crit Care. 2022;26:150.
16. Guyton AC, Lindsey AW, Abernathy B, Richardson T. Venous return at various right atrial pressures and the normal venous return curve. Am J Physiol. 1957;189:609–15.
17. Lai C, Adda I, Teboul JL, et al. Effects of prone positioning on venous return in patients with acute respiratory distress syndrome. Crit Care Med. 2021;49:781–9.
18. Jabot J, Teboul JL, Richard C, Monnet X. Passive leg raising for predicting fluid responsiveness: importance of the postural change. Intensive Care Med. 2009;35:85–90.
19. Mezidi M, Parrilla FJ, Yonis H, et al. Effects of positive end-expiratory pressure strategy in supine and prone position on lung and chest wall mechanics in acute respiratory distress syndrome. Ann Intensive Care. 2018;8:86.
20. Mekontso Dessap A, Boissier F, Charron C, et al. Acute cor pulmonale during protective ventilation for acute respiratory distress syndrome: prevalence, predictors, and clinical impact. Intensive Care Med. 2016;42:862–70.
21. Huang S, Vignon P, Mekontso Dessap A, et al. Echocardiography findings in COVID-19 patients admitted to intensive care units: a multi-national observational study (the ECHO-COVID study). Intensive Care Med. 2022;48:667–78.
22. Lhéritier G, Legras A, Caille A, et al. Prevalence and prognostic value of acute cor pulmonale and patent foramen ovale in ventilated patients with early acute respiratory distress syndrome: a multicenter study. Intensive Care Med. 2013;39:1734–42.
23. Vieillard-Baron A, Schmitt JM, Augarde R, et al. Acute cor pulmonale in acute respiratory distress syndrome submitted to protective ventilation: incidence, clinical implications, and prognosis. Crit Care Med. 2001;29:5–1555.

24. Sylvester JT, Shimoda LA, Aaronson PI, Ward JPT. Hypoxic pulmonary vasoconstriction. Physiol Rev. 2012;92:367–520.
25. Pandolfi R, Barreira B, Moreno E, et al. Role of acid sphingomyelinase and IL-6 as mediators of endotoxin-induced pulmonary vascular dysfunction. Thorax. 2017;72:460–71.
26. Ryan D, Frohlich S, McLoughlin P. Pulmonary vascular dysfunction in ARDS. Ann Intensive Care. 2014;4:28.
27. Fougères E, Teboul JL, Richard C, Osman D, Chemla D, Monnet X. Hemodynamic impact of a positive end-expiratory pressure setting in acute respiratory distress syndrome: importance of the volume status. Crit Care Med. 2010;38:802–7.
28. Mahmood SS, Pinsky MR. Heart-lung interactions during mechanical ventilation: the basics. Ann Transl Med. 2018;6:349.
29. West JB, Dollery CT, Naimark A. Distribution of blood flow in isolated lung; relation to vascular and alveolar pressures. J Appl Physiol. 1964;19:713–24.
30. Orchard CH, Sanchez de Leon R, Sykes MK. The relationship between hypoxic pulmonary vasoconstriction and arterial oxygen tension in the intact dog. J Physiol. 1983;338:61–74.
31. Gattinoni L, Caironi P, Cressoni M, et al. Lung recruitment in patients with the acute respiratory distress syndrome. N Engl J Med. 2006;354:1775–86.
32. Fossali T, Pavlovsky B, Ottolina D, et al. Effects of prone position on lung recruitment and ventilation-perfusion matching in patients with COVID-19 acute respiratory distress syndrome: a combined CT scan/electrical impedance tomography study. Crit Care Med. 2022;50:723–32.
33. Whittenberger JL, McGregor M, Berglund E, Borst HG. Influence of state of inflation of the lung on pulmonary vascular resistance. J Appl Physiol. 1960;15:878–82.
34. Albert RK, Keniston A, Baboi L, Ayzac L, Guérin C. Prone position–induced improvement in gas exchange does not predict improved survival in the acute respiratory distress syndrome. Am J Respir Crit Care Med. 2014;189:494–6.
35. Borelli M, Lampati L, Vascotto E, Fumagalli R, Pesenti A. Hemodynamic and gas exchange response to inhaled nitric oxide and prone positioning in acute respiratory distress syndrome patients. Crit Care Med. 2000;28:2707–12.
36. Michelet P, Roch A, Gainnier M, Sainty J-M, Auffray JP, Papazian L. Influence of support on intra-abdominal pressure, hepatic kinetics of indocyanine green and extravascular lung water during prone positioning in patients with ARDS: a randomized crossover study. Crit Care. 2005;9:R251–7.
37. McAuley D, Giles S, Fichter H, Perkins G, Gao F. What is the optimal duration of ventilation in the prone position in acute lung injury and acute respiratory distress syndrome? Intensive Care Med. 2002;28:414–8.
38. Rialp G, Betbesé AJ, Pérez-Márquez M, Mancebo J. Short-term effects of inhaled nitric oxide and prone position in pulmonary and extrapulmonary acute respiratory distress syndrome. Am J Respir Crit Care Med. 2001;164:243–9.
39. Matejovic M, Rokyta R, Radermacher P, Krouzecky A, Sramek V, Novak I. Effect of prone position on hepato-splanchnic hemodynamics in acute lung injury. Intensive Care Med. 2002;28:1750–5.
40. Hering R, Vorwerk R, Wrigge H, et al. Prone positioning, systemic hemodynamics, hepatic indocyanine green kinetics, and gastric intramucosal energy balance in patients with acute lung injury. Intensive Care Med. 2002;28:53–8.
41. Hering R, Wrigge H, Vorwerk R, Brensing KA. The effects of prone positioning on intraabdominal pressure and cardiovascular and renal function in patients with acute lung injury. Anesth Analg. 2001;92:1226–31.
42. Ruste M, Bitker L, Yonis H, et al. Hemodynamic effects of extended prone position sessions in ARDS. Ann Intensive Care. 2018;8:120.
43. Takata M, Wise RA, Robotham JL. Effects of abdominal pressure on venous return: abdominal vascular zone conditions. J Appl Physiol. 1990;69:1961–72.
44. Kitano Y, Takata M, Sasaki N, Zhang Q, Yamamoto S, Miyasaka K. Influence of increased abdominal pressure on steady-state cardiac performance. J Appl Physiol. 1999;86:1651–6.

45. Chiumello D, Cressoni M, Racagni M, et al. Effects of thoraco-pelvic supports during prone position in patients with acute lung injury/acute respiratory distress syndrome: a physiological study. Crit Care. 2006;10:R87.
46. Kirkpatrick AW, Pelosi P, De Waele JJ, et al. Clinical review: intra-abdominal hypertension: does it influence the physiology of prone ventilation? Crit Care. 2010;14:232.
47. Brun-Buisson C, Minelli C, Bertolini G, et al. Epidemiology and outcome of acute lung injury in European intensive care units. Results from the ALIVE study. Intensive Care Med. 2004;30:51–61.
48. Michard F, Teboul JL. Predicting fluid responsiveness in ICU patients: a critical analysis of the evidence. Chest. 2002;121:2000–8.
49. Silversides JA, Major E, Ferguson AJ, et al. Conservative fluid management or deresuscitation for patients with sepsis or acute respiratory distress syndrome following the resuscitation phase of critical illness: a systematic review and meta-analysis. Intensive Care Med. 2017;43:155–70.
50. Jozwiak M, Silva S, Persichini R, et al. Extravascular lung water is an independent prognostic factor in patients with acute respiratory distress syndrome. Crit Care Med. 2013;41: 472–80.
51. Monnet X, Shi R, Teboul JL. Prediction of fluid responsiveness. What's new? Ann Intensive Care. 2022;12:46.
52. Monnet X, Teboul JL. Passive leg raising: five rules, not a drop of fluid! Crit Care. 2015;19:18.
53. Monnet X, Marik P, Teboul JL. Passive leg raising for predicting fluid responsiveness: a systematic review and meta-analysis. Intensive Care Med. 2016;42:1935–47.
54. Cherpanath TGV, Hirsch A, Geerts BF, et al. Predicting fluid responsiveness by passive leg raising: a systematic review and meta-analysis of 23 clinical trials. Crit Care Med. 2016;44:981–91.
55. Yonis H, Bitker L, Aublanc M, et al. Change in cardiac output during Trendelenburg maneuver is a reliable predictor of fluid responsiveness in patients with acute respiratory distress syndrome in the prone position under protective ventilation. Crit Care. 2017;21:295.
56. Luo J, Su Y, Dong L, et al. Trendelenburg maneuver predicts fluid responsiveness in patients on veno-arterial extracorporeal membrane oxygenation. Ann Intensive Care. 2021;11:16.
57. Gavelli F, Teboul JL, Monnet X. The end-expiratory occlusion test: please, let me hold your breath! Crit Care. 2019;23:274.
58. Messina A, Dell'Anna A, Baggiani M, et al. Functional hemodynamic tests: a systematic review and a metanalysis on the reliability of the end-expiratory occlusion test and of the mini-fluid challenge in predicting fluid responsiveness. Crit Care. 2019;23:264.
59. Messina A, Montagnini C, Cammarota G, et al. Assessment of fluid responsiveness in prone neurosurgical patients undergoing protective ventilation: role of dynamic indices, tidal volume challenge, and end-expiratory occlusion test. Anesth Analg. 2020;130:752–61.
60. Shi R, Ayed S, Moretto F, et al. Tidal volume challenge to predict preload responsiveness in patients with acute respiratory distress syndrome under prone position. Crit Care. 2022; 26:219.
61. Gavelli F, Shi R, Teboul J-L, Azzolina D, Monnet X. The end-expiratory occlusion test for detecting preload responsiveness: a systematic review and meta-analysis. Ann Intensive Care. 2020;10:65.
62. Teboul JL, Monnet X, Chemla D, Michard F. Arterial pulse pressure variation with mechanical ventilation. Am J Respir Crit Care Med. 2019;199:22–31.
63. Yang X, Du B. Does pulse pressure variation predict fluid responsiveness in critically ill patients? A systematic review and meta-analysis. Crit Care. 2014;18:650.
64. Michard F, Boussat S, Chemla D, et al. Relation between respiratory changes in arterial pulse pressure and fluid responsiveness in septic patients with acute circulatory failure. Am J Respir Crit Care Med. 2000;162:134–8.
65. Ali A, Abdullah T, Sabanci PA, Dogan L, Orhan-Sungur M, Akinci IO. Comparison of ability of pulse pressure variation to predict fluid responsiveness in prone and supine position: an observational study. J Clin Monit Comput. 2019;33:573–80.

66. Biais M, Bernard O, Ha JC, Degryse C, Sztark F. Abilities of pulse pressure variations and stroke volume variations to predict fluid responsiveness in prone position during scoliosis surgery. Br J Anaesth. 2010;104:407–13.
67. Yang SY, Shim JK, Song Y, Seo SJ, Kwak YL. Validation of pulse pressure variation and corrected flow time as predictors of fluid responsiveness in patients in the prone position. Br J Anaesth. 2013;110:713–20.
68. Monnet X, Bleibtreu A, Ferré A, et al. Passive leg-raising and end-expiratory occlusion tests perform better than pulse pressure variation in patients with low respiratory system compliance. Crit Care Med. 2012;40:152–7.
69. Alvarado Sánchez JI, Caicedo Ruiz JD, Diaztagle Fernández JJ, Amaya Zuñiga WF, Ospina-Tascón GA, Cruz Martínez LE. Predictors of fluid responsiveness in critically ill patients mechanically ventilated at low tidal volumes: systematic review and meta-analysis. Ann Intensive Care. 2021;11:28.
70. De Backer D, Heenen S, Piagnerelli M, Koch M, Vincent JL. Pulse pressure variations to predict fluid responsiveness: influence of tidal volume. Intensive Care Med. 2005;31:517–23.
71. Myatra SN, Prabu NR, Divatia JV, Monnet X, Kulkarni AP, Teboul JL. The changes in pulse pressure variation or stroke volume variation after a "tidal volume challenge" reliably predict fluid responsiveness during low tidal volume ventilation. Crit Care Med. 2017;45:415–21.
72. Muller L, Toumi M, Bousquet PJ, et al. An increase in aortic blood flow after an infusion of 100 ml colloid over 1 minute can predict fluid responsiveness: the mini-fluid challenge study. Anesthesiology. 2011;115:541–7.
73. Mallat J, Meddour M, Durville E, et al. Decrease in pulse pressure and stroke volume variations after mini-fluid challenge accurately predicts fluid responsiveness. Br J Anaesth. 2015;115:449–56.

# Part IV

# Ventilatory Support

# Update on the Management of Acute Respiratory Failure Using Non-invasive Ventilation and Pulse Oximetry

# 13

T. Abe, T. Takagi, and T. Fujii

## 13.1 Introduction

The coronavirus disease 2019 (COVID-19) pandemic has been the biggest challenge to intensive care providers globally since the invention of ventilators in the 1930s to support patients with polio [1]. The huge number of patients with COVID-19 urged us to investigate better and safer strategies for managing respiratory failure. Given the limited resources for the large number of patients presenting with acute respiratory failure, we used non-invasive devices, i.e., pulse oximeters and non-invasive ventilation (NIV), to monitor and manage patients outside the ICU. This raised attention regarding the uncertainties of using such devices in the management of critically ill patients.

NIV emerged as a respiratory support system to reduce the need for endotracheal intubation and the risk of death. More patients than ever received respiratory support with NIV during the COVID-19 pandemic, in part also because of the limited availability of invasive mechanical ventilation. Clinicians and researchers have attempted to determine the optimal management of respiratory failure using NIV.

In this review, we summarize recent clinical research findings on the management of acute respiratory failure using NIV and pulse oximetry. For the purposes of this article, NIV includes non-invasive positive pressure ventilation (NPPV) and high-flow nasal cannula oxygen (HFNC).

T. Abe · T. Takagi · T. Fujii (✉)
Intensive Care Unit, Jikei University Hospital, Tokyo, Japan
e-mail: tofujii-tky@umin.net



J.-L. Vincent (ed.), *Annual Update in Intensive Care and Emergency Medicine 2023*, Annual Update in Intensive Care and Emergency Medicine,
https://doi.org/10.1007/978-3-031-23005-9_13

## 13.2 Effectiveness and Utility of NIV

In their systematic review published in 2020, Ferreyro et al. reported that NPPV was associated with a lower risk of mortality, particularly with helmet type (risk ratio (RR) 0.40 [95% CI 0.24–0.63]), and also with face mask type (RR 0.83 [95% CI 0.68–0.99]) in acute hypoxemic respiratory failure [2]. NPPV was also associated with lower risks of intubation (helmet type, RR 0.26 [95% CI 0.14–0.46], face mask type, RR 0.76 [95% CI 0.62–0.90]) when compared with conventional oxygen therapy. In contrast, HFNC was not significantly associated with a lower risk of mortality (RR 0.87 [95% CI 0.62–1.15]); however, it was associated with a reduced risk of intubation (RR 0.76 [95% CI 0.55–0.99]). Thus, the best probability of reducing all-cause mortality and intubation was with helmet NPPV.

Another systematic review, published in 2021, evaluated ventilation modes in addition to respiratory support devices and compared continuous positive airway pressure (CPAP), pressure support ventilation (PSV), HFNC, and conventional oxygen therapy using a network meta-analysis [3]. Only CPAP was associated with improved mortality compared to conventional oxygen therapy (RR 0.55 [95% CI 0.31–0.95]), and CPAP and PSV were associated with a lower risk of intubation (CPAP, RR 0.48 [95% CI 0.30–0.79]; PSV RR 0.67 [95% CI 0.51–0.89]). HFNC was not associated with a significantly lower risk of mortality or intubation. Thus, the best probability of reducing all-cause mortality and intubation was with CPAP.

## 13.3 Key Clinical Trials from the Systematic Reviews

Frat et al. conducted a randomized clinical trial (RCT) to assess the efficacy of HFNC for acute hypoxemic respiratory failure compared to conventional oxygen therapy and NPPV [4]. The trial revealed that intubation at 28 days was not significantly different between HFNC (38% [40/106]), conventional oxygen therapy (47% [44/94]), and NPPV (50% [55/110]) (p for the three-group comparison = 0.18). However, the risk of death at 90 days was significantly higher with conventional oxygen therapy (hazard ratio (HR) 2.01 [95% CI 1.01–3.99]) and NPPV (HR 2.50 [95% CI 1.31–4.78]) compared to HFNC. HFNC might reduce mortality at 90 days because the large tidal volume in the NPPV group (median 9.2 ± 3.0 ml/kg) may lead to *de novo* lung injury (Table 13.1).

NIV is preferred in immunocompromised patients as it may mitigate the risk of ventilator-associated pneumonia (VAP). Several trials have been conducted in immunocompromised patients. One trial compared NPPV vs. conventional oxygen therapy (n = 374), and another compared HFNC vs. conventional oxygen therapy (n = 776); neither trial found any significant difference in mortality or intubation rates at 28 days. Given that the meta-analysis suggested clinical benefits of NPPV and HFNC in non-restricted patient populations [2], Coudroy et al. conducted a multicenter RCT comparing NPPV interspaced with HFNC during the interruption period to prolong the duration of respiratory support with HFNC alone in 300 adult immunocompromised patients (50% had hematological malignancy) [8]. The

**Table 13.1** Summary of key randomized clinical trials of non-invasive ventilation (NIV) and high-flow nasal cannula oxygen (HFNC)

| Study | No. of patients | Cause of AHRF | P/F | Interventions ($cmH_2O$) | $V_T$ (ml/kg) | Comparator | Primary outcome | Results | Time to intubation |
|---|---|---|---|---|---|---|---|---|---|
| Frat, 2015 [4] | 310 | CAP (63.5%) | 155 | NPPV-PS, face mask, PS 5, PEEP 8 | 9.2 | HFNC, COT | Intubation at 28 day | 38% with HFNC, 47% with COT, and 50% with NPPV (p = 0.18 for all comparisons) | 23 h |
| Lemiale, 2015 [5] | 374 | Pneumonia (68.7%) | 142 | NPPV-PS, face mask, PS 2–10, PEEP N/A | 9.1 | COT | Mortality at 28 day | 24.1% vs. 27.3%, p = 0.47 | Half of the intubation events occurred in 1 day |
| Azoulay, 2018 [6] | 776 | Pneumonia (77.6%) | 132 | HFNC | – | COT | Mortality at 28 day | 35.6% vs. 36.1%, p = 0.94 | Half of the intubation events occurred in 1 day |
| He, 2019 [7] | 200 | CAP (94%) | 231 | NPPV-PS, face mask, PS 6, PEEP 8 | 8.1 | COT | Intubation | 10.8% vs. 9.2%, p = 0.72 | 3.65 days |
| Coudroy, 2022 [8] | 299 | Pneumonia (74.5%) | 147 | NPPV-PS alternating with HFNC, face mask, PS 7, PEEP 7 | 9.6 | HFNC alone | Mortality at 28 day | 35% vs. 36%, p = 0.83 | 24 h |
| Ospina-Tascon, 2021 [9] | 220 | COVID-19 | 104 | HFNC | – | COT | Intubation within 28 days | 34.3% vs. 51.0%, HR 0.62 (0.39–0.96), p = 0.03 | 25.75 h |
| Perkins, 2022 [10] | 1273 | COVID-19 | 114 | NPPV-CPAP, mostly face mask, PS 8.3, PEEP N/A | N/A | COT | Intubation or mortality within 30 days | 36.3% vs. 44.4%, p = 0.02 | 1.5 days |
| | | | | HFNC | – | COT | Intubation or mortality within 30 days | 44.3% vs. 45.1%, p = 0.69 | 1 day |

*AHRF* acute hypoxemic respiratory failure, *P/F* $PaO_2$ $FiO_2$ ratio, $V_T$ tidal volume, *COT* conventional oxygen therapy, *NPPV* non-invasive positive pressure ventilation, *PEEP* positive end-expiratory pressure, *CPAP* continuous positive airway pressure, *PS* pressure support, *CAP* community-acquired pneumonia, *COVID* coronavirus disease, *HR* hazard ratio results, published in 2022, showed that mortality rates at day 28 did not differ between the two groups (35% [51/145] in the NIV + HFNC group, 36% [56/154] in the HFNC alone group, $p = 0.83$).

With preserved spontaneous breathing, a mechanism called patient self-inflicted lung injury (p-SILI) can cause further alveolar damage [11, 12]. In lungs affected by the acute respiratory distress syndrome (ARDS), typified by dorsal collapse and ventral hyperinflation, strong inspiratory efforts would cause greater local strain, damaging the alveoli histologically and physiologically. In addition, some studies have suggested that a tidal volume of 9 ml/kg or more could increase the probability of NIV failure [4, 13], which may explain the lack of benefit in these trials [4, 5, 8, 13].

## 13.4 Current Knowledge of NIV for Respiratory Failure in the ICU

In respiratory failure requiring intensive care unit (ICU) admission, NPPV or HFNC probably reduce the risk of death or intubation compared to conventional oxygen therapy. In particular, NPPV has a well-established effect on acute exacerbations of chronic obstructive pulmonary disease (COPD) and cardiogenic pulmonary edema [14–16]. Additionally, the European Respiratory Society recommends using HFNC for acute hypoxemic respiratory failure in its recent clinical practice guideline [17]. NPPV can be effective if it manages to prevent increases in inspiratory effort and tidal volume while ensuring tolerance. When managing acute hypoxemic respiratory failure with NPPV, the ventilation mode may need attention to minimize the risk of p-SILI.

However, more information is required to inform clinical practice on how to manage acute hypoxemic respiratory failure using NIV. First, it is unclear how differences in the NPPV interface may affect clinical outcomes. For example, helmet NPPV might be more comfortable, and air leaks may be minimized. However, the most recent systematic review, which included 16 RCTs and 8 observational studies, found that the mortality benefit of helmet NPPV over face mask NPPV was of low certainty despite the statistically significant effect estimates (RR 0.56 [95% CI 0.33–0.95]) [18]. Furthermore, the effect of helmet NPPV compared to HFNC was uncertain [18]. Therefore, further well-designed and adequately powered clinical trials are needed to determine the optimal intervention with NIV. Second, preservation of spontaneous breathing may worsen existing lung injury and lead to p-SILI. However, there is not sufficient evidence on its clinical significance.

## 13.5 NIV for COVID-19

The COVID-19 pandemic has forced the use of NIV outside the ICU, such as in general wards [19]. HFNC was also used for acute hypoxemic respiratory failure related to COVID-19 worldwide, even before its efficacy and safety were established [20]. A recent systematic review identified nine observational studies and only one RCT that compared HFNC and NPPV by June 2021. Due to the paucity of adequately powered RCTs, it would be premature to conclude whether NIV is clinically beneficial for patients with COVID-19 or if HFNC or NPPV is superior to the other.

## 13.6 Key Clinical Trials and RECOVERY-RS

The HiFLo-Covid trial in Colombia (n = 220) compared HFNC and conventional oxygen therapy for respiratory failure due to COVID-19. HFNC was shown to reduce the rate of intubation at 28 days (34.3% vs. 51.0%, HR 0.62 [95% CI 0.39–0.96]) [9]. HFNC may reduce respiratory workload and improve gas exchange, leading to the improved intubation rate. However, physiological parameters, such as transpulmonary pressures or tidal volumes, which support the mechanisms of HFNC, were not available in this trial.

The HENIVOT trial was a RCT conducted in four ICUs in Italy (n = 110) comparing helmet NPPV and HFNC for respiratory failure in COVID-19 [21]. There was no statistically significant difference in the primary outcome, 28-day mechanical respiratory support free-days (20 days vs. 18 days, median difference (MD), 2 days, [95% CI, −2 to 6]); however, one of the secondary outcomes, the 28-day intubation rate, was reduced with helmet NPPV compared to HFNC (30% vs. 51%, HR 0.41 [95% CI 0.18–0.89]). Given the small sample sizes of the two trials, the available evidence is insufficient to conclude a positive effect of NIV or futility in patients with COVID-19.

In 2022, an awaited trial result was published. The RECOVERY-RS trial is the largest RCT of NIV strategy for respiratory failure due to COVID-19 [10]. RECOVERY-RS was a randomized, 3-arm study that compared HFNC, CPAP, and conventional oxygen therapy. Although it was terminated early, in May 2021 when 1278 patients had been enrolled, due to the decrease in numbers of hospitalized patients with COVID-19, the results showed that CPAP reduced intubation or death within 30 days compared to conventional oxygen therapy (36.3% vs. 44.4%, absolute difference −8% [95% CI −15% to −1%]). In contrast, HFNC was not significantly different compared to conventional oxygen therapy (44.3% vs. 45.1%, absolute difference −1% [95% CI −8% to 6%]). Although early termination of a trial could provide a risk of bias that overestimates the effect in general, the decision was made solely by the trial committee, which was blinded to the result of an interim analysis, thus mitigating the risk. Regrettably, the early termination made the trial underpowered to detect any clinically meaningful difference.

## 13.7 Current Knowledge About Use of NIV for COVID-19

Schmid et al. [22] updated a systematic review and meta-analysis and analyzed three RCTs comparing HFNC to NPPV, including RECOVERY-RS. The result showed that HFNC use may increase the composite outcome of intubation or mortality rate (RR 1.22 [95% CI 1.03–1.45]). However, the available evidence was insufficient to conclude the effectiveness of NPPV or HFNC because of the low level of evidence and possible bias.

Furthermore, extra considerations are needed in managing COVID-19 respiratory failure: the risk of virus transmission through aerosol dispersed from the equipment, depletion of medical resources due to pandemics, changes in standard of care, and viral mutations [23].

## 13.8 Timing of Intubation When Patients Are Receiving NIV

Delayed intubation has a poor prognosis for patients who need invasive ventilatory management. Kang et al. conducted an observational study to describe the characteristics of patients requiring tracheal intubation after HFNC failure [24]. They reported that patients who had intubation after 48 h had a higher mortality rate than those who had intubation within 48 h (66.7% [30/45] vs. 39.2% [51/130], $p = 0.001$).

Kangelaris et al. reported that 34% of patients with respiratory failure in multicenter ICUs who were managed without intubation at the time of meeting criteria for ARDS ($PaO_2/FiO_2 < 300$ or $SpO_2/FiO_2 < 315$) required intubation within the next 3 days [25]. Sixty-day mortality of the late intubation group was higher than that of patients intubated early (56% [20/36] vs. 36% [128/351]).

A recent systematic review, published in 2021, assessed whether early intubation of patients with COVID-19 was effective [26]. Twelve observational studies, representing 8944 patients with COVID-19, were included. In the pooled analysis there was no significant difference in mortality among those who had intubation early (within 24 h of ICU admission) and those intubated late (45.4% vs. 39.1%, $p = 0.08$).

The British Thoracic Society recommends evaluating patients 4–6 h after initiating NIV [27]. However, current clinical practice seems more conservative. RCTs that have assessed the effects of NIV reported that most intubation events occurred around 1–2 days after the initiation of NIV [4–6, 8]. As there are not sufficient data on the optimal timing of intubation for patients receiving NIV, close monitoring of respiratory workload and gas exchange are vital in these patients. Furthermore, optimal parameters that can inform clinicians about the best timing for intubation have yet to be determined.

## 13.9 Predicting Successful Treatment with HFNC

A strong interest has developed into predicting treatment success for HFNC. To avoid delaying intubation, Roca et al. proposed the ratio of oxygen saturation to respiratory rate (ROX) index as an early predictor of HFNC treatment failure so that intubation can be performed in a timely manner [28, 29]. The ROX index is calculated as ($SpO_2/FiO_2$)/respiratory rate. The numerator ($SpO_2/FiO_2$) is a measure of oxygenation that is positively correlated with successful high-flow oxygen therapy. The denominator (respiratory rate) is inversely correlated to high-flow oxygen therapy success. Although the predictive performance of the ROX index has been increasingly studied in recent years, there are still only a few high-quality studies [30–32].

A systematic review of eight observational studies of COVID-19-associated pneumonia found that the summary area under the curve (SAUC) of the ROX-index to predict high-flow oxygen therapy failure was 0.81 (95% CI 0.77–0.84), with a sensitivity of 0.70 (95% CI 0.59–0.80) and specificity of 0.79 (95% CI 0.67–0.88) [33]. HFNC failure was defined as the use of either invasive or non-invasive mechanical ventilation. The results indicated that the ROX index had good discriminatory power to predict HFNC failure [33]. In a subgroup analysis in which only studies that examined the ROX index within 6 h of HFNC initiation were considered, there was no change in predictive accuracy [33].

Another subgroup analysis looked at the cut-off value of the ROX index. Studies with an ROX index cut-off value greater than 5 had higher predictive accuracy (SAUC, 0.87 [0.83, 0.89]) than those with a cut-off value of 5 or less (SAUC, 0.76 [0.72, 0.80]) [33].

### 13.9.1 ROX Index in COVID-19

The utility of the ROX index in COVID-19 patients was explored in another systematic review of eight observational studies and one RCT [34]. The causes of respiratory failure were categorized as COVID-19-related pneumonia in four studies, pneumonia in two studies, hypoxic respiratory failure mainly due to pneumonia in two studies, and respiratory failure in immunocompromised patients in one study. The meta-analysis showed that the ROX index had moderate accuracy and, in a subgroup analysis, that it had higher predictive accuracy in studies of COVID-19-associated pneumonia than in studies of other diseases (COVID-19, AUC, 0.78 [0.74, 0.82]; others, 0.72 [0.68, 0.76]) [34].

The most recently updated systematic review of 13 observational studies, of which 10 included COVID-19-related pneumonia and 3 included pneumonia, found similar findings [35]. Successful withdrawal from high-flow oxygen therapy was accurately predicted by the ROX index measured within 12 h of its initiation with an area under the hierarchical summary receiver operating characteristic curve (AUHSROC) of 0.81 (95% CI, 0.77–0.84), a diagnostic odds ratio of 8.3 (95% CI 6.4–10.8), a sensitivity of 0.71 (95% CI 0.64–0.78), and a specificity of 0.78 (95% CI 0.70–0.84). The mean cut-off value was 4.8 (95% CI 4.2–5.4) and, in subgroup analysis, the predictive accuracy was high in COVID-19-related pneumonia, as previously reported [34]. Assessing the ROX index within 6 h or 6–12 h was associated with similarly good predictive ability [35].

The three systematic reviews [33–35] suggest that the ROX index measured within 12 h of initiation is a useful predictor of high-flow oxygen therapy success. However, the overall quality of the included studies was limited, and the heterogeneity observed in the pooled effects would need further exploration. Furthermore, the utility of the ROX index for NPPV is unknown as it has been developed and validated only with HFNC.

## 13.10 Monitoring Respiratory Failure Using $SpO_2$: The Risk of Inaccuracy

Dr. Takuo Aoyagi, a Japanese medical engineering specialist, invented the pulse oximeter in 1974 [36]. Since pulse oximeters use light absorption to estimate the $SaO_2$, it was acknowledged early that skin color might affect the readings [37].

Jubran et al. conducted a prospective observational study of 54 ventilator-assisted patients (29 black and 25 white) at two USA institutions in 1990 [38]. In this study, the $FiO_2$ of the ventilator was adjusted, and the $SpO_2$ and arterial partial pressure of oxygen ($PaO_2$) were recorded. The results suggested that pulse oximeters missed hypoxemia twice as often in black subjects than in white subjects. The value of $SpO_2$ required to maintain $PaO_2 > 60$ mmHg varied depending on the skin color. Based on an early experiment showing that the use of black nail polish reduced the difference in absorbance of red and infrared lights, and caused the pulse oximeter to falsely record a lower oxygen saturation, the disparity in the accuracy of $SpO_2$ could be attributable to skin color [39]. However, this issue of measurement errors in pulse oximeters has not been pursued or sufficiently investigated until recently.

### 13.10.1 Inaccuracy of Pulse Oximeters and Skin Color: New Investigations

Since the COVID-19 pandemic outbreak in 2020, measurement errors from pulse oximeters have been revisited and studied worldwide. Sjoding et al. conducted an observational study in the USA to determine the frequency of potential hypoxemia (with $SaO_2 < 88\%$ despite a pulse oximeter $SpO_2$ of 92–96%) in 10,001 individuals (8675 white and 1326 black) [40]. Latent hypoxemia undetected by the pulse oximeter occurred about three times more frequently in black subjects than in white subjects, suggesting that pulse oximeters are unreliable for triaging patients and adjusting oxygen levels. The study was published in 2020 and received worldwide attention, especially because of its important potential implications in the midst of the COVID-19 pandemic.

In 2021, Wong et al. conducted a large retrospective observational study using an American database of 87,971 individuals, including Asians, blacks, Hispanics, and whites. They reported the prevalence of potential hypoxemia ($SpO_2 > 88\%$ but $SaO_2 < 88\%$) as well as clinical outcomes [41]. With more than 80,000 participants, the precision of the study increased compared to that in the smaller study by Sjoding et al. [40]. Potential hypoxemia occurred in all racial subgroups, but there were racial differences in prevalence, being present in 6.8% of blacks, 6.0% of Hispanics, 4.8% of Asians, and 4.9% of whites ($p < 0.001$) [41]. These authors also noted a greater variability in $SaO_2$ for any given $SpO_2$ value in black subjects and reported that the risk of potential hypoxemia at 92% $SpO_2$ was 15.2% for white subjects, 18.4% for Hispanics, 18.4% for Asians, and 20.2% for black subjects [41]. Clinical outcomes showed that patients with subclinical hypoxemia had higher serum creatinine and lactate levels than those without subclinical hypoxemia and higher sequential organ failure assessment (SOFA) scores and hospital mortality [41].

These studies consistently reported that skin color differences cause pulse oximeter measurement errors, and the errors are particularly pronounced in people with darker skin, increasing the risk of potential hypoxia, organ damage, and worse clinical outcomes. Such disparities occur since most of the data that manufacturers obtain to develop pulse oximeters were derived from white subjects [42].

Following these reports, the Food and Drug Administration (FDA) has announced that to test the minimum mean accuracy of pulse oximeters, the $SpO_2$ readings must be compared with directly measured $SaO_2$ levels between 70 and 100% [43]. The FDA approves the pulse oximeter's accuracy if 66% of $SpO_2$ values are within 2–3% of $SaO_2$ values and about 95% of $SpO_2$ values are within 4–6% of $SaO_2$ values, emphasizing that $SpO_2$ values do not always agree with $SaO_2$ [43].

The pulse oximeter has become an essential monitoring device in clinical practice because it is a non-invasive and simple tool to measure oxygen saturation. However, it is fraught with potential health hazards due to misinterpretation of the numbers. Therefore, clinicians need to be aware of the limitations of pulse oximeters and make careful clinical decisions.

## 13.11 Conclusion

NPPV has a well-established beneficial effect in acute exacerbations of COPD and cardiogenic pulmonary edema and probably reduces mortality in patients with acute hypoxemic respiratory failure. In COVID-19 respiratory failure, NPPV is favored over HFNC. HFNC may also reduce mortality in patients with acute hypoxemic respiratory failure and is recommended in recent guidelines. Questions remain regarding the best NPPV interface, the clinical impact of p-SILI, and the timing of and indications for intubation when NIV is started. All clinical practitioners use pulse oximetry despite its potential inaccuracies, particularly in patients with darker skin colors. Clinicians need to be aware of the unreliability of pulse oximeters to avoid exposing those patients to harmful clinical decision making.

## References

1. Bause G. Emerson respirator or "iron lung". Anesthesiology. 2009;110:812.
2. Ferreyro BL, Angriman F, Munshi L, et al. Association of noninvasive oxygenation strategies with all-cause mortality in adults with acute hypoxemic respiratory failure: a systematic review and meta-analysis. JAMA. 2020;324:57–67.
3. Sakuraya M, Okano H, Masuyama T, Kimata S, Hokari S. Efficacy of non-invasive and invasive respiratory management strategies in adult patients with acute hypoxaemic respiratory failure: a systematic review and network meta-analysis. Crit Care. 2021;25:414.
4. Frat JP, Thille AW, Mercat A, et al. High-flow oxygen through nasal cannula in acute hypoxemic respiratory failure. N Engl J Med. 2015;372:2185–96.

5. Lemiale V, Mokart D, Resche-Rigon M, et al. Effect of noninvasive ventilation vs oxygen therapy on mortality among immunocompromised patients with acute respiratory failure: a randomized clinical trial. JAMA. 2015;314:1711–9.
6. Azoulay E, Lemiale V, Mokart D, et al. Effect of high-flow nasal oxygen vs standard oxygen on 28-day mortality in immunocompromised patients with acute respiratory failure: the HIGH randomized clinical trial. JAMA. 2018;320:2099–107.
7. He H, Sun B, Liang L, et al. A multicenter RCT of noninvasive ventilation in pneumonia-induced early mild acute respiratory distress syndrome. Crit Care. 2019;23:300.
8. Coudroy R, Frat JP, Ehrmann S, et al. High-flow nasal oxygen alone or alternating with non-invasive ventilation in critically ill immunocompromised patients with acute respiratory failure: a randomised controlled trial. Lancet Respir Med. 2022;10:641–9.
9. Ospina-Tascon GA, Calderon-Tapia LE, Garcia AF, et al. Effect of high-flow oxygen therapy vs conventional oxygen therapy on invasive mechanical ventilation and clinical recovery in patients with severe COVID-19: a randomized clinical trial. JAMA. 2021;326:2161–71.
10. Perkins GD, Ji C, Connolly BA, Couper K, et al. Effect of noninvasive respiratory strategies on intubation or mortality among patients with acute hypoxemic respiratory failure and COVID-19: the RECOVERY-RS randomized clinical trial. JAMA. 2022;327:546–58.
11. Yoshida T, Uchiyama A, Matsuura N, Mashimo T, Fujino Y. The comparison of spontaneous breathing and muscle paralysis in two different severities of experimental lung injury. Crit Care Med. 2013;41:536–45.
12. Cruces P, Retamal J, Hurtado DE, et al. A physiological approach to understand the role of respiratory effort in the progression of lung injury in SARS-CoV-2 infection. Crit Care. 2020;24:494.
13. Frat JP, Ragot S, Coudroy R, et al. Predictors of intubation in patients with acute hypoxemic respiratory failure treated with a noninvasive oxygenation strategy. Crit Care Med. 2018;46:208–15.
14. Brochard L, Isabey D, Piquet J, et al. Reversal of acute exacerbations of chronic obstructive lung disease by inspiratory assistance with a face mask. N Engl J Med. 1990;323:1523–30.
15. Masip J, Roque M, Sanchez B, Fernandez R, Subirana M, Exposito JA. Noninvasive ventilation in acute cardiogenic pulmonary edema: systematic review and meta-analysis. JAMA. 2005;294:3124–30.
16. Rochwerg B, Brochard L, Elliott MW, et al. Official ERS/ATS clinical practice guidelines: noninvasive ventilation for acute respiratory failure. Eur Respir J. 2017;50:1602426.
17. Oczkowski S, Ergan B, Bos L, et al. ERS clinical practice guidelines: high-flow nasal cannula in acute respiratory failure. Eur Respir J. 2022;59:2101574.
18. Chaudhuri D, Jinah R, Burns KEA, et al. Helmet noninvasive ventilation compared to face-mask noninvasive ventilation and high-flow nasal cannula in acute respiratory failure: a systematic review and meta-analysis. Eur Respir J. 2022;59:2101269.
19. Cammarota G, Esposito T, Azzolina D, et al. Noninvasive respiratory support outside the intensive care unit for acute respiratory failure related to coronavirus-19 disease: a systematic review and meta-analysis. Crit Care. 2021;25:268.
20. Weerakkody S, Arina P, Glenister J, et al. Non-invasive respiratory support in the management of acute COVID-19 pneumonia: considerations for clinical practice and priorities for research. Lancet Respir Med. 2022;10:199–213.
21. Grieco DL, Menga LS, Cesarano M, et al. Effect of helmet noninvasive ventilation vs high-flow nasal oxygen on days free of respiratory support in patients with COVID-19 and moderate to severe hypoxemic respiratory failure: the HENIVOT randomized clinical trial. JAMA. 2021;325:1731–43.
22. Schmid B, Griesel M, Fischer AL, et al. Awake prone positioning, high-flow nasal oxygen and non-invasive ventilation as non-invasive respiratory strategies in COVID-19 acute respiratory failure: a systematic review and meta-analysis. J Clin Med. 2022;11:391.
23. Ogawa K, Asano K, Ikeda J, Fujii T. Non-invasive oxygenation strategies for respiratory failure with COVID-19: a concise narrative review of literature in pre and mid-COVID-19 era. Anaesth Crit Care Pain Med. 2021;40:100897.

24. Kang BJ, Koh Y, Lim CM, et al. Failure of high-flow nasal cannula therapy may delay intubation and increase mortality. Intensive Care Med. 2015;41:623–32.
25. Kangelaris KN, Ware LB, Wang CY, et al. Timing of intubation and clinical outcomes in adults with acute respiratory distress syndrome. Crit Care Med. 2016;44:120–9.
26. Papoutsi E, Giannakoulis VG, Xourgia E, Routsi C, Kotanidou A, Siempos II. Effect of timing of intubation on clinical outcomes of critically ill patients with COVID-19: a systematic review and meta-analysis of non-randomized cohort studies. Crit Care. 2021;25:121.
27. Bristish Thoracic Society Standards of Care Committee. Non-invasive ventilation in acute respiratory failure. Thorax. 2002;57:192–211.
28. Roca O, Messika J, Caralt B, et al. Predicting success of high-flow nasal cannula in pneumonia patients with hypoxemic respiratory failure: the utility of the ROX index. J Crit Care. 2016;35:200–5.
29. Roca O, Caralt B, Messika J, et al. An index combining respiratory rate and oxygenation to predict outcome of nasal high-flow therapy. Am J Respir Crit Care Med. 2019;199:1368–76.
30. Goh KJ, Chai HZ, Ong TH, Sewa DW, Phua GC, Tan QL. Early prediction of high flow nasal cannula therapy outcomes using a modified ROX index incorporating heart rate. J Intensive Care. 2020;8:41.
31. Hu M, Zhou Q, Zheng R, et al. Application of high-flow nasal cannula in hypoxemic patients with COVID-19: a retrospective cohort study. BMC Pulm Med. 2020;20:324.
32. Rodriguez M, Thille AW, Boissier F, et al. Predictors of successful separation from high-flow nasal oxygen therapy in patients with acute respiratory failure: a retrospective monocenter study. Ann Intensive Care. 2019;9:101.
33. Prakash J, Bhattacharya PK, Yadav AK, Kumar A, Tudu LC, Prasad K. ROX index as a good predictor of high flow nasal cannula failure in COVID-19 patients with acute hypoxemic respiratory failure: a systematic review and meta-analysis. J Crit Care. 2021;66:102–8.
34. Junhai Z, Jing Y, Beibei C, Li L. The value of ROX index in predicting the outcome of high flow nasal cannula: a systematic review and meta-analysis. Respir Res. 2022;23:33.
35. Zhou X, Liu J, Pan J, Xu Z, Xu J. The ROX index as a predictor of high-flow nasal cannula outcome in pneumonia patients with acute hypoxemic respiratory failure: a systematic review and meta-analysis. BMC Pulm Med. 2022;22:121.
36. Aoyagi T. Pulse oximetry: its invention, theory, and future. J Anesth. 2003;17:259–66.
37. Ries AL, Farrow JT, Clausen JL. Accuracy of two ear oximeters at rest and during exercise in pulmonary patients. Am Rev Respir Dis. 1985;132:685–9.
38. Jubran A, Tobin MJ. Reliability of pulse oximetry in titrating supplemental oxygen therapy in ventilator-dependent patients. Chest. 1990;97:1420–5.
39. Coté CJ, Goldstein EA, Fuchsman WH, Hoaglin DC. The effect of nail polish on pulse oximetry. Anesth Analg. 1988;67:683–6.
40. Sjoding MW, Dickson RP, Iwashyna TJ, Gay SE, Valley TS. Racial bias in pulse oximetry measurement. N Engl J Med. 2020;383:2477–8.
41. Wong AI, Charpignon M, Kim H, et al. Analysis of discrepancies between pulse oximetry and arterial oxygen saturation measurements by race and ethnicity and association with organ dysfunction and mortality. JAMA Netw Open. 2021;4:e2131674.
42. Tobin MJ, Jubran A. Pulse oximetry, racial bias and statistical bias. Ann Intensive Care. 2022;12:2.
43. FDA. Pulse oximeter accuracy and limitations: FDA Safety Communication 2022. Available at: https://www.fda.gov/medical-devices/safety-communications/pulse-oximeter-accuracy-and-limitations-fda-safety-communication. Accessed 21 Oct 2022.

# Managing the Physiologically Difficult Airway in Critically Ill Adults

# 14

C. S. Jabaley

## 14.1 Introduction

Airway management (i.e., tracheal intubation) in critically ill adults has long been recognized as technically difficult [1]. Myriad patient and environment-specific factors conspire to increase the difficulty of conventional laryngoscopy and other approaches to the airway [2]. However, intubation in critical care settings has benefitted from advances in equipment and techniques originally developed for application in procedural environments: algorithmic approaches, video laryngoscopy, supraglottic airways, and other adjuncts. Their application to critical care settings has helped to increase the accessibility and safety of airway management.

Among this mitigation of technical difficulties, the latent physiologic difficulties of tracheal intubation in critically ill adults have become a new focus. These patients typically require definitive airway management due to organ dysfunction or other manifestations of critical illness, including altered consciousness, respiratory failure, and shock. These and other pathophysiological states increase the risks associated with sedative hypnotic (i.e., induction) agents and their hemodynamic sequelae, apnea during tracheal intubation, and/or transition to positive pressure mechanical ventilation. Therefore, successful airway management in critically ill adults requires planning and execution of strategies that mitigate potential technical and physiological difficulties.

C. S. Jabaley (✉)
Department of Anesthesiology, Emory University, Atlanta, GA, USA

Emory Critical Care Center, Atlanta, GA, USA
e-mail: csjabaley@emory.edu



J.-L. Vincent (ed.), *Annual Update in Intensive Care and Emergency Medicine 2023*, Annual Update in Intensive Care and Emergency Medicine,
https://doi.org/10.1007/978-3-031-23005-9_14

## 14.2 Adverse Outcomes and Risk Factors

Although clinicians have long been intuitively familiar with the challenges and outcomes of tracheal intubation in critically ill adults, high-quality prospective evidence has emerged to help advance our understanding of global practices and outcomes.

### 14.2.1 What Are the Outcomes of Tracheal Intubation in Critically Ill Adults?

Until recently, estimates of adverse event rates have relied on extrapolation from a heterogeneous pool of sometimes retrospective and/or single-center studies [3, 4]. Recognizing these limitations, the literature has suggested that tracheal intubation in critically ill adults is associated with an approximate 30% risk of cardiovascular instability, 20% risk of hypoxemia, and 2–4% risk of cardiac arrest. The Fourth National Audit Project (NAP4) of the Royal College of Anaesthetists examined airway complications in the United Kingdom from September 2008 to August 2009 and was the largest study of airway management complications at the time of its publication [5]. Among other findings, NAP4 identified intensive care units (ICUs) as the setting associated with the most potentially avoidable deaths related to airway management.

In 2021, the long-awaited results of the International Observational Study to Understand the Impact and Best Practices of Airway Management in Critically Ill Patients (INTUBE), a prospective study of tracheal intubation in critically ill adults over 8 consecutive weeks in 197 centers across 29 countries with observations between October 1, 2018 and July 31, 2019, were published [4]. Among the 2964 patients included, the most frequent indications for tracheal intubation were respiratory failure (52.3%), neurological impairment (30.5%), and cardiovascular instability (9.4%). Cardiovascular instability—defined as systolic blood pressure (SBP) < 65 mmHg at least once, SBP < 90 mmHg for >30 min, new or increased need for vasopressors, and/or need for fluid bolus >15 ml/kg—was the most common adverse event, occurring in 42.6% of intubations. This was followed by severe hypoxemia—defined as oxygen saturation ($SpO_2$) < 80%—in 9.3%, and cardiac arrest in 3.1%. Of the 1172 occurrences of cardiovascular instability, 1053 (89.9%) involved the need for new or increased vasopressors.

### 14.2.2 Which Patients Are at Risk?

Recognizing that the risks associated with airway management may be due to technical and/or physiological difficulty, predicting adverse outcomes requires consideration of both factors. This was exemplified by the MACOCHA score, which includes both anatomical and physiological features to predict difficult intubation and has been incorporated into relevant guidelines (Table 14.1) [6, 7]. Although the

**Table 14.1** MACOCHA score variables [6]

| Factor | Points |
|---|---|
| Mallampati III or IV | 5 |
| Obstructive sleep apnea | 2 |
| Reduced cervical spine mobility | 1 |
| Mouth opening <3 cm | 1 |
| Coma | 1 |
| $SpO_2 < 80\%$ | 1 |
| Non-anesthesiologist | 1 |

The MACOCHA score includes seven factors: Mallampati score, sleep apnea, cervical spine mobility, mouth opening, coma, hypoxemia, and non-anesthesiologist

MACOCHA score has been validated, it was not associated with adverse events in the INTUBE study when dichotomized into <3 or ≥3 [4]. In multivariate analysis, factors associated with adverse events included age, history of heart failure, history of hematologic malignancy, cardiovascular instability as an indication for intubation, and other features of hemodynamic compromise.

Risk factors for cardiovascular collapse (e.g., cardiac arrest) have also been explored. In a secondary analysis of the cohort used to derive and validate the MACOCHA score, Perbet et al. identified advanced age and more severe critical illness as risk factors for cardiovascular collapse [8]. Subsequently, De Jong et al. identified hypotension, hypoxemia, lack of pre-oxygenation, obesity, and age > 75 years as relevant risk factors for cardiac arrest [9]. Halliday et al. identified hypotension, the need for vasopressors prior to intubation, age, and cirrhosis as the top four risk factors in a secondary analysis of trial data [10–13]. Right ventricular (RV) dysfunction is also an increasingly appreciated risk factor as perturbations in gas exchange, acid/base status, and intrathoracic pressure may all lead to cardiovascular collapse [14, 15]. In a secondary analysis of INTUBE, the risk factors for cardiovascular instability included age, lower blood pressure, lower oxygen saturation, and propofol administration [16].

## 14.3 Hemodynamic Optimization

Given that cardiovascular instability is the primary risk of tracheal intubation in critically ill adults in the contemporary era, its prevention and management is a natural clinical focus. Furthermore, cardiovascular instability, among other adverse peri-intubation events, has been independently associated with ICU mortality [4, 9, 16–19].

### 14.3.1 Is There an Optimal Induction Agent?

The optimal induction agent, if any, for tracheal intubation in critically ill adults remains controversial. Clinical experience suggests that any agent has the potential for hemodynamic trespass, highlighting the importance of clinical judgement. However, extrapolated pharmacokinetic modeling from animal studies reveals that some agents (e.g., etomidate) require less dose reduction than others (e.g., propofol) in the presence of shock [20]. Propofol was the induction agent administered most frequently in INTUBE (41.5%), followed by midazolam (36.4%), etomidate (17.8%), and ketamine (14.2%) [4]. Totaling 109.9% of encounters, approximately 10% of patients received more than one induction agent. In the aforementioned secondary analysis of INTUBE, an inverse probability of treatment weighting approach to causal effect inference suggested that propofol administration was the sole variable independently associated with cardiovascular instability or collapse [16]. This finding parallels previous investigations and clinical experience, and etomidate and ketamine have been recommended as first-line induction agents in critically ill adults [7].

Etomidate, anecdotally more so than any other induction agent, continues to prompt spirited debate [21, 22]. Matchett et al. recently reported the results of the Etomidate Versus Ketamine for Emergency Endotracheal Intubation (EvK) trial in which 801 patients were randomized to receive either etomidate or ketamine for emergency tracheal intubation [23]. The resulting Kaplan-Meier curve was divergent so that patients randomized to etomidate had a significantly higher risk of mortality at day 7 and a non-significantly higher risk at day 28. Etomidate advocates inferred non-inferior outcomes from this convergence on day 28 while its detractors inferred risk of avoidable harm.

Among patients who received ketamine in the EvK trial, 25% sustained post-induction cardiovascular collapse versus 17.4% who received etomidate (mean difference 7.6%, 95% CI 2–13). Highlighting the clinical judgement involved in selecting the induction agent and dose, there was substantial heterogeneity in induction agent dose in the EvK trial, which may have influenced outcomes as dosage was not standardized. Ketamine has sympathomimetic properties but has also been found to exert dose-dependent negative inotropy *in vitro* [24]. Ketamine may be gaining popularity as it represented 68% of induction agents administered in a European bougie trial, but geographically influenced clinical practice patterns seem to also influence induction agent selection as, for example, ketamine represented only 24% of induction agents in a related North American trial [25, 26].

### 14.3.2 What Is the Role of Fluids?

While tracheal intubation is one of the most common ICU procedures, fluid administration is among the most common interventions. Recognizing the risk of hypotension due to induction agents and/or transition to positive pressure ventilation, fluid administration prior to intubation has a reasonable physiological rationale. Vasodilation from induction agents may be offset, and venous return to the heart can be increased even amid increased intrathoracic pressure. However, favorable clinical effects have not been borne out in two trials [12, 27]. In PrePARE, the impact of a 500 ml crystalloid bolus on the primary outcome of cardiovascular collapse was examined; there was no significant effect, but there was a suggestion of benefit in patients who received positive pressure during intubation with non-invasive ventilation (NIV) or bag-mask ventilation [12]. This population was specifically studied in a pragmatic follow-up trial enrolling 1067 patients, and again a 500 ml crystalloid bolus did not impact the primary outcome of cardiovascular collapse [27].

### 14.3.3 What Is the Role of Vasopressors?

Evidence to inform optimal selection and approach to vasopressor administration is lacking. However, given that cardiovascular instability accompanies a substantial proportion of tracheal intubations, it follows that the immediate availability of vasopressors should be included as part of routine preparation. Whether administered preventively or in response to hypotension, the immediate readiness of these agents guarantees a short time between the development of instability and treatment. Vasopressors have been included and studied as elements of peri-intubation bundles [28], and a trial is underway to compare the efficacy of preemptive vasopressors against a fluid bolus (ClinicalTrials.gov Identifier: NCT05318066).

## 14.4 Mitigating Hypoxemia

Hypoxemia is the second most common adverse event associated with tracheal intubation in critically ill adults. Maintaining adequate oxygenation between induction and intubation, sometimes called the apneic interval, is a key element of safe airway management. Acute or chronic lung disease coupled with concerns about aspiration serve to limit the efficacy of traditional pre-oxygenation strategies and diminish enthusiasm for certain rescue approaches.

### 14.4.1 Are Standard Pre-oxygenation Strategies Adequate?

Conventional pre-oxygenation approaches often do not meaningfully extend the safe apneic interval, particularly in patients with impaired gas exchange at baseline [29]. Secondary analysis of airway management trial data has revealed a nearly linear, proportionate relationship between $SpO_2$ at induction and the lowest $SpO_2$ during tracheal intubation [30]. This was exemplified in a study by Mort et al. in which 34 consecutive critically ill patients were pre-oxygenated prior to tracheal intubation with 100% inspired oxygen fraction ($FiO_2$) through an adult resuscitator bag for 8 min with serial arterial blood gas analysis [31]. From 0 to 4 min, the mean $PaO_2$ increased from approximately 62 mmHg to 84 mmHg, and from 4 to 8 min the mean increase was only 9 mmHg, with a quarter of patients demonstrating a reduction in $PaO_2$, likely due to atelectasis.

### 14.4.2 What About Non-invasive Ventilation?

NIV has been associated with improved oxygenation during tracheal intubation with fewer adverse events compared to conventional pre-oxygenation [32, 33]. Positive pressure likely helps overcome the absorption atelectasis that develops during pre-oxygenation with high $FiO_2$ and unsupported spontaneous breathing. Despite these advantages, INTUBE showed that NIV use was infrequent in clinical practice, although not all patients may require advanced approaches to pre-oxygenation [4]. From a speculative standpoint, there are several potential barriers to wider adoption. One may be the time required to initiate support *de novo* or other barriers to easy implementation. Another is that the mask interface must be removed prior to airway instrumentation, at which point oxygen delivery is interrupted. Finally, NIV may risk gastric insufflation and aspiration, which will be discussed subsequently.

### 14.4.3 What About Apneic Oxygenation?

High flow nasal oxygen offers the advantage of an unobtrusive nasal interface that can be maintained during airway management. Therefore, high flow nasal oxygen is one modality by which to accomplish both pre-oxygenation and apneic oxygenation during airway management. This dual functionality also complicates literature interpretation, as most studies continue high flow nasal oxygen during airway management. Similarly, studies have used different equipment, each with varying maximal flow capabilities (e.g., 15 versus 60 l/min).

Having acknowledged those potential limitations, meta-analyses suggest that pre-oxygenation with high flow nasal oxygen is at least non-inferior to conventional approaches [34–36]. Meta-analyses have also suggested that the efficacy of high flow nasal oxygen is relative to the severity of respiratory failure with limited impact as the severity of respiratory failure increases, for example, as measured by the $PaO_2/FiO_2$ (P/F) ratio (Fig. 14.1) [36]. When comparing the efficacy of high flow nasal oxygen with NIV, therefore, the severity of baseline hypoxemia must be considered. In the FLORALI-2 trial, Frat et al. reported that 24% of patients pre-oxygenated with NIV developed a $SpO_2 < 80\%$ versus 35% who were pre-oxygenated with high flow nasal oxygen (adjusted odds ratio of 0.56 [95% CI 0.32–0.99]) [37]. The OPTINIV trial explored the combination of high flow nasal oxygen and NIV in 50 patients with a mean P/F ratio of 122 and found that patients receiving the combination intervention maintained a higher $SpO_2$ during intubation than those in the NIV only group [38].

### 14.4.4 Should Mask Ventilation Be Avoided?

Critically ill patients are at risk for aspiration and for potentially severe sequelae of aspiration in the presence of acute respiratory failure. Rapid sequence intubation (RSI), which avoids mask ventilation, has long been thought to help minimize the

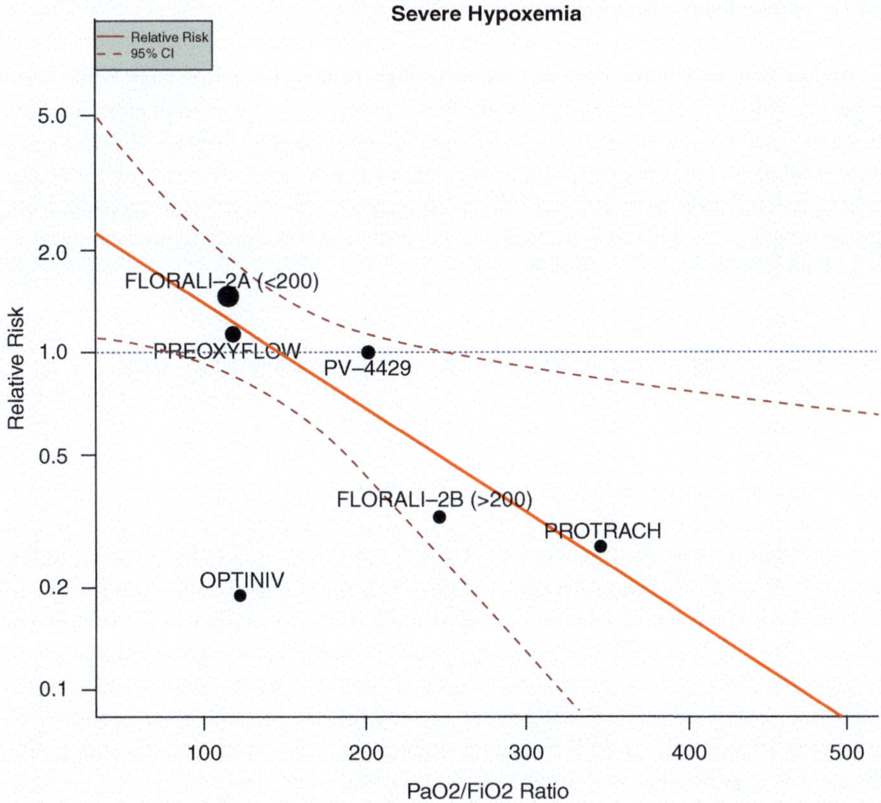


**Fig. 14.1** Efficacy of high-flow nasal oxygen for apneic oxygenation relative to the severity of respiratory failure. Relative risk indicates reduction in the incidence of severe hypoxemia, defined as $SpO_2 < 80\%$. (Reproduced from [36] under the Creative Commons Attribution 4.0 International License)

risk of aspiration, although the supporting evidence is limited. Furthermore, RSI itself may confer risks related to induction agent selection and dose and risk of hypoxemia in patients with severe respiratory failure.

The PreVent trial compared bag-mask ventilation versus its avoidance during the interval between induction and tracheal intubation in 401 critically ill adults with a primary outcome of lowest $SpO_2$ [13]. $SpO_2$ was higher in the bag-mask ventilation group (96% vs. 93%), and the incidence of a $SpO_2 < 80\%$ was lower compared to the control group (10.9% vs. 22.8%). The overall rate of reported aspiration was 3.2%. Although not designed or powered to critically examine safety outcomes, such as aspiration, the PreVent results challenge the dogma that mask ventilation must be strictly avoided and supports clinicians who choose to employ bag-mask ventilation to safely temporize hypoxemia during the apneic interval. Secondary analysis of trial data also suggests that bag-mask ventilation may be associated with higher oxygen saturation during intubation than apneic oxygenation [39].

## 14.5 First Pass Success

No matter how robust the preparation, time for tracheal intubation may be limited. In the era before video laryngoscopy, multiple attempts at airway management were found to place patients at higher risk for adverse outcomes [40]. In INTUBE, two or more intubation attempts were likewise associated with an increased risk for major adverse events [4]. In particular, the risk of severe hypoxemia increased from approximately 5% with one attempt, to more than 20% with two attempts, and to more than 30% with three attempts.

### 14.5.1 Is It Time to Universally Adopt Video Laryngoscopy?

After approximately a century of direct laryngoscopy, video laryngoscopy has increased in popularity, its advocates hailing an emerging standard of care and its detractors bemoaning loss of familiarity with other approaches. Video laryngoscopy is a catchall term for a somewhat heterogeneous group of devices: (1) those with a conventional curved blade profile; (2) those with a hyperangulated blade profile; and (3) those with integral channels for tube passage. Proficiency with one device or category is not necessarily immediately transferrable to another [41]. An updated meta-analysis of 222 video laryngoscopy trials in multiple settings found that video laryngoscopy of any design reduces the probability of failed intubation and complications, with hyperangulated designs performing favorably in those with features of a difficult airway [42]. In ICU video laryngoscopy trials, video laryngoscopy also appears to be associated with improved first pass success [43].

Although an extended discussion about the capabilities and limitations of video laryngoscopy is beyond the scope of this review, three key points are worthy of emphasis. Video laryngoscopy generally gives a superior view of the glottic aperture [42]. However, superior visualization of the airway does not eliminate the need for training and practice to establish expertise. Among trainees using a conventional profile video laryngoscopy device, both the level of training and dedicated video laryngoscopy experience (that is, 15 vs. >15 intubations) were identified as independent predictors of first pass success when intubating critically ill adults [44]. Using experience from anesthesiology, hyperangulated devices may have a steeper learning curve, with mastery requiring upwards of 70 intubations [45]. Channeled designs inherently aid in tube placement; however, both conventional profile and, more so, hyperangulated devices require a stylet to reliably facilitate endotracheal tube placement. In the absence of a stylet or adequate device-specific expertise, any advantages associated with video laryngoscopy may not materialize, resulting in prolonged airway management and increased risk of adverse events despite superior glottic visualization [46].

### 14.5.2 What About Intubation Adjuncts and Checklists?

Despite the growing popularity of video laryngoscopy, direct laryngoscopy remains commonplace worldwide, accounting for 81.5% of intubations included in INTUBE [4]. There also remains international variation in the routine use of endotracheal tube stylets due to their associated risks, which, while uncommon, are potentially severe. The recent STYLETO trial reported a first pass success rate of 78.2% in patients intubated with direct laryngoscopy and a stylet and 71.5% in those intubated without a stylet [25]. Among the 999 included patients, in the stylet group there were two laryngeal injuries, one mediastinal injury, and two esophageal injures, while in the control group there were two laryngeal injuries and one tracheal injury. For clinicians accustomed to using a stylet, the results of the BOUGIE follow-up trial suggest that a tracheal tube introducer (i.e., bougie) may not offer an advantage under usual conditions [26].

Checklists and other similar cognitive aids have been found to increase adherence to complex multistep processes in stressful clinical contexts [47]. ICU intubation checklists that incorporate physiological optimization have been shown to improve outcomes in small studies [28, 48]. Janz et al. conducted the only randomized trial of an intubation checklist and demonstrated no differences in lowest oxygen saturation or blood pressure during intubation; however, that checklist did not include preparatory steps relevant to physiologic optimization [11]. Similarly, a recent meta-analysis of 11 studies, including 3261 patients, found no association between airway checklists and improved clinical outcomes [49]. Although these findings are somewhat discouraging, given the seemingly ever-growing complexity of critical illness and the serious risks posed to patients by airway management in the ICU, further development and assessment of checklists incorporating preparation for physiological difficulties is an important avenue of investigation.

## 14.6 Is It Time for New Approaches?

Some patients in physiological extremis may not tolerate some or all elements of traditional approaches to emergency airway management, including sedative hypnotic agents, apnea, and positive pressure ventilation. Patients with severe respiratory failure, advanced shock, RV failure, and refractory acidosis are at particularly high risk. In such instances, awake intubation may be considered; however, related techniques may be unfamiliar to some intensivists without practical experience in other contexts (e.g., procedural environments). Training for awake tracheal intubation, awake transition to extracorporeal support, and other such avenues represents a potentially fruitful and important avenue for continued evolution in our management of physiologically challenging scenarios.

## 14.7 Conclusion

Tracheal intubation in the ICU is a commonplace and short procedure that poses risks to patients and challenges to intensivists. Time and dedication have led to the evolution and refinement of technical approaches to airway management. In this modern era, physiological compromise poses a greater risk to patient safety during airway management in critically ill adults than outright failure of intubation [4]. Therefore, airway management in the ICU has expanded to include preparation for and management of physiologic trespass during tracheal intubation. With this expanded scope comes additional complexity and nuance that require the integration and clinical application of multiple key concepts to each airway management encounter (Table 14.2).

**Table 14.2** Summary points for management of the physiologically difficult airway

| |
|---|
| Risks and risk prediction |
| Cardiovascular instability, hypoxemia, and cardiac arrest are the most common adverse events associated with tracheal intubation |
| Risk factors for cardiovascular collapse include age, shock, hypoxemia, advanced critical illness, and propofol administration |
| Hemodynamic optimization |
| Etomidate and ketamine may impact hemodynamics less than propofol |
| A crystalloid bolus prior to intubation has not been associated with improved hemodynamics, even in patients receiving positive pressure ventilation |
| Given the frequency of cardiovascular instability, vasopressors should be readied as part of preparation for tracheal intubation |
| Mitigating hypoxemia |
| Standard pre-oxygenation strategies are inadequate to safely extend the apneic interval in patients with moderate to severe respiratory failure |
| Non-invasive ventilation can be used with or without high flow nasal oxygen and is more effective than high flow nasal oxygen alone |
| While historically avoided, bag-mask ventilation improves oxygenation during airway management and can be employed either preemptively or for rescue |
| First pass success |
| Multiple attempts at intubation increase the risk of adverse events |
| Depending on the preferences and expertise of the intubating clinician, video laryngoscopy or direct laryngoscopy with adjuncts may improve first pass success |
| Checklists improve adherence to complex, multi-step processes and may help prompt preparation for physiologic trespass |

## References


1. Mort TC. The incidence and risk factors for cardiac arrest during emergency tracheal intubation: a justification for incorporating the ASA guidelines in the remote location. J Clin Anesth. 2004;16:508–16.
2. Taboada M, Doldan P, Calvo A, et al. Comparison of tracheal intubation conditions in operating room and intensive care unit: a prospective, observational study. Anesthesiology. 2018;129:321–8.
3. Nolan JP, Kelly FE. Airway challenges in critical care. Anaesthesia. 2011;66(Suppl 2):81–92.
4. Russotto V, Myatra SN, Laffey JG, et al. Intubation practices and adverse peri-intubation events in critically ill patients from 29 countries. JAMA. 2021;325:1164–72.
5. Cook TM, Woodall N, Harper J, Benger J. Major complications of airway management in the UK: results of the fourth National Audit Project of the Royal College of Anaesthetists and the Difficult Airway Society. Part 2: intensive care and emergency departments. Br J Anaesth. 2011;106:632–42.
6. De Jong A, Molinari N, Terzi N, et al. Early identification of patients at risk for difficult intubation in the intensive care unit: development and validation of the MACOCHA score in a multicenter cohort study. Am J Respir Crit Care Med. 2013;187:832–9.
7. Higgs A, McGrath BA, Goddard C, et al. Guidelines for the management of tracheal intubation in critically ill adults. Br J Anaesth. 2018;120:323–52.
8. Perbet S, De Jong A, Delmas J, et al. Incidence of and risk factors for severe cardiovascular collapse after endotracheal intubation in the ICU: a multicenter observational study. Crit Care. 2015;19:257.
9. De Jong A, Rolle A, Molinari N, et al. Cardiac arrest and mortality related to intubation procedure in critically ill adult patients: a multicenter cohort study. Crit Care Med. 2018;46:532–9.
10. Halliday SJ, Casey JD, Rice TW, et al. Risk factors for cardiovascular collapse during tracheal intubation of critically iii adults. Ann Am Thorac Soc. 2020;17:1021–4.
11. Janz DR, Semler MW, Joffe AM, et al. A multicenter randomized trial of a checklist for endotracheal intubation of critically ill adults. Chest. 2018;153:816–24.
12. Janz DR, Casey JD, Semler MW, et al. Effect of a fluid bolus on cardiovascular collapse among critically ill adults undergoing tracheal intubation (PrePARE): a randomised controlled trial. Lancet Respir Med. 2019;7:1039–47.
13. Casey JD, Janz DR, Russell DW, et al. Bag-mask ventilation during tracheal intubation of critically ill adults. N Engl J Med. 2019;380:811–21.
14. Kornas RL, Owyang CG, Sakles JC, Foley LJ, Mosier JM. Evaluation and management of the physiologically difficult airway: consensus recommendations from Society for Airway Management. Anesth Analg. 2021;132:395–405.
15. Al-Saadi MA, Heidari B, Donahue KR, Shipman EM, Kinariwala KN, Masud FN. Pre-existing right ventricular dysfunction as an independent risk factor for post intubation cardiac arrest and hemodynamic instability in critically ill patients: a retrospective observational study. J Intensive Care Med. 2023;38:169–78.
16. Russotto V, Tassistro E, Myatra SN, et al. Peri-intubation cardiovascular collapse in patients who are critically ill: insights from the INTUBE study. Am J Respir Crit Care Med. 2022;206:449–58.
17. Heffner AC, Swords D, Kline JA, Jones AE. The frequency and significance of postintubation hypotension during emergency airway management. J Crit Care. 2012;27:e9–13.
18. Heffner AC, Swords DS, Nussbaum ML, Kline JA, Jones AE. Predictors of the complication of postintubation hypotension during emergency airway management. J Crit Care. 2012;27:587–93.

19. Smischney NJ. Predictors of hemodynamic derangement during intubation in the critically ill: a nested case-control study of hemodynamic management - part II. J Crit Care. 2017;42:374.
20. Shafer SL. Shock values. Anesthesiology. 2004;101:567–8.
21. Katz J, Greenberg S. Etomidate is not a first-line induction agent in critically ill patients: primum non nocere-above all, do no harm. Crit Care Med. 2018;46:1495–6.
22. Lynde GC, Jabaley CS. Etomidate is a first-line induction agent in critically ill patients. Crit Care Med. 2018;46:1492–4.
23. Matchett G, Gasanova I, Riccio CA, et al. Etomidate versus ketamine for emergency endotracheal intubation: a randomized clinical trial. Intensive Care Med. 2022;48:78–91.
24. Sprung J, Schuetz SM, Stewart RW, Moravec CS. Effects of ketamine on the contractility of failing and nonfailing human heart muscles in vitro. Anesthesiology. 1998;88:1202–10.
25. Jaber S, Rollé A, Godet T, et al. Effect of the use of an endotracheal tube and stylet versus an endotracheal tube alone on first-attempt intubation success: a multicentre, randomised clinical trial in 999 patients. Intensive Care Med. 2021;47:653–64.
26. Driver BE, Semler MW, Self WH, et al. Effect of use of a bougie vs endotracheal tube with stylet on successful intubation on the first attempt among critically ill patients undergoing tracheal intubation: a randomized clinical trial. JAMA. 2021;326:2488–97.
27. Russell DW, Casey JD, Gibbs KW, et al. Effect of fluid bolus administration on cardiovascular collapse among critically ill patients undergoing tracheal intubation: a randomized clinical trial. JAMA. 2022;328:270–9.
28. Jaber S, Jung B, Corne P, et al. An intervention to decrease complications related to endotracheal intubation in the intensive care unit: a prospective, multiple-center study. Intensive Care Med. 2010;36:248–55.
29. Mosier JM, Hypes CD, Sakles JC. Understanding preoxygenation and apneic oxygenation during intubation in the critically ill. Intensive Care Med. 2017;43:226–8.
30. McKown AC, Casey JD, Russell DW, et al. Risk factors for and prediction of hypoxemia during tracheal intubation of critically ill adults. Ann Am Thorac Soc. 2018;15:1320–7.
31. Mort TC, Waberski BH, Clive J. Extending the preoxygenation period from 4 to 8 mins in critically ill patients undergoing emergency intubation. Crit Care Med. 2009;37:68–71.
32. Baillard C, Fosse JP, Sebbane M, et al. Noninvasive ventilation improves preoxygenation before intubation of hypoxic patients. Am J Respir Crit Care Med. 2006;174:171–7.
33. Baillard C, Prat G, Jung B, et al. Effect of preoxygenation using non-invasive ventilation before intubation on subsequent organ failures in hypoxaemic patients: a randomised clinical trial. Br J Anaesth. 2018;120:361–7.
34. Chaudhuri D, Granton D, Wang DX, et al. Moderate certainty evidence suggests the use of high-flow nasal cannula does not decrease hypoxia when compared with conventional oxygen therapy in the peri-intubation period: results of a systematic review and meta-analysis. Crit Care Med. 2020;48:571–8.
35. Fong KM, Au SY, Ng GWY. Preoxygenation before intubation in adult patients with acute hypoxemic respiratory failure: a network meta-analysis of randomized trials. Crit Care. 2019;23:319.
36. Jhou HJ, Chen PH, Lin C, Yang LY, Lee CH, Peng CK. High-flow nasal cannula therapy as apneic oxygenation during endotracheal intubation in critically ill patients in the intensive care unit: a systematic review and meta-analysis. Sci Rep. 2020;10:3541.
37. Frat JP, Ricard JD, Quenot JP, et al. Non-invasive ventilation versus high-flow nasal cannula oxygen therapy with apnoeic oxygenation for preoxygenation before intubation of patients with acute hypoxaemic respiratory failure: a randomised, multicentre, open-label trial. Lancet Respir Med. 2019;7:303–12.
38. Jaber S, Monnin M, Girard M, et al. Apnoeic oxygenation via high-flow nasal cannula oxygen combined with non-invasive ventilation preoxygenation for intubation in hypoxaemic patients in the intensive care unit: the single-centre, blinded, randomised controlled OPTINIV trial. Intensive Care Med. 2016;42:1877–87.

39. Vaughan EM, Seitz KP, Janz DR, et al. Bag-mask ventilation versus apneic oxygenation during tracheal intubation in critically ill adults: a secondary analysis of 2 randomized trials. J Intensive Care Med. 2022;37:899–907.
40. Mort TC. Emergency tracheal intubation: complications associated with repeated laryngoscopic attempts. Anesth Analg. 2004;99:607–13.
41. Aziz MF, Abrons RO, Cattano D, et al. First-attempt intubation success of video laryngoscopy in patients with anticipated difficult direct laryngoscopy: a multicenter randomized controlled trial comparing the C-MAC D-blade versus the GlideScope in a mixed provider and diverse patient population. Anesth Analg. 2016;122:740–50.
42. Hansel J, Rogers AM, Lewis SR, Cook TM, Smith AF. Videolaryngoscopy versus direct laryngoscopy for adults undergoing tracheal intubation: a Cochrane systematic review and meta-analysis update. Br J Anaesth. 2022;4:CD011136.
43. Arulkumaran N, Lowe J, Ions R, Mendoza M, Bennett V, Dunser MW. Videolaryngoscopy versus direct laryngoscopy for emergency orotracheal intubation outside the operating room: a systematic review and meta-analysis. Br J Anaesth. 2018;120:712–24.
44. Amalric M, Larcher R, Brunot V, et al. Impact of videolaryngoscopy expertise on first-attempt intubation success in critically ill patients. Crit Care Med. 2020;48:e889–e96.
45. Cortellazzi P, Caldiroli D, Byrne A, Sommariva A, Orena EF, Tramacere I. Defining and developing expertise in tracheal intubation using a GlideScope for anaesthetists with expertise in Macintosh direct laryngoscopy: an in-vivo longitudinal study. Anaesthesia. 2015;70:290–5.
46. Lascarrou JB, Boisrame-Helms J, Bailly A, et al. Video laryngoscopy vs direct laryngoscopy on successful first-pass orotracheal intubation among icu patients: a randomized clinical trial. JAMA. 2017;317:483–93.
47. Arriaga AF, Bader AM, Wong JM, et al. Simulation-based trial of surgical-crisis checklists. N Engl J Med. 2013;368:246–53.
48. Corl KA, Dado C, Agarwal A, et al. A modified Montpellier protocol for intubating intensive care unit patients is associated with an increase in first-pass intubation success and fewer complications. J Crit Care. 2018;44:191–5.
49. Turner JS, Bucca AW, Propst SL, et al. Association of checklist use in endotracheal intubation with clinically important outcomes: a systematic review and meta-analysis. JAMA Netw Open. 2020;3:e209278.

# Dyspnea in Patients Receiving Invasive Mechanical Ventilation

# 15

M. Decavèle, C. Bureau, and A. Demoule

## 15.1 Introduction

Over the past decades, attention has increasingly been paid to the detection and management of pain in intensive care unit (ICU) patients. Interestingly, during the same period, very little attention has been paid to dyspnea, which remains significantly under-assessed and under-treated in patients receiving invasive mechanical ventilation. Although sharing many similarities with pain, dyspnea is far worse because of its associated dimension, the fear of dying. Inappropriate ventilator settings, mainly underassist, combined with communication impairment and feelings of loss of control and/or helplessness, are likely to contribute to the onset of serious psychological consequences such as post-traumatic stress disorder (PTSD). Dyspnea should therefore be a major preoccupation for ICU stakeholders, whose mission is not only to treat diseases, but also to relieve unpleasant symptoms and improve comfort.

The aim of the present chapter is to provide information regarding the prevalence and risk factors of dyspnea in patients receiving invasive mechanical ventilation, to depict its relation to ventilator settings, to review the spectrum of its consequences and to highlight the extent of its invisibility and under-evaluation in clinical practice.

M. Decavèle (✉) · C. Bureau · A. Demoule
Sorbonne Université, INSERM, UMRS1158 Neurophysiologie Respiratoire Expérimentale et Clinique, Paris, France

AP-HP, Groupe Hospitalier Universitaire APHP-Sorbonne Université, Site Pitié-Salpêtrière, Service de Médecine Intensive-Réanimation, Paris, France
e-mail: maxens.decavele@aphp.fr



J.-L. Vincent (ed.), *Annual Update in Intensive Care and Emergency Medicine 2023*, Annual Update in Intensive Care and Emergency Medicine,
https://doi.org/10.1007/978-3-031-23005-9_15

## 15.2 Definition, Prevalence and Intensity of Dyspnea

### 15.2.1 Definition

The American Thoracic Society defines dyspnea as "a subjective experience of breathing discomfort that consists of qualitatively distinct sensations that vary in intensity" [1]. The main characteristics of dyspnea sensation are: (1) air hunger, generally associated with increased respiratory drive (hypercapnia) and marked unpleasantness; (2) labored breathing, mostly observed in the case of increased respiratory muscle load; and (3) chest tightness, generally associated with increased bronchial resistance. These three sensations can be observed in endotracheally intubated patients, alone or in combination [2, 3].

Although possibly associated with it, the definition of dyspnea does not include observable signs of respiratory distress (e.g., tachypnea, use of neck muscles, rise in clavicle, chest retractions, or abdominal paradox during inspiration), and the 2012 American Thoracic Society statement strongly emphasizes that, as with other symptoms such as pain, dyspnea *per se* can only be perceived by the person experiencing it. Consequently, to assess dyspnea the clinician first needs to ask patients for the presence or absence of dyspnea by a simple dichotomous trigger question, such as "is your breathing comfortable?", "do you feel breathless?", "are you getting enough air?". Second, if dyspnea is detected, the physician asks the patient to self-report the intensity of dyspnea on a scale (visual analog, numerical, Borg, categorical, or Likert scales) [1].

Dyspnea shares many clinical and neurophysiological features with pain [1, 4]. However, in contrast to pain, dyspnea reflects a critical threat to a vital function, namely breathing. As reported by patients who experience dyspnea, its association with the fear of dying makes dyspnea a much more terrifying experience than pain: "It is a frightened feeling where you don't think you'll get another breath…it is accompanied by fear and panic"; "when the shortness of breath was at its extreme, I thought I was going to die...I did have thoughts about suicide…".

Subsequently, the 2012 definition of dyspnea [1] appears to understate the constant and marked adverse emotional response reported by patients experiencing dyspnea. A more operational definition may describe dyspnea as "an unpleasant and frightening awareness of abnormal breathing".

### 15.2.2 Prevalence and Intensity

In contrast with pain, little attention has been given to the monitoring of dyspnea in patients receiving invasive mechanical ventilation. There are no clinical guidelines in this sense, and available data suggest that dyspnea is not routinely assessed and recorded in most ICUs worldwide. Dyspnea is seemingly listed as the primary or secondary outcome of no more than 50 studies conducted in patients receiving invasive mechanical ventilation. These studies can be classified into: (1) retrospective recall studies (survivors were asked to recall their breathing experience); (2) prospective observational studies; and (3) prospective interventional studies that assessed the impact of ventilator setting modifications on dyspnea (Table 15.1).

**Table 15.1** Relationship between ventilator settings and dyspnea in patients receiving invasive mechanical ventilation

| Ventilator setting that was changed | n | Dyspnea rating scale | Dyspnea intensity (% of full rating scale) | | Study design and main results |
|---|---|---|---|---|---|
| *Pressure support level* | | | | | |
| Vitacca (2004) [5] | 24 | VAS | 25–5: 62<br>5–5: 42 | 15–5: 35<br>0–5: 65 | Explored the effect of different levels of PS-PEEP levels on dyspnea (U-shaped relationship) |
| Schmidt (2011) [2] | 96 | VAS | Baseline: 50 (40–70)<br>Median reduction of 46 after ventilator adjustments | | Ventilator settings (PSV mode switch, increase in PS) alleviated dyspnea in 35% of cases. Dyspnea associated with weaning failure |
| Schmidt (2013) [6] | 12 | VAS | H-LowET: 5<br>H-HighET: 20<br>L-LowET:51<br>L-HighET: 51 | | Compared dyspnea between High (H) and Low (L) pressure support associated with high or low expiratory triggering (ET). Correlation with surface respiratory muscle electromyography |
| Raux (2019) [7] | 12 | VAS | Baseline: 30 (25–40)<br>Increased PS: 0 (0–10) | | Dyspnea assessed before and after increase in PS. Continuous monitoring of EEG |
| Bureau (2021) [8] | 34 | VAS | Baseline: 62 (22–75)<br>Increased PS: 37 (20–55) | | Increase in pressure support (100% increase) relieved clinically significant dyspnea |
| *PEEP* | | | | | |
| Petrof (1990) [9] | 7 | Likert from 0 (no) to +100 (improvement) | PEEP 5: +28 ± 10<br>PEEP 10: +53 ± 8<br>PEEP 15: +48 ± 13 | | Explored the effect of different PEEP levels to reduce intrinsic PEEP load in severe chronic obstructive pulmonary disease patients |
| Vovk (2007) [10] | 6 | VAS | ΔEELV 200 ml: 10% relief<br>ΔEELV 1000 ml: 40% relief | | Increased EELV using PEEP. Increasing EELV by 350 ml relieved air hunger by 10% (healthy volunteers) |
| *Inspiratory flow slope/rate* | | | | | |
| Chiumello (2001) [11] | 10 | mBorg | Lowest: 38<br>High: 27 | Low: 16<br>Highest: 33 | Explored the effect of different inspiratory flow slope levels on dyspnea (U-shaped relationship) |

(continued)

**Table 15.1** (continued)

| Ventilator setting that was changed | n | Dyspnea rating scale | Dyspnea intensity (% of full rating scale) | Study design and main results |
|---|---|---|---|---|
| Manning (1995) [12] | 10 | mVAS (40 cm) | 0.35 l/s: 30<br>0.6–1.2 l/s: 10<br>1.6 l/s: 20 | Explored the effect of different inspiratory flow rates levels on dyspnea (U-shaped relationship) in AVC ventilatory mode (healthy volunteers) |
| *$FiO_2$* | | | | |
| Volta (2006) [13] | 13 | VAS | $FiO_2$ 21%: 68<br>$FiO_2$ 80%: 24 | Dyspnea assessed between different $FiO_2$ levels. Dyspnea correlated with P0.1 ($R^2 = 0.89$) |
| *Tidal volume* | | | | |
| Manning (1992) [14] | 5 | VAS (air hunger) | 600 ml: no-mild dyspnea<br>1200 ml: extreme dyspnea | Explored the effect of tidal volume on dyspnea at constant $PetCO_2$ in quadriplegic patients |

*n* number of patients, *PSV* pressure support ventilation mode, *PS* pressure support, *SBT* spontaneous breathing trial, *PEEP* positive end-expiratory pressure, *VAS* visual analog scale, *NRS* numerical rating scale, *EELV* end-expiratory lung volume, *ΔEELV* variation of EELV, *P0.1* airway occlusion pressure, *SIMV* synchronized intermittent mandatory ventilation, *EEG* electroencephalogram, *$FiO_2$* fraction of inspired oxygen

Among the 16 retrospective recall studies (not all reported here), four [15–18] reported both prevalence and intensity of dyspnea in patients receiving invasive mechanical ventilation (“not enough air” “suffocation” or “choked”), compiling interviews from 548 patients. In these studies, dyspnea affected 33–100% of patients and was rated moderate to severe in 52–92% of cases. However, recall design has major bias, since the ability to recall symptoms is known to depend on depth of sedation during the ICU stay [17], the presence of brain injury, and patient age [19]. In addition, recall can only be elicited in ICU survivors, which induces a potential underestimation of dyspnea in the most severely ill patients, those who will die in the ICU.

Among the 20 observational prospective studies, 8 reported both prevalence and intensity of dyspnea in patients receiving invasive mechanical ventilation, compiling assessments from 1250 patients [2, 3, 20–26]. In these studies, dyspnea affected 34–100% of patients. Patients rated the intensity of dyspnea at between 29% and 63% on a full dyspnea rating scale. In addition to their small sample sizes and single-center design for the vast majority, these studies were largely heterogeneous in term of patients (post-operative, medical, difficult to wean or not, ready to wean or not), scale used to rate dyspnea intensity (visual analog, numerical, modified

Borg, categorical or Likert scales), frequency of assessment (once or repeated), and time point of assessment. Some data suggest that the prevalence and intensity of dyspnea may vary during the ICU stay. In the 24 h following ICU admission, dyspnea affects 50% of patients and is rated at 50% on a full numerical rating scale [26], whereas it concerns 25% of ready-to-wean patients before a spontaneous breathing trial (SBT), rated at 25% on a full scale [25, 27–30]. The most robust data regarding the epidemiology of dyspnea in patients receiving invasive mechanical ventilation have been provided by a recent French observational prospective multicenter cohort study that included 612 patients. In this study, dyspnea was measured as soon as patients were able to communicate (first awakening). Dyspnea was reported by 35% of patients, who rated it at 50 (40–70) mm on a visual analog scale from 0 (no dyspnea) to 100 (worse possible dyspnea) [3]. As a comparison, similar pain ratings constitute a clear and consensual indication for prompt analgesia [31].

## 15.3 Risk Factors for Dyspnea and Relation to Ventilator Settings

### 15.3.1 Pathophysiology of Dyspnea

Extensive reviews of dyspnea pathophysiology can be found elsewhere [e.g., 4]. Briefly, respiratory sensations are integrated and processed in the brain cortex and result from interactions between afferent sensory signals/inputs from numerous receptors (e.g., chemoreceptors, pulmonary stretch receptors and C-fibers, trigeminal nerve sensory branches), and efferent signals from the medullary and cortical centers to the respiratory muscles. It has been proposed that the efferent neural drive to breathe containing the expected sensory consequences (the corollary discharge) is continuously compared within the cortex with the incoming flux of respiratory-related afferents. Dyspnea arises in the event of a mismatch between the expected (corollary discharge) and real (afferent) sensory information carried by the achieved ventilation. According to this neuromechanical uncoupling theory, dyspnea can be seen as an imbalance between the 'demand for breathing and the capacity to satisfy this demand', the latter also depending on respiratory load and ventilatory assistance (Fig. 15.1). Nourishing the sensory cortex with respiratory-related afferents (e.g., high tidal volume, high inspiratory flow rate) has a considerable influence on the mitigation of dyspnea sensation.

One convincing piece of evidence supporting this theory of neuromechanical uncoupling is the occurrence of dyspnea when tidal volume is constrained (decreased capacity/reafferents) in the presence of hypercapnia (increased ventilatory drive/demand) [32]. In this case, the impossibility to increase tidal volume and generate adequate sensory reafferents results in an imbalance in the increase in respiratory drive related to hypercapnia.

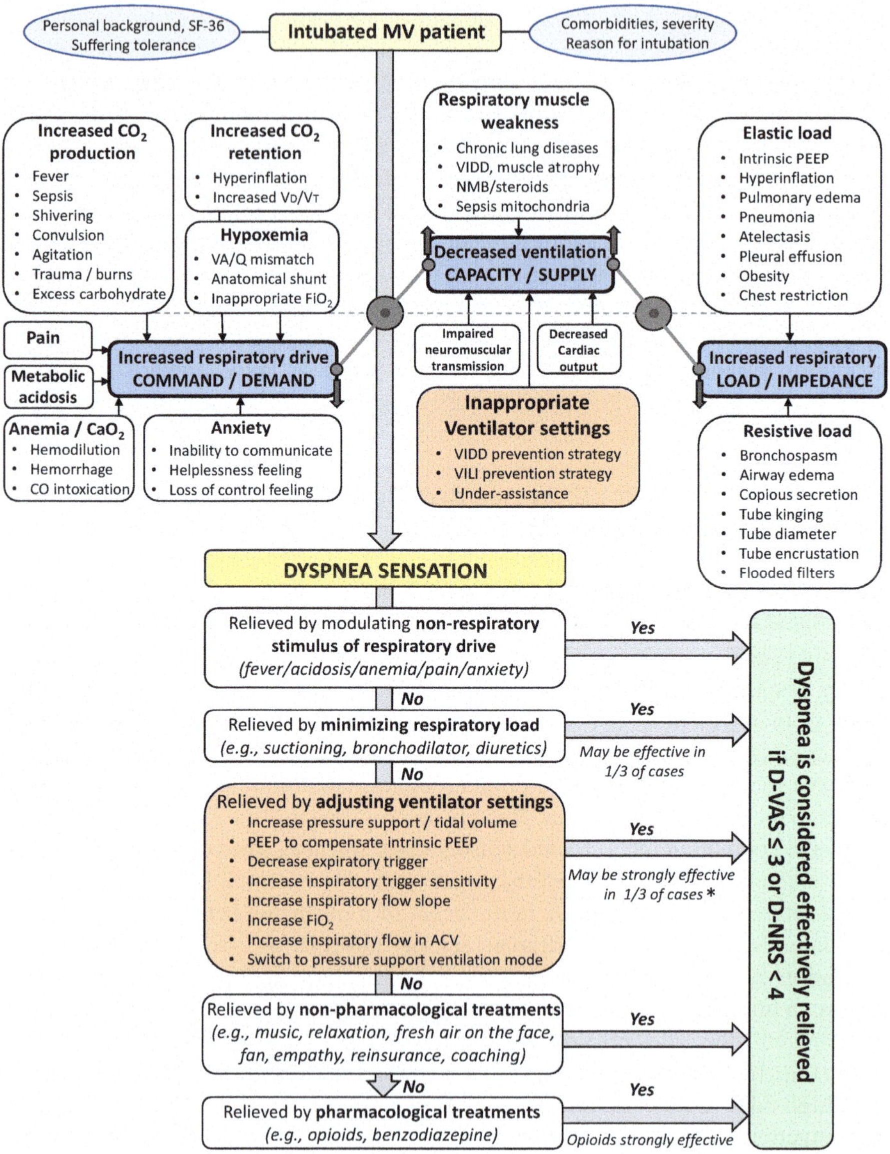


**Fig. 15.1** Pathophysiology of dyspnea in patients receiving invasive mechanical ventilation and how ventilator settings may play a part in both generating and alleviating dyspnea. *MV* mechanically ventilated, $V_D/V_T$ dead volume/tidal volume, *PEEP* positive end-expiratory pressure, *VIDD* ventilator-induced diaphragm dysfunction, *VILI* ventilator-induced lung injury, *CO* carbon monoxide, $Ca\text{-}O_2$ oxygen content of arterial blood, *ACV* assist control ventilation mode, *D-VAS* dyspnea visual analog scale, *D-NRS* dyspnea numerical rating scale, *NMD* neuromuscular blockade, $FiO_2$ fraction of inspired oxygen, $CO_2$ carbon dioxide; *SF-36* short form-36. *Ventilator setting adjustments proposed here do not correspond to all patient-centered situations and must be adapted to each patient

### 15.3.2 Risk Factors Not Related to Ventilator Settings

Factors not related to ventilator settings that are associated with dyspnea in patients receiving invasive mechanical ventilation are health-related quality of life (Short Form-36, mood state) at ICU admission [3], chronic respiratory and heart diseases [3], intubation for a respiratory cause, severity of the acute episode (respiratory and heart rate, severity scores) [3, 26], acidosis (respiratory or metabolic), fever [26], anemia, pain or anxiety [2, 3, 26], and low exposure to opioids during the ICU stay [33]. Altered respiratory mechanics (elevated resistance and low compliance) and altered gas exchange (hypoxemia and hypercapnia) are well-established causes of dyspnea. In addition, healthcare-related activities, such as bed transfers, bathing, and positioning may also contribute to the repetition of dyspnea episodes during the ICU stay. This is also the case for procedures such as ventilator disconnection, tracheal suctioning, and fiberoptic bronchoscopy [22].

### 15.3.3 How Often Do Ventilator Settings Contribute to Dyspnea?

In addition to confirming the prevalence and intensity of dyspnea reported in observational studies, interventional studies that have included changes in ventilator settings provide crucial information regarding the relationship between ventilator settings and dyspnea. Seventeen studies [2, 5–9, 11, 13, 14, 25, 27–30, 34, 35] have prospectively described the variation in dyspnea in response to ventilator setting adjustments in patients receiving invasive mechanical ventilation. Table 15.1 summarizes some of these studies, including two relevant studies in healthy volunteers [10, 12]. In three studies, ventilator setting adjustments were performed with the intention of alleviating dyspnea in dyspneic patients [2, 7, 8]. These three studies show that ventilator setting adjustments alleviate dyspnea in one third of patients, providing stakeholders with a simple opportunity to relieve dyspnea. In the remaining fourteen studies, dyspnea was measured after each change in ventilator settings, irrespective of the presence of dyspnea before ventilator setting adjustments.

The past two decades have seen a paradigm shift from 'how best to mechanically assist a patient's breathing' to 'how to avoid harm'. In this regard, prevailing lung- and diaphragm-protective ventilation (as well as reduced-sedation strategies), likely to induce underassist, may have shifted the respiratory comfort goal of care into the background, and contributed significantly to dyspnea onset in a substantial proportion of patients. Figure 15.1 shows how ventilator settings may play a part in both generating and alleviating dyspnea.

Assist control ventilation mode exposes patients to a fivefold increased risk of experiencing dyspnea [2], especially when inspiratory flow is <40 l/min [2, 12] and tidal volume is low [14]. In this regard, recommended ventilation strategies of low tidal volume are likely to increase the risk of dyspnea onset.

With pressure support ventilation, a 'reasonable' increase in pressure support level is associated with a decrease in dyspnea intensity [2, 6–8]. However, overassist may also induce dyspnea, especially in patients with chronic obstructive pulmonary disease (COPD), due to hyperinflation and ineffective triggering. It has been demonstrated that reducing pressure support or inspiratory duration with a corollary reduction in tidal volume from 10 to 6 ml/kg of predicted body weight eliminated ineffective triggering in two thirds of patients receiving invasive mechanical ventilation without inducing excessive work of breathing [36]; unfortunately, dyspnea was not measured in this study. In any case, additional studies support a U-shaped relationship between the level of assistance, the subsequent tidal volume generated, and dyspnea; when assistance is either too high or too low, respiratory discomfort increases [5, 37] (Fig. 15.2). A similar U-shaped relationship has also been observed

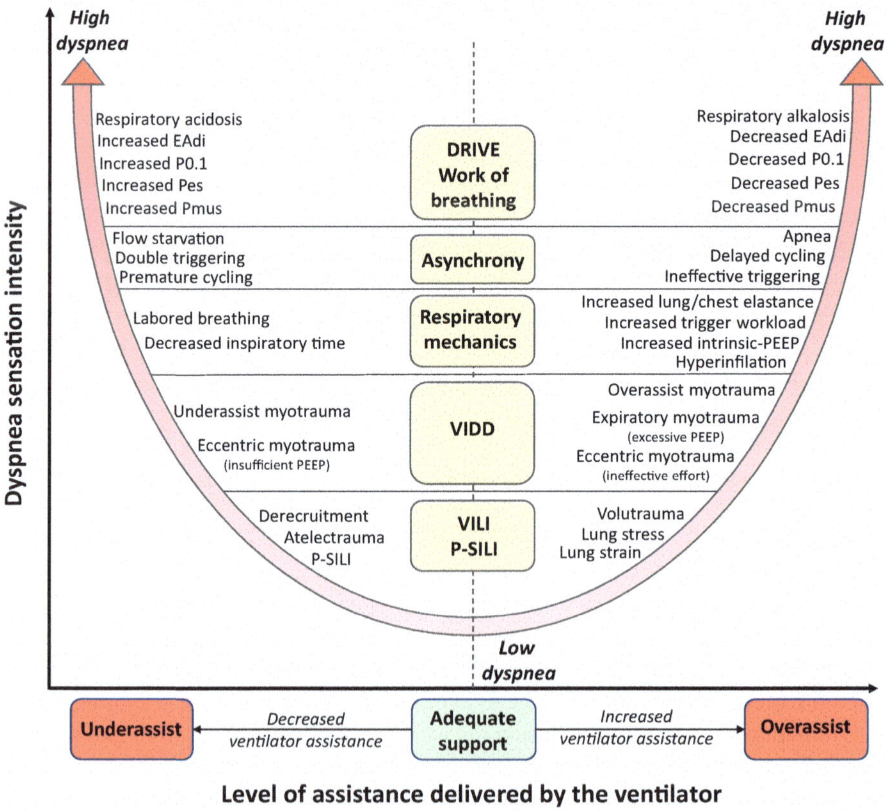


**Fig. 15.2** Relationship between dyspnea sensation and level of ventilatory assistance. Red U-shaped arrow shows that when ventilatory assistance level is either too high or too low, dyspnea intensity may increase [5, 37]. Light pink boxes represent the modifications in drive, patient-ventilator asynchronies, respiratory mechanics, ventilator-induced diaphragm dysfunction (VIDD), and ventilator-induced lung injury (VILI) that could be observed following ventilatory assistance level modification. These should be also considered during the clinical decision-making of ventilator setting adjustments. *PEEP* positive end-expiratory pressure, *P-SILI* patient self-inflicted lung injury, *EAdi* diaphragm electrical activity, *P0.1* airway occlusion pressure, *Pmus* the pressure generated by the respiratory muscles to inflate both the lung and the chest wall, *Pes* inspiratory swing in esophageal pressure

between dyspnea and the inspiratory flow slope in pressure support ventilation mode [11]. Decreasing cycling-off in patients with increased respiratory elastance (obesity, pulmonary fibrosis) increases inspiratory time, which in turn reduces inspiratory muscle workload and reduces double triggering, a patient-ventilator asynchrony. Combined with increase in pressure support, decreasing cycling-off contributes to the reduction of dyspnea in patients receiving invasive mechanical ventilation [6].

No data have specifically investigated the relationship between dyspnea and inspiratory trigger sensitivity in patients receiving invasive mechanical ventilation. Of note, ventilator setting adjustments aimed at reducing dyspnea in these patients generally involved a substantial increase in inspiratory trigger sensitivity [2, 7, 8].

Positive-end expiratory pressure (PEEP) adjustments may also reduce dyspnea by offsetting respiratory load generated by intrinsic PEEP [9] and increasing end-expiratory lung volume [10], which stimulates pulmonary stretch receptors.

Although $PaCO_2$ remains the main determinant of central respiratory drive, a study of 13 patients receiving pressure support invasive mechanical ventilation demonstrated that increasing $FiO_2$ (even generating hyperoxemia) was very effective in reducing dyspnea, which was in turn positively correlated to the reduction in respiratory drive (airway occlusion pressure [P0.1], $R^2 = 0.89$ with dyspnea) [13]. Considering the possible negative effects of hyperoxemia on outcomes, this should at least encourage healthcare professionals not to minimize the influence of hypoxemia in the genesis of dyspnea.

A major limitation of interventional studies that have investigated the impact of ventilator setting adjustments on dyspnea relief is that each change is generally part of a care bundle made up of multiple and various adjustments. Consequently, it is extremely difficult to isolate the respective effect of each ventilator setting change. Only a few interventional studies changed only one independent dyspnea driver while keeping the others constant [14]. For example, increasing the pressure support level may increase tidal volume, a stimulus for pulmonary stretch receptors, and also decrease $PaCO_2$, a stimulus for chemoreceptors.

The ideal dose of ventilatory support during pressure support ventilation in general is unknown, and when a decision is made to relieve dyspnea in patients receiving invasive mechanical ventilation, a balance between dyspnea relief and the potential harmful effects of ventilator overassist should be considered to gain a better understanding of personalized ventilation (Fig. 15.2).

## 15.4 Clinical Consequences of Dyspnea in Patients Receiving Invasive Mechanical Ventilation

There is growing evidence suggesting that dyspnea may have a deleterious impact on the outcome of patients receiving invasive mechanical ventilation. The consequences of dyspnea may occur either immediately during the ICU stay or be delayed.

### 15.4.1 Immediate Fear and Panic Related to Dyspnea

When questioned 2–48 months after ICU discharge, one half of patients who had been mechanically ventilated during their ICU stay reported having experienced anxiety, fear, panic, or insecurity during mechanical ventilation [16, 19, 38]. The interplay between anxiety and dyspnea is complex, and causal relationships may exist in both directions, suggesting that anxiety-relieving interventions may also have positive effects on dyspnea. In a prospective study of 171 ICU patients (only 34% of whom were receiving invasive mechanical ventilation), dyspnea was rated as the most distressing symptom encountered during the ICU stay [22]. A significant association is observed between dyspnea and anxiety in patients receiving invasive mechanical ventilation [2, 3, 26, 28], with a Spearman correlation coefficient of about 0.60. In a study of 612 patients receiving invasive mechanical ventilation, the prevalence of anxiety was higher among dyspneic patients than among non-dyspneic patients (72% vs. 26%, $p < 0.001$) [3]. In another study, dyspnea was independently associated with anxiety in multivariate analysis (odds ratio [OR] 8.84, 95% confidence interval [CI] 3.26–24.0, $p < 0.001$) and ventilator setting adjustments that effectively reduced dyspnea also reduced anxiety [2].

### 15.4.2 Impact of Dyspnea on Weaning

Nine studies have evaluated the relationship between dyspnea and weaning outcome. Dyspnea was measured during a SBT [23, 27–29, 34, 39, 40] or not [2, 41]. Among these studies, a significant association was observed between dyspnea and SBT failure [27, 29, 34], extubation failure [28, 41], and time from SBT to successful extubation [2, 23]. Whether dyspnea is the cause of weaning failure or simply an indicator of weaning failure remains unknown.

### 15.4.3 Association Between Dyspnea and Mortality

Although dyspnea is strongly and independently associated with mortality in various populations [42], the association between dyspnea and mortality in patients receiving invasive mechanical ventilation remains unclear [2, 3, 23]. Of note, in patients receiving non-invasive ventilation for the treatment of acute respiratory failure, the persistence of dyspnea after the first non-invasive ventilation session was independently associated with mortality [43].

### 15.4.4 Delayed Psychological Consequences, Post-traumatic Stress Disorder

Within the months following an ICU stay, PTSD affects approximately 15% of patients. Mechanical ventilation seems to play an important role in the pathogenesis of PTSD, since PTSD is associated with the duration of mechanical ventilation [44], the length of ICU stay [45], and the recall and repetition of experiencing traumatic events, including dyspnea, while being ventilated [17, 38]. In a prospective multicenter study on 612 patients receiving invasive mechanical ventilation, among the 153 patients interviewed on day 90 after ICU discharge, the proportion of patients with probable PTSD was higher among patients who self-reported dyspnea (at first awakening) than among those who did not report dyspnea (29% vs. 13%, p = 0.017). The cumulative incidence of dyspnea (number of episodes of dyspnea between inclusion and the end of mechanical ventilation) and the density of dyspnea (cumulative incidence of dyspnea divided by the number of days from inclusion to the end of invasive mechanical ventilation) were independently associated with probable PTSD [3]. It is not surprising to see such an association between dyspnea and trauma, since dyspnea during invasive mechanical ventilation shares at least three common circumstances observed during trauma [46], which are: (1) intense fear of dying as discussed above; (2) unpredictability; "The breathlessness may come to me at any time", "Sometimes, I had a feeling that it was coming, but, most of the time it was unpredictable" [47]; and (3) powerlessness/lack of control since patients cannot escape from or modulate the source of dyspnea (the ventilator) and are frequently unable to communicate their suffering to their stakeholders—"I had the feeling that I was trapped" [48].

In light of these data, addressing dyspnea in patients receiving invasive mechanical ventilation should be an important aspect of routine practice. However, to be addressed, dyspnea must be detected and measured.

## 15.5 Underestimation of Dyspnea in Patients Receiving Invasive Mechanical Ventilation

### 15.5.1 Patients Are Not Asked

There are a number of data suggesting that patients receiving invasive mechanical ventilation are not routinely asked about their dyspnea. First, compared with pain, the lack of guidelines and the small number of publications on dyspnea in patients receiving invasive mechanical ventilation explain the low level of academic and clinical interest in dyspnea. Second, very few centers report systematically assessing dyspnea in patients [42]. Third, the main questionnaires on the perception of stressors by ICU patients, such as the Intensive Care Unit Environmental Stressor Scale or the Intensive Care Experience questionnaire, do not include assessment of dyspnea. Fourth, clinical trials that aimed to improve the comfort of patients receiving invasive mechanical ventilation did not include dyspnea relief among the various interventions that were evaluated [49]. Fifth, there is no well-validated dyspnea observation scale, compared with the pain observation scale [26].

Patients receiving invasive mechanical ventilation cannot easily self-report their symptoms, which could be a reason why stakeholders do not search for dyspnea on a regular basis. However, the inability to communicate does not mean that patients do not actually experience dyspnea.

### 15.5.2 Discrepancies Between Patient Self-Reporting and Stakeholders' Observations

Unfortunately, stakeholders cannot reliably predict dyspnea in patients. Three studies in the ICU setting reported a serious discrepancy between the perception of dyspnea by the patient and the estimation of dyspnea by the stakeholder [23, 24, 50]. In addition, when nurses were detecting dyspnea, it was not followed by a therapeutic intervention, whereas pain detection was often associated with opioid delivery [24].

## 15.6 Conclusion

There is an increasing body of data showing that dyspnea is one of the most common and distressing experiences in patients receiving invasive mechanical ventilation. Worse than pain, the unquenchable thirst for air summons up an existential fear of dying, which, if repeated during the ICU stay, exposes patients to PTSD. The past two decades have seen a paradigm shift from 'how best to mechanically assist a patient's breathing' to 'how to avoid harm'. In this regard, prevailing lung- and diaphragm-protective ventilation (as well as reduced sedation strategies), likely to induce underassist, may have shifted the respiratory comfort goal of care into the background, and contributed significantly to dyspnea onset in a substantial proportion of patients. The decision to increase ventilator assistance is challenging and should consider the time-point of the patient during the ICU (acute or recovering status) and the potential harmful effects of overassist. On the other hand, leaving a patient dyspneic despite the existence of simple and efficient means of relief (e.g., ventilator settings) raises an ethical care question. As with pain, dyspnea should be listed among the symptoms to be routinely assessed, and dyspnea self-reporting should be elicited from patients receiving invasive mechanical ventilation as soon as possible during the ICU stay. Further studies should determine the feasibility and efficacy of strategies designed to minimize dyspnea, ranging from improved ventilation strategies to pharmacological and non-pharmacological interventions.

## References

1. Parshall MB, Schwartzstein RM, Adams L, et al. An official American Thoracic Society statement: update on the mechanisms, assessment, and management of dyspnea. Am J Respir Crit Care Med. 2012;185:435–52.
2. Schmidt M, Demoule A, Polito A, et al. Dyspnea in mechanically ventilated critically ill patients. Crit Care Med. 2011;39:2059–65.
3. Demoule A, Hajage D, Messika J, et al. Prevalence, intensity and clinical impact of dyspnea in critically ill patients receiving invasive ventilation. Am J Respir Crit Care Med. 2022;205:917–26.
4. Lansing RW, Gracely RH, Banzett RB. The multiple dimensions of dyspnea: review and hypotheses. Respir Physiol Neurobiol. 2009;167:53–60.

5. Vitacca M, Bianchi L, Zanotti E, et al. Assessment of physiologic variables and subjective comfort under different levels of pressure support ventilation. Chest. 2004;126:851–9.
6. Schmidt M, Kindler F, Gottfried SB, et al. Dyspnea and surface inspiratory electromyograms in mechanically ventilated patients. Intensive Care Med. 2013;39:1368–76.
7. Raux M, Navarro-Sune X, Wattiez N, et al. Adjusting ventilator settings to relieve dyspnoea modifies brain activity in critically ill patients: an electroencephalogram pilot study. Sci Rep. 2019;9:16572.
8. Bureau C, Decavèle M, Campion S, et al. Proportional assist ventilation relieves clinically significant dyspnea in critically ill ventilated patients. Ann Intensive Care. 2021;11:177.
9. Petrof BJ, Legaré M, Goldberg P, Milic-Emili J, Gottfried SB. Continuous positive airway pressure reduces work of breathing and dyspnea during weaning from mechanical ventilation in severe chronic obstructive pulmonary disease. Am Rev Respir Dis. 1990;141:281–9.
10. Vovk A, Binks AP. Raising end-expiratory volume relieves air hunger in mechanically ventilated healthy adults. J Appl Physiol. 2007;103:8.
11. Chiumello D, Pelosi P, Croci M, Bigatello LM, Gattinoni L. The effects of pressurization rate on breathing pattern, work of breathing, gas exchange and patient comfort in pressure support ventilation. Eur Respir J. 2001;18:107–14.
12. Manning HL, Molinary EJ, Leiter JC. Effect of inspiratory flow rate on respiratory sensation and pattern of breathing. Am J Respir Crit Care Med. 1995;151:751–7.
13. Volta CA, Alvisi V, Bertacchini S, et al. Acute effects of hyperoxemia on dyspnoea and respiratory variables during pressure support ventilation. Intensive Care Med. 2006;32:223–9.
14. Manning HL, Shea SA, Schwartzstein RM, Lansing RW, Brown R, Banzett RB. Reduced tidal volume increases 'air hunger' at fixed PCO2 in ventilated quadriplegics. Respir Physiol. 1992;90:19–30.
15. Pennock BE, Crawshaw L, Maher T, Price T, Kaplan PD. Distressful events in the ICU as perceived by patients recovering from coronary artery bypass surgery. Heart Lung. 1994;23:323–7.
16. Rotondi AJ, Chelluri L, Sirio C, et al. Patients' recollections of stressful experiences while receiving prolonged mechanical ventilation in an intensive care unit. Crit Care Med. 2002;30:746–52.
17. Samuelson KAM, Lundberg D, Fridlund B. Stressful memories and psychological distress in adult mechanically ventilated intensive care patients - a 2-month follow-up study. Acta Anaesthesiol Scand. 2007;51:671–8.
18. Khalaila R, Zbidat W, Anwar K, Bayya A, Linton DM, Sviri S. Communication difficulties and psychoemotional distress in patients receiving mechanical ventilation. Am J Crit Care. 2011;20:470–9.
19. Bergbom-Engberg I, Haljamäe H. Assessment of patients' experience of discomforts during respirator therapy. Crit Care Med. 1989;17:1068–72.
20. Powers J, Bennett SJ. Measurement of dyspnea in patients treated with mechanical ventilation. Am J Crit Care. 1999;8:254–61.
21. Li DT, Puntillo K. A pilot study on coexisting symptoms in intensive care patients. Appl Nurs Res. 2006;19:216–9.
22. Puntillo KA, Arai S, Cohen NH, et al. Symptoms experienced by intensive care unit patients at high risk of dying. Crit Care Med. 2010;38:2155–60.
23. Haugdahl HS, Storli SL, Meland B, Dybwik K, Romild U, Klepstad P. Underestimation of patient breathlessness by nurses and physicians during a spontaneous breathing trial. Am J Respir Crit Care Med. 2015;192:1440–8.
24. Gentzler ER, Derry H, Ouyang DJ, et al. Underdetection and undertreatment of dyspnea in critically ill patients. Am J Respir Crit Care Med. 2019;199:1377–84.
25. Nelson JE, Meier DE, Litke A, Natale DA, Siegel RE, Morrison RS. The symptom burden of chronic critical illness. Crit Care Med. 2004;32:1527–34.
26. Persichini R, Gay F, Schmidt M, et al. Diagnostic accuracy of respiratory distress observation scales as surrogates of dyspnea self-report in intensive care unit patients. Anesthesiology. 2015;123:830–7.

27. Chen Y-J, Hwang S-L, Li C-R, et al. Vagal withdrawal and psychological distress during ventilator weaning and the related outcomes. J Psychosom Res. 2017;101:10–6.
28. Knebel AR, Janson-Bjerklie SL, Malley JD, Wilson AG, Marini JJ. Comparison of breathing comfort during weaning with two ventilatory modes. Am J Respir Crit Care Med. 1994;149:14–8.
29. Bureau C, Dres M, Morawiec E, et al. Dyspnea and the electromyographic activity of inspiratory muscles during weaning from mechanical ventilation. Ann Intensive Care. 2022;12:50.
30. Leung P, Jubran A, Tobin MJ. Comparison of assisted ventilator modes on triggering, patient effort, and dyspnea. Am J Respir Crit Care Med. 1997;155:1940–8.
31. Devlin JW, Skrobik Y, Gélinas C, et al. Clinical practice guidelines for the prevention and management of pain, agitation/sedation, delirium, immobility, and sleep disruption in adult patients in the ICU. Crit Care Med. 2018;46:e825–73.
32. Banzett RB, Lansing RW, Brown R, et al. "Air hunger" from increased PCO2 persists after complete neuromuscular block in humans. Respir Physiol. 1990;81:1–17.
33. Decavèle M, Rivals I, Persichini R, et al. Prognostic value of the intensive care respiratory distress observation scale on ICU admission. Respir Care. 2022;67:823–32.
34. Stroetz RW, Hubmayr RD. Tidal volume maintenance during weaning with pressure support. Am J Respir Crit Care Med. 1995;152:1034–40.
35. Vitacca M, Ambrosino N, Clini E, et al. Physiological response to pressure support ventilation delivered before and after extubation in patients not capable of totally spontaneous autonomous breathing. Am J Respir Crit Care Med. 2001;164:638–41.
36. Thille AW, Cabello B, Galia F, Lyazidi A, Brochard L. Reduction of patient-ventilator asynchrony by reducing tidal volume during pressure-support ventilation. Intensive Care Med. 2008;34:1477–86.
37. Mols G, Vetter T, Haberthür C, Geiger K, Guttmann J. Breathing pattern and perception at different levels of volume assist and pressure support in volunteers. Crit Care Med. 2001;29:982–8.
38. Schelling G, Stoll C, Haller M, et al. Health-related quality of life and posttraumatic stress disorder in survivors of the acute respiratory distress syndrome. Crit Care Med. 1998;26:651–9.
39. Wysocki M, Cracco C, Teixeira A, et al. Reduced breathing variability as a predictor of unsuccessful patient separation from mechanical ventilation. Crit Care Med. 2006;34:2076–83.
40. Twibell R, Siela D, Mahmoodi M. Subjective perceptions and physiological variables during weaning from mechanical ventilation. Am J Crit Care. 2003;12:101–12.
41. Moody LE, Lowry L, Yarandi H, Voss A. Psychophysiologic predictors of weaning from mechanical ventilation in chronic bronchitis and emphysema. Clin Nurs Res. 1997;6:311–30, discussion 330–3.
42. Stevens JP, Dechen T, Schwartzstein RM, O'Donnell CR, Baker K, Banzett RB. Association of dyspnoea, mortality and resource use in hospitalised patients. Eur Respir J. 2021;58:1902107.
43. Dangers L, Montlahuc C, Kouatchet A, et al. Dyspnoea in patients receiving noninvasive ventilation for acute respiratory failure: prevalence, risk factors and prognostic impact: a prospective observational study. Eur Respir J. 2018;52:1702637.
44. Cuthbertson BH, Hull A, Strachan M, Scott J. Post-traumatic stress disorder after critical illness requiring general intensive care. Intensive Care Med. 2004;30:450–5.
45. Davydow DS, Zatzick D, Hough CL, Katon WJ. A longitudinal investigation of posttraumatic stress and depressive symptoms over the course of the year following medical-surgical intensive care unit admission. Gen Hosp Psychiatry. 2013;35:226–32.
46. Başoğlu M. Effective management of breathlessness: a review of potential human rights issues. Eur Respir J. 2017;49:1602099.
47. Shih FJ, Chu SH. Comparisons of American-Chinese and Taiwanese patients' perceptions of dyspnea and helpful nursing actions during the intensive care unit transition from cardiac surgery. Heart Lung. 1999;28:41–54.

48. Iosifyan M, Schmidt M, Hurbault A, et al. "I had the feeling that I was trapped": a bedside qualitative study of cognitive and affective attitudes toward noninvasive ventilation in patients with acute respiratory failure. Ann Intensive Care. 2019;9:134.
49. Kalfon P, Baumstarck K, Estagnasie P, et al. A tailored multicomponent program to reduce discomfort in critically ill patients: a cluster-randomized controlled trial. Intensive Care Med. 2017;43:1829–40.
50. Binks AP, Desjardin S, Riker R. ICU clinicians underestimate breathing discomfort in ventilated subjects. Respir Care. 2017;62:150–5.

# The Potential Risks of Pressure Support Ventilation

# 16

A. Proklou, V. Karageorgos, and K. Vaporidi

## 16.1 Introduction

Pressure support ventilation (PSV) is a mode of assisted ventilation in which all breaths are triggered by the patient and the ventilator, when triggered, provides a constant level of pressure. PSV was first introduced in the early 1980s as a weaning mode. Nowadays, PSV is the most commonly used mode of assisted ventilation, not only during weaning, but also, increasingly, in the acute phase of critical illness [1]. Setting the ventilator in pressure support mode may appear to be easy, as selecting a level of support to achieve a tidal volume of about 6–8 ml/kg will often result in a stable breathing pattern, and arterial blood gasses within the target range. The aim in this chapter is to illustrate that, despite this apparent convenience, PSV conceals significant risks.

## 16.2 Principles of Operation of Pressure Support Ventilation

In PSV, a pre-adjusted, fixed pressure is applied to each patient's breathing effort that is recognized by the ventilator. To further understand how this mode of ventilation actually works we will analyze it in three phases: triggering, pressurization, and

A. Proklou
Department of Intensive Care, University Hospital of Heraklion, Heraklion, Crete, Greece

V. Karageorgos
Department of Anesthesiology, University Hospital of Heraklion, Heraklion, Crete, Greece

K. Vaporidi (✉)
Department of Intensive Care, University Hospital of Heraklion, Heraklion, Crete, Greece

University of Crete, School of Medicine, Heraklion, Crete, Greece
e-mail: vaporidi@uoc.gr



J.-L. Vincent (ed.), *Annual Update in Intensive Care and Emergency Medicine 2023*,
Annual Update in Intensive Care and Emergency Medicine,
https://doi.org/10.1007/978-3-031-23005-9_16

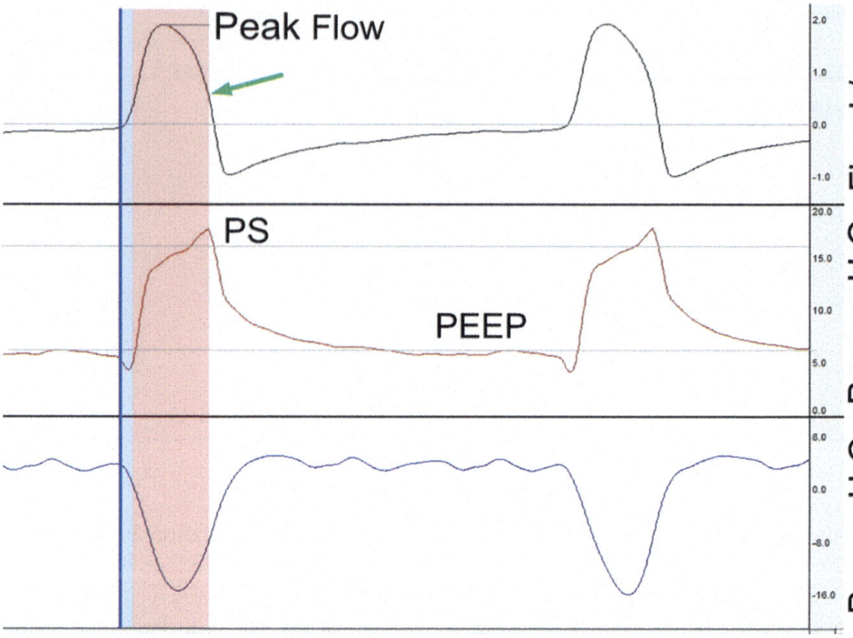


**Fig. 16.1** Triggering, pressurization, and cycling-off phases during pressure support (PS) ventilation. The blue line indicates the beginning of neural inspiration, and the blue shaded area the triggering phase, which is followed by the pressurization phase (red shaded area). The beginning of the expiratory phase is signaled by the cycling-off criterion (green arrow) as a drop of flow to the user-set percentage of its peak value. *Paw* airway pressure, *Pes* esophageal pressure

cycling-off (Fig. 16.1). Triggering is the initial phase of the ventilatory cycle, when the patient's breathing effort is detected by a pressure or flow sensor of the ventilator. The change in pressure or flow that triggers the inspiration is termed trigger sensitivity, and is set by the operator. The response time of the sensor, that is the interval between the initiation of patient effort and the beginning of the pressurization phase, is termed triggering delay; this response time varies between 50 and 250 ms, and depends on the characteristics of the ventilator and the patient's effort [2, 3]. It is important to acknowledge that a fraction varying between 1 and 10% of a patient's effort is consumed for triggering [3], and it may be much greater in patients with dynamic hyperinflation [4].

During the pressurization phase, the preset pressure support is applied throughout the mechanical inspiratory time. The ventilator, by a servo regulatory mechanism, provides the inspiratory flow required to maintain the set level of pressure support, until the cycling-off criterion is met. During the pressurization phase, the pressure available for inspiratory flow (V′) and volume (V) generation is the sum of the pressure generated by the patient's muscles (Pmus) and the set level of pressure support provided by the ventilator (Pvent): Pmus + Pvent = V′ x R + V x E (where R and E are the resistance and elastance of the respiratory system respectively).

The pressurization phase is followed by the cycling-off phase, controlling the end of mechanical inspiration and beginning of expiration, and determined by cycling-off criteria. When the patient's effort ends, muscle pressure becomes zero, leading to a decrease in inspiratory flow. The most commonly used cycling-off criterion in PSV is the decrease in inspiratory flow to an operator-selected percentage of peak inspiratory flow (usually 25% of peak flow). Most ventilators include alternative cycling-off criteria for safety purposes, such as a decrease of inspiratory flow to an absolute value, usually between 2 and 6 l/min, an increase in pressure by 1–3 $cmH_2O$ above the set level of pressure (usually caused by the abrupt relaxation of inspiratory muscles) [5], or a set duration of mechanical inspiratory time (Ti; usually greater than 2 s). The commonly used cycling-off criterion, that is the decrease in inspiratory flow to a fixed percentage of its peak value, results in a mechanical Ti that is dependent not only on the duration of the patient's effort (neural Ti), but also on the magnitude of effort, the set level of pressure support, and the respiratory system mechanics, because all these variables affect peak inspiratory flow.

The tidal volume delivered in each breath assisted with PSV, as indicated by the equation of motion, is determined by the patient effort (Pmus), the set level of pressure provided by the ventilator (Pvent), the inspiratory time (as determined by the cycling-off criterion), and the respiratory system mechanics. Two important aspects on how PSV affects tidal volume should be acknowledged. First, not all of a patient's effort contributes to generation of inspiratory flow and tidal volume (Pmus in the equation of motion), but only the part that occurs during the mechanical Ti. The effort to trigger the ventilator, as well as any effort continued after the opening of the exhalation valve (in cases of premature cycling-off, detailed below) is wasted, and does not contribute to generation of tidal volume. Second, during PSV the ventilator provides a minimum tidal volume ($V_{Tmin}$) that is delivered without any patient effort (after triggering), and depends, similar to a pressure control mode, on the set level of inspiratory pressure, the Ti (determined by the cycling-off criterion), and the respiratory system mechanics (Fig. 16.2). The greater the level of pressure support and the lower the values of E and R (normal mechanics), the higher is the resulting $V_{Tmin}$. An increase above this $V_{Tmin}$, if the patient's ventilatory demands increase, can be achieved solely by an increase in patient effort. The magnitude of increase in tidal volume (above $V_{Tmin}$) depends on the patient's effort and respiratory system mechanics. A decrease in patient effort, in response to decreased ventilatory demands, as long as it triggers the ventilator, will not decrease tidal volume below the $V_{Tmin}$.

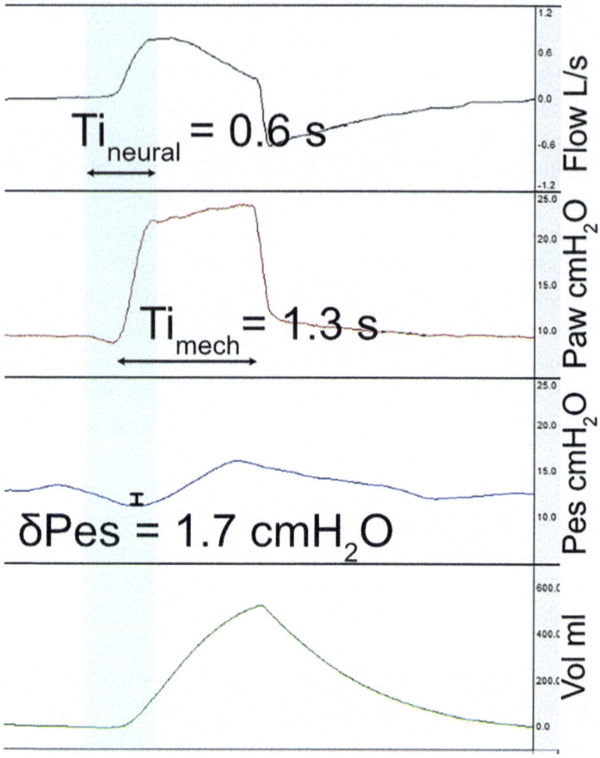


**Fig. 16.2** Minimum tidal volume ($V_{Tmin}$): The shaded area highlights a weak inspiratory effort, ending just 0.3 s after the initiation of the pressurization phase, which creates a sufficient flow due to the high pressure support level (14 $cmH_2O$), and resulting long mechanical inspiratory time (Ti), to achieve a tidal volume of 530 ml. This 530 ml is, in this case, the $V_{Tmin}$, delivered with almost no patient effort during pressure support ventilation. *Paw* airway pressure, *Pes* esophageal pressure

## 16.3 Respiratory Drive, Rate and Effort During Pressure Support Ventilation

Respiratory drive is defined as the intensity of the output by the respiratory centers which determines the effort per breath. The respiratory center output is shaped after the integration of signals from central and peripheral chemoreceptors, sensing changes in arterial blood gases, but also from stretch and irritant receptors in the lungs, and from several cortical afferents, modulating ventilation in response to sensory stimuli. In critically ill patients receiving mechanical ventilation, the chemical feedback (regulation of arterial $CO_2$, $PaCO_2$) is a main determinant of respiratory drive. The eupneic $PaCO_2$, that is the $PaCO_2$ at steady state 'desired' by the respiratory center, is determined by the intersection of two curves: the metabolic hyperbola and the $CO_2$-response curve (Fig. 16.3). The metabolic hyperbola

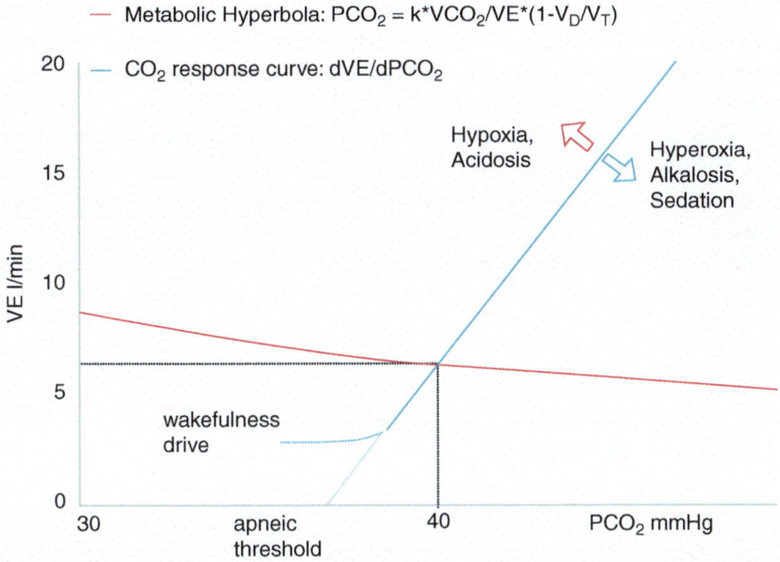


**Fig. 16.3** Graphical representation of the metabolic hyperbola (red) and the $CO_2$-response curve (blue). Their intercept indicates the steady-state $PaCO_2$, while the x-intercept of the $CO_2$-response curve indicates the apneic threshold. $V_T$ tidal volume, *VE* minute ventilation

describes $PaCO_2$ as a function of minute ventilation (VE), while the $CO_2$-response curve describes VE as a function of $PaCO_2$. The $CO_2$-response curve is linear (over the clinically relevant range) and is characterized by its slope and x-intercept. The slope, described as 'chemosensitivity', is affected by $PaO_2$, pH, and sedation. The x-intercept, is referred to as 'apneic threshold', the $PaCO_2$ level below which apnea occurs, and is normally present only during sleep (or sedation). In awake individuals below the resting $PaCO_2$, the slope of the $CO_2$-response curve becomes almost horizontal at a minimum level of ventilation, maintained despite hypocapnia (known as wakefulness drive to breathe). Similarly to chemosensitivity, the apneic threshold and minimum ventilation vary among individuals, and are affected by $PaO_2$, pH, and sedation. A change in $PaCO_2$ triggers a change in ventilation that tends to return the $PaCO_2$ levels to the steady state.

Normally the changes in ventilation are primarily achieved through changes in effort and thus tidal volume, and to a lesser extent by changes in breathing frequency. Nonetheless, in the presence of an increase in ventilatory demands, when further increase in tidal volume is limited, such as when respiratory system compliance is decreased (e.g., near total lung capacity), or in the presence of inspiratory muscle weakness, breathing frequency may increase disproportionately to tidal volume. Importantly, when ventilatory demands decrease, respiratory rate changes only minimally (10–20%), contrary to a much greater change in effort per breath

[6–8]. Several risks associated with the use of PSV are linked to this 'insensitivity' of respiratory rate to decreasing ventilatory demands.

Assisted ventilation using PSV affects the ventilatory responses and thus modifies the patient's respiratory drive and effort (Fig. 16.3). The increase in tidal volume and thus minute ventilation for a given patient effort by pressure support decreases $PaCO_2$. A patient with respiratory failure and distress may be relieved by this decrease in $PaCO_2$. Yet, if the level of pressure support is such that the increase in ventilation decreases $PaCO_2$ more than that desired by the respiratory centers (due to the insensitivity of respiratory rate to decreasing demands), the patient's effort will decrease, and if $PaCO_2$ decreases below the apneic threshold, the patient will develop apneas and periodic breathing.

## 16.4 Patient-Ventilator Interaction During Pressure Support Ventilation

Optimizing patient-ventilator interaction aiming to achieve the goals of lung- and diaphragm-protective ventilation can be challenging during PSV due to the inherent limitations of the mode. Understanding the potential risks of sub-optimal patient-ventilator interaction during PSV can facilitate prompt recognition and management.

### 16.4.1 Risk of Periodic Breathing

Periodic breathing includes a spectrum of respiratory patterns with the common feature of repeated ventilatory oscillations of central apneas/hypopneas with alternating periods of deeper and faster breaths [9]. First described by Cheyne and Stokes in the nineteenth century in patients with heart failure, periodic breathing has been described in neonates, at high altitude, in patients with pulmonary hypertension, and in patients on mechanical ventilation. The common pathogenic mechanism in all these conditions is destabilization of the control-of-breathing system. PSV can induce periodic breathing even in healthy subjects [10]. Relatively high levels of pressure support may decrease $PaCO_2$ below that desired by the respiratory center, or even below the apneic threshold, resulting in a decrease in inspiratory effort (hypopnea) or central apnea [10]. Apnea (or hypopnea) will result in an increase in $PaCO_2$ and recurrence of respiratory effort. Patients with predisposing factors for periodic breathing, such as heart failure, are more prone to the occurrence of periodic breathing during mechanical ventilation [11]. Characteristic ventilator waveforms in cases of periodic breathing are shown in Fig. 16.4. Periodic breathing adversely affects the cardiovascular system and disrupts patients' sleep [9]. Additionally, if not promptly recognized, central apneas may be considered an indication for controlled mechanical ventilation, thereby unduly delaying the weaning process. The management of periodic breathing phenomena during PSV is relatively easy once recognized, as all that is required is a reduction in the level of

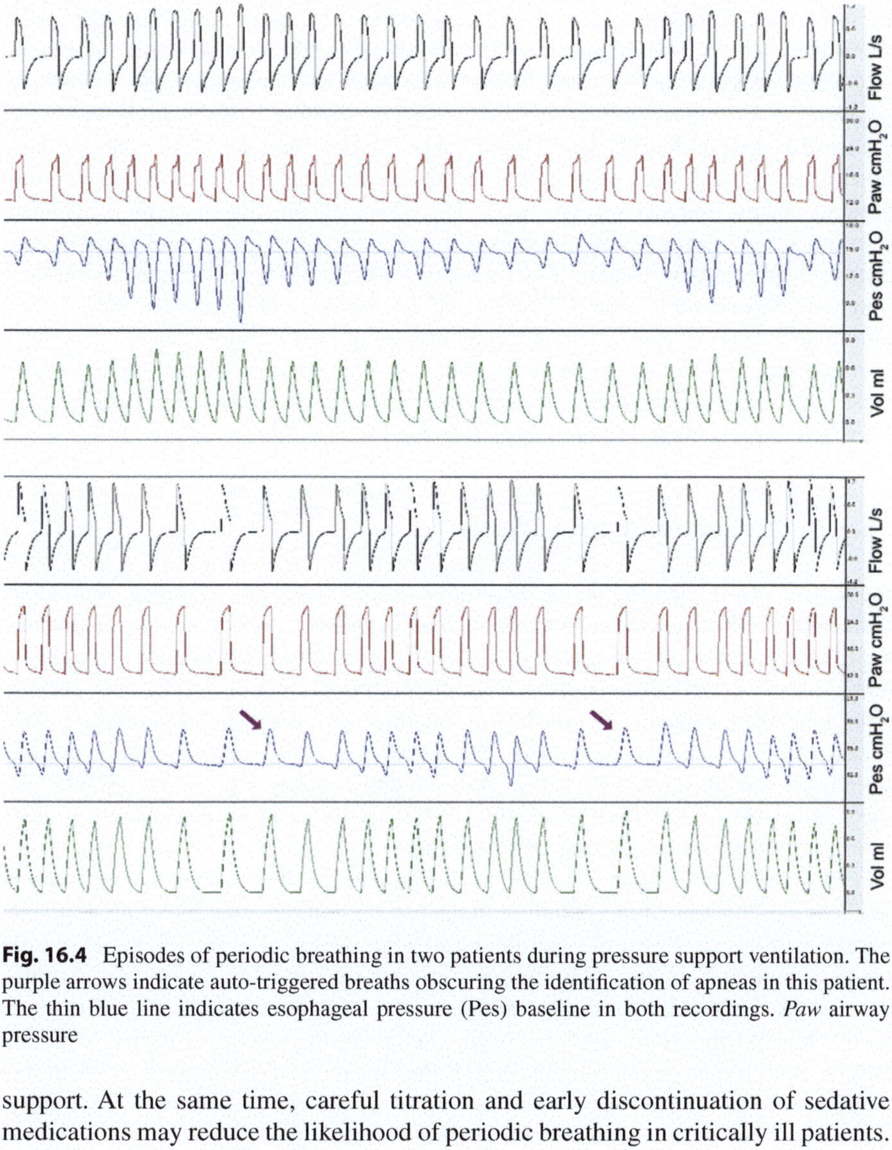


**Fig. 16.4** Episodes of periodic breathing in two patients during pressure support ventilation. The purple arrows indicate auto-triggered breaths obscuring the identification of apneas in this patient. The thin blue line indicates esophageal pressure (Pes) baseline in both recordings. *Paw* airway pressure

support. At the same time, careful titration and early discontinuation of sedative medications may reduce the likelihood of periodic breathing in critically ill patients.

### 16.4.2 Risk of Diaphragm Weakness

Diaphragm disuse atrophy was initially described in patients ventilated in controlled modes [12]. Yet, subsequent studies revealed that not just absent but also weak inspiratory efforts, as may occur with high levels of pressure support, can result in diaphragm atrophy [13], and that the mere triggering of the ventilator does not suffice to prevent diaphragm atrophy [14]. Decrease in diaphragmatic contractility has been associated with increased ventilatory assist [15], while an ultrasound study showed a linear relationship between the rate of development of diaphragmatic atrophy and the level of assist under PSV [16]. Indeed, PSV may turn into a synchronized pressure control mode when the level of support is quite high and $V_{Tmin}$ suffices to maintain $PaCO_2$ within target range. Studies have shown that overestimation of the needed level of pressure support and excessive unloading of the diaphragm occurs frequently (Fig. 16.2) [14]. The lack of clinical signs to identify over-assist and routine measurements of inspiratory effort likely contribute to this result. Diaphragmatic weakness is associated with prolonged mechanical ventilation and intensive care unit (ICU) stay, and development of complications [17]. To minimize the risk of diaphragmatic weakness, frequent titration of the level of support is mandated. Identification of the instantaneous needs of the patient and application of the lowest allowable pressure support level (to avoid distress) is the best approach in preventing diaphragmatic atrophy.

### 16.4.3 Risk of Ineffective Efforts

Ineffective effort, defined as an inspiratory effort unable to trigger a ventilator-delivered breath, is the most common form of asynchrony observed during assisted ventilation, particularly during PSV [18, 19]. Ineffective efforts occur frequently and in clusters, particularly in patients with prolonged weaning, and are associated with prolonged mechanical ventilation and increased hospital mortality [20, 21]. Weak inspiratory efforts, as a result of low respiratory drive or respiratory muscle weakness, and presence of intrinsic positive end-expiratory pressure (PEEPi) are the main causes of ineffective efforts. PSV may promote both weak inspiratory efforts and PEEPi through different mechanisms.

PEEPi refers to the positive elastic recoil pressure at the beginning of inspiration as a result of dynamic hyperinflation. In the presence of dynamic hyperinflation, the patient's effort can trigger the ventilator only after overcoming PEEPi. Patients with obstructive lung diseases and high time constants (increased resistance and compliance), may develop dynamic hyperinflation and ineffective efforts, not only when high levels of support are used, but even when pressure support is titrated to a tidal volume within the normal range [20, 21]. Prolongation of mechanical Ti when the default cycling-off criterion is used, as a result of the slow decrease in inspiratory flow due to increased resistance, can lead to increased tidal volume.

Weak inspiratory efforts occur as a result of weak respiratory muscles, caused by diaphragm weakness, as detailed above, or low respiratory drive, caused by a relatively low level of $PaCO_2$ due to excessive pressure support [18, 22]. The lack of clinical signs of excessive support, as opposed to the conspicuous symptoms of insufficient support, often prompt the caregivers to increase the level of pressure support, and, when a patient's ventilatory demands decrease, this level of support decreases $PaCO_2$ below the level desired by the respiratory centers, leading to weak, potentially ineffective inspiratory efforts. In the presence of sedation or metabolic alkalosis which decrease chemosensitivity and thus respiratory drive, the $PaCO_2$

level desired by the brain may be much higher than normal. In such cases, a level of pressure support titrated to normal tidal volume and low-normal $PaCO_2$ (36–40 mmHg), may promote weak inspiratory efforts and ineffective efforts [22].

Recognition and management of ineffective efforts is important. During an ineffective effort, the diaphragm is subject to eccentric contraction, which may promote further injury [23]. Ineffective efforts can be observed during either mechanical inspiration or expiration, and can be recognized by careful inspection of the ventilator waveforms. A distortion in the airway pressure (Paw) and an abrupt increase in inspiratory flow and decrease in expiratory flow are indicative of ineffective efforts during mechanical inspiratory or expiratory phases, respectively (Fig. 16.5a). Prevention and management of ineffective efforts includes frequent trials of reduction of the level of pressure support, correction of metabolic alkalosis, interruption of sedation, and use of external PEEP to overcome PEEPi in patients with dynamic hyperinflation.

### 16.4.4 Risk of Expiratory Asynchrony

Ideally, during assisted mechanical ventilation, mechanical and neural inspiratory times are matched and the cycling-off occurs at the end of the patient's inspiratory effort [24]. As detailed above, the determinants of the mechanical Ti in PSV include, apart from the patient's effort (Pmus, directly linked to the neural Ti), the level of pressure support, the cycling-off percentage (set by the operator), and the respiratory system mechanics. Therefore, because mechanical Ti in PSV is modified by several other variables, independent of neural Ti, there is significant risk for expiratory asynchronies due to premature or delayed cycling-off.

When the neural Ti is shorter than the mechanical Ti, inspiratory muscle contraction stops well before the end of ventilator insufflation, so the cycling-off is delayed. Delayed cycling-off occurs in patients with high time constant (obstructive lung diseases), high levels of pressure support, and brief/weak inspiratory efforts [24, 25]. Delayed cycling-off, particularly in the presence of increased airway resistance, results in prolongation of inspiratory time and increase in the delivered tidal volume, which may promote dynamic hyperinflation and PEEPi, and thus delayed or ineffective triggering [25]. Delayed cycling-off can be recognized by the shape of the inspiratory flow waveform: after the relaxation of the inspiratory muscles before the end of the mechanical inspiration, the flow waveform changes from curved to linear decay, similar to the one observed with passive ventilation [25] (Fig. 16.5a). Management of this type of asynchrony includes general measures targeting elimination of dynamic hyperinflation and increased airway resistance, simultaneously with decreasing of the assist level, and increasing the flow threshold of cycling-off.

When the neural Ti is longer than the mechanical Ti, the exhalation valve of the ventilator opens prematurely, and inspiratory muscle contraction continues after the end of ventilator insufflation (Fig. 16.5b) [25]. Premature cycling-off is mainly promoted by a low level of assist, a short time constant, and/or a relatively high threshold for cycling-off, all resulting in a short inflation time. Patients with short time

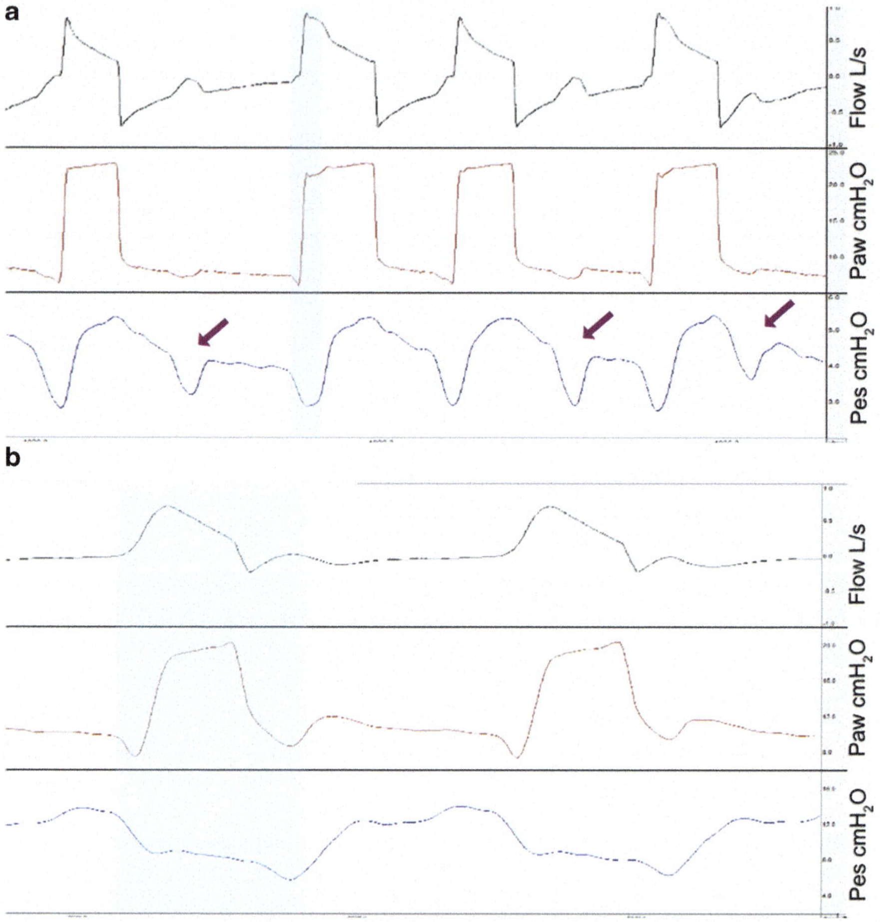


**Fig. 16.5** Expiratory asynchronies and ineffective efforts. Purple arrows on the esophageal pressure (Pes) waveform (**a**) show three ineffective efforts, which can be recognized also by the distortion in flow and airway pressure (Paw) waveforms. The blue shaded area highlights the neural inspiratory time (Ti), which in the upper panel (**a**) is much shorter than the mechanical Ti, while in the lower panel (**b**) is longer than the mechanical Ti

constants of the respiratory system and/or high respiratory drive, such as those with acute respiratory distress syndrome (ARDS), are prone to premature cycling-off and double triggering [22, 26]. As inspiratory muscles continue to contract after the end of mechanical inspiration, premature cycling-off can be recognized by the presence of low or even absent inspiratory flow after opening of the exhalation valve. Moreover, a peak in the expiratory flow waveform after a sharp drop that lasts a few milliseconds and then a gradual decrease to zero toward the end of expiration is strongly indicative of premature cycling-off. Double triggering occurs whenever the inspiratory muscle contraction is adequate enough to overcome the elastic recoil pressure of the respiratory system and a new triggering process can be initiated with a second mechanical breath before full deflation of the first one [25]. Opening of the exhalation valve during the ongoing diaphragmatic contraction results in a potentially injurious eccentric contraction of the diaphragm. Double triggering results in unpredictably high tidal volume, which increases the risk of ventilator-induced lung injury (VILI) [27]. Premature cycling-off and double triggering during PSV can be managed by addressing both the mechanical Ti and the patient's high respiratory drive. An increase in the mechanical Ti can be achieved by lowering the flow threshold for cycling-off, increasing the level of support and the rising time [25]. The management of high respiratory drive includes interventions targeting underlying diseases, such as pulmonary edema or sepsis, and metabolic acidosis, pain and delirium, as well as sedation, until the resolution of the disease process. Opioids should be titrated cautiously to avoid the opioid-induced prolongation of neural Ti.

### 16.4.5 Risk of Lung Injury

Increasing appreciation of the risk of diaphragm disuse atrophy associated with passive mechanical ventilation has prompted clinicians to use assisted modes of ventilation, such as PSV, early in the course of critical illness [1]. The early phase of critical illness, when the disease process is not yet resolved, is often characterized by metabolic acidosis due to shock and acute kidney injury, impaired lung compliance due to lung inflammation and high permeability pulmonary edema, but preserved respiratory muscle strength. In this clinical setting, patients may exhibit high respiratory drive and strong inspiratory efforts. Strong inspiratory efforts in patients with low lung compliance may lead to high tidal volumes, injurious high lung distending pressures, and lung injury through overdistention of alveoli and cyclic recruitment of collapsed lung areas [22, 28]. Negative pressure-induced pulmonary edema [29] and diaphragm fiber injury [30] may also occur as a result of strenuous efforts.

Normally the control of breathing system prevents lung over-stretch by reflex mechanisms limiting inspiratory time (Hering-Breuer reflex), and by progressively decreasing the ability of inspiratory muscles to generate pressure at increasing lung volumes, due to the change in the force–length relationship of flattened diaphragm, and decrease in respiratory system compliance [31]. During assisted ventilation with PSV, these protective mechanisms may be overridden. Mechanical Ti, as detailed above, is only partially dependent on neural Ti, so the Hering-Breuer reflex has minimal effects on tidal volume. Moreover, the decrease in inspiratory effort will not affect the delivery of the $V_{Tmin}$, which, if pressure support is high, as often needed to match patient's high respiratory drive, may be quite substantial. Additionally, severe metabolic acidosis and decreased lung compliance can overwhelm these lung-protective reflexes [32, 33]. Thus, monitoring for potentially injurious lung stress is essential in this clinical setting. Theoretically, monitoring of the driving pressure ($\Delta P$) during PSV, similarly to passive ventilation [23, 34], could help identify injurious high tidal volume and facilitate lung-protective ventilation. Nonetheless, accurate measurement of $\Delta P$ requires passive conditions, which are not present during assisted ventilation. Additionally, during PSV the end of the mechanical Ti does not coincide with the end of neural Ti, so inspiratory muscle activity may still be present during the pause, making the measurement invalid. Moreover, expiratory muscle contraction may occur, falsely increasing the measured plateau pressure. It has been shown that the mere inspection of the airway pressure waveform cannot accurately exclude the presence of respiratory muscle activity during the pause [35].

The risk for high distending pressures can be assessed indirectly through indicators of respiratory drive and effort, such as P0.1 and Pocc [36, 37], although optimal thresholds remain to be determined [38]. Patients at high risk for injurious transpulmonary pressures, such as those with low compliance [33] or high ventilatory demands [39], could be monitored closely, possibly using esophageal pressure to directly measure inspiratory efforts and lung distending pressures.

## 16.5 Conclusion

The development of PSV signified a major improvement from controlled modes in terms of patient-ventilator interactions in spontaneously breathing patients. Now, 40 years later, we have 'raised the bar' for PSV, and aim to provide lung- and diaphragm-protective ventilation. Acknowledging the potential risks of PSV, such as weak inspiratory efforts and diaphragm atrophy, ineffective efforts and periodic breathing, or high distending pressures and risk of lung injury, and the clinical setting in which these problems may arise, can help physicians promptly recognize and address them, by close monitoring and titration of pressure support.

## References


1. van Haren F, Pham T, Brochard L, et al. Spontaneous breathing in early acute respiratory distress syndrome: insights from the large observational study to UNderstand the Global Impact of Severe Acute Respiratory FailurE Study. Crit Care Med. 2019;47:229–38.
2. Thille AW, Lyazidi A, Richard JCM, Galia F, Brochard L. A bench study of intensive-care-unit ventilators: new versus old and turbine-based versus compressed gas-based ventilators. Intensive Care Med. 2009;35:1368–76.
3. Akoumianaki E, Prinianakis G, Kondili E, Malliotakis P, Georgopoulos D. Physiologic comparison of neurally adjusted ventilator assist, proportional assist and pressure support ventilation in critically ill patients. Respir Physiol Neurobiol. 2014;203:82–9.
4. Prinianakis G, Kondili E, Georgopolous D. Patient-ventilator interaction: an overview. Respir Care Clin N Am. 2005;11:201–24.
5. Prinianakis G, Plataki M, Kondili E, Klimathianaki M, Vaporidi K, Georgopoulos D. Effects of relaxation of inspiratory muscles on ventilator pressure during pressure support. Intensive Care Med. 2008;34:70–4.
6. Georgopoulos D, Mitrouska I, Bshouty Z, Webster K, Patakas D, Younes M. Respiratory response to CO2 during pressure-support ventilation in conscious normal humans. Am J Respir Crit Care Med. 1997;156:146–54.
7. Lilitsis E, Stamatopoulou V, Andrianakis E, et al. Inspiratory effort and breathing pattern change in response to varying the assist level: a physiological study. Respir Physiol Neurobiol. 2020;280:103474.

8. Akoumianaki E, Vaporidi K, Georgopoulos D. The injurious effects of elevated or nonelevated respiratory rate during mechanical ventilation. Am J Respir Crit Care Med. 2019;199:149–57.
9. Randerath W, Schiza S, Deleanu O, Pepin JL. Central sleep apnoea and periodic breathing in heart failure: prognostic significance and treatment options. Eur Respir Rev. 2019;28:190084.
10. Meza S, Mendez M, Ostrowski M, Younes M. Susceptibility to periodic breathing with assisted ventilation during sleep in normal subjects. J Appl Physiol. 1985;1998(85):1929–40.
11. Parthasarathy S, Tobin MJ. Effect of ventilator mode on sleep quality in critically ill patients. Am J Respir Crit Care Med. 2002;166:1423–9.
12. Levine S, Nguyen T, Taylor N, et al. Rapid disuse atrophy of diaphragm fibers in mechanically ventilated humans. N Engl J Med. 2008;358:1327–35.
13. Hudson MB, Smuder AJ, Nelson WB, Bruells CS, Levine S, Powers SK. Both high level pressure support ventilation and controlled mechanical ventilation induce diaphragm dysfunction and atrophy. Crit Care Med. 2012;40:1254–60.
14. Urner M, Mitsakakis N, Vorona S, et al. Identifying subjects at risk for diaphragm atrophy during mechanical ventilation using routinely available clinical data. Respir Care. 2021;66:551–8.
15. Goligher EC, Fan E, Herridge MS, et al. Evolution of diaphragm thickness during mechanical ventilation. Impact of inspiratory effort. Am J Respir Crit Care Med. 2015;192:1080–8.
16. Zambon M, Beccaria P, Matsuno J, et al. Mechanical ventilation and diaphragmatic atrophy in critically ill patients: an ultrasound study. Crit Care Med. 2016;44:1347–52.
17. Goligher EC, Dres M, Fan E, et al. Mechanical ventilation-induced diaphragm atrophy strongly impacts clinical outcomes. Am J Respir Crit Care Med. 2018;197:204–13.
18. Carteaux G, Cordoba-Izquierdo A, Lyazidi A, Heunks L, Thille AW, Brochard L. Comparison between neurally adjusted ventilatory assist and pressure support ventilation levels in terms of respiratory effort. Crit Care Med. 2016;44:503–11.
19. Terzi N, Pelieu I, Guittet L, et al. Neurally adjusted ventilatory assist in patients recovering spontaneous breathing after acute respiratory distress syndrome: physiological evaluation. Crit Care Med. 2010;38:1830–7.
20. Vaporidi K, Babalis D, Chytas A, et al. Clusters of ineffective efforts during mechanical ventilation: impact on outcome. Intensive Care Med. 2017;43:184–91.
21. Blanch L, Villagra A, Sales B, et al. Asynchronies during mechanical ventilation are associated with mortality. Intensive Care Med. 2015;41:633–41.
22. Vaporidi K, Akoumianaki E, Telias I, Goligher EC, Brochard L, Georgopoulos D. Respiratory drive in critically ill patients. Pathophysiology and clinical implications. Am J Respir Crit Care Med. 2020;201:20–32.
23. Goligher EC, Dres M, Patel BK, et al. Lung- and diaphragm-protective ventilation. Am J Respir Crit Care Med. 2020;202:950–61.
24. Yamada Y, Du HL. Analysis of the mechanisms of expiratory asynchrony in pressure support ventilation: a mathematical approach. J Appl Physiol (1985). 2000;88:2143–50.
25. Georgopoulos D, Prinianakis G, Kondili E. Bedside waveforms interpretation as a tool to identify patient-ventilator asynchronies. Intensive Care Med. 2006;32:34–47.
26. Liu L, Xu XT, Yu Y, Sun Q, Yang Y, Qiu HB. Neural control of pressure support ventilation improved patient-ventilator synchrony in patients with different respiratory system mechanical properties: a prospective, crossover trial. Chin Med J. 2021;134:281–91.
27. Karageorgos V, Proklou A, Vaporidi K. Lung and diaphragm protective ventilation: a synthesis of recent data. Expert Rev Respir Med. 2022;16:375–90.
28. Yoshida T, Fujino Y, Amato MBP, Kavanagh BP. Fifty years of research in ARDS. Spontaneous breathing during mechanical ventilation. Risks, mechanisms, and management. Am J Respir Crit Care Med. 2017;195:985–92.
29. Brochard L, Slutsky A, Pesenti A. Mechanical ventilation to minimize progression of lung injury in acute respiratory failure. Am J Respir Crit Care Med. 2017;195:438–42.
30. Jiang TX, Reid WD, Belcastro A, Road JD. Load dependence of secondary diaphragm inflammation and injury after acute inspiratory loading. Am J Respir Crit Care Med. 1998;157:230–6.
31. Vaporidi K. NAVA and PAV+ for lung and diaphragm protection. Curr Opin Crit Care. 2020;26:41–6.

32. Mascheroni D, Kolobow T, Fumagalli R, Moretti MP, Chen V, Buckhold D. Acute respiratory failure following pharmacologically induced hyperventilation: an experimental animal study. Intensive Care Med. 1988;15:8–14.
33. Vaporidi K, Psarologakis C, Proklou A, et al. Driving pressure during proportional assist ventilation: an observational study. Ann Intensive Care. 2019;9:1.
34. Amato MBP, Meade MO, Slutsky AS, et al. Driving pressure and survival in the acute respiratory distress syndrome. N Engl J Med. 2015;372:747–55.
35. Soundoulounaki S, Akoumianaki E, Kondili E, et al. Airway pressure morphology and respiratory muscle activity during end-inspiratory occlusions in pressure support ventilation. Crit Care. 2020;24:467.
36. Telias I, Spadaro S. Techniques to monitor respiratory drive and inspiratory effort. Curr Opin Crit Care. 2020;26:3–10.
37. Bertoni M, Telias I, Urner M, et al. A novel non-invasive method to detect excessively high respiratory effort and dynamic transpulmonary driving pressure during mechanical ventilation. Crit Care. 2019;23:346.
38. Tobin MJ, Jubran A, Laghi F. Respiratory drive measurements do not signify conjectural patient self-inflicted lung injury. Am J Respir Crit Care Med. 2021;203:142–3.
39. Proklou A, Papadakis E, Kondili E, et al. Ventilatory ratio threshold for unassisted breathing: a retrospective exploratory analysis. Respir Care. 2021;66:1699–703.

# Advancing Sedation Strategies to Improve Clinical Outcomes in Ventilated Critically Ill Patients

# 17

Y. Shehabi, W. Al-Bassam, and D. Antognini

## 17.1 Introduction

Sedation strategies for critically ill patients receiving mechanical ventilation have radically evolved over the past 20 years. The Clinical Practice Guidelines from the Society of Critical Care Medicine of 2002, 2013, and 2018 witnessed a major transition from sustained sedation to an analgesia first and light sedation paradigm to recommendations to avoid benzodiazepines in favor of propofol and dexmedetomidine [1–3]. Over the last 2 years, the coronavirus disease 2019 (COVID-19) pandemic created a set of new realities and challenges in the provision of sedation to hundreds of thousands of ventilated patients with severe pneumonia and hypoxemia [4, 5]. For the bedside caregivers, the clock rapidly turned back in time and sustained deep sedation with benzodiazepines and high dose opiates became normal practice [5]. In a cohort of ventilated patients in 64 intensive care units (ICUs), 64%

Y. Shehabi (✉)
School of Clinical Sciences, Monash University, Clayton, VIC, Australia

Monash Health – Monash Medical Centre, Clayton, VIC, Australia

School of Clinical Medicine, University New South Wales and Prince of Wales Hospitals, Sydney, Australia
e-mail: Yahya.shehabi@monashhealth.org

W. Al-Bassam
School of Clinical Sciences, Monash University, Clayton, VIC, Australia

Monash Health – Monash Medical Centre, Clayton, VIC, Australia

D. Antognini
School of Clinical Sciences, Monash University, Clayton, VIC, Australia

Monash Health – Monash Medical Centre, Clayton, VIC, Australia

School of Medicine, University of Queensland, Brisbane, QLD, Australia



J.-L. Vincent (ed.), *Annual Update in Intensive Care and Emergency Medicine 2023*, Annual Update in Intensive Care and Emergency Medicine,
https://doi.org/10.1007/978-3-031-23005-9_17

received benzodiazepine infusions for a median of 7 days, with a median Richmond Agitation-Sedation Scale RASS [6] score of −4 (responsive only to painful stimuli) while ventilated, 80% of patients were in a coma for >10 days, and 55% suffered delirium for >3 days [7].

The above observations, albeit thought-provoking, should not incite frustration but rather invite a rethink of the currently recommended strategies and the evidence behind current practice guideline recommendations for sedation of critically ill patients treated with mechanical ventilation.

The 2018 clinical practice guidelines for the prevention and management of pain, agitation/sedation, delirium, immobility, and sleep disruption (PADIS) in adult patients in the ICU [3] uncovered a dearth of high level evidence to inform sedation strategies in critically ill patients. They highlighted the considerable reliance on observational data and trials with high risk of bias in the absence of definitive high quality randomized clinical trials. Many of these studies, despite their flaws, induced a paradigm shift in the practice of sedation and shaped contemporary thinking of sedation strategies and research priorities.

Understanding the limitations of these studies and the evolution in practice over the last 20 years is imperative to advance modern sedation strategies to improve clinically relevant patient-centered outcomes. Many of these studies were observational cohorts, single center, conducted many years ago, compared sedation practices with outdated sedatives in selected populations, and did not report long-term patient-centered outcomes [8–14]. Furthermore, these studies formed the cornerstone of different sedation paradigms and frameworks [15, 16].

In this chapter, we examine the evidence behind current recommended strategies for sedation, such as sedative interruption, light sedation, no sedation or analgosedation, and early mobilization. We also evaluate the evidence behind current strategies for delirium management. We provide suggestions, supported by the best available evidence, for targeted strategies in different populations of ventilated critically ill patients to improve patient-centered clinical outcomes, such as mortality, ventilation duration, and delirium.

## 17.2 Evolution of Sedation Strategies and Evidence Evaluation

### 17.2.1 Daily Sedative Interruption

One of the early trials to highlight potential problems, such as longer ventilation duration and ICU and hospital stays, with continuous intravenous sedation was a single center observational trial in 1998 [17]. These findings were confirmed in a randomized trial in 1999 at the same center [18]. In these two studies, lorazepam, fentanyl, and morphine were the dominant sedative and analgesic agents. In a landmark trial in 2000, the concept of "daily wake up" was promoted by Kress et al., who reported shorter ventilation duration and ICU stay with this approach [8]. Major study limitations included the single center open label design, small sample size, enrollment after 48 h of sedative infusion, and the use of midazolam and morphine as the primary sedative and analgesic combination, thus reducing the internal and external validity of the results. The accumulation of benzodiazepines, morphine, and their active metabolites [19] following continuous infusions in critically ill patients was likely the main reason for these findings. Alternative sedatives, to overcome the negative kinetic profile of benzodiazepines and associated adverse effects, such as propofol and dexmedetomidine, were not yet widely available or used.

In concert, the above studies promoted a healthy awareness of adverse events associated with sustained sedation, which led to recommendations to monitor sedation level and lessen sedative load with daily sedative interruption in the 2002 clinical practice guidelines [1, 20].

A sedative interruption and spontaneous breathing trial of 336 patients conducted in four ICUs showed a significant increase in the primary outcome of ventilator-free days at day 28, a reduction in ICU stay and 1 year mortality, but not in 28-day mortality [11]. In addition to the limitations, including late enrollment (median 2.2 days), non-comparable sedation level (the control group had longer coma and deep sedation), and unexplainable late mortality, the results of this trial have never been replicated with contemporary sedation practice.

Subsequent trials using daily sedative interruption revealed inconsistent results [21, 22]. A sedation protocol incorporating sedative interruption in a pilot trial in Australian and New Zealand ICUs failed to replicate the benefits seen with sedation interruption [23]. A meta-analysis conducted in 2011 highlighted the absence of adequate evidence for the universal adoption of sedative interruption with a non-significant pooled estimate for mortality and ventilation time [24]. In a pivotal adequately powered, multicenter randomized trial by Mehta et al. in 2012, sedative interruption did not shorten ventilation time or ICU stay despite the use of midazolam and fentanyl as the primary sedative analgesic agents [25].

These findings suggest that sedation interruption may not be as critical to sedation outcomes in contemporary sedation practice, especially with the use of shorter acting sedative agents.

### 17.2.2 Light Sedation

Given the recognition of possible adverse events associated with sustained sedation, albeit with circumstantial evidence, light sedation became a recommended sedation strategy in multiple clinical practice sedation guidelines [3, 26, 27].

There are, however, important aspects of sedation depth that should be considered. First, most sedation trials did not report sedation practice or depth in the critical and acute early phase of critical illness, specifically in the first 48–72 h following commencement of mechanical ventilation. The trials that reported early sedation depth, even when light sedation was mandated and protocolized, showed that a high proportion of patients are deeply sedated for 2–4 days following initiation of mechanical ventilation [28–30] (Fig. 17.1). This important observation implies that clinicians believe that deep sedation in the acute phase of critical illness is necessary. Second, observational data reporting the independent association of early deep sedation with mortality [12, 31, 32] is, therefore, subject to selection bias. Thus, the

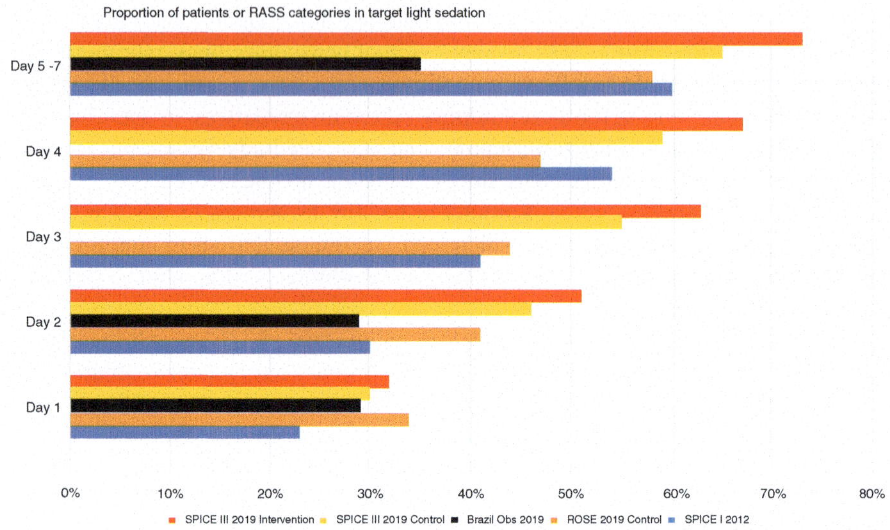


**Fig. 17.1** Proportion of patients or Richmond Agitation-Sedation Scale (RASS) in target light sedation. Trials that recorded early sedation depth in the first 1–3 days of mechanical ventilation showing a consistently low proportion of patients or RASS [6] categories within light sedation target for the first few days following initiation of mechanical ventilation. Sedation target in SPICE III [30] was RASS −2 to +1, Brazil Obs [29] was RASS −3 and above, and in the ROSE trial [28] was a RASS of −1 to +1

interpretation of observational data must be filled with caution. Third, there are few [13, 14] randomized clinical trials that have compared light vs. deep sedation in critically ill patients. These trials shared significant limitations including small sample size, selected homogeneous populations, and short-term outcomes, thus providing very weak evidence to endorse light sedation. Finally, despite all the above, sedation opinion leaders, guideline writers and, to a lesser extent, mainstream ICU clinicians continue to promote a light sedation strategy, because of the belief that it is always beneficial for most patients, ignoring proven clinical behavior to the contrary in the first 2–4 days of critical illness.

It is highly likely that deep sedation mediates significant harm if prolonged and therefore should be avoided [33]. It is, however, plausible, and acceptable, that short, timely and reversible deeper sedation to facilitate life-saving therapeutic interventions, is both safe and justified.

### 17.2.3 No Sedation or Analgo-Sedation

Following the theme that light sedation should always be targeted in all patients, the concept of not using any sedatives at all was tested in Denmark. The strategy of "no sedation" essentially replaced sedative agents with morphine and supplemental haloperidol, in essence using an analgo-sedation strategy. In a single center, open label pilot trial, a protocol of no sedation delivered more days without ventilation, and shorter ICU and hospital stays compared with a standard sedation protocol including sedative interruption [9]. The small sample size, the addition of midazolam at 48 h post-randomization in the standard care group, and the exclusion of patients who either died or were extubated within 48 h are among many of the acknowledged limitations. Despite such limitations, the "no sedation" concept gained popularity, particularly, in Scandinavian ICUs.

A pivotal multicenter trial led by Olsen et al., evaluated the "no sedation" protocol in mainly Danish ICUs and failed to replicate the results of the single center pilot with no benefits on either the primary or any of the secondary outcomes [34]. Despite the limited power for the primary outcome of 90-day mortality, a non-significant 5.4% increase in mortality was observed in the no sedation group. Furthermore, the no sedation group had more agitation, self-extubation, and device removals [34]. These results highlight the importance of adequately powered and well-designed randomized trials to validate the results of single center studies with multiple limitations.

### 17.2.4 Early Mobilization

In an observational cohort, Bailey et al. demonstrated the potential feasibility and safety of early physical activity in patients who were receiving mechanical ventilation for more than 4 days, with less than 1% related adverse events [35]. The impact of early physical and occupational therapy in ventilated critically ill patients was evaluated by Schweickert et al., who reported a greater return to independent functional status at hospital discharge, shorter duration of delirium, and more ventilator-free days, when compared with standard care [10]. This trial, however, was in two affiliated ICUs with a small sample size and included patients 72 h following the initiation of mechanical ventilation in the ICU.

Early goal-directed mobilization in surgical ICU patients was evaluated in a multicenter randomized controlled trial of 200 patients who were ventilated for less than 48 h [36]. The study showed improvement in the primary outcome of surgical mobility score and secondary outcome of functional independence at hospital discharge. Although not powered for mortality, the trial observed a non-significant increase in mortality with the intervention.

Systematic reviews and meta-analyses showed substantial heterogeneity amongst the included randomized controlled trials. While early mobilization appears to reduce ICU-acquired weakness and increase ventilator free days and functional independence, it seems to be associated with a non-significant increase in mortality and increase in adverse events [37, 38]. These findings highlight the urgent need for well-designed multicenter randomized trials to evaluate the safety and efficacy of early mobilization in critically ill surgical and medical patients before wide adoption in clinical practice and recommendation in practice guidelines.

A noticeable feature of the above strategies was the sedative agnostic nature of these clinical trials. The evaluation of these strategies occurred in an era when benzodiazepines, lorazepam, and midazolam were the most commonly used sedatives. Alternative sedatives such as propofol and dexmedetomidine were not widely used in clinical practice (Table 17.1).

**Table 17.1** Randomized trials evaluating different sedation strategies—characteristics of single vs. multicenter trials

| Author, date [ref] | Design | Number | Intervention | Control | Primary outcome | Findings | Remarks |
|---|---|---|---|---|---|---|---|
| *Single center/institution RCTs* | | | | | | | |
| Kress 2000 [8] | Open label | 168 | Daily sedative interruption | Standard sedation | Ventilation time | Shorter ventilation, ICU stay | Midazolam and morphine |
| Girard 2008 [11] (4 ICUs) | Open label | 335 | Sedative interruption and spontaneous breathing trial (SBT) | Clinician directed sedation + SBT | VFDs at day-28 | More VFDs, shorter ICU and hospital stay, lower 90-day mortality | Benzodiazepines and opioids. More propofol in intervention |
| Pandharipande 2007 [39] (2 affiliated ICUs) | Double-blind | 106 | Dexmedetomidine | Lorazepam | Days alive and delirium- and coma-free | More days alive, coma- and delirium-free | High dose fentanyl in intervention |
| De Wit 2008 [21] | Open label | 74 | Daily sedative interruption | Nurse implemented sedation protocol | VFDs at day-29 and duration of ventilation | Longer ventilation time and higher mortality | Terminated early by data safety committee |
| Schweickert 2009 [10] (2 affiliated ICUs) | Open label | 104 | Early physical and occupational therapy + sedative interruption | Sedative interruption | Independent functional status at hospital discharge | Higher functional status, less delirium, and more VFD | Propofol, lorazepam and morphine. Patients ventilated >72 h |
| Treggiari 2009 [13] | Open label | 129 | Awake and cooperative | Deep sedation | PTSD, anxiety and depression at 4 weeks | Less PTSD and more VFD | Midazolam and opioids |
| Strøm 2010 [10] | Open label | 113 | No sedation | Standard sedation | Days without ventilation | Shorter ventilation, ICU stay | Midazolam and propofol |
| *Multicenter RCTs* | | | | | | | |
| Mehta 2012 [25] (16 ICUs) | Open label | 423 | Daily sedative interruption + protocolized sedation | Protocolized sedation | Time to successful extubation | No difference in primary outcome and other secondary outcomes | Midazolam and fentanyl |

| | | | | | | | |
|---|---|---|---|---|---|---|---|
| Schaller 2016 [36] (5 ICUs) | Single blind | 200 | Early goal-directed mobilization | Standard care | Surgical optimal mobilization score (SOMS) | Higher SOMS, other outcomes no difference, but higher non-significant mortality | Surgical patients ventilated >48 h |
| Kawazoe 2017 [40] (8 ICUs) | Open label | 201 | Dexmedetomidine | Midazolam or propofol | 28-day mortality and VFDs | No significant difference in primary or secondary outcomes | Sepsis cohort. Underpowered for mortality |
| Shehabi 2019 [30] (74 ICUs) | Open label | 4000 | Dexmedetomidine | Usual care | 90-day mortality, significant age-related heterogeneity | No difference over all | Usual care mainly propofol and less so midazolam |
| Olsen 2020 [34] (8 ICUs) | Open label | 710 | No sedation | Light sedation (RASS −2 to −3) | 90-day mortality | Non-significant increase 5.4% with no sedation | All secondary outcomes were comparable. Used midazolam |
| Hughes 2021 [41] (13 medical centers) | Double blind | 422 | Dexmedetomidine | Propofol | Days alive and delirium- and coma-free at day 14 | No significant difference in primary or secondary outcomes | Ventilated sepsis patients |

Trials showing significant difference in sedation-related outcomes are usually single center, open label, small sample size and benzodiazepines were commonly used. Results of these trials could not be replicated in multicenter randomized controlled trials (RCTs) where contemporary sedation practice or non-benzodiazepine sedation was used. *RASS* Richmond Agitation-Sedation Scale, *VFDs* ventilator-free days, *PTSD* post-traumatic stress disorder

## 17.3 Comparative Trials of Commonly Used Sedatives

The introduction of propofol and dexmedetomidine as potential alternative sedatives to benzodiazepines in ventilated ICU patients [42, 43] and the recognition of delirium as a major morbidity in ICU patients [44], triggered a cascade of comparative trials of these sedatives.

Although these trials were mostly sponsored and for registration purposes with different regulatory agencies, they have added substantially to the body of knowledge and the practice of sedation. In a double-blind randomized controlled trial conducted in 106 adults ventilated >24 h in two ICUs, dexmedetomidine significantly increased number of days alive and free of coma and delirium, with treated patients spending more time in target sedation compared with lorazepam [39]. This was followed by the global SEDCOM multicenter double-blind randomized controlled trial comparing midazolam and dexmedetomidine in 375 adults ventilated for >24 h [45]. Dexmedetomidine treatment reduced the prevalence of delirium and shortened time to extubation but was more likely to cause bradycardia. Two parallel non-inferiority double-blind randomized controlled trials compared propofol with dexmedetomidine (n = 247 vs. 251) and midazolam with dexmedetomidine (n = 251 vs. 249) in adults ventilated for >24 h [46]. These trials, conducted in Europe, showed that dexmedetomidine shortened ventilation time when compared with midazolam but not propofol and treated patients were more interactive when compared with either midazolam or propofol. However, more adverse events, such as bradycardia and hypotension, were observed with dexmedetomidine treatment.

While these trials were double-blind and multicenter, they were not powered for mortality and the sample sizes did not allow meaningful subgroup analysis or heterogeneity of treatment effect evaluation. Nonetheless, in concert, these trials led to a conditional recommendation of the use dexmedetomidine and propofol as the preferred sedatives, over benzodiazepines, in patients needing mechanical ventilation in the ICU [3].

The evidence for clinical practice guideline recommendations remains weak despite the above trials and the progress made over the last 20 years. Sedative administration in ICU patients receiving mechanical ventilation is a ubiquitous intervention, like fluids and antibiotics. While large scale trials evaluating common ICU interventions have been conducted [47, 48], similar trials evaluating the impact of different sedatives in ventilated critically ill patients remained lacking until recently [30].

## 17.4 Sedation Practice in Intensive Care Evaluation, the SPICE-III Trial

The 2018 PADIS clinical practice guidelines issued a weak conditional recommendation for the use of dexmedetomidine and propofol as the preferred sedatives for ventilated critically ill patients [3]. The recommendation uncovered a significant evidence gap in many areas of sedation related practices and outcomes.

The SPICE-III trial [30], was the first investigator initiated, large scale, multinational randomized controlled trial in this field and addressed many limitations of previous studies. The SPICE-III trial had a sample size approximately ten times larger than any other sedation randomized controlled trial. Patients were randomized within a few hours of initiation of mechanical ventilation; thus, the trial captured the early phase of critical illness and ventilation, a unique feature in comparison with most other sedation randomized controlled trials. The trial was powered for 90-day mortality and stratified for the presence of sepsis at randomization with six pre-specified subgroups including young vs. old patients dichotomized at the median age of the cohort. A high level of external and internal validity was reflected by the global nature of the trial and a high internal fidelity and minimal loss to follow up. The trial was an open label design, comparing early dexmedetomidine use with usual care as dictated by treating clinicians.

While the primary outcome of 90-day mortality was comparable between early dexmedetomidine treatment and usual care, there was a modest increase in days alive free of coma and delirium, and ventilator-free days at day-28. In addition, early dexmedetomidine sedation was associated with more bradycardia, episodes of asystole and hypotension.

The sample size, 4000 patients, and the study robustness as outlined above, allowed further evaluation of many aspects of early sedation with dexmedetomidine and propofol, the most used sedative in the usual care arm, within the construct of a randomized trial, with direct implications for sedation practice and patient outcomes.

### 17.4.1 Early Sedation Depth in Ventilated Critically Ill Patients

Most previous sedation trials ignored the early phase of critical illness and missed a fundamental component of clinician determined sedation practice. The global SPICE-III trial [30] and sedation trials in the United States [28] and Brazil [29] have all collected important information on early sedation depth. Although protocol mandated, the proportion of patients achieving a light sedation target in the first 48 h of initiation of mechanical ventilation was 50%, 40%, and 30%, respectively in these trials. The concordance of these data worldwide strongly suggests that many patients appropriately need moderate to deep sedation in the early phase of critical illness, as chosen by treating clinicians.

### 17.4.2 Improving Patient-Centered Outcomes in Ventilated Critically Ill Adults

The pre-specified subgroup analysis in the SPICE-III trial revealed a significant age-related interaction in mortality with dexmedetomidine treatment with a divergent effect in younger vs. older patients [30]. This heterogeneity of treatment effect was further evaluated using Bayesian analysis and showed data with direct relevance to clinical practice and patient-centered outcomes [49].

Albeit exploratory, the SPICE-III secondary analyses provide an unparalleled insight into the potential benefits and adverse events of commonly used and recommended sedatives, dexmedetomidine and propofol, in different critically ill patient populations.

### 17.4.3 The Age Interaction with Early Dexmedetomidine Treatment

Despite achieving comparable level sedation in the first 14 days post-randomization, older patients required a significantly lower dose of all sedatives, regardless of group disposition. Despite comparable APACHE II scores (excluding the age component), as expected, 90-day mortality was much higher in older patients overall at 38.4% compared with 20.9% in younger patients [49]. In addition, older patients had reduced number of days alive and free of coma and delirium and ventilator-free days at day 28, compared with younger patients. There was, however, heterogeneity of dexmedetomidine treatment in these outcomes with obvious implications, considering the above context.

#### 17.4.3.1 Critically Ill Older Patients

In the SPICE-III trial [49], 1825 (46.7%) patients included in the primary analysis, were over 65 years old, of whom 913 and 912 were randomized to early dexmedetomidine sedation or usual care, respectively. In this group of patients, the probability of reduced 90-day mortality with early dexmedetomidine sedation was 99.5%. This was highest at the lower end of APACHE II scores, less than 25, with a low probability of benefit at APACHE II scores >25. In addition, early dexmedetomidine sedation was associated with a high probability (>93%) of increased days alive and free of coma and delirium and increased ventilator-free days (>96%) at day 28.

#### 17.4.3.2 Critically Ill Younger Patients

Conversely, 2079 (53.3%) of those included in the primary analysis were younger than 65 years with 1035 randomized to early dexmedetomidine sedation and 1044 to the usual care arm. In this group of patients, early dexmedetomidine treatment was associated with a very high probability of increased mortality and a low probability of increased delirium- and coma-free days or ventilator-free days.

These data are compelling and imply that younger patients should not receive early dexmedetomidine sedation outside an approved research protocol. The European Medicine Agency and the Federal Institute for Drugs and Medical Devices issued a direct healthcare professional alert about the increased mortality with dexmedetomidine treatment in patients younger than 65 years old [50].

#### 17.4.3.3 Ventilated Critically Ill Surgical Patients

One of the pre-specified subgroup analyses in the SPICE-III trial was surgical vs. non-surgical patients. In a Bayesian analysis of the heterogeneity of dexmedetomidine treatment in surgical vs. non-surgical patients [49], 976 (29.4%) of patients included in the primary analysis were classified as a surgical cluster vs. 2346

(70.6%) as a non-surgical cluster. The probability of lower mortality in the surgical cluster, regardless of age, was greater than 84% with >88% probability of increased days alive and free of coma and delirium but a much lower probability, 70%, of increased ventilator-free days. Conversely, the probability of lower mortality in the cluster of non-surgical patients was 33%; however, the probabilities of increased delirium- and coma-free days and increased ventilator-free days were 77% and 58%, respectively.

If we consider age heterogeneity within the clustering of surgical vs. non-surgical patients, the probability of increased mortality in younger non-surgical patients was very high while the probability of reduced mortality in younger surgical patients remained reasonably high. In essence, this implies that extreme caution is warranted for the use of dexmedetomidine sedation in non-surgical patients who are younger than 65 years.

#### 17.4.3.4 Critically Ill Patients with Sepsis

The impact of sedation on patients with sepsis has been the subject of many clinical trials. Albeit underpowered for mortality (n = 201 in Japan), dexmedetomidine was comparable to usual care in the DESIRE randomized trial with comparable mortality and ventilator-free days [40]. Similarly, dexmedetomidine and propofol had a comparable effect on days alive and free of coma and delirium 14 days post-randomization [41] in the double-blind randomized MENDS2 trial of 422 patients in the United States.

Patients in the SPICE-III trial were stratified according to the presence or absence of sepsis at randomization with 1248 septic patients randomized to early sedation with dexmedetomidine and 1256 patients to usual care, making this the largest sedation trial of critically ill ventilated septic patients. While the 90-day mortality was comparable, 32.9% vs. 31.8% between dexmedetomidine treatment and usual care, the subgroup analysis of the SPICE-III septic cohort showed significant age-related heterogeneity with younger patients showing a significant 5.5% increase and older patients showing a non-significant 2.9% decrease in 90-day mortality.

In addition, while DESIRE [40] and MENDS2 [41] failed to show any difference in delirium-related outcomes, the SPICE-III septic cohort demonstrated significantly more days alive, free of coma and delirium (median difference +2) in older septic patients treated with dexmedetomidine with an overall mean difference of +1 day.

#### 17.4.3.5 Critically Ill Cardiovascular Patients

Within the construct of SPICE-III, 579 patients were critically ill with a cardiovascular diagnosis, of whom 300 were randomized into the early dexmedetomidine sedation arm. In this post-hoc analysis, early sedation with dexmedetomidine appeared to be associated with a significant reduction in 90-day mortality (risk difference −9.2%, p = 0.017) and more days alive free of delirium and coma (mean difference +2, p = 0.012). While these findings are exploratory, they imply that further research is urgently needed in this area and they affirm the view that ventilated critically ill patients react differently to sedative medications and may have differing clinically important clinical outcomes.

## 17.5 Reducing the Burden of Delirium with Dexmedetomidine

One of the major issues facing contemporary intensive care is the emergence of delirium as a significant morbidity in critically ill adults with associated increase in mortality, hospital stay, and cognitive decline. While the results of the SPICE-III trial are primarily related to the early use of dexmedetomidine and the apparent harm in specific populations, the positive role of dexmedetomidine administration for agitation and delirium has been demonstrated in a meta-analysis and systematic review of randomized trials including more than 11,000 patients [51]. These findings, however, should not detract from the importance of non-pharmacological interventions aimed at reducing the risk of delirium.

## 17.6 Conclusion

Sedation practice has progressed significantly over the last 25 years, albeit with slow but steady steps. Paradigm shifting trials led to the adoption of practices such as daily sedative interruption, light sedation, analgesia first, and early mobilization. These trials, however, were fit for purpose 20 years ago and the COVID-19 pandemic uncovered the need for a different approach. The introduction and widespread use of the short-acting non-benzodiazepine sedatives propofol and dexmedetomidine into clinical practice, led to a major shift in research priorities. Adopted principles from 20 years ago became outdated with failure to replicate their positive effect in multicenter trials. Large scale sedation trials, conducted for the first time, have provided an unparalleled insight into the role of the two recommended sedatives, propofol and dexmedetomidine. Sedative administration and sedation strategies should be tailored to specific populations rather than prescribed with a one size fits all principle. Propofol seems to be the sedative of choice for the younger non-surgical critically ill patient, while dexmedetomidine seems the sedative of choice for older critically ill patients, those with cardiovascular disease and for delirium management in general. It is time to take bigger steps to advance sedation practice with well-designed clinical trials of population-specific sedation strategies, and newer sedatives to improve patient-centered outcomes.

## References

1. Jacobi J, Fraser GL, Coursin DB, et al. Clinical practice guidelines for the sustained use of sedatives and analgesics in the critically ill adult. Crit Care Med. 2002;30:119–41.
2. Barr J, Fraser GL, Puntillo K, et al. Clinical practice guidelines for the management of pain, agitation, and delirium in adult patients in the intensive care unit. Crit Care Med. 2013;41:263–306.

3. Devlin J, Skrobik Y, Gelinas C, et al. Clinical practice guidelines for the prevention and management of pain, agitation/sedation, delirium, immobility, and sleep disruption in adult patients in the ICU. Crit Care Med. 2018;46:e825–73.
4. Hanidziar D, Bittner EA. Sedation of mechanically ventilated COVID-19 patients: challenges and special considerations. Anesth Analg. 2020;131:e40–1.
5. Payen JF, Chanques G, Futier E, Velly L, Jaber S, Constantin JM. Sedation for critically ill patients with COVID-19: which specificities? One size does not fit all. Anaesth Crit Care Pain Med. 2020;39:341–3.
6. Sessler CN, Gosnell MS, Grap MJ, et al. The Richmond agitation–sedation scale validity and reliability in adult intensive care unit patients. Am J Respir Crit Care Med. 2002;166:1338–44.
7. Pun BT, Badenes R, La Calle GH, et al. Prevalence and risk factors for delirium in critically ill patients with COVID-19 (COVID-D): a multicentre cohort study. Lancet Respir Med. 2021;9:239–50.
8. Kress JP, Pohlman AS, O'Connor MF, Hall JB. Daily interruption of sedative infusions in critically ill patients undergoing mechanical ventilation. N Engl J Med. 2000;342:1471–7.
9. Strøm T, Martinussen T, Toft P. A protocol of no sedation for critically ill patients receiving mechanical ventilation: a randomised trial. Lancet. 2010;375:475–80.
10. Schweickert WD, Pohlman MC, Pohlman AS, et al. Early physical and occupational therapy in mechanically ventilated, critically ill patients: a randomised controlled trial. Lancet. 2009;373:1874–82.
11. Girard TD, Kress JP, Fuchs BD, et al. Efficacy and safety of a paired sedation and ventilator weaning protocol for mechanically ventilated patients in intensive care (awakening and breathing controlled trial): a randomised controlled trial. Lancet. 2008;371:126–34.
12. Shehabi Y, Bellomo R, Reade MC, et al. Early intensive care sedation predicts long-term mortality in ventilated critically ill patients. Am J Respir Crit Care Med. 2012;186:724–31.
13. Treggiari MM, Romand JA, Yanez ND, et al. Randomized trial of light versus deep sedation on mental health after critical illness. Crit Care Med. 2009;37:2527–34.
14. Samuelson K, Lundberg D, Fridlund B. Light vs. heavy sedation during mechanical ventilation after oesophagectomy–a pilot experimental study focusing on memory. Acta Anaesthesiol Scand. 2008;52:1116–23.
15. Pandharipande P, Banerjee A, McGrane S, Ely EW. Liberation and animation for ventilated ICU patients: the ABCDE bundle for the back-end of critical care. Crit Care. 2010;14:1.
16. Riker RR, Fraser GL. Altering intensive care sedation paradigms to improve patient outcomes. Crit Care Clin. 2009;25:527–38.
17. Kollef MH, Levy NT, Ahrens TS, Schaiff R, Prentice D, Sherman G. The use of continuous iv sedation is associated with prolongation of mechanical ventilation. Chest. 1998;114:541–8.
18. Brook AD, Ahrens TS, Schaiff R, et al. Effect of a nursing-implemented sedation protocol on the duration of mechanical ventilation. Crit Care Med. 1999;27:2609–15.
19. Bauer TM, Ritz R, Haberthür C, et al. Prolonged sedation due to accumulation of conjugated metabolites of midazolam. Lancet. 1995;346:145–7.
20. Nasraway SA, Jacobi J, Murray MJ, Lumb PD. Sedation, analgesia, and neuromuscular blockade of the critically ill adult: revised clinical practice guidelines for 2002. Crit Care Med. 2002;30:117–8.
21. De Wit M, Gennings C, Jenvey WI, Epstein SK. Randomized trial comparing daily interruption of sedation and nursing-implemented sedation algorithm in medical intensive care unit patients. Crit Care. 2008;12:R70.
22. Carson SS, Kress JP, Rodgers JE, et al. A randomized trial of intermittent lorazepam versus propofol with daily interruption in mechanically ventilated patients. Crit Care Med. 2006;34:1326–32.

23. Elliott R, McKinley S, Aitken LM, Hendrikz J. The effect of an algorithm-based sedation guideline on the duration of mechanical ventilation in an Australian intensive care unit. Intensive Care Med. 2006;32:1506–14.
24. Augustes R, Ho K. Meta-analysis of randomised controlled trials on daily sedation interruption for critically ill adult patients. Anaesth Intensive Care. 2011;39:401–9.
25. Mehta S, Burry L, Cook D, et al. Daily sedation interruption in mechanically ventilated critically ill patients cared for with a sedation protocol. A randomized controlled trial. JAMA. 2012;308:1985–92.
26. Martin J, Heymann A, Bäsell K, et al. Evidence and consensus-based German guidelines for the management of analgesia, sedation and delirium in intensive care–short version. Ger Med Sci. 2010;8:Doc02.
27. Girard TD, Alhazzani W, Kress JP, et al. An official American Thoracic Society/American College of Chest Physicians Clinical Practice Guideline: liberation from mechanical ventilation in critically ill adults. Rehabilitation protocols, ventilator liberation protocols, and cuff leak tests. Am J Respir Crit Care Med. 2017;195:120–33.
28. National Heart L, Network BIPCT. Early neuromuscular blockade in the acute respiratory distress syndrome. N Engl J Med. 2019;380:1997–2008.
29. Nassar AP, Zampieri FG, Salluh JI, et al. Organizational factors associated with target sedation on the first 48 h of mechanical ventilation: an analysis of checklist-ICU database. Crit Care. 2019;23:1–8.
30. Shehabi Y, Howe B, Bellomo R, et al. Early sedation with dexmedetomidine in critically ill patients. N Engl J Med. 2019;380:2506–17.
31. Shehabi Y, Chan L, Kadiman S, et al. Sedation depth and long-term mortality in mechanically ventilated critically ill adults: a prospective longitudinal multicentre cohort study. Intensive Care Med. 2013;39:910–8.
32. Balzer F, Weiß B, Kumpf O, et al. Early deep sedation is associated with decreased in-hospital and 2-years follow-up survival. Crit Care. 2015;19:197.
33. Devlin JW. The pharmacology of over sedation in mechanically ventilated adults. Curr Opin Crit Care. 2008;14:5–407.
34. Olsen HT, Nedergaard HK, Strøm T, et al. Nonsedation or light sedation in critically ill, mechanically ventilated patients. N Engl J Med. 2020;382:1103–11.
35. Bailey P, Thomsen GE, Spuhler VJ, et al. Early activity is feasible and safe in respiratory failure patients. Crit Care Med. 2007;35:139–45.
36. Schaller SJ, Anstey M, Blobner M, et al. Early, goal-directed mobilisation in the surgical intensive care unit: a randomised controlled trial. Lancet. 2016;388:1377–88.
37. Zhang L, Hu W, Cai Z, et al. Early mobilization of critically ill patients in the intensive care unit: a systematic review and meta-analysis. PLoS One. 2019;14:e0223185.
38. Zang K, Chen B, Wang M, et al. The effect of early mobilization in critically ill patients: a meta-analysis. Nurs Crit Care. 2020;25:360–7.
39. Pandharipande PP, Pun BT, Herr DL, et al. Effect of sedation with dexmedetomidine vs lorazepam on acute brain dysfunction in mechanically ventilated patients. JAMA. 2007;298:2644–53.
40. Kawazoe Y, Miyamoto K, Morimoto T, et al. Effect of dexmedetomidine on mortality and ventilator-free days in patients requiring mechanical ventilation with sepsis: a randomized clinical trial. JAMA. 2017;317:1321–8.
41. Hughes CG, Mailloux PT, Devlin JW, et al. Dexmedetomidine or propofol for sedation in mechanically ventilated adults with sepsis. N Engl J Med. 2021;384:1424–36.
42. Bhana N, Goa KL, McClellan KJ. Dexmedetomidine. Drugs. 2000;59:263–8.
43. Fulton B, Sorkin EM. Propofol. Drugs. 1995;50:636–457.
44. Ely EW, Shintani A, Truman B, et al. Delirium as a predictor of mortality in mechanically ventilated patients in the intensive care unit. JAMA. 2004;291:10.
45. Riker RR, Shehabi Y, Bokesch PM, et al. Dexmedetomidine vs midazolam for sedation of critically ill patients: a randomized trial. JAMA. 2009;301:489–99.

46. Jakob SM, Ruokonen E, Grounds RM, et al. Dexmedetomidine vs midazolam or propofol for sedation during prolonged mechanical ventilation: two randomized controlled trials. JAMA. 2012;307:1151–60.
47. Myburgh JA, Finfer S, Bellomo R, et al. Hydroxyethyl starch or saline for fluid resuscitation in intensive care. N Engl J Med. 2012;367:1901–11.
48. Venkatesh B, Finfer S, Cohen J, et al. Adjunctive glucocorticoid therapy in patients with septic shock. N Engl J Med. 2018;378:797–808.
49. Shehabi Y, Neto AS, Howe BD, et al. Early sedation with dexmedetomidine in ventilated critically ill patients and heterogeneity of treatment effect in the SPICE III randomised controlled trial. Intensive Care Med. 2021;47:455–66.
50. European Medicines Agency (EMA) and the Federal Institute for Drugs and Medical Devices (BfArM): Direct Healthcare Professional Communication (DHPC) on dexmedetomidine: risk of increased mortality in intensive care patients ≤ 65 years of age. Available at: https://www.bfarm.de/SharedDocs/Risikoinformationen/Pharmakovigilanz/EN/RHB/2022/rhb-dexmedetomidin.html. Accessed 8 Sept 2022.
51. Lewis K, Alshamsi F, Carayannopoulos KL, et al. Dexmedetomidine vs other sedatives in critically ill mechanically ventilated adults: a systematic review and meta-analysis of randomized trials. Intensive Care Med. 2022;48:811–40.

# Part V

# Extracorporeal Support

# Setting and Monitoring of Mechanical Ventilation During Venovenous ECMO

# 18

B. Assouline, A. Combes, and M. Schmidt

## 18.1 Introduction

In patients with the acute respiratory distress syndrome (ARDS), mechanical ventilation can cause ventilator-induced lung injury (VILI) through multiple mechanisms, including volutrauma, barotrauma, atelectrauma, myotrauma, and biotrauma [1]. In the most severe forms of ARDS, the smaller the baby lung, the greater the potential for unsafe ventilation despite mechanical ventilation volume and pressure limitation. To further limit the energy transmitted to the lungs by the mechanical ventilator, "ultra-lung-protective" ventilation reducing tidal volume (≤4 ml/kg), respiratory rate (<20/min), and airway (plateau pressure <25 $cmH_2O$ and driving pressure ≤15 $cmH_2O$) pressures has been proposed [2]. However, this strategy can result in severe respiratory acidosis without extracorporeal gas exchange using extracorporeal life support (ECLS) devices. Venovenous extracorporeal membrane oxygenation (VV-ECMO) is a form of ECLS that provides full extracorporeal blood oxygenation and carbon dioxide removal, which can replace pulmonary function. VV-ECMO allows marked reductions in tidal volume, respiratory rate, plateau and driving pressures [3, 4]. It has been associated with survival benefits in randomized controlled trials (RCTs) and meta-analyses [3–6]. However, optimal mechanical

B. Assouline
Médecine Intensive Réanimation, Institut de Cardiologie, Assistance Publique-Hôpitaux de Paris, Paris, France

A. Combes (✉) · M. Schmidt
Médecine Intensive Réanimation, Institut de Cardiologie, Assistance Publique-Hôpitaux de Paris, Paris, France

Sorbonne Université, GRC 30, RESPIRE, UMRS 1166, ICAN Institute of Cardiometabolism and Nutrition, Paris, France
e-mail: alain.combes@aphp.fr



J.-L. Vincent (ed.), *Annual Update in Intensive Care and Emergency Medicine 2023*, Annual Update in Intensive Care and Emergency Medicine,
https://doi.org/10.1007/978-3-031-23005-9_18

ventilation settings on ECMO are still debated. In this narrative review, we summarize the current knowledge, rationale, and evidence for mechanical ventilation management and monitoring in patients receiving VV-ECMO for severe ARDS. We will also discuss the research agenda in this field.

## 18.2 Historical Perspective

### 18.2.1 Ventilation Strategies in ECMO Landmark Trials

There is a paucity of data regarding optimal mechanical ventilation settings during ECLS (Table 18.1). Current recommendations are thus based on expert opinion [7] and the results of very few landmark trials [3, 4]. The concept of lung rest during ECLS was first proposed by Gattinoni et al. in a non-controlled series [8], in which ARDS patients were ventilated with peak inspiratory pressures limited to less than 35–45 $cmH_2O$, low respiratory rates (<5/min), and positive end-expiratory pressure (PEEP) set to 15–25 $cmH_2O$. In the CESAR trial [4], patients were randomized to receive either conventional management at their center (90 patients) or to be referred for consideration for ECMO at an ECMO center (90 patients), where a "lung-rest" strategy was applied under ECMO (pressure control mode, peak inspiratory pressure limited to 20–25 $cmH_2O$, PEEP 10–15 $cmH_2O$, respiratory rate 10/min, and fraction of inspired oxygen [$FiO_2$] 0.3). Although the rate of mortality or severe disability was lower at 6 months in the ECMO group, the study was criticized for several methodological limitations. Specifically, only 75% of the referred patients received ECMO, and protective mechanical ventilation was applied in only 70% of the control group. In the EOLIA trial [3], patients with severe ARDS were randomly assigned to receive immediate VV-ECMO or conventional protective mechanical ventilation. Ultra-protective ventilation was provided to the ECMO group either by assisted-control mode (tidal volume reduced to obtain plateau pressure $\leq$24 $cmH_2O$, PEEP $\geq$10 $cmH_2O$, respiratory rate 10 to 30 cycles/min, and $FiO_2$ 0.3) or by airway pressure release ventilation (APRV; high pressure $\leq$24 $cmH_2O$, PEEP $\geq$10 $cmH_2O$, ratio of inspiratory to expiratory time 1:2, and $FiO_2$ 0.3). In the hours following randomization, ECMO patients had a significant decrease in tidal volume (6.0 ± 1.3 vs. 3.5 ± 1.0 ml/kg), plateau pressure (30 ± 6 vs. 24 ± 3 $cmH_2O$), driving pressure (18 ± 7 vs. 13 ± 2 $cmH_2O$), respiratory rate (30 ± 5 vs. 23 ± 2 breaths/min), while PEEP (12 ± 4 vs. 11 ± 3 $cmH_2O$) remained unchanged. Mortality was lower in the ECMO group (35% vs. 46%) although this difference did not reach statistical significance ($p = 0.07$).

**Table 18.1** Mechanical ventilation settings in landmark trials and cohorts in patients with acute respiratory distress syndrome (ARDS) treated with venovenous-extracorporeal membrane oxygenation (VV-ECMO)

| | Design | Number of patients | Mechanical ventilation strategy on ECMO | Mean mechanical power reduction | Main findings |
|---|---|---|---|---|---|
| CESAR [4] | RCT | 180 | **PC mode with:**<br>• PIP 20–25 $cmH_2O$<br>• PEEP 10–15 $cmH_2O$<br>• RR 10/min<br>• $FiO_2$ 0.3 | Not available | Referral to an ECMO center for severe ARF (Murray score > 3.0 or pH <7.20):<br>• Improves survival without severe disability (RR 0.69; 95% CI 0.05–0.97, p = 0.03)<br>• Cost-effective strategy |
| EOLIA [3] | RCT | 249 | **ACV mode with:**<br>• $V_T$ to obtain Pplat ≤24 $cmH_2O$<br>• PEEP ≥10 $cmH_2O$<br>• RR 10 to 30/min<br>• $FiO_2$ 0.3<br>**APRV mode with:**<br>• High pressure ≤ 24 $cmH_2O$<br>• Low pressure ≥ 10 $cmH_2O$<br>• $FiO_2$ 0.3 | From 28 to 10 J/min | On day 60:<br>• 11% absolute mortality reduction in favor of the ECMO group (35% vs. 46%, p = 0.07)<br>• 28% of the control group required crossover and emergent cannulation |
| LIFEGARDS [10] | Prospective cohort | 350 | • $V_T$ 3.7 ± 2.0 ml/kg<br>• Pplat 24 ± 7 $cmH_2O$<br>• ΔP 14 ± 4 $cmH_2O$<br>• RR 14 ± 6/min | From 26 to 6.6 J/min | A combination of $V_T$ (≤4 ml/kg) and a ΔP ≤15 $cmH_2O$ during the first two days of ECMO was obtained in 45% of patients<br>Lack of association between mechanical ventilation settings during the first two days of ECMO and survival |

(continued)

**Table 18.1** (continued)

| | Design | Number of patients | Mechanical ventilation strategy on ECMO | Mean mechanical power reduction | Main findings |
|---|---|---|---|---|---|
| Serpa Neto et al. [19] | Meta-analysis | 545 | • $V_T$ 4.0 ± 1.7 ml/kg PBW<br>• Pplat 26.2 ± 4.6 $cmH_2O$<br>• ΔP 13.7 ± 5.3 $cmH_2O$<br>• RR 17.8 ± 8/min | Not available | In hospital mortality = 35.2%<br>ΔP was the only ventilatory parameter that showed an independent association with in-hospital mortality |
| Wang et al. [32] | RCT | 104 | • $V_T$ 4.0 ± 1.3 ml/kg PBW<br>• Pplat 24.0 ± 2.6 $cmH_2O$<br>• PEEP 13.1 ± 2.4 $cmH_2O$<br>• RR 17.7 ± 4.8/min | From 26 to 7.5 J/min | The Ptp-guided group had:<br>• Higher rate of successful weaning ($p = 0.017$)<br>• Lower 60-day mortality rate compared to the lung rest group (32.7% vs. 54%, $p = 0.030$)<br>• Shorter ECMO duration ($p = 0.004$) |

*RCT* randomized controlled trial, *PC* pressure-control, *ACV* assist-control ventilation, *APRV* airway pressure release ventilation, *PIP* peak inspiratory pressure, $V_T$ tidal volume, *Pplat* plateau pressure, *PBW* predicted body weight, *PEEP* positive end-expiratory pressure, *Ptp* transpulmonary pressure, *RR* respiratory rate, *ΔP* driving pressure, $FiO_2$ the fraction of inspired oxygen, *ARF* acute respiratory failure

### 18.2.2 Current Practice in ECMO-Experienced Centers

An international cross-sectional survey [9] conducted in 2013 among 141 medical directors and ECMO program coordinators from 283 Extracorporeal Life Support Organization (ELSO)-registered centers, revealed that only 27% of centers had an explicit mechanical ventilation protocol for patients on VV-ECMO. The majority of these centers (77%) reported "lung rest" to be the primary goal of mechanical ventilation, whereas 9% reported "lung recruitment" to be their ventilation strategy. A tidal volume of 6 ml/kg or less was targeted by 76% of respondents, but only 34% of them were setting tidal volumes to less than 4 ml/kg. PEEP was ≤10 $cmH_2O$ in 77% of the patients. More recently, the LIFEGARDS (ventiLatIon management oF patients with Extracorporeal membrane oxyGenation for Acute Respiratory Distress Syndrome) was the first prospective study specifically designed to describe the ventilatory management of ECMO-treated patients with ARDS [10]. LIFEGARDS included an international, multicenter cohort of 350 patients supported by ECMO in 23 medium- to high-volume ECMO intensive care units (ICUs) across 10 countries. It confirmed the widespread adoption of ultra-protective ventilation after ECMO initiation, with marked reduction in tidal volume (6.4 ± 2.0 vs. 3.7 ± 2.0 ml/kg), plateau pressure (32 ± 7 vs. 24 ± 7 $cmH_2O$), driving pressure (20 ± 7 vs. 14 ± 4 $cmH_2O$), respiratory rate (26 ± 8 vs. 14 ± 6 breaths/min), and mechanical power (26.1 ± 12.7 vs. 6.6 ± 4.8 J/min), while PEEP (12 ± 4 vs. 11 ± 3 $cmH_2O$) was kept greater than 10 $cmH_2O$ in most patients. No association was however found in multivariable analysis between ventilator settings during the first 2 days of ECMO and survival.

## 18.3 Targeting Ultra-Lung-Protective Mechanical Ventilation During ECMO

### 18.3.1 Tidal Volume

Decreasing tidal volume is the cornerstone of limiting the stress and strain applied by the mechanical ventilator to the lungs and the resulting VILI. Using a rat model of acid-induced lung injury, a tidal volume reduction from 12 to 6 to 3 ml/kg, with the same level of PEEP (10 $cmH_2O$), decreased pulmonary edema and lung injury and increased protection of the alveolar epithelium [11]. Indeed, the limited tidal volume reduction (6.3 to 4.5 ml/kg) due to insufficient $CO_2$ removal to control respiratory acidosis by the extracorporeal carbon dioxide removal ($ECCO_2R$) device may explain the failure of the REST trial to improve the outcomes of ARDS patients [12]. By contrast, ECMO enabled larger tidal volume reduction (<4 ml/kg) in patients randomized to the ECMO group of the EOLIA trial and in those of the LIFEGARDS cohort. Targeting a tidal volume of less than 4 ml/kg is recommended in the guidelines of the Extracorporeal Life Support Organization (ELSO) [7].

### 18.3.2 Plateau Pressure

Plateau pressure is easily measurable at the bedside and received considerable attention after publication of the ARMA trial [13]. The REVA Network study on $H_1N_1$ influenza-related ARDS reported that the mean plateau pressure after initiation of VV-ECMO was significantly lower in survivors than in non-survivors (25 ± 3 vs. 29 ± 5 $cmH_2O$; $p < 0.01$) [14]. In that study, higher plateau pressures (>25 $cmH_2O$) on the first day of VV-ECMO were significantly associated with mortality (odds ratio [OR] = 1.33, 95% confidence interval [CI] 1.14 to 1.59, $p < 0.01$). A plateau pressure <25 $cmH_2O$ was targeted in the most recent VV-ECMO series [15, 16] and is also recommended by the ELSO [7].

### 18.3.3 Driving Pressure

The driving pressure is the plateau airway pressure minus PEEP. It can also be expressed as the ratio of tidal volume to respiratory system compliance ($\Delta P = V_T/C_{RS}$), indicating the decreased functional size of the lung observed in patients with ARDS (i.e., baby lung). Driving pressure is a strong predictor of mortality in patients with ARDS as demonstrated by a *post hoc* analysis of previous RCTs and subsequent studies [10, 17, 18], with driving pressure >14 $cmH_2O$ being associated with a higher risk of mortality [17]. An individual patient data meta-analysis of observational studies in adult patients with ARDS receiving ECMO reported that driving pressure was the only ventilatory parameter that showed an independent association with in-hospital mortality [19]. In that context, targeting a driving pressure <14 $cmH_2O$ on VV-ECMO appears desirable and is currently applied in centers with high ECMO volume [10].

### 18.3.4 Respiratory Rate

The frequency of lung collapse and expansion, i.e., the respiratory rate, contributes to VILI. In a pig model of ARDS, Grasso et al. assessed the benefit of respiratory rate reduction combined with $ECCO_2R$ [20]. At a fixed tidal volume (6 ml/kg), lower respiratory rate was associated with reduced biotrauma while lung aeration was preserved [20]. A secondary analysis of the LUNG SAFE study [21] also confirmed that higher respiratory rate was independently associated with increased in-hospital mortality. More recently, Costa et al. demonstrated, in a retrospective pooled database of 4549 patients with ARDS, that only the driving pressure and respiratory rate had significant associations with mortality [22]. In that study, the impact of the driving pressure on mortality was four times as large as that of the respiratory rate. While the ELSO recommends a respiratory rate of 4–15 breaths/min [7], higher respiratory rates on ECMO were reported in EOLIA (23 ± 2) [3] and in the LIFEGARDS study (14 ± 6) [10]. A minimal respiratory rate (4/min) may however be needed to maintain lung volume and to avoid derecuitement during ultra-lung-protective ventilation [8].

### 18.3.5 Mechanical Power

Mechanical power represents the energy delivered by the ventilator to the respiratory system [23]. It is a function of transpulmonary pressure, tidal volume, and respiratory rate and was shown to be independently associated with mortality in ARDS patients when >17 J/min [24]. By applying ultra-lung-protective ventilation during ECMO, the mechanical power can be dramatically reduced. Indeed, it was significantly lower (10 J/min vs. 28 J/min) in the ECMO compared to the control group in the EOLIA trial, an effect mediated by a 43% and 23% reduction in tidal volume and respiratory rate, respectively [25]. Similarly, the mean mechanical power was reduced from 26 J/min to 6.6 J/min after ECMO initiation in the LIFEGARDS cohort study [10]. Although the mechanical power concept has several limitations, it may enable the contribution of all modifiable mechanical ventilation settings (tidal volume, respiratory rate, driving pressure, PEEP, inspiratory to expiratory ratio, inspiratory flow) to VILI to be quantified. Although its computation may help to guide current practice (Fig. 18.1), the extent to which mechanical power should be reduced in ECMO patients remains undetermined.

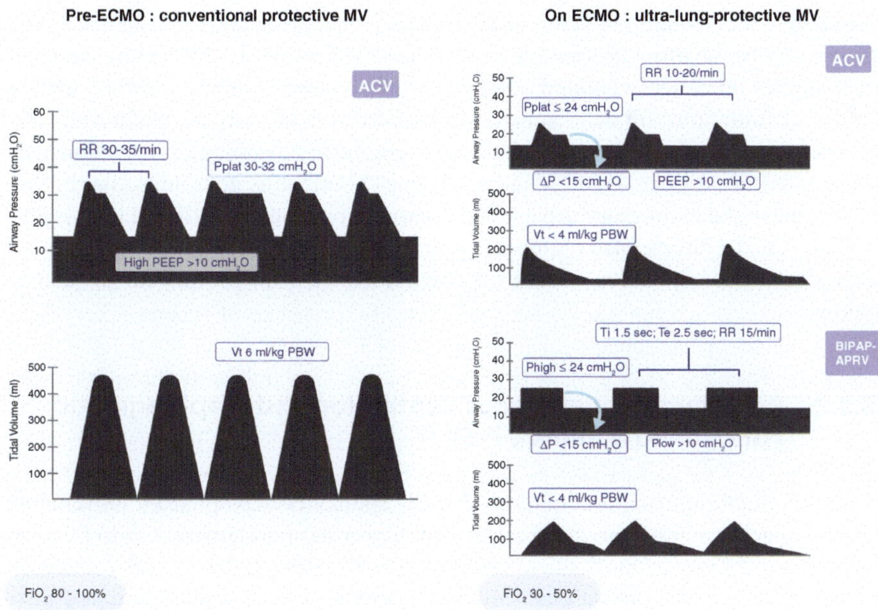


**Fig. 18.1** Pre-extracorporeal membrane oxygenation (ECMO) conventional protective ventilation compared to ultra-lung protective mechanical ventilation during ECMO. *ACV* assist-control ventilation, *BIPAP-APRV* bilevel positive airway pressure-airway pressure release ventilation, *RR* respiratory rate, *PEEP* positive end-expiratory pressure, *PBW* predicted body weight, *Vt* tidal volume, $FiO_2$ inspired fraction in $O_2$, *Pplat* plateau pressure, $\Delta P$ driving pressure, $P_{high}$ high pressure, $P_{low}$ low pressure, *Ti* inspiratory time, *Te* expiratory time

### 18.3.6 Applying Apneic Ventilation?

Decreasing tidal volume to less than 4 ml/kg may not be sufficient to prevent excess strain (defined as tidal volume/end-expiratory lung volume) delivered by mechanical ventilation to inflamed and inhomogeneous lungs, as recently suggested in a randomized crossover physiological study in 10 patients with ARDS receiving VV-ECMO [18]. In this study, a substantial risk of biotrauma and VILI persisted despite a mean tidal volume of 2.4 ml/kg in patients with low respiratory system compliance. Specifically, a linear relationship existed between changes in inspiratory pressure and concentrations of plasma biomarkers (soluble receptor for advanced glycation endproducts [S-RAGE], interleukin [IL]-6, tumor necrosis factor [TNF]-alpha) during mechanical ventilation. Biotrauma was lowest in the absence of tidal ventilation in the continuous positive airway pressure (CPAP) mode (10 cm$H_2O$). Similarly, Graf et al. compared lung protective with apneic ventilation in 24 patients with severe ARDS receiving VV-ECMO in a prospective, monocenter physiological study [26]. Ultra-lung-protective ventilation was associated with increased stress, strain, and mechanical power, despite a low driving pressure (11.9 ± 5.8 cm$H_2O$). In a large animal model of ARDS supported with VV-ECMO, near apneic ventilation (driving pressure 10 cm $H_2O$, PEEP 10 cm $H_2O$, and respiratory rate 5/min) was also associated with decreased lung injury and fibroproliferation compared to a conventional ventilation strategy [27]. Although (near) apneic ventilation might be the ultimate strategy to decrease VILI during ECMO, more data and larger studies on patient-centered outcomes are now needed before it can be widely adopted. Limitations of near apneic ventilation should also be evaluated. The absence of lung cycling may have short- and long-term physiological consequences and may require deeper sedation and sometimes continuous neuromuscular blockade to control the respiratory drive and subsequent patient self-inflicted lung injury (P-SILI). The technique also requires higher blood flow in the VV-ECMO circuit to reach adequate oxygenation, which may be associated with complications such as hemolysis.

### 18.3.7 Preserving Spontaneous Ventilation and Diaphragmatic Function to Minimize P-SILI?

Preserving diaphragmatic function by allowing spontaneous respiratory movements may facilitate weaning from mechanical ventilation, as short periods (18 to 69 h) of diaphragm inactivity on mechanical ventilation were associated with a 55% decrease in transdiaphragmatic pressure and marked atrophy of both slow-twitch and fast-twitch diaphragm fibers in humans [28]. On the other hand, spontaneous breathing could be associated with strong respiratory efforts and elevated transpulmonary pressure in patients with high respiratory drive and low pulmonary compliance and cause P-SILI [29, 30]. Although switching from controlled to assisted-spontaneous ventilation has several benefits (muscle function preservation, decreased sedation, hemodynamic improvement), minimizing P-SILI while maintaining (part of) the diaphragm activity is challenging in patients with the most severe forms of ARDS receiving ECMO. In that context, the APRV mode that combines the control of plateau and driving pressures while allowing non-synchronized spontaneous breathing may be valuable.

## 18.4 How to Set the Optimal PEEP on ECMO?

As with any intervention, the ultra-lung-protective ventilation strategy does not come without risks. Indeed, the resultant decrease in mean airway pressure could cause lung derecruitment, atelectrauma, and biotrauma. Lung collapse and overdistension may also occur simultaneously in severely injured lungs. Interestingly, PEEP was ≤10 $cmH_2O$ in 77% of the patients in an international survey of ECMO specialists and the ELSO guidelines recommend a modest level of PEEP (10 $cmH_2O$) during ECMO support [7]. However, the optimal PEEP in ARDS may vary between patients and depend on several factors (alveolar recruitability, pleural pressure, body weight, and hemodynamics) and may also evolve rapidly during the disease process. Selecting the adequate PEEP for a specific patient and at a specific time point is therefore challenging and a 'one-size fits all' strategy would likely not be of any clinical benefit. Several methods have been recently described to guide clinicians in the individualization of PEEP levels during ultra-protective ventilation on ECMO (Fig. 18.2).

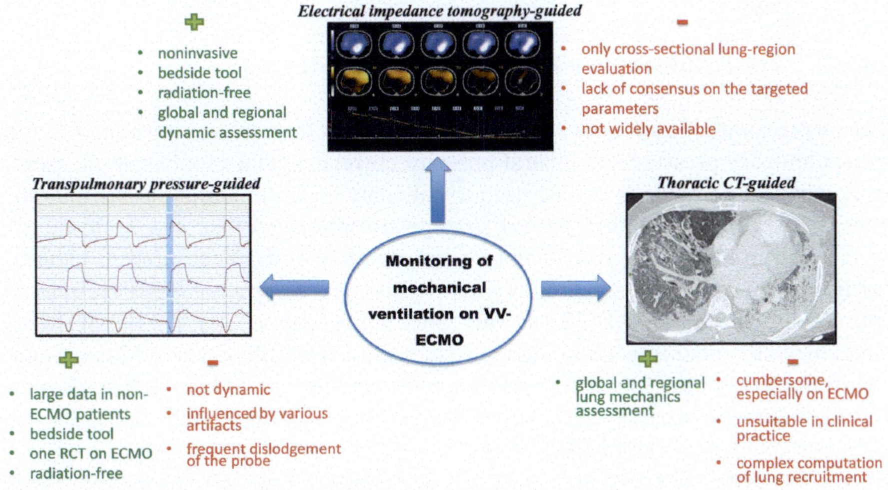


**Fig. 18.2** Tools to set positive end-expiratory pressure on venovenous extracorporeal membrane oxygenation (VV-ECMO). *RCT* randomized controlled trial, *CT* computed tomography

### 18.4.1 Electrical Impedance Tomography-Guided Strategy

Electrical impedance tomography (EIT) provides individual, noninvasive, radiation-free imaging of the lungs at the bedside, with global and regional dynamic lung analyses. This technique displays a graphic representation of the regional distribution of lung ventilation and provides real-time information regarding ventilation including heterogeneity of ventilation distribution, regional tidal volume, and gravitational distribution of respiratory system compliance. It identifies impedance changes in the lungs and enables distinction between ventilated and non-ventilated alveolar units. PEEP titration can therefore be guided by EIT, to determine the optimal setting that minimizes lung collapse and overdistension. Franchineau et al. showed the wide diversity in patients' EIT-derived "best compromise" PEEPs in a series of 15 ECMO patients, with values of 15, 10, and 5 $cmH_2O$ for 7, 6, and 2 patients, respectively, whereas PEEP 20 and PEEP 0 were never selected [31]. Assessment of the distribution of airway opening and closure by EIT within each lung and between the two lungs is ventilation. Biotrauma AiCLOSE Study (ClinicalTrials.gov Identifier: NCT05196074).

Several limitations of EIT should be mentioned. First, the technique only provides a cross-sectional evaluation of a specific lung region, which may differ from the whole lungs, and only captures the ventral-to-dorsal regional ventilation distribution. Second, it requires specific equipment, which is still not widely available and the acquisition of data is time-consuming. Lastly, there is still a lack of consensus on the EIT target parameters to define the optimal PEEP level. The benefit of such an EIT-guided ventilation strategy to further decrease VILI during ECMO deserves further investigation.

### 18.4.2 Transpulmonary Pressure-Guided Strategy

Plateau pressure is a surrogate of the pressure gradient that stresses the lung, i.e., the transpulmonary pressure. As pleural pressure correlates with esophageal pressure, an esophageal manometer can be used to calculate the end-expiratory transpulmonary pressure. This pressure-guided strategy to optimize PEEP can limit atelectrauma and minimize the risk of lung overdistention. It has been used to identify candidates for ECMO (i.e., refractory hypoxemia despite optimal PEEP) [20] or to optimize PEEP on ECMO [32]. In this latter study, patients on VV-ECMO were randomized to either transpulmonary pressure-guided ventilation ($n = 52$) or a lung rest strategy ($n = 52$) [32]. The transpulmonary pressure-guided group had a higher rate of successful weaning, a significantly lower 60-day mortality rate (33% vs. 54%, $p = 0.03$), and shorter ECMO duration ($p = 0.004$) compared to the lung rest group. However, the transpulmonary pressure-guided strategy remains controversial in patients with ARDS and is not supported by the results of the EPVent-2 trial [33].

### 18.4.3 Other Methods

Lung ultrasound can be used to guide the setting of mechanical ventilation in ARDS patients and assess bedside lung recruitment [34]. Changes in the lung ultrasound score correlated with PEEP-induced increases in end-expiratory lung volume in a series of ARDS patients receiving conventional mechanical ventilation [35] and also correlated significantly with computed tomography (CT) scan data in a series of 18 patients receiving ECMO [36].

The recruitment-to-inflation (R/I) ratio is a recent tool that has been developed to evaluate the potential for lung recruitment. It is calculated as the ratio between the compliance of the recruited lung following the application of a high PEEP to that of the respiratory system measured at a lower PEEP. This parameter can be easily measured at the bedside with any ICU ventilator and may help to optimize ventilator settings, particularly PEEP [37]. As of today, this parameter has not been studied during ECMO with very low tidal volume.

## 18.5 Prone Positioning During ECMO

Prone position is an effective first-line intervention in moderate to severe ARDS [38] that should be considered mandatory before ECMO consideration. However, this procedure during ECMO is still controversial, despite its increasing use, especially during the coronavirus disease 2019 (COVID-19) pandemic [39]. Several observational studies and a recent meta-analysis have shown that prone positioning during ECMO was feasible, safe, and could enhance ECMO weaning and improve outcomes [39, 40]. To date, the lack of RCTs, the fear of accidental decannulation, and the difficulties of routinely training the nursing staff in this procedure are still barriers to generalizing its use in ECMO patients, especially in centers with low ECMO volume. The results of the ongoing randomized controlled PRONECMO trial (ClinicalTrials.gov Identifier: NCT04607551) may help clarify the indications for prone positioning of ECMO patients.

## 18.6 Gas Exchange Targets on ECMO

There are no evidence-based guidelines for the management of oxygenation, carbon dioxide, or pH in patients with ARDS supported with ECMO, and safe limits of hypoxemia and hypercapnia have not been well established, although both hypoxemia and hyperoxemia have been associated with increased mortality [41]. Gas exchange targets implemented in the EOLIA trial ($PaO_2$ 65–90 mmHg; $PaCO_2 < 45$ mmHg) [3] are most frequently recommended until more data become available. Because current ECMO membranes allow a significant reduction in mechanical ventilation intensity and can ensure adequate gas exchange despite minimal residual lung function, the ventilator $FiO_2$ should be reduced to its minimal value. Additionally, a high fraction of $FiO_2$ in lung areas with a low ventilation-perfusion ratio might cause denitrogenation atelectasis, especially if PEEP is low [42]. Lastly, rapid correction of hypercapnia after the initiation of ECMO should be avoided since it was associated with the development of neurological complications [43].

## 18.7 Mechanical Ventilation During ECMO Weaning

Mechanical ventilation during the weaning of ECMO has received little attention so far. In the EOLIA trial, patients were switched to volume-assist controlled ventilation with tidal volume set at 6 ml/kg when "clinical, radiological, gasometric, and pulmonary compliance had improved" [3]. More recently, in a series of 83 patients undergoing weaning of ECMO, those with higher tidal volume, heart rate, ventilatory ratio, and esophageal pressures swings during a sweep gas-off trial were less likely to achieve safe liberation from VV-ECMO [44]. As mentioned above, prone positioning during ECMO may also facilitate weaning from the device.

## 18.8 Conclusion

Mechanical ventilation during ECMO for ARDS should aim to reduce VILI by decreasing its intensity. However, further studies are needed to determine how particular ventilator variables should be adjusted during the course of ECMO and during its weaning phase. Pending the results of such studies, EOLIA ventilator settings [3] are a reasonable option.

## References

1. Slutsky AS, Ranieri VM. Ventilator-induced lung injury. N Engl J Med. 2013;369:2126–36.
2. Rozencwajg S, Guihot A, Franchineau G, et al. Ultra-protective ventilation reduces biotrauma in patients on venovenous extracorporeal membrane oxygenation for severe acute respiratory distress syndrome. Crit Care Med. 2019;47:1505–12.
3. Combes A, Hajage D, Capellier G, et al. Extracorporeal membrane oxygenation for severe acute respiratory distress syndrome. N Engl J Med. 2018;378:1965–75.
4. Peek GJ, Mugford M, Tiruvoipati R, et al. Efficacy and economic assessment of conventional ventilatory support versus extracorporeal membrane oxygenation for severe adult respiratory failure (CESAR): a multicentre randomised controlled trial. Lancet. 2009;374:1351–63.
5. Brodie D, Slutsky AS, Combes A. Extracorporeal life support for adults with respiratory failure and related indications: a review. JAMA. 2019;322:557–68.
6. Combes A, Peek GJ, Hajage D, et al. ECMO for severe ARDS: systematic review and individual patient data meta-analysis. Intensive Care Med. 2020;46:2048–57.
7. Tonna JE, Abrams D, Brodie D, et al. Management of adult patients supported with venovenous extracorporeal membrane oxygenation (VV ECMO): Guideline from the Extracorporeal Life Support Organization (ELSO). ASAIO J. 2021;67:601–10.
8. Gattinoni L, Pesenti A, Mascheroni D, et al. Low-frequency positive-pressure ventilation with extracorporeal CO2 removal in severe acute respiratory failure. JAMA. 1986;256:881–6.

9. Marhong JD, Telesnicki T, Munshi L, Del Sorbo L, Detsky M, Fan E. Mechanical ventilation during extracorporeal membrane oxygenation. An international survey. Ann Am Thorac Soc. 2014;11:956–61.
10. Schmidt M, Pham T, Arcadipane A, et al. Mechanical ventilation management during extracorporeal membrane oxygenation for acute respiratory distress syndrome. An international multicenter prospective cohort. Am J Respir Crit Care Med. 2019;200:1002–12.
11. Frank JA, Gutierrez JA, Jones KD, Allen L, Dobbs L, Matthay MA. Low tidal volume reduces epithelial and endothelial injury in acid-injured rat lungs. Am J Respir Crit Care Med. 2002;165:242–9.
12. McNamee JJ, Gillies MA, Barrett NA, et al. Effect of lower tidal volume ventilation facilitated by extracorporeal carbon dioxide removal vs standard care ventilation on 90-day mortality in patients with acute hypoxemic respiratory failure: The REST randomized clinical trial. JAMA. 2021;326:1013–23.
13. Brower RG, Matthay MA, Morris A, Schoenfeld D, Thompson BT, Wheeler A. Ventilation with lower tidal volumes as compared with traditional tidal volumes for acute lung injury and the acute respiratory distress syndrome. N Engl J Med. 2000;342:1301–8.
14. Pham T, Combes A, Rozé H, et al. Extracorporeal membrane oxygenation for pandemic influenza A(H1N1)-induced acute respiratory distress syndrome: a cohort study and propensity-matched analysis. Am J Respir Crit Care Med. 2013;187:276–85.
15. Schmidt M, Langouet E, Hajage D, et al. Evolving outcomes of extracorporeal membrane oxygenation support for severe COVID-19 ARDS in Sorbonne hospitals, Paris. Crit Care. 2021;25:1–11.
16. Barbaro RP, MacLaren G, Boonstra PS, et al. Extracorporeal membrane oxygenation for COVID-19: evolving outcomes from the international Extracorporeal Life Support Organization Registry. Lancet. 2021;398:1230–8.
17. Amato MBP, Meade MO, Slutsky AS, et al. Driving pressure and survival in the acute respiratory distress syndrome. N Engl J Med. 2015;372:747–55.
18. Del Sorbo L, Goffi A, Tomlinson G, et al. Effect of driving pressure change during extracorporeal membrane oxygenation in adults with acute respiratory distress syndrome: a randomized crossover physiologic study. Crit Care Med. 2020;48:1771–8.
19. Serpa Neto A, Schmidt M, Azevedo LCP, et al. Associations between ventilator settings during extracorporeal membrane oxygenation for refractory hypoxemia and outcome in patients with acute respiratory distress syndrome: a pooled individual patient data analysis: mechanical ventilation during ECMO. Intensive Care Med. 2016;42:1672–84.
20. Grasso S, Stripoli T, Mazzone P, et al. Low respiratory rate plus minimally invasive extracorporeal CO2 removal decreases systemic and pulmonary inflammatory mediators in experimental acute respiratory distress syndrome. Crit Care Med. 2014;42:e451–60.
21. Bellani G, Laffey JG, Pham T, et al. Epidemiology, patterns of care, and mortality for patients with acute respiratory distress syndrome in intensive care units in 50 countries. JAMA. 2016;315:788–800.
22. Costa EL V, Slutsky AS, Brochard LJ, et al. Ventilatory variables and mechanical power in patients with acute respiratory distress syndrome. Am J Respir Crit Care Med. 2021;204:303–11.
23. Gattinoni L, Tonetti T, Cressoni M, et al. Ventilator-related causes of lung injury: the mechanical power. Intensive Care Med. 2016;42:1567–75.
24. Serpa Neto A, Deliberato RO, Johnson AEW, et al. Mechanical power of ventilation is associated with mortality in critically ill patients: an analysis of patients in two observational cohorts. Intensive Care Med. 2018;44:1914–22.
25. Quintel M, Busana M, Gattinoni L. Breathing and ventilation during extracorporeal membrane oxygenation: how to find the balance between rest and load. Am J Respir Crit Care Med. 2019;200:954–6.
26. Graf PT, Boesing C, Brumm I, et al. Ultraprotective versus apneic ventilation in acute respiratory distress syndrome patients with extracorporeal membrane oxygenation: a physiological study. J Intensive Care. 2022;10:1–11.

27. Araos J, Alegria L, Garcia P, et al. Near-apneic ventilation decreases lung injury and fibroproliferation in an acute respiratory distress syndrome model with extracorporeal membrane oxygenation. Am J Respir Crit Care Med. 2019;199:603–12.
28. Levine S, Nguyen T, Taylor N, et al. Rapid disuse atrophy of diaphragm fibers in mechanically ventilated humans. N Engl J Med. 2008;358:1327–35.
29. Yoshida T, Amato MBP, Kavanagh BP, Fujino Y. Impact of spontaneous breathing during mechanical ventilation in acute respiratory distress syndrome. Curr Opin Crit Care. 2019;25:192–8.
30. Crotti S, Bottino N, Spinelli E. Spontaneous breathing during veno-venous extracorporeal membrane oxygenation. J Thorac Dis. 2018;10:S661–9.
31. Franchineau G, Bréchot N, Lebreton G, et al. Bedside contribution of electrical impedance tomography to setting positive end-expiratory pressure for extracorporeal membrane oxygenation-treated patients with severe acute respiratory distress syndrome. Am J Respir Crit Care Med. 2017;196:447–57.
32. Wang R, Sun B, Li X, et al. Mechanical ventilation strategy guided by transpulmonary pressure in severe acute respiratory distress syndrome treated with venovenous extracorporeal membrane oxygenation. Crit Care Med. 2020;48:1280–8.
33. Beitler JR, Sarge T, Banner-Goodspeed VM, et al. Effect of titrating positive end-expiratory pressure (PEEP) with an esophageal pressure-guided strategy vs an empirical high PEEP-FiO2 strategy on death and days free from mechanical ventilation among patients with acute respiratory distress syndrome: a randomized clinical trial. JAMA. 2019;321:846–57.
34. Mojoli F, Bouhemad B, Mongodi S, Lichtenstein D. Lung ultrasound for critically ill patients. Am J Respir Crit Care Med. 2019;199:701–14.
35. Bouhemad B, Brisson H, Le-Guen M, Arbelot C, Lu Q, Rouby JJ. Bedside ultrasound assessment of positive end-expiratory pressure-induced lung recruitment. Am J Respir Crit Care Med. 2011;183:341–7.
36. Curry S, Tan A, Gargani L, et al. Lung ultrasound and the role of lung aeration score in patients with acute respiratory distress syndrome on extracorporeal membrane oxygenation. Int J Artif Organs. 2021;44:854–60.
37. Chen L, Del Sorbo L, Grieco DL, et al. Potential for lung recruitment estimated by the recruitment-to-inflation ratio in acute respiratory distress syndrome. A clinical trial. Am J Respir Crit Care Med. 2020;201:178–87.
38. Guérin C, Reignier J, Richard J-C, et al. Prone positioning in severe acute respiratory distress syndrome. N Engl J Med. 2013;368:2159–68.
39. Zaaqoq AM, Barnett AG, Griffee MJ, et al. Beneficial effect of prone positioning during venovenous extracorporeal membrane oxygenation for coronavirus disease 2019. Crit Care Med. 2022;50:275–85.
40. Petit M, Fetita C, Gaudemer A, et al. Prone-positioning for severe acute respiratory distress syndrome requiring extracorporeal membrane oxygenation. Crit Care Med. 2022;50:264–74.
41. Mikkelsen ME, Christie JD, Lanken PN, et al. The adult respiratory distress syndrome cognitive outcomes study: long-term neuropsychological function in survivors of acute lung injury. Am J Respir Crit Care Med. 2012;185:1307–15.
42. Santos C, Ferrer M, Roca J, Torres A, Hernández C, Rodriguez-Roisin R. Pulmonary gas exchange response to oxygen breathing in acute lung injury. Am J Respir Crit Care Med. 2000;161:26–31.
43. Cavayas YA, Munshi L, Del Sorbo L, Fan E. The early change in Pa(CO(2)) after extracorporeal membrane oxygenation initiation is associated with neurological complications. Am J Respir Crit Care Med. 2020;201:1525–35.
44. Al-Fares AA, Ferguson ND, Ma J, et al. Achieving safe liberation during weaning from VV-ECMO in patients with severe ARDS: the role of tidal volume and inspiratory effort. Chest. 2021;160:1704–13.

# Early Mobilization in Patients Receiving ECMO for Respiratory Failure

# 19

K. E. Melville, D. Brodie, and D. Abrams

## 19.1 Introduction

Critically ill patients are at risk for neuromuscular weakness and physical deconditioning following an intensive care unit (ICU) admission, known as ICU-acquired weakness, with immobility and use of invasive mechanical ventilation among the well-recognized risk factors [1–3]. Participation in physical therapy programs has been shown to be safe and feasible in a large majority of ICU patients, and has been associated with decreases in ICU and hospital lengths of stay, decreased rates of delirium, and improvement in return to independent function with increased mobility [4–8]. Patients receiving extracorporeal membrane oxygenation (ECMO) for severe respiratory failure are at significant risk for ICU-acquired weakness [9], and it is reasonable to extrapolate that these patients would gain benefit from early mobilization and physical therapy. However, concerns remain regarding the ability to safely mobilize these patients, both due to the severity of their clinical presentation, as well as device malfunction, especially cannula dislodgment. Recently, studies addressing these concerns in patients receiving ECMO have identified barriers and facilitators to early mobilization, and explored patient-centered outcomes related to physical therapy.

K. E. Melville · D. Brodie · D. Abrams (✉)
Division of Pulmonary, Allergy, and Critical Care Medicine, Department of Medicine, Columbia University College of Physicians and Surgeons, New York, NY, USA

Center for Acute Respiratory Failure, New York-Presbyterian Hospital, New York, NY, USA
e-mail: da2256@cumc.columbia.edu



J.-L. Vincent (ed.), *Annual Update in Intensive Care and Emergency Medicine 2023*, Annual Update in Intensive Care and Emergency Medicine,
https://doi.org/10.1007/978-3-031-23005-9_19

## 19.2 Evidence

The role of early mobilization in patients receiving ECMO for respiratory failure differs depending on whether ECMO is used as a bridge to recovery in acute forms of respiratory failure, such as the acute respiratory distress syndrome (ARDS), or as a bridge to lung transplantation in the setting of chronic lung disease. These patient populations differ in their clinical characteristics; approach to management, including degree of sedation; presence of concurrent invasive mechanical ventilation; and involvement of other organ system failures; along with differences that may be seen in ECMO configurations and use. Additionally, the requirement in some lung transplant programs for lung transplant candidates to maintain physical activity to avoid deconditioning and debility – in order to remain actively listed for lung transplantation – is another important factor. There is evidence that mobilization and ambulation in the bridge to lung transplantation population improves outcomes. In a 2019 study that explored outcomes of patients who received ECMO as a bridge to lung transplantation, ambulation was found to be the only independent predictor of successful bridging [10]. All 121 patients in this cohort participated in physical therapy and 68% were ambulatory. When comparing patients who were ultimately transplanted to those where bridge to lung transplantation was not successful (i.e., patients who were delisted or died prior to lung transplantation), a significantly greater number of those who were transplanted had ambulated (76% compared to 57%). Additionally, in a related cohort of patients with interstitial lung disease and concurrent pulmonary hypertension who were receiving ECMO as a bridge to transplant, ambulation during ECMO prior to transplant was associated with an 80% reduction in the risk of death (HR 0.2; 95% CI 0.08–0.48) [11]. The feasibility and benefit of early mobilization in the bridge to recovery patient population is less well defined in the literature.

One of the earlier retrospective studies of early mobilization of patients receiving ECMO details a single center's experience in bridge to recovery and bridge to lung transplantation populations and showed that mobilization was safe and feasible [12]. In 100 consecutive patients who were managed with ECMO starting in 2009, 26 were initiated with the intention of bridge to lung transplantation and 74 with the intention of bridge to recovery. Of these 100 patients, 35 participated in active physical therapy during their time receiving ECMO support. Given differences in severity of illness and other clinical parameters, the 19 bridge to transplant and 16 bridge to recovery patients who were mobilized were analyzed separately in the study. Twenty-seven of the patients mobilized had purely upper body configurations, either via a dual lumen catheter for venovenous ECMO (VV-ECMO) or with internal jugular drainage and subclavian artery reinfusion in patients receiving venoarterial ECMO (VA-ECMO). The remaining eight patients had at least one femoral cannula. Following cannulation to ECMO, two-thirds of patients in the cohort receiving physical therapy were able to be liberated from invasive mechanical ventilation, with about equal rates in the bridge to recovery and bridge to transplant groups. Aside from logistical considerations, there are several other benefits to liberation when considering ability and feasibility of mobilization, including decreased sedative requirements in most patients, increased patient comfort, and the potential ability to receive oral nutrition.

Patients in this study [12] participated in a median of five physical therapy sessions. The degree of mobilization achieved during physical therapy was graded using a validated ordinal scale, ranging from one (no mobilization or passive range of motion only) to eight (ambulation). In total, 51% of all patients were able to ambulate, including two who had femoral cannulae. Across the entire cohort, the median maximum score achieved was eight (ambulation), with a median of eight in the bridge to transplant group compared with a median of two (active range of motion while in bed) in the bridge to recovery group. The vast majority of the patients either maintained the same level of activity or increased their level of activity across the physical therapy sessions they participated in while on ECMO. The physical therapy sessions were tolerated well, with no patient- or circuit-related complications reported as a result of mobilization. Overall, no significant changes to ECMO blood flow rate, sweep gas flow rate, vasopressor dosing, or supplemental oxygen were needed during or following the sessions.

A study by Munshi et al. evaluated the effect of physical therapy consultation specifically in a bridge to recovery population, given the relative lack of data regarding safety, feasibility, and outcomes in this subset of patients [13]. This retrospective cohort study included 61 patients with ARDS between 2010 and 2015 and focused on the frequency and nature of physical therapy performed, as well as whether there was an association with ICU mortality. The vast majority (93%) of the patients underwent VV-ECMO, whereas four patients received veno-arterial support. Most (53%) of these patients were cannulated with upper body dual-lumen bicaval cannulas, and the remainder had at least one femoral cannula in place.

Of these 61 patients, the physical therapy team was consulted for 50 (82%). The best score on the ICU mobility scale was recorded for each patient undergoing physical therapy. Thirty-nine percent of the patients were able to achieve at least in-bed exercises and 17% of the patients were able to at least actively sit on the edge of the bed. For the primary outcome of association with mortality, ICU and in-hospital mortality was significantly lower (22% compared with 64%) among those who underwent physical therapy when compared with those that did not (OR 0.19; 95% CI 0.04–0.98). This association is likely confounded by selection bias, in that sicker patients, who were ultimately less likely to survive, were less often recommended for physical therapy. Regarding factors associated with achieving higher intensity physical therapy, only Sedation Agitation Scale (SAS) score on the day following ECMO cannulation was found to be associated, reflecting increased alertness.

In both of these studies [12, 13], over the years they were conducted, a higher percentage of patients were referred for physical therapy over time, despite relatively stable clinical characteristics, likely reflecting an increased level of comfort mobilizing these patients based on institutional experience as well as more established protocols.

In 2017, a study from the University of Maryland detailed that center's experience with early mobilization and physical therapy for patients receiving VV- or VA-ECMO for bridge to lung transplantation or bridge to recovery, mainly focusing on safety and feasibility, especially in the presence of femoral cannulation, as well as a patient-centered outcome of discharge location [14]. This was a retrospective cohort study, which included 254 patients who received ECMO support, 167 of whom participated in a total of 607 physical therapy sessions. Of those patients who participated in physical therapy, 80% had at least one femoral cannula, 40% had bifemoral cannulae, and arterial support was present in 26% of patients. Twenty-five of these patients (15%) were able to complete standing exercises or full ambulation with physical therapy, including those with one or two femoral cannulae, with VV- and VA-ECMO support.

When comparing discharge locations for survivors who received physical therapy during ECMO with those who received physical therapy only after decannulation, a higher percentage in the former group were able to be discharged home or to acute rehabilitation (93% vs. 81%). Those patients who received physical therapy during their time on ECMO achieved higher scores on the ICU mobility scale, both during their time on ECMO and following decannulation, than their counterparts who received physical therapy only following decannulation.

Throughout the 607 sessions, only three individual safety events were reported, which included two episodes of arrhythmia and one hypotensive event. These were considered minor and therapy sessions were able to resume that same day. No major events, including cannulae- or circuit-related events, were reported.

A study conducted in Germany detailed safety, feasibility, and resource utilization in patients being supported with different modalities of extracorporeal life support (ECLS) for severe cardiopulmonary disease [15]. In a cohort of 115 patients receiving ECLS, a majority of whom were receiving venoarterial support (64%), with a large incidence of femoral cannulation (94%), active mobilization with at least edge-of-bed activity was achieved in 43 patients (37.4%). Ambulation was infrequent, with only two episodes of walking out of a total of 332 mobilizations (0.6%); the majority of the active mobilizations consisted of standing and walking a short distance to a chair. Of the 332 mobilizations, 313 (94.3%) occurred in the presence of at least one femoral cannula. The clinical characteristics of the patients and the goals of ECLS support in this population differed in some ways from those previously discussed, with greater frequency of arterial support and less overall time receiving ECLS support. Only 12 of the 115 patients (10.4%) in the cohort were not receiving concurrent mechanical ventilation, however, a disproportionately large number of mobilizations occurred in this group (70.2%). The patients who were able to achieve active mobilization had lower severity of illness than those who were not.

The primary outcome of interest was complications during mobilization. There were three incidents of major bleeding requiring transfusions and/or surgical intervention in the mobilized patients (6.9%), all from femoral catheter sites, compared with a higher number of similar bleeding events in the patients who were not mobilized (15.3%). Minor bleeding, which did not require surgical intervention, transfusion, or cessation of therapy occurred in a higher frequency in the mobilized compared with the non-mobilized group (20.9% v 1.4%). A major event of femoral cannula displacement occurred during one mobilization session (0.3% of all sessions) and was managed with effective re-cannulation. All other adverse clinical events that occurred during mobilization, such as desaturation events, hypotension, or decrease in ECLS blood flow, were brief and either self-limited, or managed without issue by the clinical team. Although major adverse events were rare, this study again highlighted the need for an experienced bedside team during mobilization efforts, such that complications are able to be handled quickly and effectively. The median number of team members present during each mobilization, including physical therapists, nurses, physicians, and perfusionists, was three, similar to what has been described elsewhere in the literature.

As early mobilization of ECMO patients has become more common, due in part to the data highlighting safety and feasibility, several questions remain unanswered. One such question is whether certain factors are predictive of a patient's ability to participate in high-intensity physical therapy during a mobilization program. In the largest cohort study to date, 177 patients supported with ECMO underwent active physical therapy at a single center [16]. The patients encompassed bridge to transplant and bridge to recovery populations; however, the majority (88%) of those mobilized were awaiting lung transplantation. These 177 patients participated in a total of 2706 physical therapy sessions. The primary outcome was the ability to stand, march in place, or ambulate, collectively referred to as out-of-bed activities, which correlated to a score of ≥4 on the ICU mobility scale. Seventy-eight percent of patients were able to achieve this level of activity, and most (61%) were able to ambulate.

Factors associated with increased likelihood of achieving out-of-bed physical therapy were: incremental year of ECMO initiation since the start of the mobilization program (2009), bridge to transplant as the indication for ECMO, venovenous cannulation (as opposed to venoarterial configurations), and higher Charlson Comorbidity Index. There are likely several factors contributing to the finding that ECMO patients being bridged to lung transplantation were more likely to perform better with physical therapy. As discussed previously, these patients are often less acutely critically ill and more frequently able to be supported without deep sedation or neuromuscular blocking agents. Additionally, there is the added imperative of maintaining strength and functional status such that they remain appropriate candidates for lung transplantation. It is also worth mentioning that the time spent on ECMO for bridge to transplant patients was significantly longer than that for bridge to recovery patients, reflecting increased opportunity to work with physical therapy. The association with higher comorbidity scores is less intuitive, but, specifically in a bridge to transplant population, may be explained by the prioritization of mobilization in a group of individuals at high likelihood of debility and at greater risk for being deemed ineligible for transplantation. At the very least, this association implies that patients with a higher burden of comorbid conditions may be mobilized successfully. Importantly, as seen in other cohorts, as programs become more experienced and comfortable mobilizing these patients safely, the percentage of patients participating in physical therapy increases.

Presence of invasive mechanical ventilation and femoral cannulation were factors associated with decreased odds of being able to perform out-of-bed physical therapy activities. The negative association with invasive mechanical ventilation is likely twofold, reflecting both the added difficulty of logistically mobilizing patients on multiple life-support devices, but also due to the fact that patients who are unable to be liberated from invasive mechanical ventilation once receiving ECMO are likely more critically ill and also more likely to be sedated and, perhaps, to be receiving neuromuscular blocking agents. Similarly, the association with femoral cannulation likely reflects relative clinician discomfort with mobilization in this population, but also potentially points to a population needing more ECMO support, by way of multiple cannulae, including arterial femoral cannulae in some patients. Similarly, one of the additional aims of this study was to address the ability to safely mobilize patients with femoral cannulae. While these patients were mobilized with lower frequency and were not as able to perform high intensity physical therapy as those without femoral cannulae, over 700 of the physical therapy sessions were performed in the presence of at least one femoral cannula, including many sessions with two femoral cannulae, including femoral arterial cannulae.

In general, this study [16] was able to demonstrate the safety of early mobilization of patients supported with ECMO on a large scale. Across all 2706 sessions, there were 59 adverse events (2%), affecting 28 (16%) of the patients. Self-limited bleeding occurred during 13 sessions, with the majority occurring in the presence of a femoral cannula, but no cannulae became dislodged during any of the sessions. Despite the low incidence of adverse events, there were three serious adverse events that occurred during physical therapy sessions, including two cerebrovascular accidents and one cardiac arrest. The cardiac arrest was due to a pulmonary embolism in a patient receiving VV-ECMO support; the patient recovered well and was able to resume participation in physical therapy during the hospitalization.

In 2020, a research letter was published describing ECMO utilization in coronavirus disease 2019 (COVID-19) associated severe ARDS at two centers in Chicago during the first several months of the pandemic [17, 18]. This retrospective observational study detailed the use of single-access, dual-stage VV-ECMO via right atrial drainage and pulmonary arterial reinfusion in 40 patients. Early extubation was prioritized in this population, in part to decrease the need for sedative medications and to facilitate mobilization. The primary outcome was survival following liberation from mechanical ventilation and ECMO support. Patients underwent extubation an average of 11 days following ECMO cannulation, receiving mechanical ventilation for an average of 15 days overall. Mortality in this cohort was 17.5%, lower than that in other analyses of patients with severe COVID-19-associated ARDS receiving ECMO support [19]. Additionally, 50% of the patients were able to be discharged directly home from the hospital without intervening rehabilitation stays. Complications were described as minimal, and no specific reference to mobilization-related complications was cited. The authors attribute the relatively low mortality and morbidity in this cohort to their cannulation approach, which avoided femoral cannulae, provided right ventricular support via reinfusion into the pulmonary artery, and may have facilitated earlier extubation and mobilization. As part of this bundled intervention, early mobilization may have had some impact on improved outcomes in this population.

Taken together, these studies highlight the safety and feasibility of early mobilization in patients receiving ECMO, be it for bridge to transplant or bridge to recovery, including those with femoral cannulation (Table 19.1). However, these studies are limited by the fact that they are all observational, largely single center, experiences.

**Table 19.1** Safety and feasibility of mobilization while receiving extracorporeal membrane oxygenation (ECMO) support; data from randomized controlled and notable observational studies

| Study author [ref] | Patients mobilized (n) | PT sessions (n) | BTT n (%) | BTR n (%) | VV-ECMO n (%) | Femoral cannulae n (%) | Ambulatory patients n (%) | Ambulations out of all mobilizations n (%) | Adverse event rate (%) |
|---|---|---|---|---|---|---|---|---|---|
| *Randomized controlled data* | | | | | | | | | |
| Hodgson [20] | 10 | 56 | 0 | 10 (100) | 3 (30) | 1 (10) | NA | NA | 2 |
| *Selected observational studies* | | | | | | | | | |
| Munshi [13] | 50 | NA | 0 (0) | 50 (100) | 49 (98) | 23 (47) | NA | NA | NA |
| Wells [14] | 167 | 607 | NA | NA | 98 (59) | 134 (80) | 8 (5) | 37 (6) | 0.5 |
| Braune [15] | 43 | 332 | 2 (5) | 41 (95) | 19 (44) | 40 (93) | NA | 2 (0.6) | 1 |
| Abrams [16] | 177 | 2706 | 124 (70) | 53 (30) | 113 (64) | 66 (37) | 108 (61) | 1284 (47) | 2 |

*NA* data not reported in publication, *VV* venovenous, *BTT* bridge to transplantation, *BTR* bridge to recovery, *PT* physical therapy

Recently, a pilot randomized controlled trial (RCT) was published, describing the results of an early mobilization intervention in patients receiving ECMO in three ICUs in Australia [20]. The patients received either early mobilization (within 72 h of initiation of ECMO) for 7 days or standard of care. The primary outcome of interest was feasibility of delivering the intervention, including whether the two groups had a degree of separation in the amount and intensity of physical therapy. Secondary outcomes included safety, differences in strength or functional status, ICU and hospital length of stay, and mortality. In the 20 patients randomized, those in the intervention group spent more time doing active physical therapy in the first seven days (median 133 v. 27.5 min) compared to the control arm, although the maximum level of activity achieved did not differ significantly. At hospital discharge, there was increased functional independence, using the Katz activities of daily living scale, in those in the early mobilization arm. There was no difference in lengths of ICU or hospital stay or mortality.

An important point regarding feasibility is the fact that this trial was originally planned for four sites, but one of the sites was unable to enroll due to the unavailability of their experienced physical therapist. This highlights the point that an experienced multidisciplinary team is of utmost importance to safely and successfully mobilize patients during ECMO.

The same group in Australia is currently preparing to enroll for a phase 2 multicenter RCT (ClinicalTrials.gov Identifier: NCT05003609). Their goal is to enroll 100 ECMO patients and randomize to early mobilization and rehabilitation or standard of care with similar patient-centered outcome measures, including functional disability and independence, muscle strength, length of ICU and hospital stay, and mortality, among other outcomes. Areas for future research on this topic should continue to address the efficacy and impact of early mobilization in this population as well as ways to identify subgroups who may derive the most benefit with the fewest complications.

## 19.3 Conclusion

Early mobilization performed at experienced centers is safe, feasible, and effective in patients receiving ECMO for respiratory failure. The indication for ECMO, whether for bridge to recovery or bridge to lung transplantation, is important when considering feasibility and potential benefits of early mobilization. Mobilization in bridge to transplant patients is important to avoid deconditioning in order to maintain transplant candidacy, and outcomes appear to be improved when patients are ambulatory prior to transplant. Taken together, these are strong arguments for mobilizing bridge to transplant patients. In the appropriate bridge to recovery ECMO patient, mobilization is also feasible, regardless of cannulation strategy, although more data are needed on the effect of functional outcomes in this population. Additionally, serious adverse events, while rare, are possible, and the risk-benefit ratio of mobilization may be patient-specific depending on patient factors as well as perceived benefit and goals of therapy. A multidisciplinary team with experience and expertise, and with screening and safety protocols in place, is perhaps the most important factor in regards to safe mobilization.

## References


1. Needham DM. Mobilizing patients in the intensive care unit: improving neuromuscular weakness and physical function. JAMA. 2008;300:1685–90.
2. Stevens RD, Dowdy DW, Michaels RK, Mendez-Tellez PA, Pronovost PJ, Needham DM. Neuromuscular dysfunction acquired in critical illness: a systematic review. Intensive Care Med. 2007;33:1876–91.
3. Fan E, Dowdy DW, Colantuoni E, et al. Physical complications in acute lung injury survivors: a 2-year longitudinal prospective study. Crit Care Med. 2014;42:849–59.
4. Waldauf P, Jiroutkova K, Krajcova A, Puthucheary Z, Duska F. Effects of rehabilitation interventions on clinical outcomes in critically ill patients: systematic review and meta-analysis of randomized controlled trials. Crit Care Med. 2020;48:1055–65.
5. Morris PE, Goad A, Thompson C, et al. Early intensive care unit mobility therapy in the treatment of acute respiratory failure. Crit Care Med. 2008;36:2238–43.
6. Tipping CJ, Harrold M, Holland A, Romero L, Nisbet T, Hodgson CL. The effects of active mobilisation and rehabilitation in ICU on mortality and function: a systematic review. Intensive Care Med. 2017;43:171–83.
7. Nydahl P, Sricharoenchai T, Chandra S, et al. Safety of patient mobilization and rehabilitation in the intensive care unit. systematic review with meta-analysis. Ann Am Thorac Soc. 2017;14:766–77.
8. Schweickert WD, Pohlman MC, Pohlman AS, et al. Early physical and occupational therapy in mechanically ventilated, critically ill patients: a randomised controlled trial. Lancet. 2009;373:1874–82.
9. Hayes K, Holland AE, Pellegrino VA, Mathur S, Hodgson CL. Acute skeletal muscle wasting and relation to physical function in patients requiring extracorporeal membrane oxygenation (ECMO). J Crit Care. 2018;48:1–8.
10. Tipograf Y, Salna M, Minko E, et al. Outcomes of extracorporeal membrane oxygenation as a bridge to lung transplantation. Ann Thorac Surg. 2019;107:1456–63.
11. Chicotka S, Pedroso FE, Agerstrand CL, et al. Increasing opportunity for lung transplant in interstitial lung disease with pulmonary hypertension. Ann Thorac Surg. 2018;106:1812–9.
12. Abrams D, Javidfar J, Farrand E, et al. Early mobilization of patients receiving extracorporeal membrane oxygenation: a retrospective cohort study. Crit Care. 2014;18:R38.
13. Munshi L, Kobayashi T, DeBacker J, et al. Intensive care physiotherapy during extracorporeal membrane oxygenation for acute respiratory distress syndrome. Ann Am Thorac Soc. 2017;14:246–53.
14. Wells CL, Forrester J, Vogel J, Rector R, Tabatabai A, Herr D. Safety and feasibility of early physical therapy for patients on extracorporeal membrane oxygenator: University of Maryland Medical Center experience. Crit Care Med. 2018;46:53–9.
15. Braune S, Bojes P, Mecklenburg A, et al. Feasibility, safety, and resource utilisation of active mobilisation of patients on extracorporeal life support: a prospective observational study. Ann Intensive Care. 2020;10:161.
16. Abrams D, Madahar P, Eckhardt CM, et al. Early mobilization during extracorporeal membrane oxygenation for cardiopulmonary failure in adults: factors associated with intensity of treatment. Ann Am Thorac Soc. 2022;19:90–8.
17. Mustafa AK, Alexander PJ, Joshi DJ, et al. Extracorporeal membrane oxygenation for patients with COVID-19 in severe respiratory failure. JAMA Surg. 2020;155:990–2.
18. Mustafa AK, Tatooles AJ. Extracorporeal membrane oxygenation and coronavirus disease 2019—reply. JAMA Surg. 2021;156:403.
19. Ramanathan K, Shekar K, Ling RR, et al. Extracorporeal membrane oxygenation for COVID-19: a systematic review and meta-analysis. Crit Care. 2021;25:211.
20. ECMO-PT Study Investigators; International ECMO Network. Early mobilisation during extracorporeal membrane oxygenation was safe and feasible: a pilot randomised controlled trial. Intensive Care Med. 2020;46:1057–9.

# Physiological Adaptations During Weaning from Venovenous ECMO

# 20

P. D. Collins, L. Giosa, and L. Camporota

## 20.1 Introduction

Venovenous extracorporeal membrane oxygenation (VV-ECMO) is a technique that can support gas exchange and enable a reduction in the mechanical power applied to the injured lung in patients with acute severe and refractory, but potentially reversible, respiratory failure.

The increasing emphasis on reducing ergotrauma, technological improvements in extracorporeal devices, and viral pandemics (i.e., $H_1N_1$ influenza and severe acute respiratory syndrome coronavirus 2 [SARS-CoV-2]) have resulted in an exponential growth in ECMO utilization over the last decade [1]. The possible applications of VV-ECMO are wide, including severe acute respiratory distress syndrome (ARDS) [2–4] near fatal asthma [5], severe air leak syndromes [6], interstitial lung disease [7], or as a bridge to lung transplantation [8].

In contrast to the abundance of data on indications, complications, and prognostic factors for ECMO survival [1, 2, 3], consensus guidelines on weaning [9] are based on limited direct evidence for the criteria to initiate a weaning trial, how to monitor patients undergoing weaning, and how to adjust mechanical ventilation to optimally support patients during this phase.

P. D. Collins
Department of Critical Care Medicine, Guy's and St. Thomas' National Health Service Foundation Trust, London, UK

L. Giosa · L. Camporota (✉)
Department of Critical Care Medicine, Guy's and St. Thomas' National Health Service Foundation Trust, London, UK

King's College London, School of Basic and Medical Biosciences, Centre for Human and Applied Physiological Sciences, London, UK
e-mail: luigi.camporota@kcl.ac.uk



J.-L. Vincent (ed.), *Annual Update in Intensive Care and Emergency Medicine 2023*, Annual Update in Intensive Care and Emergency Medicine,
https://doi.org/10.1007/978-3-031-23005-9_20

Identifying strategies that can accelerate the safe liberation of patients from ECMO is essential to reduce length of stay and risk of complications, as well as ensuring equity of access at times of strain on healthcare resources [10]. This is also important, as international surveys have highlighted wide intercenter variations in the approach to mechanical ventilation and weaning during VV-ECMO [11] and-perhaps consequently- in outcome [1].

A sound understanding of the physiological interactions between the extracorporeal circuit, the patient, and the ventilator is required to guide physicians throughout the process of weaning. Accordingly, after a summary of current approaches to VV-ECMO liberation reported in the literature, in this chapter we describe a possible physiological approach to weaning from VV-ECMO.

## 20.2 Intercenter Variability in the Approach to Weaning

In Table 20.1 [3, 9, 12–24], we summarize possible approaches to weaning from VV-ECMO reported in the literature.

### 20.2.1 Different Preconditions for Weaning

Expert opinion suggests that a weaning trial should be considered in patients whose cardiovascular state is stable and who show clinical and radiological improvement with reducing extracorporeal blood flow (ECBF) and sweep gas flow (SGF) requirements [9]. Traditionally, the oxygen exchange capability of the natural lung ($V'O_{2NL}$) should be evaluated for a rise in $PaO_2$ > 30 kPa (>225 mmHg) on a ventilator $FiO_2$ 1.0 under stable mechanical ventilation and ECBF (Cilley's test). However, the magnitude of response to this test is a poor predictor of successful decannulation from VV-ECMO when used in isolation [25]. Recent studies have demonstrated the feasibility of a proactive daily trial off VV-ECMO for patients who fulfil pre-weaning criteria [20, 21]. Indeed, the successful weaning of patients requiring up to 4 l/min SGF at baseline suggests that liberation from VV-ECMO may be safely accelerated in some cases. Analogous to mechanical ventilation, a daily weaning trial (similar to a spontaneous breathing trial) can provide objective evidence of ECMO dependency and has the potential to shorten length of stay.

### 20.2.2 Different Ventilatory Strategies During Weaning

Another source of variation is the titration of mechanical ventilation (modes and settings) prior to or during weaning. Some centers opt to wean patients on assisted or spontaneous/assisted modes rather than mandatory mechanical ventilation. This is consistent with evidence suggesting a lack of mortality benefit for deep sedation and neuromuscular blockade over light sedation in ARDS [26]. However, most centers have prioritized the weaning of ECMO prior to mechanical ventilation and maintain patients on controlled or assist-control ventilation until ECMO decannulation [10].

**Table 20.1** Varied approaches to weaning from venovenous extracorporeal membrane oxygenation (VV-ECMO) in the literature

| Source | Preconditions for weaning | Preferred ventilation | Targeted parameters during weaning: ECBF (l/min) | $FdO_2$ | SGF (l/min) | Duration (h) | Measured effort/drive | Monitoring criteria for successful trial |
|---|---|---|---|---|---|---|---|---|
| Sen et al. 2016 [12] | PEEP 5–10, peak pressure 20–25, $V_T$ 6 ml/kg, RR ~15, $PaO_2$ 50–80, radiological improvement | Controlled or spontaneous | 2 | 0.21 | 0 | Unspecified | – | Clinician discretion |
| Reeb et al. 2017 [13] | Sats >88% ($PaO_2$ > 60), $FiO_2$ ≤ 0.6, PEEP ≤15, RR ≤35 | Not specified | Not specified | 1.0 | 0 | 4 | – | Stable ABG |
| Combes et al. 2018 [3] | Clinical + radiological improvement | Controlled | Not specified | 1.0 | 0 | ≥1 | – | $PaO_2$ > 70 mmHg on $FiO_2$ < 0.6 Plateau pressure < 30. No acute cor pulmonale |
| Broman et al. 2018[a] [14] | $FiO_2$ 0.35–0.55, minimal $V'CO_{2ML}$ with 5% $CO_2$ added to SGF <2 l/min | Controlled or spontaneous | Not specified | 1.0 | 0 | ≥2–12 | – | Clinician discretion |
| Broman et al. 2018[b] [14] | $FiO_2$ < 0.45, PEEP <10, peak pressure <27 | Not specified | 1.5 | 1.0 | 0 | 0.5–1 | – | Stable ABG and absence of dyspnea |
| Broman et al. 2018[c] [14] | Clinical + radiological improvement | Spontaneous | 2.5–3 | 1.0 | 0 | Unspecified | – | Absence of dyspnea |
| Grant et al. 2018 [15] | Sats >90%, $FiO_2$ ≤ 0.5, PEEP ≤10, plateau pressure ≤ ₂5, $V_T$ ≤ 6–8 ml/kg | Controlled | 3–4 | 0.21 | ≤1 1 | Unspecified | – | Stable ABG, maintain preconditions |
| Seiler et al. 2018 [16] | Clinician discretion | Controlled | 2 | 1.0 | 0 | 1 | – | Stable ABG |
| Chaves et al. 2019 [17] | $FiO_2$ ≤ 0.6, PEEP ≤15, peak pressure ≤ 30, $V_T$ ≤ 6 ml/kg, RR ≤35 and radiological improvement | Spontaneous | Unspecified | 1.0 | 0 | 6 | – | Clinical stability, normal pH and $PaO_2$ |

(continued)

**Table 20.1** (continued)

| Source | Preconditions for weaning | Preferred ventilation | Targeted parameters during weaning | | | | Measured effort/drive | Monitoring criteria for successful trial |
|---|---|---|---|---|---|---|---|---|
| | | | ECBF (l/min) | $FdO_2$ | SGF (l/min) | Duration (h) | | |
| Vasques et al. 2019 [18] | Sats >88% on $FiO_2$ 0.6, $PaO_2 > 225$ on Cilley test, $V'CO_{2NL} > 50\%$ of total, $V_T \leq 6$–8 ml/kg | Spontaneous | Unspecified | 0.21 | 0 | Unspecified | Yes | P 0.1 > −10, RR ≤35, ratio of $V'CO_{2NL}$ to minute ventilation >80% of baseline, absence of distress |
| Li et al. 2020 [19] | Clinical + radiological improvement | Controlled | 2.5 | 1.0 | 0 | 24–48 | – | RR ≤20, P:F ratio > 150, Murray Index 2–3, $PaCO_2 \leq 50$, temperature <38 °C |
| Gannon et al. 2021 [20] | SGF ≤3, Sats ≥88% ($PaO_2 \geq 60$) with $FiO_2 \leq 0.6$, PEEP ≤15. RR ≤35, HR <120, systolic BP ≥180 or <90, pH ≥7.35 | Controlled or spontaneous | <3 | 0.5 | 0 | 0.5 | – | Maintain non-ECMO preconditions, ≤20% change in HR |
| Tonna et al. (ELSO guideline), 202 [19] | $PaO_2 \geq 70$ $FiO_2 \leq 0.6$, PEEP ≤10, plateau pressure ≤28, $V_T \leq 6$ ml/kg, RR ≤28, improved CXR | Controlled or spontaneous | 1–1.5[d] | 0.21 | 0 | ≥2–3 | – | Normocapnia, $PaO_2 > 70$, no respiratory distress |
| Teijeiro et al. 2021 [21] | No air leak, No NMB >24 h, $FiO_2 \leq 0.6$ Sats >88% $PaO_2 > 60$ peak pressure ≤ 20, $V_T \leq 9$ ml/kg, hemodynamically stable, SGF <5, ECBF <5 | Spontaneous | <5 | 1.0 | 0 | 2–24 | – | Respiratory distress, $V_T > 9$ ml/kg, sats <88% (or requiring $FiO_2 > 0.6$, PEEP ≥20) pH <7.25, hemodynamic instability, agitation or drowsiness |

| | | | | | | | | |
|---|---|---|---|---|---|---|---|---|
| Belliato et al. 2021 [22] | Clinical and radiological improvement, PEEP ≤10–15, hemodynamic stability | Controlled or spontaneous | Not specified | 1.0 | 0 | 6–12 | – | Clinician discretion |
| Al-Fares et al., 2021 [23] | Clinician discretion | Controlled or Spontaneous | >3 | 1.0 | 0 | Not specified | Yes | Clinician discretion |
| Lazarri et al. 2022 [24] | ΔPes ≤15, RR ≤30, pH >7.25, $PaCO_2 \leq 60$, $PaO_2 > 70$ with $FiO_2 \leq 0.6$ | Controlled or spontaneous | Not specified | 1.0 | 0 | Not specified | Yes | Maintain preconditions |

*ECBF* extracorporeal blood flow, *$FdO_2$* fraction of oxygen of the sweep gas flow (SGF), *PEEP* positive end expiratory pressure, $V_T$ tidal volume (per kilogram of predicted body weight), *RR* respiratory rate, *ABG* arterial blood gas, *$PaO_2$* partial pressure of arterial oxygen, *$PaCO_2$* the partial pressure of arterial carbon dioxide, $V'CO_{2ML}$ carbon dioxide cleared by the membrane lung, $V'CO_{2NL}$ carbon dioxide cleared by the native lung, $\Delta Pes$ the change in esophageal pressure, *P:F ratio* ratio of $PaO_2$ to $FiO_2$. All airway pressures measured in centimeters of water. All non-airway pressures (including partial pressures) measured in millimeters of mercury

[a]Broman et al. reported an approach from the Karolinska Institute

[b]Broman et al. reported an approach from the Regensburg Hospital

[c]Broman et al. reported an approach from the San Raffaele Hospital

[d]A reduction in ECBF is considered optional within the guidelines

### 20.2.3 Different Targeted Parameters During Weaning

There are no studies that compared the relative benefit of targeting different parameters during a trial off VV-ECMO, and weaning was not tightly protocolized in the landmark randomized trials in ARDS [2, 3]. Indeed, there is significant variation among centers on how weaning is performed. Most commonly, weaning follows a gradual reduction in SGF rate to zero, generally with an oxygen fraction through the membrane lung ($FdO_2$) of 1.0 [3, 13, 14, 16, 17, 19, 21–24]. Some centers wean the $FdO_2$ prior to reducing SGF to test the dependency on oxygenation before testing the ability to maintain $CO_2$ clearance consequent to the SGF reduction [9, 12, 15, 18, 20]. A minority of centers preferentially wean the ECBF during weaning [10]. Interestingly, one center proposed to add 5% $CO_2$ to the SGF once flow was ≤2 l/min and to stop SGF when the pre- and post-membrane $CO_2$ difference was minimal [14].

The duration of a weaning trial is another parameter that is quite variable between centers. In the EOLIA trial, a 1-hour trial off ECMO [3] was used, but the extracorporeal life support organization (ELSO) recommends at least a 2–3 h trial [9], and other groups have used a trial of 30 min [20]. However, recently Al-Fares et al. found that patients who were liberated inappropriately (i.e., failed decannulation defined as re-cannulation within 48 h or a significant escalation in respiratory or cardiovascular support) could not be identified until at least four hours after a trial off SGF [23]. This may be the reason why some centers- including ours- opt for a longer period of assessment off SGF (12–24 h or longer, especially in complex patients or with longer ECMO runs) [18].

### 20.2.4 Different Evaluation Criteria for a Weaning Trial

Conceptually, weaning success is defined by the ability to maintain gas exchange via the natural lung with protective ventilatory parameters and without excessive respiratory effort. Although recent studies suggest that invasive measurements of effort, such as the esophageal pressure swing, provide useful information during VV-ECMO weaning [23, 24], the majority of the reported literature relies on clinical signs (such as respiratory rate and heart rate) and blood gas analysis (see Table 20.1).

Given this variation in practice, in the next section we will outline an understanding of the interactions between the circuit, patient, and ventilator that underpin a physiological approach to weaning.

## 20.3 Physiology of Weaning from VV-ECMO

### 20.3.1 The Extracorporeal Circuit

#### 20.3.1.1 $V'O_{2ML}$, $V'CO_{2ML}$ and the Effects of Weaning

The extracorporeal circuit is depicted in Fig. 20.1. Table 20.2 summarizes the effects of weaning different ECMO parameters on the oxygen delivery ($V'O_{2ML}$) and the

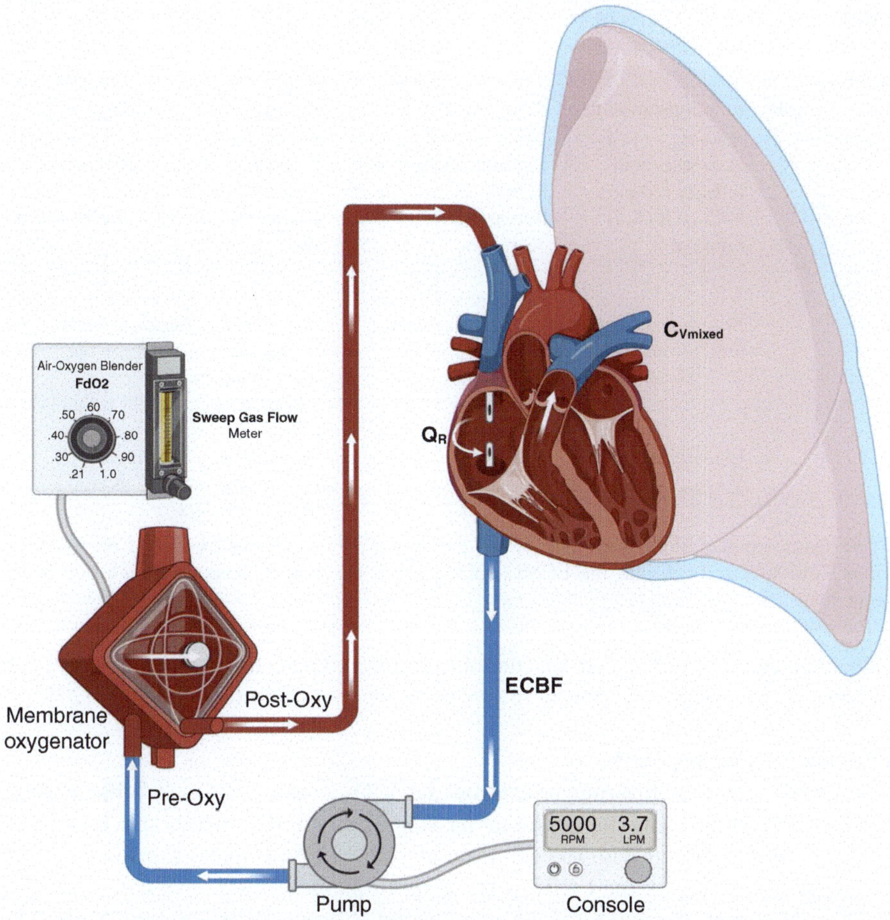


**Fig. 20.1** The anatomy and physiology of the extracorporeal circuit, depicted in a femoral-jugular configuration. Blood is drained from the central venous system ($C_V$) via a cannula and centrifugal pump which generates extracorporeal blood flow (ECBF). Pre-oxygenator blood is a mixture of central venous ($C_v$) and recirculating ($Q_R$) blood. It is pumped across hollow fibers within the membrane oxygenator across which there is sweep gas flow (SGF). Post-oxygenator blood is passes through the return lumen where it becomes mixed with the $C_V$ blood in the right ventricle and pulmonary arteries to form the mixed venous blood ($C_{Vmixed}$) before being distributed through the native pulmonary circulation. Mixed central venous blood oxygen content ($C_{Vmixed}O_2$) will be determined by the central venous oxygen content ($C_{vO2}$), the post-oxygenator blood's oxygen content ($C_{post\text{-}oxy\ O2}$), the ECBF, recirculation flow ($Q_R$) and overall cardiac output (Qt) according to the formula: $C_{Vmixed}O_2 \cdot Qt = [C_vO_2 \cdot (Qt - ECBF + Qr)] + [C_{post\text{-}oxy}O_2 \cdot (ECBF\text{-}QR)]$. Although the ECBF contributes to the calculation of the overall $CO_2$ clearance of the membrane lung [$V'CO_{2ML} = (C_{post\text{-}oxy}\ CO_2 \text{-} C_{post\text{-}oxy}CO_2) \cdot ECBF \cdot 25)$], during usual VV-ECMO ECBF levels (>2.5 L), the primary determinant of $V'CO_2ML$ is the SGF rate which generates the gradient for $CO_2$ diffusion and resulting difference in pre- and post-oxygenator $CO_2$ content. (Figure created with BioRender.com, adapted from a template created by Dr. Yevgeniy Brailovsky from Sidney Kimmel School of Medicine)

**Table 20.2** Titratable extracorporeal membrane oxygenation (ECMO) parameters during weaning and their effects

| Parameter which can be weaned | Relationship with $V'O_{2ML}$ | Relationship with $VCO_{2ML}$ | Downsides of weaning in isolation |
|---|---|---|---|
| ECBF | Decreases will linearly reduce $V'O_{2ML}$ if $Q_R$ is minimal | Minimal change >1 l ECBF<br>Between 0.5–1 l decreases logarithmically decrease $V'CO_{2ML}$ | Low ECBF flows may increase circuit thrombosis<br>Changes in ECBF will also affect $Q_R$ |
| SGF | Minimal change until almost zero | Linearly decrease $V'CO_{2ML}$ | When SGF is turned to zero $V'O_{2ML}$ ceases suddenly but hypoxic pulmonary vasoconstriction takes minutes to react |
| $FdO_2$ | Linearly decrease $V'O_{2ML}$ | No effect | Weaning may alter the respiratory quotient and reduce alveolar oxygen |

*ECBF* extracorporeal blood flow, *SGF* sweep gas flow, $FdO_2$ fraction of oxygen of the SGF, $Q_R$ blood flow directly back into the ECMO circuit which has already passed through the membrane lung

$CO_2$ clearance ($V'CO_{2ML}$) of the membrane lung. There are three main settings which can be manipulated during the weaning from or trial off VV-ECMO [27]:

### Effects of Reducing ECBF

The ECBF rate has differing effects on the $V'O_{2ML}$ and $V'CO_{2ML}$. With a well-functioning circuit, any hemoglobin passing through the membrane lung will become fully saturated with oxygen even at very low SGF rates. Consequently, if the $FdO_2$ is unchanged, the ECBF is the main titratable variable that can affect the $V'O_{2ML}$. However, the nature of the relationship between ECBF and the $V'O_{2ML}$ is affected by the amount of recirculated blood flow ($Q_R$).

1. Recirculation occurs when arterialized blood (post oxygenator) returned to the venous system after passing through the membrane lung is aspirated straight back into the circuit (see Fig. 20.1). Given that the recirculated blood is already fully saturated with oxygen, the greater the $Q_R$ relative to the ECBF, the lower the gradient between the pre- and post-membrane bloods' oxygen content and so the lower the $V'O_{2ML}$. Effective ECBF, equal to total ECBF minus $Q_R$, is linearly related to $V'O_{2ML}$ [27] but $Q_R$ cannot be easily quantified at the bedside.
2. The proportion of $Q_R$ may be higher at higher blood flow rates. If a given decrease in ECBF during weaning disproportionately reduces $Q_R$ then the change in $V'O_{2ML}$ may not be as anticipated. For example, if the $Q_R$ reduces from 1 l to 250 ml when the ECBF is weaned by 25% from 4 to 3 l/min, then the effective ECBF has only changed from 3 l to 2.75 l. Conversely, where $Q_R$ is minimal, decreasing the total ECBF will decrease the effective ECBF and so the $V'O_{2ML}$ in a linear fashion [27].

The effect of weaning the ECBF on systemic oxygenation will depend mainly on the patient's cardiac output and venous admixture. As the proportion of the total cardiac output captured in the ECBF falls, the mixed venous oxygen content will decrease. The final effect on systemic oxygenation will be determined by native lung function and the venous admixture.

In contrast to $V'O_{2ML}$, the relationship between ECBF and $V'CO_{2ML}$ is not linear, but follows a natural logarithmic curve with ECBF >0.5 ml/min, which plateaus at >1.0 l/min [28–30]. The impact of the ECBF on $V'CO_{2ML}$ is also affected by the ratio of SGF:ECBF and the surface area of the membrane lung [28]. Accordingly, step-wise decreases in ECBF have a minimal independent effect on the $V'CO_{2ML}$ until reaching very low levels, which are generally avoided in VV-ECMO to prevent circuit thrombosis. Consequently, although ECBF is often reduced prior to weaning as native lung function improves, reductions <2.5–3 l/min during a trial off VV-ECMO are generally not advisable.

### Effects of Reducing SGF Rate Without Altering the $FdO_2$

Complete saturation of hemoglobin can be achieved even with very low SGF rates (<0.5 l/min) particularly when $FdO_2$ is maintained at 1.0 [27]. For this reason, step-wise decreases in SGF do not affect $V'O_{2ML}$ until SGF is almost off. Moreover, even the small amount of SGF required to saturate hemoglobin can affect ECMO dependency for another reason: VV-ECMO causes a mixed venous 'hyperoxia', blunting or abolishing the physiological hypoxic pulmonary vasoconstriction [31] (which normally optimizes ventilation/perfusion matching). This results in an increased native lung venous admixture, with lower than expected ventilation to perfusion ratio [31–33]. Accordingly, when the SGF is turned to zero at the last step of a weaning trial, patients are abruptly totally dependent on the native lung's capacity to transfer oxygen ($V'O_{2NL}$), but the biphasic response of the pulmonary vasculature to hypoxia requires several minutes to occur, with other slower changes over hours [34]. For this reason, the assessment of the oxygen exchange capacity of the natural lung might be confounded by this sudden change. Indeed, delayed hypoxic vasoconstriction increases the effective venous admixture, making any residual lung abnormality have a disproportionate effect on gas exchange [35]. This may also be why ~30% of patients in a recent prospective study experienced frank hypoxemia after a stepwise decrease in SGF to zero without altering the $FdO_2$ [24].

In contrast to oxygenation, stepwise decreases in SGF are associated with a progressive reduction in $V'CO_{2ML}$ [27, 28]. Analogous to the minute ventilation for the native lung, SGF drives bulk transfer of $CO_2$ out of the artificial membrane and increases the gradient for $CO_2$ in the venous blood to diffuse across the membrane. Accordingly, stepwise decreases in SGF result in a higher $CO_2$ in the pulmonary vasculature and greater load to the native lung ($V'CO_{2NL}$), whose exchange capacity will affect $PaCO_2$. Although in clinical practice the oxygen exchange capability is usually assessed simply through the $PaO_2/FiO_2$ ratio (rarely implemented by venous admixture calculation), several indices have been proposed for bedside evaluation of the $CO_2$ clearance capacity of the natural lung (Table 20.3 [23, 24, 36, 37]). Interestingly, the end-tidal to partial pressure of arterial $PCO_2$ ratio ($P_{ET}/PaCO_2$), an

**Table 20.3** Evaluation of carbon dioxide ($CO_2$) clearance by native lung ($V'CO_{2NL}$) during weaning from venovenous extracorporeal membrane oxygenation (VV-ECMO)

| Parameter | Formula | Downsides/specifics |
|---|---|---|
| Ventilatory ratio [30] | $(VE \cdot PaCO_2)/(PBW \cdot 100 \cdot 37.5)$ | Assumes constant $V'CO_{2NL}$ |
| Enghoff index | $(PaCO_2 - PECO_2)/PaCO_2$ | Evaluates shunt and dead space |
| Ratio of endtidal to partial pressure of carbon dioxide | $EtCO_2/PaCO_2$ | Evaluates shunt and dead space [20, 32] |
| Bohr alveolar dead space | $(PACO_2 - PECO_2)/PACO_2$ | Evaluates pure alveolar dead space but requires analysis of volumetric capnography curve [31] |
| Ventilatory efficiency | $VE/V'CO_{2NL}$ | No available data during ECMO |
| Ventilatory efficiency | $\Delta P_{es}/V'CO_{2NL}$ | Influenced by lung elastance |

*PBW* predicted body weight, *VE* minute ventilation, *$PECO_2$* mean expired $CO_2$ partial pressure, *$PACO_2$* alveolar $CO_2$ partial pressure

index of global gas-exchange efficiency [38], was the best predictor of weaning outcome in a recent study [24]. The same study also showed that the baseline ventilatory efficiency (the ratio of effort to $V'CO_{2NL}$) was lower in patients who failed a weaning trial.

When SGF is set to zero, VV-ECMO makes no contribution to gas exchange and, after the restoration of hypoxic pulmonary vasoconstriction, a true assessment of native lung function can occur. A special case in which a sudden reduction in arterial oxygenation is unrelated to lung function and severe hypoxemia following switching off SGF– which is refractory to increasing $FiO_2$ on ventilation– occurs when there is an intracardiac shunt: in this case, the flow from the return cannula can force blood through the shunt, bypassing the native lung and potentially leading to profound desaturation when SGF (and, thereby, $VO_{2ML}$) falls to zero. Indeed, if ECBF is not concomitantly reduced to <1 l/min, the deleterious effects of blood passing through the anatomical shunt will become evident when no compensatory oxygen is added from the extracorporeal circuit [39].

### Effects of Reducing the $FdO_2$ Prior to Reducing the SGF

A gradual reduction in the $FdO_2$ at constant SGF rate allows the two components of gas exchange to be separated: $V'O_{2ML}$ is sequentially decreased, while $V'CO_{2ML}$ remains unaltered. The progressive, rather than abrupt, decrease in $FdO_2$ has the advantage of gaining time for some physiological recovery hypoxic pulmonary vasoconstriction [27], thereby allowing a more accurate assessment of the oxygen exchange capacity of the native lung. The effect on systemic oxygenation of a reduction in $V'O_{2ML}$ through stepwise decreases in $FdO_2$ will depend on the ratio of ECBF to cardiac output and on the venous admixture of the native lung. Counterintuitively, decreasing the $V'O_{2ML}$ without changing the $V'CO_{2ML}$ at constant $V'CO_{2NL}$ will lead to a progressive decrease in the respiratory quotient of the native lung ($RQ_{NL} = V'CO_{2NL}/V'O_{2NL}$) [40]. Indeed, $RQ_{NL}$ is an important component of the alveolar gas equation:

$$PAO_2 = FiO_2 \cdot \left(P_{atm} - P_{H_2O}\right) - \frac{PACO_2}{RQ_{NL}}$$

where $PAO_2$ and $PACO_2$ are the alveolar partial pressures of oxygen and carbon dioxide respectively, $P_{atm}$ and $PH_2O$ are the atmospheric pressure and the vapor pressure of water respectively, and $FiO_2$ is the inspired oxygen fraction.

According to this equation, any decrease in $RQ_{NL}$ is associated with a decrease in $PAO_2$, worsening systemic oxygenation. However, the quantitative importance of this effect during weaning from VV-ECMO should be put into context:

1. The extended alveolar equation has a supplementary term (in bold here below) which, accounting for changes in alveolar gas volume during breathing, blunts the deleterious effect of low RQ on $PAO_2$, especially if the $FiO_2$ from the native lung is high [41].

$$PAO_2 = FiO_2 \cdot \left(P_{atm} - P_{H_2O}\right) - \frac{PACO_2}{RQ} + \mathbf{FiO_2 \cdot PACO_2 \cdot \frac{1 - RQ_{NL}}{RQ_{NL}}}$$

2. The reduction in $PAO_2$ at low $RQ_{NL}$ has been previously described during extracorporeal $CO_2$ removal ($ECCO_2R$), where ECBF is <1 l/min. However, this will be less evident during weaning from VV-ECMO where the ECBF is much higher: indeed, even at $FdO_2$ $0._{21}$, there may still be a substantial $V'O_{2ML}$. This would blunt the effects of the reduction in $RQ_{NL}$ [40].

### 20.3.2 The Patient

The patient's response to a weaning trial is dictated by the physiology of breathing control and, particularly, by the effects of variations in gas-exchange on the output of the respiratory centers.

#### 20.3.2.1 Physiology of Breathing Control

A simple, yet effective model describing the control of breathing was proposed by Vaporidi et al. [42] and subsequently adopted by others [43]. As depicted in Fig. 20.2 [42–45], this model describes the interdependence between the arterial partial pressure of $CO_2$ ($PaCO_2$) and the minute ventilation (VE) by plotting them in the same graph according to three different curves: (1) the metabolic hyperbola, describing the relationship between $PaCO_2$ and VE at a given $V'CO_{2NL}$ and dead space; (2) the $CO_2$ sensitivity curve (also called the brain curve), describing the change in VE that the respiratory centers desire when $PaCO_2$ deviates from its set-point; (3) the ventilation curve, depicting the corresponding change in VE that the respiratory system can actually achieve for a given $PaCO_2$. The intersection between the brain curve and the metabolic hyperbola gives the "eupneic $PaCO_2$", i.e., the $PaCO_2$ set-point of the respiratory centers. Conversely, the intersection between the ventilation curve and the metabolic hyperbola gives the "actual $PaCO_2$" of the patient. Panel a in Fig. 20.2 describes physiological and pathological determinants of the slopes and positions of these three curves [42, 43].

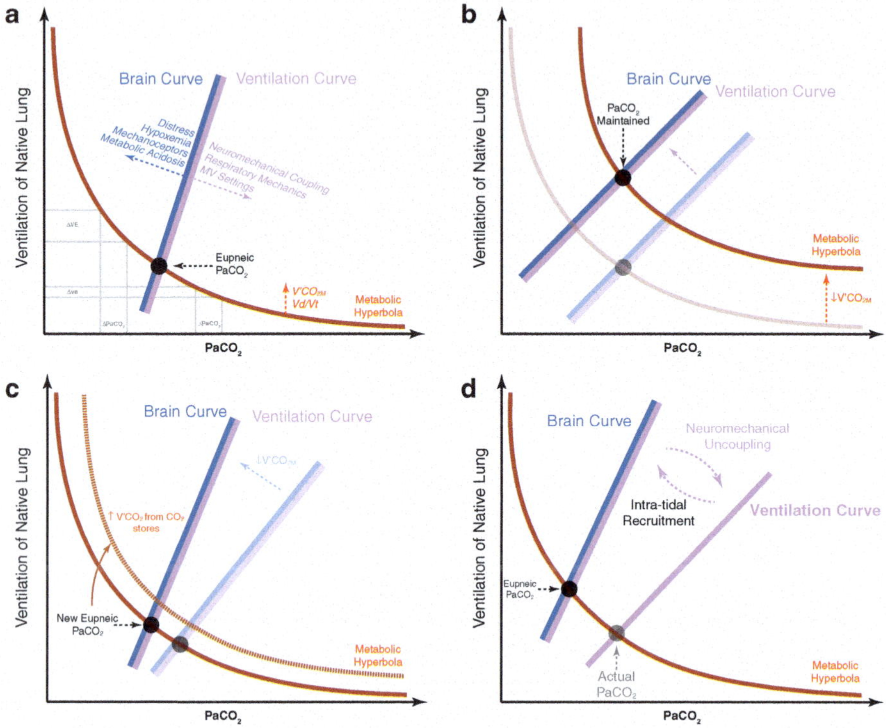


**Fig. 20.2** Model of breathing control during weaning. Panel **a** reflects health, where the brain and ventilation curves are the same, thereby eupneic and actual partial pressure of arterial carbon dioxide ($PaCO_2$) coincide. Possible contributors to the position of the brain curve, ventilation curve, and metabolic hyperbola, and the varying slope of the latter (larger $\Delta VE$ required to achieve a given $\Delta PaCO_2$ when ventilation is higher) are also shown. Panel **b** represents a possible sweep gas flow (SGF) weaning trial: as the $CO_2$ cleared by the membrane lung ($V'CO_{2ML}$) is reduced, the metabolic hyperbola shifts upwards and to the right, while the brain and ventilation curves shift in parallel to the left to maintain the eupneic $PaCO_2$. Panel **c** represents a possible fraction of oxygen of the SGF ($FdO_2$) or extracorporeal blood flow (ECBF) weaning trial: as the oxygen provided by the membrane lung ($V'O_{2ML}$) is reduced during weaning, any hypoxemia would shift the position and slope of the brain curve to a new eupneic $PaCO_2$. This new equilibration point will drive non-metabolic $CO_2$ from body stores into the bloodstream possibly shifting the metabolic hyperbola upward and to the right. Panel **d** depicts possible weaning-induced changes in the relative position of the brain and ventilation curves (maintained synonymous for simplicity in all other Panels): note that any deviation between the two curves induces a difference between the actual and eupneic $CO_2$. $V'CO_{2NL}$ the total $CO_2$ to be cleared by the natural lung, *Vd/Vt* the dead space fraction of the tidal volume. (Figure created using with BioRender.com)

#### 20.3.2.2 Effects of Weaning on Respiratory Center Output

According to the aforementioned model of breathing control, weaning may affect respiratory center output through the following mechanisms.

**Stepwise Decreases in SGF May Change the Position of the Metabolic Hyperbola**

Normally, around 6–7 l/min of VE is sufficient to maintain a $PaCO_2$ of 40 mmHg at physiologic $VCO_{2NL}$. During VV-ECMO, whereby the membrane lung contributes to $CO_2$ clearance, $VCO_{2NL}$ decreases, and the metabolic hyperbola shifts downward and to the left (i.e., lower VE is required to maintain the same $PaCO_2$). Conversely, during weaning, stepwise decreases in SGF rate reduce $V'CO_{2ML}$ and the total metabolic $V'CO_2$ increases at higher work of breathing. For both reasons, $V'CO_{2NL}$ is expected to increase, shifting the metabolic hyperbola upward and to the right (see Panel b in Fig. 20.2).

**Stepwise Decreases in $FdO_2$ or ECBF May Change the Set-Point of the Brain Curve**

Normally, the brain is set to maintain a $PaCO_2$ around 40 mmHg. However, chemical ($PaO_2$ and pH), reflex (lung and chest wall receptors), and cortical (wakefulness, sedation, agitation) inputs can change the set-point to lower or higher values. In ARDS, VV-ECMO may correct hypoxemia, but stimulation of lung mechanoceptors and inflammation contribute to maintaining a low $PaCO_2$ set point. For this reason, even with maximal $V'CO_{2ML}$ it is uncommon to induce apnea in ARDS [46]. During weaning, step decreases in $FdO_2$ or ECBF, by reducing $VO_{2ML}$, may induce hypoxemia, thereby lowering the $PaCO_2$ set point. To achieve a lower set-point, during hypoxemia the brain curve shifts to the left and increases its slope (see Panel c in Fig. 20.2).

**Changes in Breathing Pattern May Affect the Ventilation Curve**

In health, ventilation satisfies the activity of the respiratory centers, thereby the ventilation and brain curve overlap and the actual $PaCO_2$ corresponds to the eupneic $PaCO_2$. In ARDS, the descending pathway from the brain to the lung is altered for several reasons (high elastance of the respiratory system, neuromechanical uncoupling, etc). Thereby, a dissociation between the two curves occurs, resulting in dyspnea and further increasing the already high respiratory center output. During weaning, elicited natural lung ventilation might decrease lung elastance (intra-tidal recruitment) [47] or resistances (inversely correlated with tidal volume [48]) thereby partially re-establishing the matching between the brain and the ventilation curve. On the other hand, neuro-mechanical uncoupling may worsen if PEEP is increased without corresponding recruitment [42, 43, 49] or if muscular fatigue is associated with inadequate support. Accordingly, the dissociation between the brain and the ventilation curve may increase (see Panel d in Fig. 20.2).

Some other interesting interrelationships between the metabolic hyperbola and the brain curve possibly occurring during weaning are worth mentioning:

1. With increasing $VCO_{2NL}$, shifting the metabolic hyperbola upward and to the right would result in increased $PaCO_2$ if the brain curve did not concomitantly change position (see Fig. 20.2, Panel b). However, it has been experimentally shown that $PaCO_2$ remains constant at decreasing SGF, unless extreme effort is reached [24]. A similar behavior of the respiratory centers has been described during exercise, where increasing $VCO_{2NL}$ is associated with a parallel leftward shift of the brain curve (at constant slope) to maintain constant $PaCO_2$ (isocapnic hyperpnea) [44]. The underlying mechanism explaining this phenomenon remains debated [50].
2. A primary change in the set point of the brain curve may also affect the position of the metabolic hyperbola (see Fig. 20.2, panel c). Indeed, when the brain curve shifts to lower $PaCO_2$ set points, the entire pool of $CO_2$ body stores must equilibrate with the new $PaCO_2$. This requires displacement of a vast amount of non-metabolic $CO_2$ from peripheral tissues, which adds to the metabolic $CO_2$ increasing $V'CO_{2NL}$ [51] and further shifting the metabolic hyperbola upward and to the right. The higher the pool of total body $CO_2$ stores (for example due to permissive hypercapnia prior to weaning), the higher the amount of $CO_2$ displaced to reach equilibrium. Accordingly, a non-negligible additional "non-metabolic" $CO_2$ load might be imposed on the natural lung during weaning.
3. The slope of the metabolic hyperbola, describing how much VE must change to obtain a given change in $PaCO_2$ (the so called "plant gain") has two characteristics which are relevant to weaning. First, it is lower at higher VE [45] (see Fig. 20.2, panel a). Therefore, during weaning, higher changes in VE (and, thereby, effort) are required to achieve a new $PaCO_2$ set-point if the patient is already hyperventilating prior to the trial. This might be one of the reasons why high breathing effort before or during a weaning trial has been recently associated with weaning failure [23, 24]. Second the slope decreases when the $V'CO_{2ML}$ is decreased [45]. Accordingly, reaching a new $PaCO_2$ set-point (e.g., because of hypoxemia) requires much more effort during the later stages of a weaning trial. For both reasons, avoiding hypoxemia, distress, or any other cause for a shift in the eupneic threshold is important during a weaning trial.

#### 20.3.2.3 Monitoring Respiratory Center Output

Respiratory centers can express their output in terms of timing or intensity: the timing is reflected by respiratory rate, while the intensity of output is referred to as respiratory drive. Respiratory rate increases significantly only when respiratory drive is 3–4 times higher than normal [42, 43]. Similarly, clinical signs of excessive effort (use of accessory muscles, diaphoresis and distress) occur when drive is already excessive. For this reason, invasive assessment of drive is necessary to predict the success or failure of weaning prior to the development of overt distress. Directly measuring the rate of change of the electrical activity of the brain centers is not feasible in routine practice, thereby surrogates need to be employed. According to their distance from the brainstem, these surrogates relate more or less directly to respiratory drive (e.g., the electrical activity of the diaphragm, EAdi [52]), others with respiratory effort (e.g., P0.1 [53], the swing in esophageal pressure and transdiaphragmatic pressure [54], or the muscle pressure and the occlusion pressure [55, 56]), others with lung stress (e.g., dynamic transpulmonary pressure [54, 55]). As previously mentioned, if the descending pathway is altered, a dissociation between these indices might occur. For example, low effort in spite of high drive suggests neuromechanical uncoupling, and low tidal volume despite high dynamic transpulmonary pressure reflects high respiratory system elastance. Both situations are typical of patients receiving VV-ECMO, thereby complicating the assessment of the respiratory centers' output.

### 20.3.3 The Ventilator

#### 20.3.3.1 Passive, Controlled Patients

In fully sedated patients in controlled modes, mechanical ventilation can help maintain gas-exchange during a weaning trial: adjusting $FiO_2$ and positive end-expiratory pressure (PEEP) to prevent hypoxemia, and minute ventilation to avoid excessive hypercapnia represent the most obvious interventions. In case of wakefulness, increased sedation may be required to maintain synchrony if ventilation is not adjusted to match the demands of the brain curve. Clearly, since one of the aims of VV-ECMO is to assure protective ventilation, any ventilatory change should be performed in the context of ventilator-induced lung injury (VILI) prevention. Overall, protective ventilation during VV-ECMO is debated [57]. The concept of mechanical power [58] has raised awareness of the importance of other parameters than the classic driving pressure [59], particularly highlighting the potential harms of respiratory rate, although clear safety thresholds are lacking [60, 61]. Associations between mortality and the use of higher driving pressure [62]· and mechanical power [63] during VV-ECMO have been made from cohort studies and a period of total lung rest with zero driving pressure was correlated with lower plasma biomarkers of lung injury in a recent small randomized trial [64]. However, whether a strategy of lung rest with ultra-low frequency and power is superior to standard care remains to be demonstrated. Furthermore, the strongest associations between ventilator settings and outcome are in the early phase of VV-ECMO: ultra-protective ventilation may be unnecessarily cautious when patients have improved to the point of a weaning trial.

#### 20.3.3.2 Spontaneously Breathing Patients

We have described how changes in ventilation induced by weaning in spontaneously breathing patients are a direct consequence of changes in respiratory center output translating into breathing effort and, consequently, lung stress. Since the latter is the main contributor to patient self-induced lung injury (P-SILI) [47, 65], strategies to reduce effort and stress are important to ensure safe weaning. The role of the ventilator in this regard is crucial and can be divided into two components.

**Maneuvers Reducing Effort and Stress**
Any maneuver shifting the $CO_2$ sensitivity curve to higher $PaCO_2$ or improving the matching between the ventilation and the brain curve has the potential to reduce breathing effort and lung stress [42, 43]. The use of sedation, shifting the $CO_2$ sensitivity curve to the right, is a typical "non-ventilatory" strategy in this regard. For the ventilator, increasing $FiO_2$ and PEEP (if associated with recruitment) may have beneficial effects. However, increasing PEEP has some downsides: it possibly worsens neuromechanical uncoupling [49] (further dissociating the ventilation and the brain curve) and it might increase the static stress to the lung contributing to the total mechanical power of ventilation [66, 58]. As the patient is challenged with increased $V'CO_{2NL}$, the change in breathing pattern may produce altered flow demands or desynchrony (such as premature cycling in more than 30% of patients in one series [21]): maneuvers improving patient-ventilator synchrony also have the potential to reduce effort and regional stress [47, 65].

**Maneuvers Reducing Effort But Not Stress**
Any maneuver simply unloading the respiratory muscles (e.g., increasing pressure support) has the potential to reduce breathing effort, but not lung stress. Indeed, when the respiratory centers are set to maintain a certain $PaCO_2$, pressure support leads to a decreased workload by the respiratory muscles (i.e., effort decreases), but the total ventilation required to maintain $PaCO_2$ does not change (i.e., stress will not decrease although its distribution may vary) [67]. Accordingly, the main benefit of increasing pressure support is to reduce muscular fatigue.

Irrespective of the maneuver performed, general principles of lung protection during a weaning trial in spontaneously breathing patients are similar to those in fully sedated patients under controlled ventilation (Table 20.4 [18, 23, 24, 65] summarizes possible stopping criteria of a weaning trial based on the possibility of maintaining acceptable gas exchange with safe ventilation). However, some important specifics must be highlighted:

1. The presence of active muscular contraction, variable between inspiration and expiration, makes it challenging to estimate a patient's chest wall compliance. One implication is that whole respiratory system indices, such as driving pressure, might less reliably reflect lung stress than during passive ventilation. Additionally, abdominal muscle contraction may reduce the static stress associated with PEEP [68, 69] and alter the estimation of effort with esophageal pressure if gastric pressure is not concomitantly measured [47, 54].
2. All measurable indices of effort represent an 'average' measurement of the stress applied to the lung. Indeed, in spontaneous breathing, highly variable regional changes in esophageal and transpulmonary pressure have been reported, especially in the solid-like consolidated lung [70]. This may elicit pendelluft and negative pressure alveolar edema which could worsen P-SILI [47, 65]. Previous

**Table 20.4** Stopping criteria during weaning from venovenous extracorporeal membrane oxygenation (VV-ECMO)

| Parameter | Values of concern | Downsides |
|---|---|---|
| Oxygen saturation | <88% | Late sign of distress |
| Heart rate | >110 | Multifactorial causes |
| $PaCO_2$ | New respiratory acidosis | Late sign of distress |
| Respiratory rate | >35 | Late sign of distress |
| Tidal volume | >8 ml/kg IBW | Depends on respiratory system elastance |
| Driving pressure | >15 $cmH_20$ | Evaluates lung and chest wall |
| P 0.1 | >10 $cmH_2O$ | May be falsely low in patients with respiratory muscle weakness |
| $\Delta P_{es}$ | <−15 $cmH_2O$ | Requires an esophageal catheter |
| $P_{occ}$ | <−20 $cmH_2O$ | Requires multiple manual maneuvers |
| $P_{mus}$[a] | >10 $cmH_2O$ | Requires measurement (or estimation) of chest wall elastance |
| $\Delta P_L$ | >20 $cmH_2O$ | Requires esophageal catheter |
| Total lung stress ($PEEP_L + \Delta P_L$) | Unknown | Difficult assessment of $PEEP_L$ in patients with abdominal contraction |

$PEEP_L$ static stress associated with positive end-expiratory pressure (PEEP), *IBW* ideal body weight, $P_L$ transpulmonary pressure

[a]Respiratory muscle pressure ($P_{mus}$) can be derived from the esophageal pressure swing ($\Delta P_{es}$) and the estimated chest wall elastance. Alternatively, it can be estimated from $-0.75 \times P_{occ}$

studies found that the ratio of esophageal pressure to transpulmonary pressure swings correlated with failure of non-invasive ventilation (NIV) and the authors suggested that a higher effort (esophageal pressure) to achieve the same stress (transpulmonary pressure) might be an index of regional differences in transpulmonary pressure [71]. However interesting, this hypothesis still needs to be verified. Finally, PEEP may increase lung homogeneity and may reduce pendelluft and regional stress [72, 73]. However, its downsides must be kept in mind.

Importantly, if the patient is breathing spontaneously, the development of hypercapnia or respiratory distress are late signs (panel b, Fig. 20.3). Accordingly, measurement of drive and effort is essential to optimize mechanical ventilation and avoid exposing the patient to P-SILI and premature decannulation. Even with 'protective' parameters measured from the airway, the spontaneous effort to maintain normocapnia can generate enormous transpulmonary pressures [74]. Increased tidal volumes (driven by increased dead space) and new tachycardia predicted unsafe decannulation in a recent case series, but change in esophageal pressure of >16 $cmH_2O$ had the greatest accuracy [23]. Furthermore, the magnitude of spontaneous effort measured by esophageal pressure swings is prognostic for the failure of respiratory support in acute hypoxic respiratory failure in other settings [71, 75].

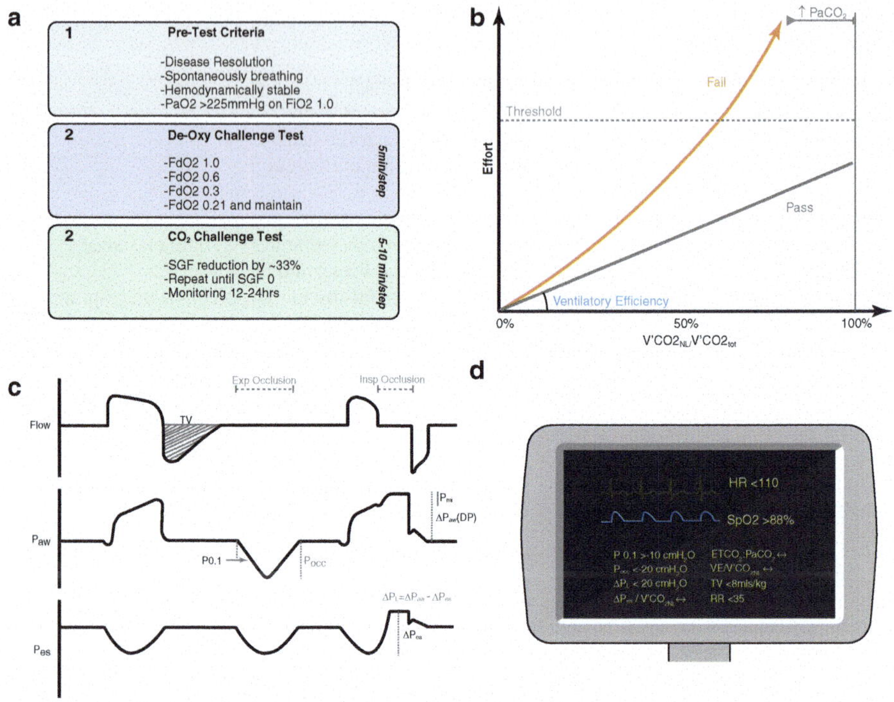


**Fig. 20.3** Our process for weaning venovenous extracorporeal membrane oxygenation (VV-ECMO). Panel **a**: sequence for VV-ECMO weaning. Throughout, monitor for stopping criteria. Panel **b**: as sweep gas flow (SGF) is weaned, the proportion of metabolically produced $CO_2$ cleared by the natural lung ($V'CO_{2NL}/V'CO_{2tot}$) increases. In patients who are not yet suitable for decannulation, this load can only be managed with excessive effort (see next panels). Ventilatory efficiency can be expressed as the ratio of the effort (or minute ventilation) to the $V'CO_{2NL}$. In patients who fail a weaning trial this efficiency is usually lower, and may worsen as the demands on the respiratory system rise. If they are not able to clear all of the metabolically produced $CO_2$, then hypercapnia ensues. Panel **c**: Monitoring drive and effort during a weaning trial. Waveforms during a pressure supported breath, an expiratory occlusion throughout an inspiratory cycle and an end inspiratory occlusion. Panel **d**: targets to maintain during a trial off VV-ECMO, including measures of drive (P0.1), effort ($P_{occ}$ or $\Delta P_{es}$ if available), stress ($\Delta P_L$ or DP if not available), and native lung ventilator efficiency ($\Delta P_{es}/V'CO_{2NL}$, endtidal $CO_2$ to arterial $CO_2$ ratio ($ETCO_2$:$PaCO_2$) or the ratio of minute ventilation to clearance ($VE/V'CO_{2NL}$). Efficiency should not worsen during a trial. *TV* tidal volume, *P0.1* pressure deflection during 100 ms of occlusion, $P_{occ}$ maximal pressure deflection during occlusion, $\Delta P_{es}$ esophageal pressure swing, $\Delta P_{aw}$ plateau after inspiratory inclusion, including the rebound pressure from relaxing inspiratory muscles, $\Delta P_L$ transpulmonary pressure, $FdO_2$ the fraction of oxygen of the SGF. (Figure created using with BioRender.com)

## 20.4 A Proposed Approach to Weaning

Our approach to weaning has been described previously [18] and is represented in Fig. 20.3. Prior to commencing weaning, comprehensive assessment of respiratory drive, effort, mechanical ventilation, and the $CO_2$ clearance capacity of the lung should take place, both to optimize mechanical assistance and as a baseline measure. The $V'CO_{2NL}$ should be at least 50% of the total metabolically produced carbon dioxide. Our preference is for patients to be on a spontaneous or assisted mode of ventilation. First the $FiO_2$ is set to 0.6 in anticipation of reducing $V'O_{2ML}$ and to avoid alveolar hypoxia as the respiratory quotient is changed during weaning. The ECBF is held static unless there is suspicion of an intracardiac shunt. Next, the $FdO_2$ is sequentially weaned in 5 min intervals, allowing for re-establishment of hypoxic pulmonary vasoconstriction and potentially increasing native ventilatory efficiency with improved V/Q matching. If an $FdO_2$ of 0.21 is tolerated, the SGF is sequentially decreased to zero in 5–10 min intervals. As the $V'CO_{2ML}$ falls, the $V'CO_2$ of the natural lung should rise if the patient is ECMO independent and monitoring continues to ensure that this is not at the cost of injurious effort or stress. In all patients, the total $V'CO_2$ will rise due to the increasing work of breathing to manage the load from the $V'CO_{2ML}$. Depending on the pulmonary mechanics and ventilatory efficiency, in some patients the native lungs will not be capable of managing this load and they will demonstrate increasing respiratory drive, effort, minute ventilation, sympathetic activation, and ultimately hypercapnia. Time to equilibrate at each step is essential in order to fully assess response and prevent P-SILI. Throughout, multimodal monitoring is continued, and the weaning test is stopped if there are indices of concern (see Table 20.3 and Fig. 20.3). As decannulation itself often produces a systemic inflammatory response in the subsequent days (which may create $V'CO_2$ and $V'O_2$ demands beyond those experienced during the weaning test) our preference is for a conservative approach to decannulation and a trial off SGF of 24 h.

## 20.5 Conclusion

The rationale for the use of VV-ECMO in ARDS and other forms of severe respiratory failure is becoming clearer. However, variation in mortality between centers [8] and a lack of prospective randomized evidence regarding the management of patients on VV-ECMO means there is a strong scientific rationale for further study. Early, safe liberation from VV-ECMO has the potential to hasten patient recovery and maintain equity of access to other patients who may benefit from this effective but scarce and intensive treatment. Although there is not yet high-grade evidence to guide clinicians, we have outlined an approach to weaning underpinned by physiology. The feasibility of weaning from VV-ECMO should be considered daily. We advocate separating the ability of the natural lung to provide $O_2$ and remove $CO_2$ by weaning the $FdO_2$ prior to the SGF. The complex interactions between the determinants of respiratory drive, patient effort, and ventilatory assistance, lung mechanics and efficiency of $V'CO_{2NL}$ will determine the outcome of a weaning trial. Care must be taken to avoid occult P-SILI in patients making spontaneous breathing effort and we advocate multimodal assessment of drive, effort, and stress throughout the weaning process.

## References


1. Barbaro RP, Odetola FO, Kidwell KM, et al. Association of hospital-level volume of extracorporeal membrane oxygenation cases and mortality. Analysis of the extracorporeal life support organization registry. Am J Respir Crit Care Med. 2015;191:894–901.
2. Peek GJ, Mugford M, Tiruvoipati R, et al. Efficacy and economic assessment of conventional ventilatory support versus extracorporeal membrane oxygenation for severe adult respiratory failure (CESAR): a multicentre randomised controlled trial. Lancet. 2009;374:1351–63.
3. Combes A, Hajage D, Capellier G, et al. Extracorporeal membrane oxygenation for severe acute respiratory distress syndrome. N Engl J Med. 2018;378:1965–75.
4. Combes A, Peek GJ, Hajage D, et al. ECMO for severe ARDS: systematic review and individual patient data meta-analysis. Intensive Care Med. 2020;46:2048–57.
5. Warren A, Chiu YD, Villar SS, et al. Outcomes of the NHS England National Extracorporeal Membrane Oxygenation Service for adults with respiratory failure: a multicentre observational cohort study. Br J Anaesth. 2020;125:259–66.
6. Odish MF, Yang J, Cheng G, et al. Treatment of bronchopleural and alveolopleural fistulas in acute respiratory distress syndrome with extracorporeal membrane oxygenation, a case series and literature review. Crit Care Explor. 2021;3:e0393.
7. Usagawa Y, Komiya K, Yamasue M, Fushimi K, Hiramatsu K, Kadota JI. Efficacy of extracorporeal membrane oxygenation for acute respiratory failure with interstitial lung disease: a case control nationwide dataset study in Japan. Respir Res. 2021;22:211.
8. Wan X, Bian T, Ye S, et al. Extracorporeal membrane oxygenation as a bridge vs. non-bridging for lung transplantation: a systematic review and meta-analysis. Clin Transpl. 2021;35:e14157.
9. Tonna JE, Abrams D, Brodie D, et al. Management of adult patients supported with venovenous extracorporeal membrane oxygenation (VV ECMO): guideline from the Extracorporeal Life Support Organization (ELSO). ASAIO J. 2021;67:601–10.
10. Gannon WD, Stokes JW, Francois SA, et al. Association between availability of extracorporeal membrane oxygenation and mortality in patients with COVID-19 eligible for extracorporeal membrane oxygenation: a natural experiment. Am J Respir Crit Care Med. 2022;205:1354–7.
11. Marhong JD, Telesnicki T, Munshi L, et al. Mechanical ventilation during extracorporeal membrane oxygenation. An international survey. Ann Am Thorac Soc. 2014;11:956–61.
12. Sen A, Callisen HE, Alwardt CM, et al. Adult venovenous extracorporeal membrane oxygenation for severe respiratory failure: current status and future perspectives. Ann Card Anaesth. 2016;19:97–111.
13. Reeb J, Olland A, Pottecher J, et al. Extracorporeal membrane oxygenation for acute respiratory distress syndrome after pneumonectomy. Ann Thorac Surg. 2017;103:881–9.
14. Broman LM, Walfertheiner MV, Montisci A, Pappalardo F. Weaning from veno-venous extracorporeal membrane oxygenation: how I do it. J Thorac Dis. 2018;10:S692–7.
15. Grant AA, Hart VJ, Lineen EB, et al. A weaning protocol for venovenous extracorporeal membrane oxygenation with a review of the literature. Artif Organs. 2018;42:605–10.
16. Seiler F, Trudzinski FC, Horsch SI, et al. Weaning from prolonged veno-venous extracorporeal membrane oxygenation (ECMO) after transfer to a specialized center: a retrospective study. J Artif Organs. 2018;21:300–7.
17. Chaves RCF, Rabello Filho R, Timenetsky KT, et al. Extracorporeal membrane oxygenation: a literature review. Rev Bras Ter Intensiva. 2019;31:410–24.

18. Vasques F, Romitti F, Gattinoni L, Camporata L. How I wean patients from veno-venous extracorporeal membrane oxygenation. Crit Care. 2019;23:316.
19. Li X, Guo Z, Li B, et al. Extracorporeal membrane oxygenation for coronavirus Disease 2019 in Shanghai, China. ASAIO J. 2020;66:475–81.
20. Gannon WD, Stokes JW, Bloom S, et al. Safety and feasibility of a protocolized daily assessment of readiness for liberation from venovenous extracorporeal membrane oxygenation. Chest. 2021;160:1693–703.
21. Teijeiro-Paradis R, Tiwari P, Spriel A, Del Sorbo L, Fan E. Standardized liberation trials in patients with COVID-19 ARDS treated with venovenous extracorporeal membrane oxygenation: when ready, let them breathe! Intensive Care Med. 2021;47:1494–6.
22. Belliato M, Cremascoli L, Epis F, et al. Carbon dioxide elimination during veno-venous extracorporeal membrane oxygenation weaning: a pilot study. ASAIO J. 2021;67:700–8.
23. Al-Fares AA, Ferguson ND, Ma J, et al. Achieving safe liberation during weaning from V-V ECMO in patients with severe ARDS: the role of tidal volume and inspiratory effort. Chest. 2021;160:1704–13.
24. Lazzari S, Romitti F, Busana M, et al. End-tidal to arterial PACO2 ratio as guide to weaning from veno-venous extra-corporeal membrane oxygenation. Am J Respir Crit Care Med. 2022;206:973–80.
25. Hartley EL, Sanderson B, Vasques F, et al. Prediction of readiness to decannulation from venovenous extracorporeal membrane oxygenation. Perfusion. 2020;35:57–64.
26. Moss M, Huant DT, Brower RG, et al. Early neuromuscular blockade in the acute respiratory distress syndrome. N Engl J Med. 2019;380:1997–2008.
27. Ficial B, Vasques F, Zhang J, et al. Physiological basis of extracorporeal membrane oxygenation and extracorporeal carbon dioxide removal in respiratory failure. Membranes (Basel). 2021;11:225.
28. Karagiannidis C, Strassmann S, Brodie D, et al. Impact of membrane lung surface area and blood flow on extracorporeal CO2 removal during severe respiratory acidosis. Intensive Care Med Exp. 2017;5:34.
29. Quintel M, Bartlett RH, Grocott MPW, et al. Extracorporeal membrane oxygenation for respiratory failure. Anesthesiology. 2020;132:1257–76.
30. Duscio E, Cipulli F, Vasques F, et al. Extracorporeal CO2 removal: The minimally invasive approach, theory, and practice. Crit Care Med. 2019;47:33–40.
31. Marshall BE, Marshall C. A model for hypoxic constriction of the pulmonary circulation. J Appl Physiol. 1985;1988(64):68–77.
32. Bishop MJ, Cheney FW. Effects of pulmonary blood flow and mixed venous O2 tension on gas exchange in dogs. Anesthesiology. 1983;58:130–5.
33. Domino KB, Wetstein L, Glasser SA, et al. Influence of mixed venous oxygen tension (PVO2) on blood flow to atelectatic lung. Anesthesiology. 1983;59:428–34.
34. Tarry D, Powell M. Hypoxic pulmonary vasoconstriction. BJA Educ. 2017;17:208–13.
35. Gierhardt M, Pak O, Walmrath D, Seeger W, Grimminger F, Ghofrani HA. Impairment of hypoxic pulmonary vasoconstriction in acute respiratory distress syndrome. Eur Respir Rev. 2021;30:210059.
36. Sinha P, Calfee CS, Beitler JR, et al. Physiologic analysis and clinical performance of the ventilatory ratio in acute respiratory distress syndrome. Am J Respir Crit Care Med. 2019;199:333–41.
37. Suarez-Sipmann F, Villar J, Fernando C, Sanchez-Giralt JA, Tusman G. Monitoring expired CO2 kinetics to individualize lung-protective ventilation in patients with the acute respiratory distress syndrome. Front Physiol. 2021;12:785014.
38. Bonifazi M, Romitti F, Busana M, et al. End-tidal to arterial PCO2 ratio: a bedside meter of the overall gas exchanger performance. Intensive Care Med Exp. 2021;9:21.
39. Gillon SA, Barrett NA, Ioannou N, et al. Intracardiac right-to-left shunt impeding liberation from veno-venous extracorporeal membrane oxygenation: two case studies. Crit Care Med. 2016;44:e583–6.

40. Cipriani E, Langer T, Bottino N, et al. Key role of respiratory quotient to reduce the occurrence of hypoxemia during extracorporeal gas exchange: a theoretical analysis. Crit Care Med. 2020;48:e1327–31.
41. Diehl JL, Mercat A, Pesenti A. Understanding hypoxemia on ECCO2R: back to the alveolar gas equation. Intensive Care Med. 2019;45:255–6.
42. Vaporidi K, Akoumianaki E, Telias I, Goligher EC, Brochard L, Georgopoulos D. Respiratory drive in critically ill patients. Pathophysiology and clinical implications. Am J Respir Crit Care Med. 2020;201:20–32.
43. Spinelli E, Mauri T, Beitler JR, Pesenti A, Brodie D. Respiratory drive in the acute respiratory distress syndrome: pathophysiology, monitoring, and therapeutic interventions. Intensive Care Med. 2020;46:606–18.
44. Asmussen E, Nielsen M. Ventilatory response to CO2 during work at normal and at low oxygen tensions. Acta Physiol Scand. 1957;39:27–35.
45. Haouzi P. Revisiting the effects of the reciprocal function between alveolar ventilation and CO2 partial pressure (PACO2) on PACO2 homeostasis at rest and in exercise. J Appl Physiol. 1985;2022(133):913–6.
46. Spinelli E, Mauri T, Lissoni A, et al. Spontaneous breathing patterns during maximum extracorporeal CO2 removal in subjects with early severe ARDS. Respir Care. 2020;65:911–9.
47. Yoshida T, Fujino Y, Amato MBP, Kavanagh BP. Fifty years of research in ARDS. spontaneous breathing during mechanical ventilation. risks, mechanisms, and management. Am J Respir Crit Care Med. 2017;195:985–92.
48. Briscoe WA, Dubois AB. The Relationship between airway resistance, airway conductance and lung volume in subjects of different age and body size. J Clin Invest. 1958;37:1279–85.
49. Jansen D, Jonkman AH, de Vries HJ, et al. Positive end-expiratory pressure affects geometry and function of the human diaphragm. J Appl Physiol (1985). 2021;131:1328–39.
50. Forster HV, Haouzi P, Dempsey JA. Control of breathing during exercise. Compr Physiol. 2012;2:743–77.
51. Giosa L, Busana M, Bonifazi M, et al. Mobilizing carbon dioxide stores. an experimental study. Am J Respir Crit Care Med. 2021;203:318–27.
52. Dres M, Demoule A. Monitoring diaphragm function in the ICU. Curr Opin Crit Care. 2020;26:18–25.
53. Sato R, Hasegawa D, Hamahata NT, et al. The predictive value of airway occlusion pressure at 100 msec (P0.1) on successful weaning from mechanical ventilation: a systematic review and meta-analysis. J Crit Care. 2021;63:124–32.
54. Kassis EB, Talmor D. Clinical application of esophageal manometry: how I do it. Crit Care. 2021;25:6.
55. Bertoni M, Telias I, Urner M, et al. A novel non-invasive method to detect excessively high respiratory effort and dynamic transpulmonary driving pressure during mechanical ventilation. Crit Care. 2019;23:346.
56. Roesthuis L, van den Berg M, van der Hoeven H. Non-invasive method to detect high respiratory effort and transpulmonary driving pressures in COVID-19 patients during mechanical ventilation. Ann Intensive Care. 2021;11:26.
57. Abrams D, Schmidt M, Pham T, et al. Mechanical ventilation for acute respiratory distress syndrome during extracorporeal life support: research and practice. Am J Respir Crit Care Med. 2020;201:514–25.
58. Gattinoni L, Tonetti T, Cressoni M, et al. Ventilator-related causes of lung injury: the mechanical power. Intensive Care Med. 2016;42:1567–75.
59. Amato MBP, Meade MO, Slutsky AS, et al. Driving pressure and survival in the acute respiratory distress syndrome. N Engl J Med. 2015;372:747–55.
60. Serpa Neto A, Deliberato RO, Johnson AEW, et al. Mechanical power of ventilation is associated with mortality in critically ill patients: an analysis of patients in two observational cohorts. Intensive Care Med. 2018;44:1914–22.
61. Romitti F, Busana M, Palumbo MM, et al. Mechanical power thresholds during mechanical ventilation: an experimental study. Physiol Rep. 2022;10:e15225.

62. Neto AS, Schmidt M, Azevedo LCP, et al. Associations between ventilator settings during extracorporeal membrane oxygenation for refractory hypoxemia and outcome in patients with acute respiratory distress syndrome: a pooled individual patient data analysis: mechanical ventilation during ECMO. Intensive Care Med. 2016;42:1672–84.
63. Chiu LC, Lin SW, Chuang LP, et al. Mechanical power during extracorporeal membrane oxygenation and hospital mortality in patients with acute respiratory distress syndrome. Crit Care. 2021;25:13.
64. Del Sorbo L, Goffi A, Tomlinson G, et al. Effect of driving pressure change during extracorporeal membrane oxygenation in adults with acute respiratory distress syndrome: a randomized crossover physiologic study. Crit Care Med. 2020;48:1771–8.
65. Goligher EC, Jonkman AH, Dianti J, et al. Clinical strategies for implementing lung and diaphragm-protective ventilation: avoiding insufficient and excessive effort. Intensive Care Med. 2020;46:2314–26.
66. Vassalli F, Pasticci I, Romitti F, et al. Does iso-mechanical power lead to iso-lung damage? An experimental study in a porcine model. Anesthesiology. 2020;132:1126–37.
67. Bellani G, Grasselli G, Teggia-Droghi M, et al. Do spontaneous and mechanical breathing have similar effects on average transpulmonary and alveolar pressure? A clinical crossover study. Crit Care. 2016;20:142.
68. Shi ZH, Jonkman A, de Vries H, et al. Expiratory muscle dysfunction in critically ill patients: towards improved understanding. Intensive Care Med. 2019;45:1061–71.
69. Chandra A, Coggeshall JW, Ravenscraft SA, Marini JJ. Hyperpnea limits the volume recruited by positive end-expiratory pressure. Am J Respir Crit Care Med. 1994;150:911–7.
70. Yoshida T, Amato MBP, Grieco DL, et al. Esophageal manometry and regional transpulmonary pressure in lung injury. Am J Respir Crit Care Med. 2018;197:1018–26.
71. Tonelli R, Fantini R, Tabbi L, Castaniere I, Pisani L, Pellegrino MR. Early inspiratory effort assessment by esophageal manometry predicts noninvasive ventilation outcome in *de novo* respiratory failure. A pilot study. Am J Respir Crit Care Med. 2020;202:558–67.
72. Sang L, Zhao Z, Yun PJ, et al. Qualitative and quantitative assessment of pendelluft: a simple method based on electrical impedance tomography. Ann Transl Med. 2020;8:1216.
73. Morais CCA, Koyama Y, Yoshida T, et al. High positive end-expiratory pressure renders spontaneous effort noninjurious. Am J Respir Crit Care Med. 2018;197:1285–96.
74. Mauri T, Langer T, Zanella A, Grasselli G, Pesenti A. Extremely high transpulmonary pressure in a spontaneously breathing patient with early severe ARDS on ECMO. Intensive Care Med. 2016;42:2101–3.
75. Coppola S, Chiumello D, Busana M, et al. Role of total lung stress on the progression of early COVID-19 pneumonia. Intensive Care Med. 2021;47:1130–9.

# Novel Strategies to Enhance the Efficiency of Extracorporeal $CO_2$ Removal

21

G. Florio, A. Zanella, and G. Grasselli

## 21.1 Introduction

Extracorporeal carbon dioxide removal ($ECCO_2R$) is an extracorporeal lung support system designed to remove carbon dioxide ($CO_2$) from the blood through an artificial membrane lung. The concept of $ECCO_2R$ was introduced in the 1970s by Kolobow et al. as a possible strategy to decrease minute ventilation and allow protective mechanical ventilation in patients with acute respiratory failure [1–3]. The original idea was to develop a treatment capable of splitting the physiological relationship between partial pressure of $CO_2$ ($PCO_2$), $CO_2$ production, and alveolar ventilation, that is described by the equation:

$$PCO_2 = \dot{V}CO_2 / VA \times k$$

where (1) $PCO_2$, in healthy people, is almost identical in the alveolar gas and the arterial blood; (2) $\dot{V}CO_2$ is the $CO_2$ eliminated with ventilation, which, at a steady state, is equal to the $CO_2$ produced by the body metabolism; (3) VA is the alveolar ventilation; and (4) k is a constant.

G. Florio
Department of Pathophysiology and Transplantation, University of Milan, Milan, Italy

A. Zanella · G. Grasselli (✉)
Department of Pathophysiology and Transplantation, University of Milan, Milan, Italy

Dipartimento di Anestesia, Rianimazione ed Emergenza-Urgenza, Fondazione IRCCS Ca' Granda Ospedale Maggiore Policlinico, Milan, Italy
e-mail: giacomo.grasselli@unimi.it



J.-L. Vincent (ed.), *Annual Update in Intensive Care and Emergency Medicine 2023*, Annual Update in Intensive Care and Emergency Medicine,
https://doi.org/10.1007/978-3-031-23005-9_21

Animal studies demonstrated that by removing the entire metabolic $CO_2$ production through a membrane lung, it was possible to obtain apnea and to keep the animal alive for hours while administering intratracheal oxygen to maintain a stable level of blood oxygen [1–3].

In the subsequent years, $ECCO_2R$ has been proposed as a treatment for acute respiratory distress syndrome (ARDS) [4], chronic obstructive pulmonary disease (COPD) exacerbation [5], acute asthma [6, 7], patients waiting for lung transplantation [8–10], and as a strategy to avoid endotracheal intubation or fasten extubation [11]; however, among the clinical community, a consensus regarding clinical indications for $ECCO_2R$ is still lacking.

Low (300–500 ml/min) and high (>800 ml/min) blood flow $ECCO_2R$ devices are currently available and are characterized by different amounts of removed $CO_2$ and different clinical applications. Specifically, devices enabling a higher level of $CO_2$ extraction seem to be required to control the respiratory drive in spontaneously breathing patients with ARDS and to limit patient self-inflicted lung injury (P-SILI) [12, 13]. Lower $CO_2$ extraction can be sufficient in patients with COPD exacerbation. Azzi et al. described that $ECCO_2R$ in patients with acute COPD exacerbations unresponsive to non-invasive ventilation (NIV) was associated with improvement in pH and $PaCO_2$ and enabled endotracheal intubation to be avoided in 85% of cases [14].

The multicenter SUPERNOVA clinical trial demonstrated that $ECCO_2R$ could be used to treat respiratory acidosis and enable ultra-protective ventilation in patients with moderate ARDS; however, it also reported a relatively high number of adverse events, mainly hemorrhagic complications, and highlighted the need for a larger trial to assess the risk/benefit ratio of this strategy [12]. The more recent REST trial [15] compared lung ultra-protective ventilation associated with $ECCO_2R$ versus conventional low tidal volume ventilation and failed to show any benefit in 90-day mortality; it was stopped early because of futility. Higher rates of adverse events, mainly intracranial hemorrhages, were reported in the $ECCO_2R$ group raising significant concerns about the safety of the treatment.

To overcome these limitations, improvements in the available technology are required. Specifically, developing clinically effective systems that do not need systemic anticoagulation could reduce the risk of hemorrhagic complications and increase clinical use of the treatment. Optimizing the biocompatibility of artificial lung membranes could solve this problem but, to date, none of the available surface-coating techniques are sufficiently effective to fully overcome the need for systemic anticoagulation. However, promising alternatives are currently undergoing preclinical evaluation and may become available in the near future [16].

Another possible solution could be the regional anticoagulation of the blood flowing through the extracorporeal circuit. Indeed, trisodium citrate-based regional anticoagulation [17, 18] is universally applied during continuous renal replacement therapy (CRRT). Unfortunately, this solution can be applied only to low blood flow treatments, which may be insufficient to reach a clinically relevant efficiency of $CO_2$ extraction. Alternative approaches for regional anticoagulation are currently being investigated, based on the concomitant administration of heparin and protamine [19] or on ion-exchange resins for calcium removal [20], but they still seem to be indicated for low blood flow devices.

Enhancing $CO_2$ removal efficiency by increasing the $CO_2$ extraction at a defined blood flow may enable effective $ECCO_2R$ treatment to be combined with the low blood flows required for regional anticoagulation. Furthermore, enhanced $CO_2$ removal efficiency may favor the integration of technologies for multiple organ support.

After a brief description of the physiological bases, we will review the strategies proposed to enhance $ECCO_2R$ efficiency.

## 21.2 Blood $CO_2$ Transportation

Carbon dioxide is transported in the blood in three forms: (1) dissolved, (2) as bicarbonate ($HCO_3^-$), and (3) combined with proteins as carbamino compounds, see Fig. 21.1, Panel a. Notably, the blood $PCO_2$ is directly proportional to the amount of dissolved $CO_2$, which is about 5% of the total $CO_2$ content in arterial blood. Most of the $CO_2$ is hydrated and is transported as bicarbonate ions. This reaction occurs primarily inside the red blood cell (RBC) due to the presence of carbonic anhydrase and is sustained by the exchange movement of bicarbonate and chloride across the RBC membrane. Interestingly, this reaction in the lungs (natural or artificial), where $CO_2$ is removed from the blood, produces an alkalization of the RBC, which facilitates the uptake of $O_2$ and the release of $CO_2$ by hemoglobin, while the opposite occurs in the tissue. The remaining $CO_2$ forms carbamino compounds reacting with the amino group of proteins, primarily hemoglobin, especially in the reduced form (Fig. 21.1, Panel b).

One liter of arterial blood of a healthy person contains about 500 ml of $CO_2$, which is about 2.5 times higher than the $O_2$ content (200 ml/l blood). Notably, the total arteriovenous $CO_2$ difference is approximately 60% attributable to the bicarbonate ion, 30% to the carbamino compounds, and the remaining 10% to the dissolved form.

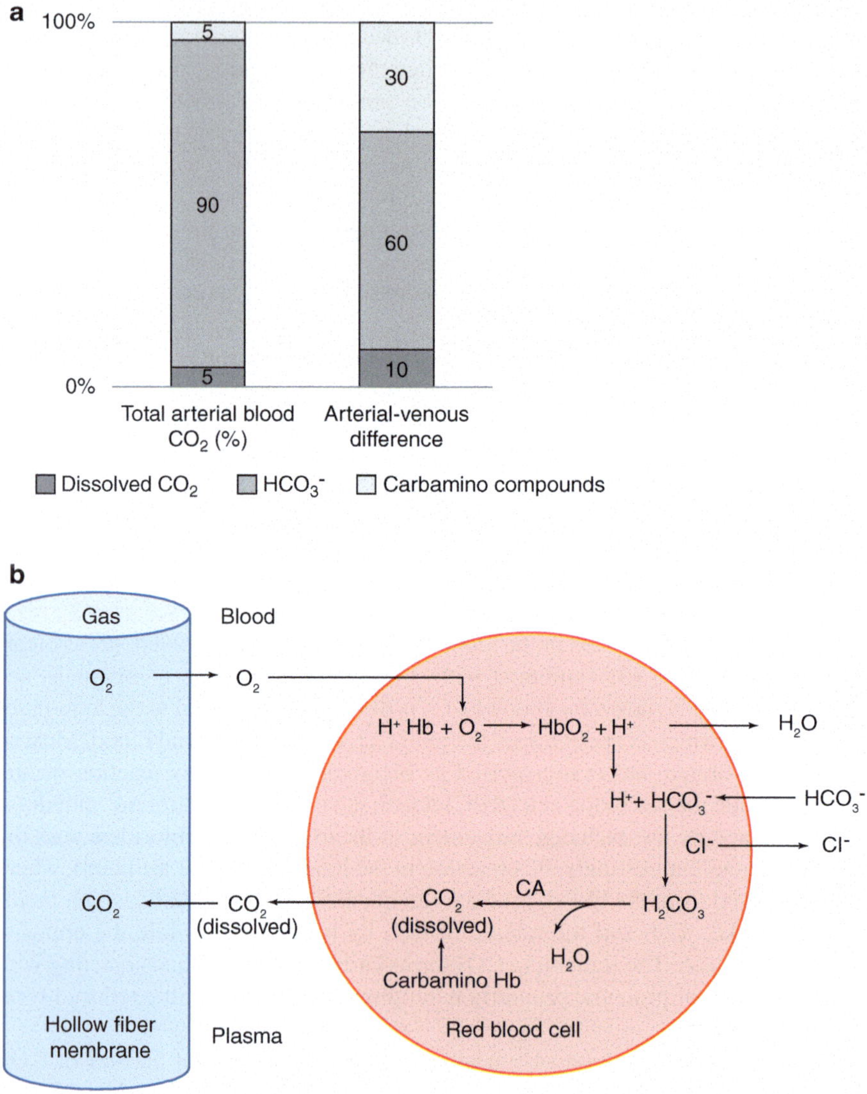


**Fig. 21.1** Blood $CO_2$ transportation. Panel (**a**). $CO_2$ is transported in the blood in three forms: (1) dissolved, (2) as bicarbonate ($HCO_3^-$), and (3) combined with proteins as carbamino compounds. Panel (**b**). Most of the $CO_2$ is hydrated and is transported as bicarbonate ions. This reaction occurs primarily inside the red blood cell due to the presence of carbonic anhydrase and is sustained by the exchange movement of bicarbonate and chloride across the red blood cell membrane

## 21.3 Factors Affecting Extracorporeal $CO_2$ Removal

$O_2$ and $CO_2$ diffuse through the lungs, both native and membrane, proportionally to the difference in partial pressure across the membrane separating the gas and blood phases and the gas exchange surface, and inversely to the distance across the membrane. Although technological development led to the availability of highly performant artificial lungs, membrane lung gas exchange efficiency remains much lower than that of the native lung. This is due to a much smaller exchange surface (<2.5 vs. >100 $m^2$) and surface area to blood volume ratio (~30 vs. ~300 $cm^{-1}$) and a greater distance between gas and blood phases (~20 vs. ~1 μm). Modern membrane lungs are constituted by microporous hollow fiber membranes made with hydrophobic polymers. The extracorporeal blood flows outside the fibers while the sweep gas flows inside the fiber lumen.

Extracorporeal $CO_2$ removal depends on several factors, such as the $PCO_2$ of the blood entering the membrane lung ($PCO_2$-in), the design of the membrane lung, the extracorporeal blood flow, and the sweep gas flow [21–24]. During venous-venous extracorporeal membrane oxygenation (VV-ECMO), a form of extracorporeal respiratory support that employs high blood flows, the sweep gas flow is commonly used to titrate $PaCO_2$ and the ratio between gas flow and blood flow is often <2:1. With low blood flow $ECCO_2R$, higher gas flow to blood flow ratios must be employed.

Pivotal data from Kolobow et al. showed that the extraction of $CO_2$ by spiral-coiled membrane lungs made with silicon rubber increased proportionally to the $PCO_2$-in and the logarithm of the blood flow [2]. Karagiannidis et al., in a porcine model with a $CO_2$ production similar to an adult human, showed that with a poly-methylpentene membrane lung, low blood flow rates (250–500 ml/min) were not sufficient to correct severe hypercapnia, neither were membrane lungs with large lung surface area (up to 1.3 $m^2$). In this model, amelioration of the respiratory acidosis was obtained only when the blood flow was increased from 750 to 1000 ml/min with a membrane lung surface area of at least 0.8 $m^2$. Low surface membrane lungs (0.4 $m^2$) were not sufficient to completely correct respiratory acidosis even with the higher blood flow used in the study (1000 ml/min) [21]. These data highlight that, with the available technology, increased $CO_2$ removal may be obtained by employing membrane lungs with a high surface area and a blood flow of at least 750 ml/min.

Similarly, Strassmann et al. investigated the impact of sweep gas flow (from 2 to 8 l/min) on $CO_2$ removal and found that it depended predominantly on blood flow rate and membrane lung area [23]. This finding was also confirmed by Duscio et al., who showed that the extracorporeal $CO_2$ extraction increased linearly with increasing blood flow and $PCO_2$-in, but had no relationship with the sweep flow [24].

It has been shown that an intermittent 'high gas flow recruitment maneuver' is an effective procedure to improve membrane lung $CO_2$ extraction by decreasing the dead space associated with water vapor trapping within the hollow fiber membrane lungs [25].

Recent studies investigated the role of hematocrit as a factor affecting extracorporeal $CO_2$ extraction, as previously documented in studies of the native lungs. In an *in vitro* model, May et al. found a significant and linear correlation between the hematocrit of the blood entering the membrane lung and the $CO_2$ extraction [26]. Specifically, a reduction in hematocrit from 33% to 8% led to a reduction in $CO_2$ removal between 32 and 42%.

## 21.4 Novel Strategies to Enhance the Efficiency of Extracorporeal $CO_2$ Removal

### 21.4.1 Blood Mixing

Some strategies promote $CO_2$ removal by increasing blood mixing within the membrane lung, which eventually helps to maximize the $PCO_2$ gradient across all hollow fiber membranes. The clinically available Hemolung RAS system (ALung, Pittsburgh, PA), although featuring a relatively small membrane surface (0.59 $m^2$), has the potential advantage of having the hollow fibers positioned around the centrifugal pump, thus increasing blood mixing. Incremental changes in sweep gas flow, up to 10 l/min, were tested in 8 patients with acute exacerbations of COPD, median $PaCO_2$ of 61 mmHg (range = 56–85 mmHg) and blood flow 390 ± 50 ml/min [27]. This study, in agreement with the literature, showed a nonlinear relationship between sweep gas flow and $CO_2$ extraction, which reached a plateau between 4 and 6 l/min. Indeed, increasing the sweep gas flow rate resulted in a loss of efficiency, thus no additional $CO_2$ clearance could be obtained above a certain level of gas flow.

Jeffries et al. developed a prototype membrane lung featuring six rotating impellers (rotation speeds up to 5000 rpm) surrounded by hollow fiber membranes able to generate active mixing and to optimize the blood flow distribution within the membrane lung [28]. The *in vitro* tests showed a conspicuous increase in $CO_2$ removal, increasing the rotation speed from 0 to 2000 rpm, while acceptable hemolysis was detected.

### 21.4.2 Bicarbonate Removal

Since most blood $CO_2$ is transported as bicarbonate ions, many researchers proposed to enhance $CO_2$ extraction through bicarbonate removal. These strategies, named respiratory dialysis, are primarily based on hemodiafiltration systems that use replacement solutions with a bicarbonate concentration lower than the blood concentration. The major challenge of removing $CO_2$ as bicarbonate is to safely replace the bicarbonate ions without incurring hydro-electrolytic and acid-base derangements.

Historical data report hypoxemia in patients with chronic renal failure undergoing acetate-bath hemodialysis (replacement solution with acetate instead of bicarbonate). This common complication was attributed to the decrease in minute ventilation due to the $CO_2$ loss through the dialyzer [29]. Recently, Cove et al. developed a dialysis system aimed at removing $CO_2$ by dialyzing the blood with a novel dialysate solution (Bicarb16) with the following composition: 140 mmol/l sodium, 111 mmol/l chloride, 3 mmol/l lactate and 16 mmol/l bicarbonate. The dialysate pH was subsequently titrated to 10 by adding hydrochloric acid [30, 31]. This system was tested for 3 hours in hypercapnic swine with blood and dialysate flows of 400 ml/min. At constant minute ventilation, $PaCO_2$ decreased from 104 ± 8 to 74 ± 8 mmHg with a calculated $CO_2$ removal of 101 ± 13 ml/min. A minimal increase in plasma sodium and chloride concentration was detected, but no hemolysis. These results were achieved at the expense of an extremely high dose of CRRT (mean dose received 390 ml/kg/h) that was required since the bicarbonate concentration of the replacement solution was 16 mmol/l.

A similar setup but with a postfilter replacement solution with no bicarbonate content (composition: NaCl 110 mmol/l, NaOH 26 mmol/l, $K^+$ 4.4 mmol/l, $PO_4^{2-}$ 3 mmol/l, $MgSO_4$ 2.1 mmol/l, glucose 80 mg/dl) was tested by the group of Kolobow in sheep. The replacement solution was infused into a dedicated centrifugal pump chamber positioned after the hemofilter to reduce the possible hemolysis due to its extremely high pH (12.04). The blood flow was 378 ± 99 ml/min. Minute ventilation was reduced to 50% while the ultrafiltrate flow (determinant of $CO_2$ extraction) was set to maintain a constant $PaCO_2 \sim 37 \pm 2$ mmHg. With a mean ultrafiltrate flow ranging from 109 ± 19 to 117 ± 23 ml/min, the average $CO_2$ removal was 60 ± 11 ml/min (0.53 ± 0.04 ml $CO_2$ per ml of ultrafiltrate) [32].

Although dialytic strategies aimed to remove bicarbonate and to employ custom-made replacement solutions with low bicarbonate concentration are still not clinically available, the combination of low blood flow $ECCO_2R$ and CRRT with standard replacement solutions (containing physiological concentrations of bicarbonate ions) has been increasingly applied in clinical practice. A more complex approach combining multiorgan support within one single hemodialysis device has been introduced with the advanced organ support (ADVOS) therapy (ADVITOS GmbH, Munich, Germany) [33]. Although initially designed for kidney and liver support and acid-base balance correction, this commercially available device, without any artificial lung, enables extracorporeal $CO_2$ extraction primarily through bicarbonate removal [34]. The ADVOS system consists of an extracorporeal blood circuit featuring a pump (blood flows 100–400 ml/min) and two parallel high-flux dialyzers along the blood stream and a closed dialysate loop circuit primed with an electrolyte solution added with albumin. The dialysate circuit splits into two paths involving the infusion of an acid or a basic solution (solution infusion rate 160–320 ml/min), respectively. Subsequently, after the pre-dilution, the dialysate is ultrafiltered within two high-flux filters before reaching, reunited, the blood hemofilter. $CO_2$ removal could be achieved on both the dialysate paths since the acid solution does not contain any form of $CO_2$ while the alkalotic solution could be provided with zero $CO_2$ (BC-Bic0) or containing low concentrations of $Na_2CO_3$ (BC-Bic20). In an *in vitro* study, Perez Ruiz de Garibay et al. showed, with a blood flow of 400 ml/min, $CO_2$ removal as high as 142 ± 17 and 77 ± 20 ml/min with

BC-Bic0 and BC-Bic20, respectively, but the inlet blood $PCO_2$ and $HCO_3^-$ concentrations were very increased [34]. In a subgroup of experiments with inlet blood gas kept within physiological ranges, the highest $CO_2$ removal was 61 ± 7 ml/min achieved with BC-Bic0 ml/min.

Allescher et al. applied the ADVOS system to nine hypercapnic patients with moderate to severe ARDS. The median blood flow was 300 ml/min (IQR: 250–300 ml/min). The median $CO_2$ removal was 49 ml/min (IQR: 27–72 ml/min) although, during some treatments, $CO_2$ removal as high as 160 ml/min was achieved [33]. Interestingly regional citrate anticoagulation was always applied alone (8%) or in combination with unfractionated heparin infusion (92%).

### 21.4.3 Carbonic Anhydrase

In the 1970s, Broun and co-workers introduced the idea of promoting the transfer of $CO_2$ across membranes by covering the membrane with carbonic anhydrase [35], which accelerates the conversion of bicarbonate to $CO_2$. This concept was applied to $ECCO_2R$, immobilizing carbonic anhydrase to the external surface (blood side) of the hollow fiber membranes of the artificial lung to promote the conversion of bicarbonate to $CO_2$, resulting in increased blood $PCO_2$ and, subsequently, enhancing $CO_2$ transfer efficiency. Several strategies of carbonic anhydrase immobilization have been tested, showing different degrees of lost carbonic anhydrase activity [36]. Arazawa et al. reported a 37% increase in $CO_2$ removal across membrane lungs coated with carbonic anhydrase (via glutaraldehyde crosslinking and chitosan tethering) compared to conventional membrane lungs [37]. Moreover, several studies have reported improved hemocompatibility of membranes with immobilized carbonic anhydrase compared to unmodified membranes [38, 39]. To date, membrane lungs coated with carbonic anhydrase are still not clinically available.

### 21.4.4 Acidification

Since the majority of blood $CO_2$ is combined with water to form bicarbonate ion according to the equation $CO_2 + H_2O \leftrightarrow H_2CO_3 \leftrightarrow H^+ + HCO_3^-$, the acidification of blood entering the membrane lung could shift the equilibrium from bicarbonate ion towards dissolved $CO_2$ with subsequent increase in blood $PCO_2$ and $CO_2$ gradient across the membrane lung, thus theoretically leading to enhanced extracorporeal $CO_2$ extraction. Pesenti et al. tested this hypothesis in an experimental *in vivo* study and demonstrated that lactic acid infusion in the blood entering the membrane lung resulted in increased $CO_2$ transfer capacity [40]. A relationship between the acid infusion rate and the $CO_2$ removal was also described. Specifically, with a blood flow set to 500 ml/min, acid infusion at 1, 2, and 5 mEq/min increased membrane lung $CO_2$ extraction up to 11, 23, and 70%, respectively, while keeping $PCO_2$-in constant (47 ± 5 mmHg) [40]. Lactic acid was initially chosen because it is quickly metabolized, and its blood concentration could easily be monitored at the bedside.

However, two different classes of acids can be used to obtain blood acidification: metabolizable and not-metabolizable. Differently from metabolizable acids, non-metabolizable acids require extracorporeal removal to prevent blood accumulation. Metabolizable acids, such as lactic, citric, and acetic acid, are energetic substrates and could be metabolized by organisms, thus affecting total $CO_2$ production [41]. In fact, without metabolic control (constant caloric intake) during metabolic acid infusion, increased $CO_2$ production is possible, thus negatively affecting the potential decrease in alveolar ventilation due to the acidification. It has been demonstrated that lactic acid infusion, compared with isocaloric glucose infusion, is associated with a slight increase in $CO_2$ production [42]. Interestingly, citric acid infusion may allow concurrent regional anticoagulation (due to the chelating power of citrate for calcium ions) and enhancement of $CO_2$ removal as demonstrated in an *in vitro* study on human blood [43]. Unfortunately, body citrate clearance does not allow high infusions of citrate, thus requiring external extracorporeal techniques to prevent systemic citrate accumulation if blood flows higher than 200–250 ml/min are employed.

To avoid direct acid infusion in the blood and allow infusion of highly concentrated acids, our group implemented a veno-venous circuit with a hemofilter and a closed dialysate loop (obtained connecting the two dialysate ports of the hemofilter) placed on the blood line before the membrane lung. The acid infusion in the dialysate enabled us to demonstrate *in vivo* the feasibility and the safety of blood acidification up to 48 h as a strategy to enhance extracorporeal $CO_2$ removal [44].

To minimize blood contact with non-biological surfaces, we tested a further strategy placing a membrane lung on the dialysate loop downstream of the dialysate acidification. This $ECCO_2R$ technique gave a substantial increase in $CO_2$ removal but was less efficient compared to dialysate acidification with membrane lung on blood (about 15% less), mainly due to the absence of carbonic anhydrase in the dialysate and subsequent decreased shift of bicarbonate towards dissolved $CO_2$ [45].

Acidification with non-metabolizable acids, such as hydrochloric acid, although highly efficient in enhancing $CO_2$ removal and not increasing $CO_2$ production, requires a dedicated system or a technique to prevent the systemic accumulation of the infused acid.

To overcome the issues associated with metabolizable and non-metabolizable acids we developed a complex system based on electrodialysis. This technique is based on a electrodialytic chamber, placed on the dialytic circuit, that exploits electric current to separate positive and negative charges, thus creating a compartment enriched with $Na^+$ ions, the alkaline side, and a compartment enriched with $Cl^-$ ions, the acid side. The acid side allowed acidification without any requirement for external acid infusion, whereas the alkaline liquid, reinfused in a central vein, maintains electrolyte equilibrium. Electrodialysis showed extremely high efficiency in $CO_2$ removal and significant decrease in minute ventilation (up to 70%) was possible, but was associated with a low safety profile because of the presence of an extremely alkalotic environment. Furthermore, this technique also required calcium removal to avoid its precipitation in the alkalotic lines, thus adding further complexity to the system, and was associated with $H_2$ and $O_2$ production [46].

Ion-exchange resins allowing acidification through sodium removal in exchange with protons were tested as a further possible strategy to enhance $CO_2$ removal without the technical complexity of electrodialysis. However, despite showing high efficiency in $CO_2$ removal (membrane lung $CO_2$ extraction increased up to 145 ml/min and minute ventilation decreased up to 70%), this strategy was also associated with a very low safety profile because of the infusion of highly alkalotic NaOH solutions to replace the removed sodium and to maintain electrolyte equilibrium [47].

Interestingly, Arazawa et al. tested the effect of ventilating a carbonic anhydrase-coated membrane lung with an acidifying sweep gas (2.2% sulfur dioxide), showing more than double $CO_2$ removal vs. conventional techniques. Although promising, further improvements are required to promote the removal of accumulating exogenous sulfites [48].

Our group also performed an *in vitro* study to test a technique to enhance $CO_2$ removal based on membrane lung ventilation with a sodium hydroxide solution with high $CO_2$ absorption [49]. The so-called "alkaline liquid ventilation" proved to be safe and was associated with significantly higher $CO_2$ removal capacity compared to conventional gas ventilation.

## 21.5 Limitations

Although enhancing the efficiency of $ECCO_2R$ may increase the overall safety profile of the treatment, it may foster some known adverse events. First, an effective $ECCO_2R$ treatment leads to a significant decrease in a patient's minute ventilation, thus promoting a reduction in alveolar $PO_2$; if this target is achieved with a highly efficient technique, i.e., with low blood flows, the risk of hypoxemia is increased, thus preventive strategies such as an increase in $FiO_2$ and or positive end-expiratory pressure (PEEP) would be mandatory. Second, at low blood flows, the risk of hemolysis is increased due to the design of the available centrifugal pumps [50]. Third, the increased transit time through the membrane lung due to the low blood flow may have a negative impact on the coagulation and inflammatory systems.

## 21.6 Conclusion

Although recent trials have highlighted some limitations associated with $ECCO_2R$ support, we believe the rationale for applying $ECCO_2R$ in patients with acute or chronic respiratory failure remains extremely solid. An enhanced $ECCO_2R$ system could help to overcome some of the technical limits now affecting the treatment. Today, effective interventions to increase the efficiency of $CO_2$ extraction are still at a preclinical stage. A synergic combination of some of the reported strategies could expedite the clinical transition of a safe and effective technology. Moreover, combining $ECCO_2R$ with regional anticoagulation could represent a critical approach to reduce the risk of hemorrhagic complications and to foster the implementation of modular multi-organ support.

## References

1. Kolobow T, Gattinoni L, Tomlinson T, White D, Pierce J, Iapichino G. The carbon dioxide membrane lung (CDML): a new concept. Trans Am Soc Artif Intern Organs. 1977;23:17–21.
2. Kolobow T, Gattinoni L, Tomlinson TAJE, Pierce JE. Control of breathing using an extracorporeal membrane lung. Anesthesiology. 1977;46:138–41.
3. Kolobow T, Gattinoni L, Tomlinson T, Pierce JE. An alternative to breathing. J Thorac Cardiovasc Surg. 1978;75:261–6.
4. Terragni PP, Del Sorbo L, Mascia L, et al. Tidal volume lower than 6 ml/kg enhances lung protection. Anesthesiology. 2009;111:826–35.
5. Crotti S, Lissoni A, Tubiolo D, et al. Artificial lung as an alternative to mechanical ventilation in COPD exacerbation. Eur Respir J. 2012;39:212–5.
6. Maqsood U, Patel N. Extracorporeal membrane oxygenation (ECMO) for near-fatal asthma refractory to conventional ventilation. BMJ Case Rep. 2018;2018:bcr-2017-223276.
7. Alzeer A, Al Otair H, Khurshid S, Badrawy S, Bakir B. A case of near fatal asthma: the role of ECMO as rescue therapy. Ann Thorac Med. 2015;10:143.
8. Olsson KM, Simon A, Strueber M, et al. Extracorporeal membrane oxygenation in nonintubated patients as bridge to lung transplantation. Am J Transplant. 2010;10:2173–8.
9. Javidfar J, Bacchetta M. Bridge to lung transplantation with extracorporeal membrane oxygenation support. Curr Opin Organ Transplant. 2012;17:496–502.
10. Fuehner T, Kuehn C, Hadem J, et al. Extracorporeal membrane oxygenation in awake patients as bridge to lung transplantation. Am J Respir Crit Care Med. 2012;185:763–8.
11. Terragni P, Maiolo G, Ranieri VM. Role and potentials of low-flow CO(2) removal system in mechanical ventilation. Curr Opin Crit Care. 2012;18:93–8.
12. Combes A, Fanelli V, Pham T, Ranieri VM. Feasibility and safety of extracorporeal CO2 removal to enhance protective ventilation in acute respiratory distress syndrome: the SUPERNOVA study. Intensive Care Med. 2019;45:592–600.
13. Combes A, Tonetti T, Fanelli V, et al. Efficacy and safety of lower versus higher CO2 extraction devices to allow ultraprotective ventilation: secondary analysis of the SUPERNOVA study. Thorax. 2019;74:1179–81.
14. Azzi M, Aboab J, Alviset S, et al. Extracorporeal CO2 removal in acute exacerbation of COPD unresponsive to non-invasive ventilation. BMJ Open Respir Res. 2021;8:e001089.
15. McNamee JJ, Gillies MA, Barrett NA, et al. Effect of lower tidal volume ventilation facilitated by extracorporeal carbon dioxide removal vs standard care ventilation on 90-day mortality in patients with acute hypoxemic respiratory failure. JAMA. 2021;326:1013.
16. Roberts TR, Leslie DC, Cap AP, Cancio LC, Batchinsky AI. Tethered-liquid omniphobic surface coating reduces surface thrombogenicity, delays clot formation and decreases clot strength ex vivo. J Biomed Mater Res Part B Appl Biomater. 2020;108:496–502.
17. Morimont P, Habran S, Desaive T, et al. Extracorporeal CO2 removal and regional citrate anticoagulation in an experimental model of hypercapnic acidosis. Artif Organs. 2019;43:719–27.
18. Sharma AS, Weerwind PW, Bekers O, Wouters EM, Maessen JG. Carbon dioxide dialysis in a swine model utilizing systemic and regional anticoagulation. Intensive Care Med Exp. 2016;4:2.
19. Tramarin J, Cortegiani A, Gregoretti C, et al. Regional anticoagulation with heparin of an extracorporeal CO2 removal circuit: a case report. J Med Case Reports. 2019;13:123.
20. Zanella A, Scaravilli V, Castagna L, et al. Ion-exchange resin anticoagulation (I-ERA): a novel extracorporeal technique for regional anticoagulation. Shock. 2016;46:304–11.
21. Karagiannidis C, Strassmann S, Brodie D, et al. Impact of membrane lung surface area and blood flow on extracorporeal CO2 removal during severe respiratory acidosis. Intensive Care Med Exp. 2017;5:34.
22. Karagiannidis C, Kampe K, Sipmann F, et al. Veno-venous extracorporeal CO2 removal for the treatment of severe respiratory acidosis: pathophysiological and technical considerations. Crit Care. 2014;18:R124.

23. Strassmann S, Merten M, Schäfer S, et al. Impact of sweep gas flow on extracorporeal CO2 removal (ECCO2R). Intensive Care Med Exp. 2019;7:17.
24. Duscio E, Cipulli F, Vasques F, et al. Extracorporeal CO2 removal: the minimally invasive approach, theory, and practice. Crit Care Med. 2019;47:33–40.
25. Castagna L, Zanella A, Scaravilli V, et al. Effects on membrane lung gas exchange of an intermittent high gas flow recruitment maneuver: preliminary data in veno-venous ECMO patients. J Artif Organs. 2015;18:213–9.
26. May AG, Omecinski KS, Frankowski BJ, Federspiel WJ. Effect of hematocrit on the CO2 removal rate of artificial lungs. ASAIO J. 2020;66:1161–5.
27. Barrett NA, Hart N, Camporota L. In vivo carbon dioxide clearance of a low-flow extracorporeal carbon dioxide removal circuit in patients with acute exacerbations of chronic obstructive pulmonary disease. Perfusion. 2020;35:436–41.
28. Jeffries RG, Lund L, Frankowski B, Federspiel WJ. An extracorporeal carbon dioxide removal (ECCO2R) device operating at hemodialysis blood flow rates. Intensive Care Med Exp. 2017;5:41.
29. Dolan MJ, Whipp BJ, Davidson WD, Weitzman RE, Wasserman K. Hypopnea associated with acetate hemodialysis: carbon dioxide-flow-dependent ventilation. N Engl J Med. 1981;305:72–5.
30. Cove ME, Vu LH, Ring T, May AG, Federspiel WJ, Kellum JA. A proof of concept study, demonstrating extracorporeal carbon dioxide removal using hemodialysis with a low bicarbonate dialysate. ASAIO J. 2019;65:605–13.
31. Cove ME, Vu LH, Ring T, Federspiel WJ, Kellum JA. Respiratory dialysis - a novel low bicarbonate dialysate to provide extracorporeal CO2 removal. Crit Care Med. 2020;48:e592–8.
32. Cressoni M, Zanella A, Epp M, et al. Decreasing pulmonary ventilation through bicarbonate ultrafiltration: an experimental study. Crit Care Med. 2009;37:2612–8.
33. Allescher J, Rasch S, Wiessner JR, et al. Extracorporeal carbon dioxide removal with the Advanced Organ Support system in critically ill COVID-19 patients. Artif Organs. 2021;45:1522–32.
34. Ruiz P, de Garibay A, Kellum JA, Honigschnabel J, Kreymann B. Respiratory and metabolic acidosis correction with the ADVanced Organ Support system. Intensive Care Med Exp. 2019;7:56.
35. Broun G, Selegny E, Minh CT, Thomas D. Facilitated transport of CO2 across a membrane bearing carbonic anhydrase. FEBS Lett. 1970;7:223–6.
36. Manap HH, Abdul Wahab AK. Extracorporeal carbon dioxide removal (ECCO2R) in respiratory deficiency and current investigations on its improvement: a review. J Artif Organs. 2017;20:8–17.
37. Arazawa DT, Kimmel JD, Federspiel WJ. Kinetics of CO2 exchange with carbonic anhydrase immobilized on fiber membranes in artificial lungs. J Mater Sci Mater Med. 2015;26:193.
38. Kaar JL, Oh H, Russell AJ, Federspiel WJ. Towards improved artificial lungs through biocatalysis. Biomaterials. 2007;28:3131–9.
39. Kimmel JD, Arazawa DT, Ye SH, Shankarraman V, Wagner WR, Federspiel WJ. Carbonic anhydrase immobilized on hollow fiber membranes using glutaraldehyde activated chitosan for artificial lung applications. J Mater Sci Mater Med. 2013;24:2611–21.
40. Zanella A, Patroniti N, Isgrò S, et al. Blood acidification enhances carbon dioxide removal of membrane lung: an experimental study. Intensive Care Med. 2009;35:1484–7.
41. Scaravilli V, Kreyer S, Linden K, et al. Enhanced extracorporeal CO2 removal by regional blood acidification: effect of infusion of three metabolizable acids. ASAIO J. 2015;61:533–9.
42. Zanella A, Giani M, Redaelli S, et al. Infusion of 2.5 meq/min of lactic acid minimally increases CO2 production compared to an isocaloric glucose infusion in healthy anesthetized, mechanically ventilated pigs. Crit Care. 2013;17:R268.
43. Scaravilli V, Di Girolamo L, Scotti E, et al. Effects of sodium citrate, citric acid and lactic acid on human blood coagulation. Perfusion. 2018;33:577–83.
44. Zanella A, Mangili P, Redaelli S, et al. Regional blood acidification enhances extracorporeal carbon dioxide removal: a 48-hour animal study. Anesthesiology. 2014;120:416–24.

45. Zanella A, Mangili P, Giani M, et al. Extracorporeal carbon dioxide removal through ventilation of acidified dialysate: an experimental study. J Heart Lung Transplant. 2014;33:536–41.
46. Zanella A, Castagna L, Salerno D, et al. Respiratory electrodialysis. a novel, highly efficient extracorporeal CO2 removal technique. Am J Respir Crit Care Med. 2015;192:719–26.
47. Zanella A, Pesenti A, Busana M, et al. A minimally invasive and highly effective extracorporeal CO2 removal device combined with a continuous renal replacement therapy. Crit Care Med. 2022;50:e468–76.
48. Arazawa DT, Kimmel JD, Finn MC, Federspiel WJ. Acidic sweep gas with carbonic anhydrase coated hollow fiber membranes synergistically accelerates CO2 removal from blood. Acta Biomater. 2015;25:143–9.
49. Vivona L, Battistin M, Carlesso E, et al. Alkaline liquid ventilation of the membrane lung for extracorporeal carbon dioxide removal ($ECCO_2R$): in vitro study. Membranes (Basel). 2021;11:464.
50. Gross-Hardt S, Hesselmann F, Arens J, et al. Low-flow assessment of current ECMO/ECCO2R rotary blood pumps and the potential effect on hemocompatibility. Crit Care. 2019;23:348.

# Extracorporeal Cardiopulmonary Resuscitation for Out-Of-Hospital Cardiac Arrest: A Systematic Approach

22

D. Rob and J. Bělohlávek

## 22.1 Introduction

Despite intensive efforts to improve out-of-hospital cardiac arrest (OHCA) outcomes, survival rates at hospital discharge are very low, on average 8%, varying from 0% to 18% in Europe [1]. Most of the resuscitated OHCA patients are refractory to standard advanced cardiac life support (ACLS) and never achieve return of spontaneous circulation (ROSC) [2]. Veno-arterial extracorporeal membrane oxygenation (VA-ECMO) implantation during ongoing resuscitation, a method called extracorporeal cardiopulmonary resuscitation (ECPR) effectively restores circulation, provides cardiopulmonary support, and serves as a bridge to recovery from multiorgan failure in patients with refractory OHCA [2, 3]. Two single center randomized trials (ARREST and Prague OHCA) have been published with results suggesting possible benefit of advanced logistics and ECPR over standard ACLS [2, 3]. Despite encouraging results from the randomized trials, published ECPR studies vary widely in terms of prehospital system of care, eligibility criteria, transport of patients, ECPR strategy (in-hospital vs. pre-hospital), and outcomes [2–7]. Implantation of VA-ECMO is only one of many steps required to achieve good outcomes in patients with refractory OHCA. A key prerequisite for a successful outcome is a systemic approach including close collaboration between the providers of care, assurance of high quality resuscitation, proper patient selection, minimizing the time delays, treatment of the cardiac arrest cause, and comprehensive intensive care [2, 4, 5]. In this chapter, we provide a summary of the most important steps of ECPR (Fig. 22.1) based on published evidence and the authors' experience.

D. Rob · J. Bělohlávek (✉)
2nd Department of Medicine, Department of Cardiovascular Medicine, First Faculty of Medicine, Charles University in Prague and General University Hospital in Prague, Prague, Czech Republic
e-mail: jan.belohlavek@vfn.cz



J.-L. Vincent (ed.), *Annual Update in Intensive Care and Emergency Medicine 2023*, Annual Update in Intensive Care and Emergency Medicine,
https://doi.org/10.1007/978-3-031-23005-9_22

| | |
|---|---|
| Step 1 – System design and quality | High rates of bystander CPR, cooperation between EMS and cardiac arrest center, ECPR model adjusted to the location and minimize time delays |
| Step 2 – Patient selection | Initial shockable rhythm, witnessed arrest, age ≤ 70 years, duration of no-flow and low-flow time |
| Step 3 - Transport | Timely decision, ensure high-quality CPR during transport, appropriate mechanical compression device use |
| Step 4 – Patient admission | Direct transport to the place of ECMO cannulation without intra-hospital delay, rapid eligibility criteria re-assessment |
| Step 5 – ECMO cannulation | Percutaneous insertion under ultrasound and/or fluoroscopic guidance, Routine distal perfusion assessment/cannulation<br>Limited number of highly experienced operators providing 24/7 service |
| Step 6 – initial diagnostic and therapeutic procedures | Immediate CAG in the absence of evident non-cardiac cause<br>Immediate PCI for culprit lesion only |
| Step 7 – Intensive care | Centralized ECMO unit with experienced team of intensivists<br>Protocols for anticoagulation, neuroprognostication, TTM<br>Psychological, palliative and spiritual care for victims of cardiac arrest/relatives |
| Step 8 – Hospital discharge and follow-up | Intensive rehabilitation, nutrition, social, psychological and palliative care after hospital discharge |

**Fig. 22.1** Systemic approach (key steps) overview for extracorporeal cardiopulmonary resuscitation (ECPR). *ECMO* extracorporeal membrane oxygenation, *CAG* coronary angiography, *TTM* therapeutic temperature management, *CPR* cardiopulmonary resuscitation, *EMS* emergency medical service, *PCI* percutaneous coronary intervention

## 22.2 System Design and Quality

Less than 10% of all OHCA patients are potential candidates for ECPR [2, 8]. Therefore, ECPR should be perceived as a complementary method provided in a well-organized system with high-quality conventional ACLS [2, 3, 5]. In such a system, ECPR represents an additional link of the chain of survival and the chain is only as strong as its weakest link [9]. Continuous efforts to achieve maximum rates of bystander and telephone-assisted cardiopulmonary resuscitation (CPR) are extremely important as these are associated with favorable long-term outcomes and are also increasing the pool of patients considered for ECPR [2, 3, 10, 11].

Another important prerequisite is close cooperation between the emergency medical service (EMS) and the cardiac arrest center. Thorough and repeated education and training of EMS crews is necessary to increase early and correct recognition of potential ECPR candidates, ensure brief and informative phone calls between EMS and cardiac center coordinator, and provide rapid transport of a patient to a cardiac arrest center under high quality CPR [12]. An additional step is to raise awareness of the benefits of ECPR and provide feedback from the cardiac arrest center to EMS crews to keep them motivated for this demanding job.

There are currently several models of ECPR provision (in-hospital, pre-hospital, hybrid approach) [2, 3, 6]. In fact, each ECPR system is different, which is probably a consequence of the resuscitation system organization, local specificities (city/area size, population, traffic, number of EMS bases, centralized or de-centralized dispatch center, cardiac arrest centers, etc.) and experience. Due to the lack of comparative data and differences between systems and regions, it is difficult to make

**Table 22.1** Pros and cons of different extracorporeal cardiopulmonary resuscitation (ECPR) systems

| System | Pros | Cons |
|---|---|---|
| In-hospital | • Evidence of benefit from observational studies and two RCTs<br>• Availability of ECMO team, fluoroscopy, ultrasound without additional delays and costs<br>• Immediate advanced imaging like CT, CAG, and PCI | • Potentially harmful intra-arrest transport<br>• Prolonged time to ECMO?<br>• Delayed selection of appropriate patients<br>• Increased workload and resources when ECPR not indicated |
| Pre-hospital | • Uninterrupted on-scene resuscitation<br>• Reducing time to ECMO?<br>• Earlier selection of appropriate patients | • Lack of evidence, no RCTs<br>• Challenging cannulation<br>• Logistic barriers (extra mobile ECMO unit, extra highly trained staff)<br>• Resource demanding |
| Hybrid system | • Tailored decision based on arrest location<br>• Reducing time to ECMO? | • Lack of evidence, no RCTs<br>• Logistic barriers<br>• Resource demanding |

*ECMO* extracorporeal membrane oxygenation, *PCI* percutaneous coronary intervention, *RCT* randomized controlled trial, *CT* computed tomography, *CAG* coronary angiography

any valid recommendation regarding the organization of ECPR services [2, 3, 6]. Although each model has strengths and limitations (Table 22.1), it is currently more important to focus on correct patient selection and time to VA-ECMO initiation, which are major determinants of ECPR outcome [2, 5, 6, 13].

In addition to a well-organized system, every cardiac arrest center should ensure the correct resuscitation and outcome data collection and benchmarking necessary for effective feedback, improvement, and experience sharing within the international scientific community [14].

## 22.3 Patient Selection

Patient selection is the cornerstone of results as only carefully chosen patients have a chance for good neurological outcome despite prolonged resuscitation times [2, 3, 13]. Unfortunately, there is great complexity and interplay of factors influencing refractory OHCA outcomes (Fig. 22.2). Our experience suggests that it is very hard to reliably predict outcome prior to VA-ECMO insertion based on prehospital and admission data. Patients with unmeasurable pH, high lactate levels, and low-flow times over 60 min have survived with good neurological outcome [2, 15], and, *vice versa*, patients with more favorable parameters on admission have not. However, criteria that are too liberal can lead to burden on the system with unsalvageable patients supported by ECMO [5]; criteria that are too restrictive may mean that good ECPR candidates are missed, thus reducing the case volume size, which is important to establish experience and expertise [16]. This concern was recently confirmed by an observational study where retrospective application of the consensus criteria would have increased the survival rate of the ECPR cohort from 26% to 48% but would have excluded 58% of survivors [17].

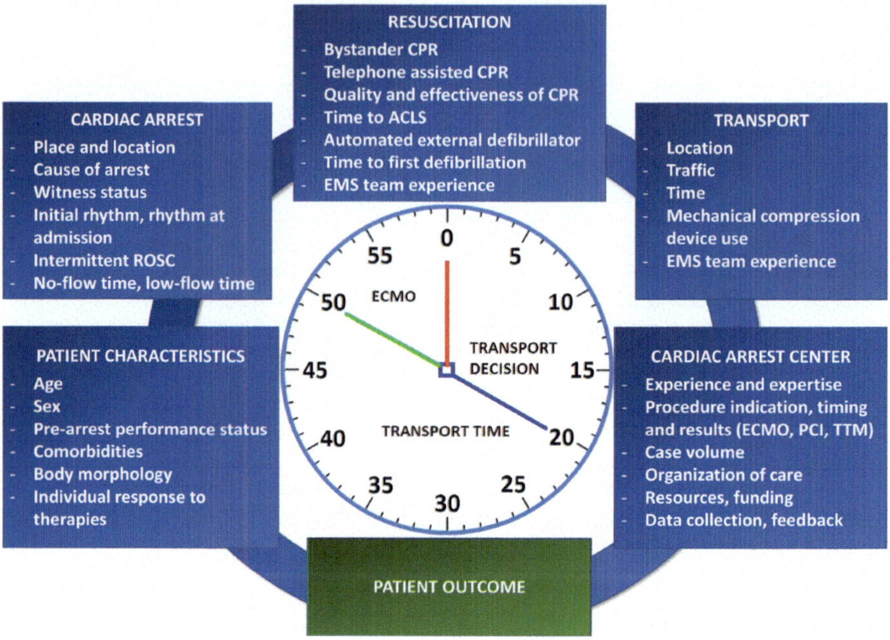


**Fig. 22.2** Complexity, interplay of factors in refractory out-of-hospital cardiac arrest (OHCA) and extracorporeal cardiopulmonary resuscitation (ECPR) and ultimate time goals to achieve favorable outcome. *ECMO* extracorporeal membrane oxygenation, *PCI* percutaneous coronary intervention, *TTM* therapeutic temperature management, *ACLS* advanced cardiac life support, *ROSC* return of spontaneous circulation, *CPR* cardiopulmonary resuscitation

Several predictors of prognosis have been consistently identified across ECPR observational studies, including age, witnessed arrest, longer duration of no-flow and low-flow time, and initial rhythm [4, 5, 6, 13]. The Prague OHCA trial provided the first randomized data confirming a huge difference in refractory OHCA outcomes between patients with shockable and non-shockable initial rhythms [2]. Survival at 180-days in the invasive arm occurred in 49% of patients with an initial shockable rhythm but in only 8% patients with a non-shockable rhythm [2]. It is also probable that the occurrence of a non-shockable rhythm after the first defibrillation or at hospital admission is associated with a worse prognosis, but this question has not yet been studied in ECPR recipients. Of note, patients with intermittent ROSC and recurrent ventricular fibrillation represent the population that probably benefits the most from the ECPR approach [2, 3, 6, 13]. Taken together, it seems reasonable to limit use of ECPR to patients with an initial shockable rhythm, witnessed arrest, presumed cardiac etiology, and age ≤70 years.

Based on the above criteria, the EMS crew can easily recognize a potential candidate for ECPR on arrival at the scene. After the initial procedures are performed according to the guidelines [14], with at least three defibrillations (in the case of ongoing shockable rhythm) and airway management and while the patient is being resuscitated by other EMS team members, the first and direct contact with the cardiac center coordinator by mobile phone should be established to discuss eligibility and ECPR team availability.

## 22.4 Transport

Time-to-ECPR is strongly associated with a favorable neurological survival [2, 3, 18], but there is a narrow window where transport to ECPR may be considered [19, 20]. It is difficult to balance the risks and benefits of early versus later transport because each case of CPR is unique, including the time required for initial procedures and initiation of transport. We must emphasize that, despite intensive efforts, a first call made too late or transport that takes too long remain major and frequent problems, even within a randomized trial environment [2, 21]. Therefore, we recommend proceeding to the first telephone contact immediately after three initial defibrillations and airway management to review eligibility criteria and reach a final decision on intra-arrest transport no later than the 15th minute of ACLS. Thereafter, every effort must be made to reach the ECPR team within 50 but no later than 60 min after the initial collapse or '911' call. The use of defibrillation or other interventions during transport should follow resuscitation guidelines [14]. Special attention must be paid to the correct use of mechanical chest compression devices, maximizing their effectiveness and minimizing the risk of trauma.

The main risk of intra-arrest transport is that resuscitation quality may deteriorate, compared to on-scene CPR [19, 20]. This concern is based on observational data and was confirmed by the Prague OHCA study, in which patients in the invasive arm undergoing intra-arrest transport less frequently arrived at hospital with ROSC compared to those with continued resuscitation on scene [2, 19, 20]. However, this potentially harmful effect of intra-arrest transport has been overcome with ECPR [2]. Based on the current evidence [2, 19, 20], we also suggest that routine intra-arrest transport without preestablished subsequent ECPR and intra-arrest transport of patients not eligible for ECPR should be strongly discouraged and all efforts must focus on high quality on-scene CPR to achieve sustained ROSC.

## 22.5 Patient Admission

Direct transport to the place where the ECPR team is prepared, without any intrahospital delays, is of utmost importance. On admission, overall status, quality of CPR, ROSC presence and institutional criteria for ECMO initiation are reevaluated. This may occur during unloading the patient from the ambulance to minimize any further delays.

There are currently several different places in the hospital where ECPR is provided (catheterization laboratory, emergency department (ED), intensive care unit (ICU), operating room) but there are no evidence-based data enabling comparison

[5]. Both ARREST and the Prague OHCA trial used the catheterization laboratory as the place to provide cannulation and initial ECPR management [2, 3]. The catheterization laboratory has several advantages over other places, namely high quality fluoroscopy, available ultrasound guidance, sterile conditions, specialists with extensive experience with large-bore percutaneous approaches, full equipment in case of troubleshooting, and the possibility of directly proceeding to diagnostic and therapeutic procedures that can reveal and reverse the underlying cause of refractory OHCA [2, 15].

The in-hospital ECPR team ideally consists of two interventionalists, two catheterization laboratory nurses, and one perfusionist who focus on rapid ECMO cannulation and launch, and one intensivist with two intensive care nurses who continue with high quality CPR, perform brief echocardiography, ensure proper ventilation and monitoring, and provide general intensive care during the initial procedures. Formal plans detailing responsibilities and task division, and clear team communication are important for proper team cooperation [5, 9, 14].

## 22.6 ECMO Cannulation

The percutaneous modified Seldinger technique with ultrasound guidance combined with fluoroscopic verification of wire positioning is the method of choice to achieve maximum rates of successful cannulation with minimal vascular complications within the in-hospital environment [12, 22]. Further, the risk of distal limb ischemia from the inserted femoral arterial cannula should be mitigated by placing a distal reperfusion cannula routinely under ultrasound and fluoroscopic guidance [2, 12, 22]. Skill and experience with large-bore sheath insertion is a recognized prerequisite for successful VA-ECMO insertion [2, 3, 13]. We suggest establishment of a small team of highly experienced specialists with extensive expertise in cannulation (number of experts should reflect the number of ECMO cases) who can provide 24/7 service [2, 3, 13, 22].

## 22.7 Initial Diagnostic and Therapeutic Procedures

Following successful VA-ECMO initiation, most centers proceed directly to coronary angiography as severe coronary artery disease is the main cause of refractory OHCA and percutaneous coronary intervention (PCI) is feasible in these patients with high success rates [2, 3, 15]. However, there is limited evidence suggesting the benefit of immediate PCI among refractory OHCA and ECPR patients [15, 23]. In recent years, many trials have failed to show any benefit of early revascularization in OHCA patients with stable spontaneous ROSC without ST elevation myocardial infarction [24]. Immediate PCI should probably be reserved for patients with acutely occluded or critically stenosed vessels with altered coronary flow only, because PCI of non-culprit lesions is associated with a risk of complications (vessel dissection, perforation, stent-thrombosis, contrast-induced nephropathy, etc), and the need for dual antiplatelet therapy which further increases the bleeding risk [24]. Moreover,

12-lead electrocardiogram (EKG) or any EKG for evaluating signs of myocardial ischemia is frequently not available in refractory OHCA patients simply due to the fact that the patients remain in cardiac arrest.

In the absence of obstructive coronary disease, based on the case presentation and rapid echocardiography evaluation, it is possible to proceed with invasive aortography, ventriculography, or pulmonary angiography bearing in mind contrast agent sparing. A low threshold for whole body computed tomography (CT) is advocated by the clinically important diagnostic yield (complications of CPR, intracranial hemorrhage, cause of arrest) and its minimal risks. Early transesophageal echocardiography may also bring useful information both during initial cannulation (wire positions) and for determining the cause of arrest (aortic dissection, tamponade, pulmonary embolism, etc.).

Currently, there are no data supporting targeted therapeutic hypothermia among ECPR patients and the result of the largest trial in OHCA patients with spontaneous ROSC did not show any benefit of hypothermia over strictly controlled normothermia [25]. We suggest active temperature management in all patients with refractory OHCA, targeting strict normothermia (<37.5 °C) or mild hypothermia of 36 °C in preference to 33 °C, as the lower temperature is associated with more complications [25]. Target core temperature should be maintained for 24 h followed by a slow rise in core temperature to normothermia of 37 °C during 8 h with a rewarming rate of 0.5 °C/h. Fever should be avoided in all cases.

## 22.8 Intensive Care

After initial diagnostic and therapeutic procedures, the vital component of success is comprehensive intensive care, as multiorgan failure, infections, and bleeding occur in most ECPR recipients [2, 3]. A high-level of expertise is necessary to overcome these complications and a centralized ECMO unit has been suggested as the preferred strategy [3, 13]. Despite the importance of intensive care recognized by all experts in the field [2, 3, 5], there is lack of data and evidence-based therapies targeting major problems faced by intensivists in ECPR patients, namely brain edema and severe systemic inflammatory response syndrome (SIRS) with multiorgan failure (Table 22.2).

Bleeding complications remain another barrier on the path to achieving better results [2, 26]. This risk can be mitigated by ECMO cannulation under ultrasound and fluoroscopy guidance by an experienced operator, strict coagulation, and platelet level control, minimizing blood loss in case of bleeding (discontinuation of heparin, plasma and coagulation factor infusions, surgery), and early ECMO weaning when appropriate. Daily monitoring is required to provide early detection and treatment of related complications. Prespecified institutional protocols should include careful monitoring of anticoagulation.

Further, there are few data on appropriate blood gas ($PaO_2$ and $PaCO_2$) targets [27]. Extreme variances in $PaO_2$ and $PaCO_2$ during the first hours and days have been linked with neurological complications and should be avoided by careful monitoring and adjustment of ventilation and ECMO gas exchange [27]. However, our

**Table 22.2** Major knowledge gaps for extracorporeal cardiopulmonary resuscitation (ECPR) and areas of possible future research

| Area | Gaps or targets |
|---|---|
| System design, coordination, and widespread use | In-hospital vs. pre-hospital vs. hybrid ECPR system comparison<br>Protocols and novel approaches to decrease time to VA-ECMO<br>Large, adequately powered, multicenter RCTs<br>Demographic definition of ECPR feasibility to assess equal access to treatment |
| Patient selection | Early predictors of conventional CPR non-responders<br>Novel predictors of outcome, stratification scores<br>Outcome of ECPR in selected refractory OHCA patients with initial PEA |
| Transport | Optimal time window for intra-arrest transport<br>Novel, improved mechanical chest compression devices<br>Intra-arrest target temperature management |
| Hospital treatment | Influence of immediate PCI and (continued) TTM on ECPR outcome<br>Novel therapies to prevent and treat brain edema, SIRS, multiorgan failure (cytokine removal, selective brain reperfusion)<br>Ventilation, anticoagulation, left ventricle venting strategies |
| Outcomes | Long-term survival, long-term neurological outcome, quality of life, organ donation, cost-effectiveness, and QALY analysis |

*VA-ECMO* veno-arterial extracorporeal membrane oxygenation, *TTM* therapeutic temperature management, *PCI* percutaneous coronary intervention, *SIRS* systemic inflammatory response syndrome, *QALY* quality-adjusted life year, *PEA* pulseless electrical activity, *RCT* randomized controlled trial

experience suggests that gas fluctuations are rather manifestation of severe SIRS with multiorgan failure than causative factors of poor neurological prognosis.

Another major complication that may occur after VA-ECMO implantation in refractory OHCA is the absence of left ventricular (LV) pulsatility and aortic valve opening despite restitution of a stable sinus rhythm [26]. ECMO retrograde blood flow increases LV afterload and LV end-diastolic pressure, which may lead to pulmonary edema, LV blood stasis, and the risk of thrombosis [26]. The presence of LV pulsatility must be monitored by arterial waveform and echocardiography. The initial approach should be to keep ECMO flow as low as necessary for sufficient end-organ perfusion. This strategy is difficult to use in ECPR patients who frequently have severe shock and multiple organ dysfunction and need full ECMO support [2, 3]. Inotropes may sometimes help to sustain LV contractility and aortic valve opening at the expense of increased oxygen demand and increased risk of arrhythmias, but their effect is rather small. There are multiple LV unloading strategies currently used (transaortic percutaneous axial left ventricular support device, intra-aortic balloon pump [IABP], septostomy etc.) but no firm evidence-based recommendations regarding the timing and method selection. Studies evaluating and comparing the most effective method for LV decompression are still missing [26].

Freely available psychological, palliative, and spiritual care should be offered to victims of cardiac arrest and to their relatives.

## 22.9 Hospital Discharge and Long-Term Follow-Up

After successful ECMO weaning and awakening of the patient, most ECPR survivors need complex care including physical and neurocognitive rehabilitation, nutrition and resocialization, to be able to leave the hospital. But the story does not end at discharge. It is necessary to provide routine outpatient visits, as many ECPR survivors face ongoing health problems ('vulnerable period') and all efforts and finances spent on the acute care may be hampered by inadequate post-discharge care. Limited experience from a single center observational study suggests that ECPR survivors have a significantly lower quality of life compared to controls at 12 months [28]. However, data regarding long term risk of cardiovascular events and survival are missing. As during intensive care, psychological, spiritual, or palliative support should be available on an ambulatory basis, or even as a home care service.

## 22.10 Conclusion

ECPR can improve survival with good neurological recovery in refractory OHCA when performed within a well-coordinated system with high-quality ACLS. Proper patient selection, time to VA-ECMO initiation, an experienced team, and comprehensive intensive care are all key factors influencing the outcome. There are many knowledge gaps and a vast need for experimental, translational, and clinical research in the field of refractory OHCA and ECPR.

## References


1. Gräsner JT, Herlitz J, Tjelmeland IB, et al. European Resuscitation Council Guidelines 2021: epidemiology of cardiac arrest in Europe. Resuscitation. 2021;161:61–79.
2. Belohlavek J, Smalcova J, Rob D, et al. Effect of intra-arrest transport, extracorporeal cardiopulmonary resuscitation, and immediate invasive assessment and treatment on functional neurologic outcome in refractory out-of-hospital cardiac arrest: a randomized clinical trial. JAMA. 2022;327:737–47.
3. Yannopoulos D, Bartos J, Raveendran G, et al. Advanced reperfusion strategies for patients with out-of-hospital cardiac arrest and refractory ventricular fibrillation (ARREST): a phase 2, single centre, open-label, randomised controlled trial. Lancet. 2020;396:1807–16.
4. Holmberg MJ, Geri G, Wiberg S, et al. Extracorporeal cardiopulmonary resuscitation for cardiac arrest: a systematic review. Resuscitation. 2018;131:91–100.
5. Abrams D, MacLaren G, Lorusso R, et al. Extracorporeal cardiopulmonary resuscitation in adults: evidence and implications. Intensive Care Med. 2021;48:1–15.
6. Bougouin W, Dumas F, Lamhaut L, et al. Extracorporeal cardiopulmonary resuscitation in out-of-hospital cardiac arrest: a registry study. Eur Heart J. 2020;41:1961–71.
7. Patricio D, Peluso L, Brasseur A, et al. Comparison of extracorporeal and conventional cardiopulmonary resuscitation: a retrospective propensity score matched study. Crit Care. 2019;23:1–10.
8. Poppe M, Weiser C, Holzer M, et al. The incidence of "load&go" out-of-hospital cardiac arrest candidates for emergency department utilization of emergency extracorporeal life support: a one-year review. Resuscitation. 2015;91:131–6.

9. Nolan J, Soar J, Eikeland H. The chain of survival. Resuscitation. 2006;71:270–1.
10. Tanaka Y, Taniguchi J, Wato Y, et al. The continuous quality improvement project for telephone-assisted instruction of cardiopulmonary resuscitation increased the incidence of bystander CPR and improved the outcomes of out-of-hospital cardiac arrests. Resuscitation. 2012;83:1235–41.
11. Kragholm K, Wissenberg M, Mortensen RN, et al. Bystander efforts and 1-year outcomes in out-of-hospital cardiac arrest. N Engl J Med. 2017;376:1737–47.
12. Belohlavek J, Kucera K, Jarkovsky J, et al. Hyperinvasive approach to out-of hospital cardiac arrest using mechanical chest compression device, prehospital intraarrest cooling, extracorporeal life support and early invasive assessment compared to standard of care. A randomized parallel groups comparative study proposal. "Prague OHCA study". J Transl Med. 2012;10:1–13.
13. Bartos JA, Grunau B, Carlson C, et al. Improved survival with extracorporeal cardiopulmonary resuscitation despite progressive metabolic derangement associated with prolonged resuscitation. Circulation. 2020;141:877–86.
14. Soar J, Böttiger BW, Carli P, et al. European resuscitation council guidelines 2021: adult advanced life support. Resuscitation. 2021;161:115–51.
15. Rob D, Kavalkova P, Smalcova J, et al. Coronary angiography and percutaneous coronary intervention in cardiac arrest patients without return of spontaneous circulation. Resuscitation. 2022;175:133–41.
16. Goh AX, Seow JC, Lai MY, et al. Association of high-volume centers with survival outcomes among patients with nontraumatic out-of-hospital cardiac arrest: a systematic review and meta-analysis. JAMA Netw Open. 2022;5:e2214639.
17. Mørk SR, Stengaard C, Linde L, et al. Mechanical circulatory support for refractory out-of-hospital cardiac arrest: a Danish nationwide multicenter study. Crit Care. 2021;25:1–13.
18. Wengenmayer T, Rombach S, Ramshorn F, et al. Influence of low-flow time on survival after extracorporeal cardiopulmonary resuscitation (eCPR). Crit Care. 2017;21:1–6.
19. Grunau B, Kime N, Leroux B, et al. Association of intra-arrest transport vs continued on-scene resuscitation with survival to hospital discharge among patients with out-of-hospital cardiac arrest. JAMA. 2020;324:1058–67.
20. Grunau B, Reynolds J, Scheuermeyer F, et al. Relationship between time-to-ROSC and survival in out-of-hospital cardiac arrest ECPR candidates: when is the best time to consider transport to hospital? Prehosp Emerg Care. 2016;20:615–22.
21. Hsu CH, Meurer WJ, Domeier R, et al. Extracorporeal cardiopulmonary resuscitation for refractory out-of-hospital cardiac arrest (EROCA): results of a randomized feasibility trial of expedited out-of-hospital transport. Ann Emerg Med. 2021;78:92–101.
22. Danial P, Hajage D, Nguyen LS, et al. Percutaneous versus surgical femoro-femoral veno-arterial ECMO: a propensity score matched study. Intensive Care Med. 2018;44:2153–61.
23. Rob D, Smalcova J, Kovarnik T, et al. Immediate percutaneous coronary intervention in patients with refractory out of hospital cardiac arrest. Circulation. 2021;144(Suppl_2):A11324 (abst).
24. Nikolaou NI, Netherton S, Welsford M, et al. A systematic review and meta-analysis of the effect of routine early angiography in patients with return of spontaneous circulation after Out-of-Hospital Cardiac Arrest. Resuscitation. 2021;163:28–48.
25. Dankiewicz J, Cronberg T, Lilja G, et al. Hypothermia versus normothermia after out-of-hospital cardiac arrest. N Engl J Med. 2021;384:2283–94.
26. Rob D, Belohlávek J. The mechanical support of cardiogenic shock. Curr Opin Crit Care. 2021;27:440–6.
27. Cashen K, Reeder R, Dalton HJ, et al. Hyperoxia and hypocapnia during pediatric extracorporeal membrane oxygenation: Associations with complications, mortality and functional status among survivors. Pediatr Crit Care Med. 2018;19:245.
28. Spangenberg T, Schewel J, Dreher A, et al. Health related quality of life after extracorporeal cardiopulmonary resuscitation in refractory cardiac arrest. Resuscitation. 2018;127:73–8.

# Temporary and Durable Mechanical Circulatory Support in the ICU

# 23

A. Pinsino, M. N. Gong, and M. Rahmanian

## 23.1 Introduction

Mechanical circulatory support has evolved dramatically in the last 30 years. Initial devices were pulsatile-flow paracorporeal pumps conceived to provide temporary support for selected hospitalized patients awaiting heart transplantation (bridge to transplant) [1], but technological advancements in the field have now resulted in continuous-flow, implantable, dischargeable left ventricular (LV) assist devices (LVADs) [2]. Contemporary, durable LVADs have shown a dramatic improvement in outcomes when compared with first-generation devices [3] and represent the only advanced therapy available to advanced heart failure patients deemed ineligible for transplantation (destination therapy). Concurrent with the evolution of long-term devices, the field has witnessed an expansion of available temporary mechanical circulatory support systems. Short-term mechanical circulatory support is used, in addition to a bridge to transplant, as rescue therapy in patients whose candidacy for durable LVAD or transplant requires additional evaluation after improvement in end-organ perfusion (bridge to decision), or in patients with a potentially reversible cause of cardiac dysfunction (bridge to recovery). Temporary mechanical circulatory support is routinely used in the setting of cardiogenic shock complicating acute myocardial infarction, *de*

A. Pinsino · M. N. Gong · M. Rahmanian (✉)
Division of Critical Care Medicine, Montefiore Medical Center, Bronx, NY, USA
e-mail: mrahmani@montefiore.org



J.-L. Vincent (ed.), *Annual Update in Intensive Care and Emergency Medicine 2023*, Annual Update in Intensive Care and Emergency Medicine,
https://doi.org/10.1007/978-3-031-23005-9_23

*novo* heart failure (e.g., myocarditis), and chronic heart failure. Other indications include post-cardiotomy shock, complications of heart transplant leading to cardiogenic shock (e.g., primary graft dysfunction), and drug overdose resulting in cardiac depression (e.g., calcium channel blockers). An expanding indication for temporary mechanical circulatory support is represented by cardiac arrest (extracorporeal cardiopulmonary resuscitation [ECPR]).

As a result of the increased uptake of mechanical circulatory support, intensivists with different degrees of training and experience in the contemporary management of advanced heart failure and cardiogenic shock are increasingly likely to participate in the care of this patient population. Herein, we review the current options for mechanical circulatory support with a focus on the available devices and on the complications associated with their use, and we highlight the most recent contributions to the field.

## 23.2 Temporary Mechanical Circulatory Support

### 23.2.1 Devices

#### 23.2.1.1 Intra-Aortic Balloon Pump

The intra-aortic balloon pump (IABP) is the most commonly used temporary mechanical circulatory support device due to its limited cost, wide availability, and facility of insertion. Using heliox to inflate a balloon placed in the proximal ascending aorta during diastole followed by a deflation in systole (Fig. 23.1a), IABP reduces LV afterload and facilitates coronary perfusion, resulting in a net improvement in the myocardial oxygen supply/demand ratio [4]. The increase in cardiac output generated by IABP support is modest (0.5–1.2 l/min) [5]. Although IABPs have been historically placed through the femoral artery, implantation of this device via the axillary artery allows ambulation and longer duration of support [6].

In the IABP-SHOCK II trial, routine use of IABP in patients with cardiogenic shock complicating myocardial infarction did not reduce mortality [7]. However, clinical equipoise persists among acute-on-chronic heart failure patients with cardiogenic shock [5]. Additionally, IABP may be beneficial in patients with myocardial infarction and cardiogenic shock who are supported with veno-arterial extracorporeal membrane oxygenation (VA-ECMO) [8].

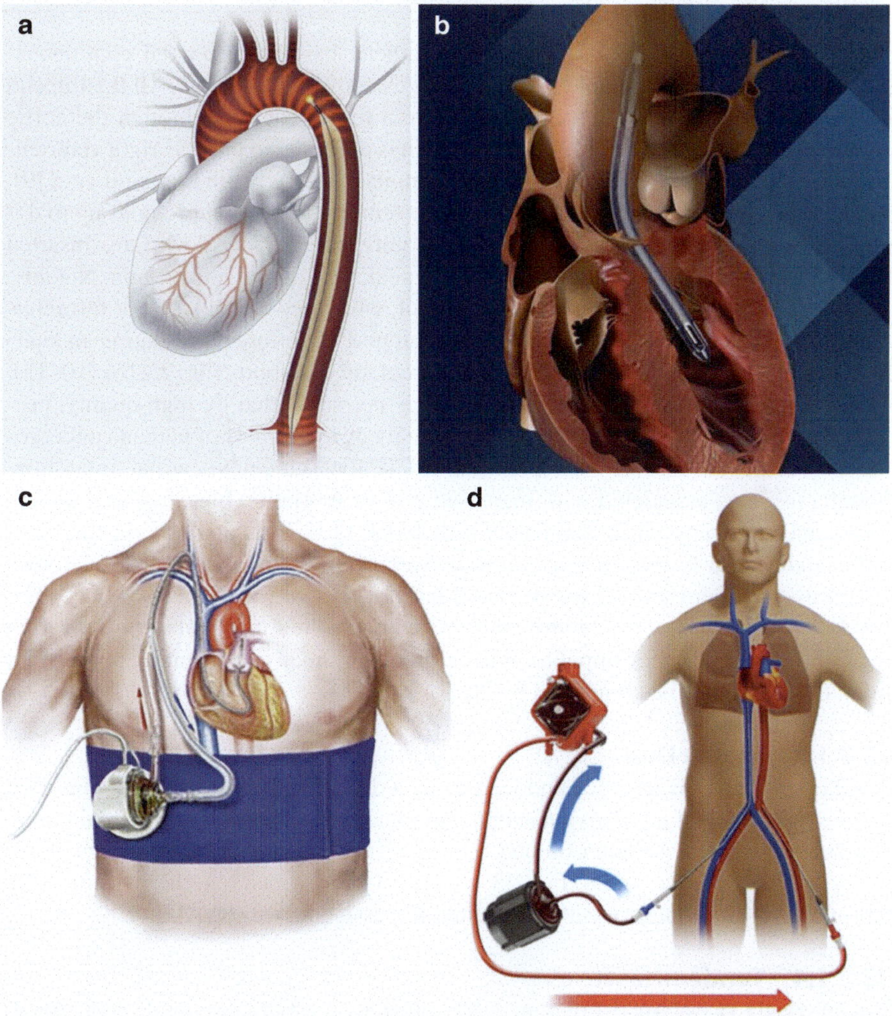


**Fig. 23.1** Temporary mechanical circulatory support devices. (**a**) Intra-aortic balloon pump. (Figure from Getinge, reproduced with permission) (**b**) Impella 5.5. (Figure from Abiomed, reproduced with permission) (**c**) Protek Duo. (Reproduced from [42] under a Creative Commons Attribution 4.0 International License) (**d**) Veno-arterial extracorporeal membrane oxygenation. (Reproduced from [43] under a Creative Commons Attribution 4.0 International License)

#### 23.2.1.2 Impella

Impella (Abiomed, Danvers, MA, USA) is a catheter-based, micro-axial, continuous-flow device, which is available in different sizes and configurations. All the Impella devices are positioned in the left ventricle in a retrograde way through the aortic valve, with the exception of Impella RP, which is designed to provide right ventricular (RV) support and is inserted into the pulmonary artery via the femoral vein [9]. Impella CP is inserted percutaneously via the femoral artery and provides up to 4 l/min of blood flow. Impella 5.0 and 5.5 require surgical cut-down, are inserted through the axillary artery, and can provide a peak flow rate of 5 to 6 l/min. Notably, Impella 5.5 has a new design without a pigtail, which reduces the risk of thrombus accumulation and allows longer duration of support, therefore representing an alternative to surgically implanted mechanical circulatory support (Fig. 23.1b) [10–12].

The use of Impella in cardiogenic shock is not supported by high-quality, prospective evidence. In a recent retrospective analysis in a cohort of patients undergoing percutaneous coronary intervention (PCI) for acute myocardial infarction, Impella use was associated with increased risk of mortality, bleeding, and kidney replacement therapy when compared with IABP [13]. This analysis, in line with prior studies that found an association between Impella use and worse outcomes [14], raises concern around the potential harm associated with these devices. The DanGer Shock study, an ongoing randomized controlled trial that is investigating the safety and efficacy of Impella CP in cardiogenic shock complicating myocardial infarction [15], will be completed by 2023.

#### 23.2.1.3 Protek Duo

The Protek Duo (LivaNova, London, UK) is a dual-lumen cannula that is inserted via the right internal jugular vein and, in combination with an extracorporeal pump, can drain more than 4 l/min of blood from the right atrium to the pulmonary artery to support the right ventricle (Fig. 23.1c) [16]. It represents, together with Impella RP, an alternative to a surgically implanted RV assist device (RVAD).

#### 23.2.1.4 TandemHeart

TandemHeart (LivaNova, London, UK) refers to an extracorporeal, centrifugal, continuous-flow mechanical circulatory support device and to a catheter produced by the same company that can be positioned in the left atrium via transseptal puncture [12]. With a configuration that entails an inflow cannula inserted from the femoral vein into the left atrium and an outflow cannula to the femoral artery, TandemHeart provides hemodynamic support up to 5 l/min. The use of TandemHeart as a percutaneous RVAD has also been described [17]. The main limitation preventing widespread use of TandemHeart is related to the need for transseptal puncture [11].

#### 23.2.1.5 Veno-Arterial Extracorporeal Membrane Oxygenation

ECMO can provide hemodynamic support when used in a VA configuration, unlike the veno-venous configuration which is used primarily for respiratory failure. With VA-ECMO, deoxygenated blood is removed through a venous inflow cannula and oxygenated blood returned to the arterial circulation through an outflow cannula (Fig. 23.1d). Cannulation for VA-ECMO can be either central or peripheral. With central cannulation, at least one cannula is placed through the chest wall, typically in the right atrium for the inflow cannula and in the aorta for the outflow cannula [18]. Central cannulation requires sternotomy and is therefore reserved for post-cardiotomy shock. Peripheral cannulation can be placed percutaneously or through surgical cut-down. While femoro-femoral cannulation is the most commonly used for peripheral VA-ECMO, cannulation via the internal jugular vein and axillary artery may allow early ambulation [19]. Unlike other forms of temporary mechanical circulatory support, VA-ECMO provides robust biventricular support and respiratory support. In addition, peripheral cannulation can be quickly performed at the bedside.

Increasingly, VA-ECMO is being evaluated for hemodynamic support during cardiac arrest (ECPR). In a recent, single-center, randomized study (ARREST trial), VA-ECMO-facilitated resuscitation improved survival among patients with out-of-hospital cardiac arrest and refractory shockable rhythm [20]. The study was performed at the University of Minnesota and randomized 30 patients with refractory shockable rhythm to VA-ECMO or standard advanced cardiac life support (ACLS). The trial was stopped at the first interim analysis due to the superiority of VA-ECMO, which resulted in a significant mortality benefit (43% rate of survival at discharge versus 7% in the standard ACLS group) and in an improvement in neurological outcomes. It should be noted that the results of the ARREST trial are not fully generalizable to clinical practice, since the study was performed in a center with extensive ECPR experience and involved trained emergency medical services providers. In addition, the early stopping of the trial may have resulted in an overestimation of the benefits of ECPR.

Unlike IABP and Impella, VA-ECMO increases LV afterload, which can lead to LV distension and pulmonary edema. Strategies which can contribute to minimize or reduce LV distension include inotropic support or concomitant use of IABP or Impella to unload the left ventricle. In a recent retrospective study including over 12,000 patients on VA-ECMO support, mechanical LV unloading by IABP or Impella was associated with lower in-hospital mortality [21]. Notably, in this analysis, mechanical unloading by IABP was associated with a lower incidence of bleeding and renal failure and a trend towards decreased mortality when compared with Impella.

#### 23.2.1.6 Surgically-Implanted Temporary Ventricular Assist Devices

Surgically-implanted temporary mechanical circulatory support devices provide excellent long duration hemodynamic support (up to 10 l/min for the most common device, Centrimag [Abbott, Plymouth, MN, USA]) to left, right, or both (biventricular assist device [BiVAD]) ventricles. However, the use of these devices is limited by the need for median sternotomy for both implantation and explantation [11]. An alternative minimally invasive configuration, which combines Centrimag and ECMO has been described [22].

### 23.2.2 Principles of Device Selection and Weaning of Temporary Mechanical Circulatory Support

Evidence guiding the selection of device and strategies for temporary mechanical circulatory support is limited. Current guidelines recommend an interdisciplinary approach to guide initiation and escalation of temporary mechanical circulatory support. In an effort to improve outcomes in cardiogenic shock through a timely use of temporary mechanical circulatory support, tertiary centers have created shock teams which include a heart failure cardiologist, a cardiothoracic surgeon, an interventional cardiologist, and an intensivist.

Several factors contribute to the selection of the appropriate option for temporary mechanical circulatory support. Patient-related factors include expected duration of support, likelihood of cardiac recovery, eligibility for heart transplantation or durable mechanical circulatory support, and specific hemodynamic profile. While the evidence supporting the use of a pulmonary artery catheter is limited to retrospective studies, invasive hemodynamic assessment using a pulmonary artery catheter is recommended [23]. Patients with isolated LV failure may benefit from IABP or Impella support. Percutaneous options for isolated RV failure include Protek Duo and Impella RP. Devices that provide biventricular support are VA-ECMO and Centrimag BiVAD. In addition, the severity of the shock should guide the device selection – as an example, a patient with profound left-sided shock is more likely to benefit from Impella 5.5 than from IABP or Impella CP. Lastly, in patients with severe respiratory failure (e.g., concomitant acute respiratory distress syndrome [ARDS]), VA-ECMO is the main option for temporary mechanical circulatory support.

Weaning from temporary mechanical circulatory support should be attempted daily [24], because longer duration of support is associated with worse outcomes. Patients with an improvement in the condition that required mechanical circulatory support (e.g., myocardial infarction), improving end-organ function, stable hemodynamics on low-dose inotropic and vasopressor support, should undergo a weaning trial. While different approaches have been proposed, stepwise weaning of the device-specific degree of support while on therapeutic anticoagulation is recommended [23]. If the patient tolerates weaning of mechanical circulatory support and the lowest support level (e.g., 1–2 l/min of flow for patients on VA-ECMO) is achieved and maintained with clinical stability as defined by a set of hemodynamic, metabolic, and echocardiographic variables, decannulation can be considered. The failure of a weaning trial should prompt a multi-disciplinary discussion to optimize reversible causes and consideration for advanced therapies (i.e., heart transplant, durable LVAD).

### 23.2.3 Complications

The use of temporary mechanical circulatory support is associated with complications that may be related to the device itself, its insertion, the effect of the device on organ function, and the use of anticoagulation. The common and device-specific complications of temporary mechanical circulatory support are summarized in Table 23.1.

**Table 23.1** Complications of temporary mechanical circulatory support

| Common to all devices | Device-specific |
|---|---|
| **Vascular** | **Intra-aortic balloon pump** |
| Limb ischemia | Spinal cord ischemia |
| Insertion site bleeding | **Impella** |
| Vessel perforation | Valvular damage |
| Retroperitoneal hematoma | Perforation |
| **Neurological** | **Tandem Heart** |
| Ischemic stroke | Perforation |
| Hemorrhagic stroke | Atrial septal defect |
| **Hematological** | **Veno-arterial ECMO** |
| Major bleeding | Air embolism |
| Hemolysis | Circuit clotting |
| Thrombocytopenia | Left ventricular distension |
| **Mechanical** | Differential hypoxemia |
| Device malposition | Drug pharmacokinetics |
| Device malfunction | **Surgical temporary VAD** |
| **Infectious** | Sternal infection |
| Sepsis | Sternotomy osseous complications |
| Insertion site infection | |

*ECMO* extracorporeal membrane oxygenation, *VAD* ventricular assist device

The incidence of these complications is influenced by several factors, which include the mechanical circulatory support device, patient-specific factors (e.g., size of the vessel), and the duration of support. Since large bore cannulas are more likely to result in vascular complications, VA-ECMO has the highest rate of limb ischemia and prophylactic distal perfusion catheters are routinely used in patients receiving VA-ECMO support [23]. Bleeding frequently complicates temporary mechanical circulatory support and often requires temporary or permanent interruption of anti-coagulation, which can result in thromboembolism and hemolysis. While hemolysis can occur with all temporary mechanical circulatory support devices, this complication is particularly frequent with Impella and has historically limited the use of these devices for longer duration of support. However, the design of the newest device of the Impella family, Impella 5.5, may result in a lower incidence of hemolysis [25]. Migration of the device is particularly dangerous in patients supported with TandemHeart, since malposition of the inflow cannula in the right atrium results in the shunting of deoxygenated blood to the systemic circulation [23]. Infectious complications are prevalent and include common sources in critically ill patients (e.g., ventilator-acquired pneumonia [VAP]) as well as access site infections for percutaneous devices and sternal infection for surgically implanted devices. Prophylactic antibiotics may be used in patients with central VA-ECMO and open chest, but are not recommended in patients with peripheral ECMO cannulation or other temporary mechanical circulatory support devices [23]. In addition to LV distension, patients supported with peripheral VA-ECMO are at risk of differential hypoxia (also known as Harlequin or North-South syndrome). In VA-ECMO with femoro-femoral cannulation, oxygenated blood flows from the femoral cannula to the left ventricle in a retrograde fashion and mixes with the blood ejected from the left ventricle. In patients with severe impairment of gas exchange and recovery of left ventricular function, deoxygenated blood from the left ventricle may represent the main blood source for right subclavian and carotid arteries and result in a marked discrepancy in the oxygen saturation between the lower extremities and the cerebral circulation [18]. The detection of differential hypoxemia requires continuous monitoring of the arterial oxygen saturation of the right radial artery and non-invasive cerebral saturation. A potential solution for differential hypoxemia is represented by the placement of a new venous outflow cannula, which brings oxygenated blood to the right atrium (veno-arterial-venous ECMO).

## 23.3 Durable Mechanical Circulatory Support

Durable LVADs are the most used form of long-term mechanical circulatory support. Total artificial heart is an alternative to a durable LVAD for patients with biventricular failure, typically as a bridge to transplant. However, this type of device is rarely used in clinical practice and is beyond the scope of this review.

### 23.3.1 Devices

While the first-generation devices were pulsatile, all the currently available durable LVADs provide continuous flow and share a similar design. Each device has a pump, an inflow cannula draining blood from the LV apex, an outflow cannula connected to the ascending aorta, and a driveline which connects the pump to an external battery and to the controller. HeartMate II (Abbott, Plymouth, MN, USA), the first continuous-flow durable LVAD approved for bridge to transplant and destination therapy in the USA [26], has an axial-flow impeller which is placed in an abdominal pocket (Fig. 23.2a).

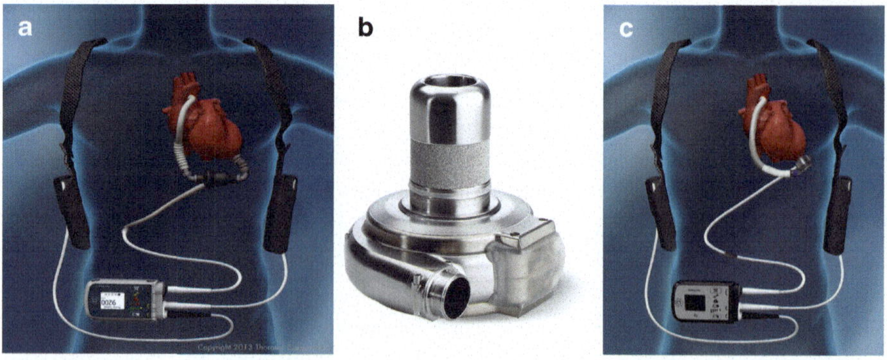


**Fig. 23.2** Durable mechanical circulatory support devices. (**a**) HeartMate II. (Figure from Abbott, reproduced with permission) (**b**) HeartWare ventricular assist device (HVAD). (Figure from Medtronic, reproduced with permission) (**c**) HeartMate 3. (Figure from Abbott, reproduced with permission)

HeartWare ventricular assist device (HVAD, Medtronic, Mounds View, MN, USA) was the first centrifugal durable LVAD approved in the USA for bridge to transplant. The HVAD is a smaller pump compared to the HeartMate II and is implanted in the pericardial space (Fig. 23.2b). Compared to HeartMate II, HVAD implantation was associated with a higher risk of cerebrovascular accidents [27]. In addition, the USA Food and Drug Administration (FDA) recalled HVADs for unexpected power source switching and pump stoppage. As a result of these safety concerns, in June 2021 the manufacturer discontinued the production of HVAD.

HeartMate 3 (Abbott, Plymouth, MN, USA) is the newest centrifugal LVAD with a design that includes a fully magnetically levitated rotor, wider blood-flow paths, and an artificial pulse which occurs asynchronously from the native cardiac cycle through fixed rotor speed changes every 2 s (Fig. 23.2c), and is currently the most used durable device worldwide. The MOMENTUM 3 trial compared HeartMate 3 with HeartMate II in 1028 patients with advanced heart failure [3]. In the final report of the MOMENTUM 3 trial, at 2-year follow-up, 77% patients implanted with HeartMate 3 were alive and free of disabling stroke or pump exchange (versus 65% in the HeartMate II group). In addition, patients implanted with HeartMate 3 had significantly lower rates of stroke of any severity and of gastrointestinal bleeding. In a subsequent analysis of a continuous access protocol post-pivotal trial [28], patients implanted with HeartMate 3 had a lower adverse event burden and reduced hospital admissions when compared to results from the MOMENTUM 3 trial, suggesting that outcomes may improve as clinical experience accumulates.

### 23.3.2 Complications

Patients implanted with a durable LVAD will often experience adverse events, which often result in a prolonged postoperative hospital stay or in intensive care unit (ICU) readmissions. The most common complications related to LVAD include RV failure, hemocompatibility-related adverse events (bleeding, stroke and pump thrombosis), driveline infection and aortic insufficiency.

#### 23.3.2.1 Right Ventricular Failure

Right heart failure is a common occurrence in the postoperative period in a population with pre-implant pulmonary hypertension and RV dysfunction, which is further exacerbated by the hemodynamic changes generated by LVAD support (i.e., increased RV preload). While most cases of postoperative RV failure require only transient inotropic support, severe cases may require temporary mechanical circulatory support, either percutaneous (e.g., ProtekDuo) or surgical.

In addition to the postoperative period, RV failure can occur months or years after implantation. In a recent analysis of a large multicenter registry, late RV failure occurring over 6 months after implantation was associated with worse outcomes compared to the early occurrence of this complication [29].

#### 23.3.2.2 Hemocompatibility-Related Adverse Events

Patients receiving LVAD support are at increased risk of bleeding and thrombotic events due to the activation of procoagulant and anticoagulant pathways. From a clinical perspective, this aberrant hemocompatibility physiological state results in a constellation of gastrointestinal bleeding, stroke, and pump thrombosis [30].

Gastrointestinal bleeding is the most common hemocompatibility-related adverse event. Up to half of the gastrointestinal bleeding occurring in patients supported by LVAD is related to arteriovenous malformation, an otherwise uncommon cause in the general population. The pathogenesis of arteriovenous malformation is multifactorial, including the use of antithrombotic therapy, enhanced angiogenesis secondary to continuous-flow, and acquired von Willebrand deficiency [31].

Among patients supported with LVAD, the incidence of stroke is approximately 15% per year and is associated with significant morbidity and mortality. Stroke can be ischemic or hemorrhagic, and the use of antithrombotic therapy may result in higher rates of hemorrhagic transformation of ischemic strokes [31]. Pump thrombosis is associated with hemolysis, evidence of reduced LV unloading, and may require urgent pump exchange [32].

Elevated blood pressure is associated with an increased risk for both stroke and pump thrombosis [33]. In the ENDURANCE Supplemental trial [27], enhanced blood pressure management that included home blood pressure monitoring and targeted a mean arterial pressure (MAP) $< 85$ mmHg successfully reduced the incidence of stroke in patients implanted with an HVAD. The incidence of stroke and pump thrombosis is significantly reduced among patients implanted with HeartMate 3 compared to HeartMate II and HVAD [3, 34]. In a recent analysis including over 6000 patients, HeartMate 3 use was associated with a sixfold decrease in the risk for cerebrovascular events when compared with HVAD use [35].

An active area of research in the field is represented by the management of antithrombotic therapy. Per the current standard care, patients on LVAD support receive both anticoagulation with vitamin K antagonists and an antiplatelet therapy (e.g., low-dose aspirin). A multicenter randomized trial, ARIES, is currently evaluating the hypothesis that withdrawal of antiplatelet therapy may reduce bleeding events without increasing thrombotic complications in a cohort of HeartMate 3 recipients [36].

#### 23.3.2.3 Driveline Infection

The percutaneous driveline represents an ideal gateway for the access of pathogens. The driveline often becomes colonized and this may result in a systemic infection that can confers significant morbidity and mortality and may require pump exchange. The driveline of HeartMate 3 has features that may increase the risk of infection compared to other devices [37]. In the final report of the MOMENTUM 3 trial [3], there was a numerically higher rate of infection in the HeartMate 3 group than in the HeartMate II group (23% versus 19%, $p = 0.60$). In a recent single-center analysis among 591 LVAD recipients [38], *Staphylococcus aureus* and *Pseudomonas aeruginosa* were the most common pathogens. Notably, in the same study, a standardized driveline care protocol was associated with a significant reduction in driveline infections.

#### 23.3.2.4 Aortic Insufficiency

LVAD support can cause *de novo* aortic insufficiency or accelerate progression, which represents a significant barrier to long-term support since it is associated with an increased risk for heart failure [32]. The proposed mechanisms for the development of aortic insufficiency in this population include the closure of the aortic valve (intermittent or continuous) resulting from LV unloading, persistent stress on the aortic side of the valve with increased turbulent flow causing endothelial changes, and aortic annular dilation [39]. The artificial pulse generated by HeartMate 3 may potentially prevent onset and progression of aortic insufficiency by increasing the frequency of valve opening. However, in a recent single-center retrospective study, the incidence of moderate to severe aortic insufficiency did not differ significantly between HeartMate II and HeartMate 3 [40].

## 23.4 Conclusion

Mechanical circulatory support has become a mainstay in the treatment of cardiogenic shock and advanced heart failure. As demand increases and technology improves, intensivists are increasingly likely to participate in the different phases of the care of patients on mechanical circulatory support, from the management of complications to percutaneous cannulation [41]. While the field has seen considerable development in a short span of time, significant knowledge gaps persist. Randomized controlled studies are warranted to provide an evidence-based foundation for temporary device selection and to improve the medical management of patients receiving durable mechanical circulatory support.

## References

1. Champsaur G, Ninet J, Vigneron M, Cochet P, Neidecker J, Boissonnat P. Use of the Abiomed BVS System 5000 as a bridge to cardiac transplantation. J Thorac Cardiovasc Surg. 1990;100:122–8.
2. Rose EA, Gelijns AC, Moskowitz AJ, et al. Long-term use of a left ventricular assist device for end-stage heart failure. N Engl J Med. 2001;345:1435–43.
3. Mehra MR, Uriel N, Naka Y, et al. A fully magnetically levitated left ventricular assist device—final report. N Engl J Med. 2019;380:1618–27.
4. Combes A, Price S, Slutsky AS, Brodie D. Temporary circulatory support for cardiogenic shock. Lancet. 2020;396:199–212.
5. Fried JA, Nair A, Takeda K, et al. Clinical and hemodynamic effects of intra-aortic balloon pump therapy in chronic heart failure patients with cardiogenic shock. J Heart Lung Transplant. 2018;37:1313–21.
6. Bhimaraj A, Agrawal T, Duran A, et al. Percutaneous left axillary artery placement of intra-aortic balloon pump in advanced heart failure patients. JACC Heart Fail. 2020;8:313–23.
7. Thiele H, Zeymer U, Neumann FJ, et al. Intraaortic balloon support for myocardial infarction with cardiogenic shock. N Engl J Med. 2012;367:1287–96.
8. Nishi T, Ishii M, Tsujita K, et al. Outcomes of venoarterial extracorporeal membrane oxygenation plus intra-aortic balloon pumping for treatment of acute myocardial infarction complicated by cardiogenic shock. J Am Heart Assoc. 2022;11:e023713.

9. Pieri M, Pappalardo F. Impella RP in the treatment of right ventricular failure: what we know and where we go. J Cardiothorac Vasc Anesth. 2018;32:2339–43.
10. Ramzy D, Soltesz E, Anderson M. New surgical circulatory support system outcomes. ASAIO J. 2020;66:746–52.
11. Zhou AL, Etchill EW, Giuliano KA, et al. Bridge to transplantation from mechanical circulatory support: a narrative review. J Thorac Dis. 2021;13:6911–23.
12. Baran DA, Jaiswal A, Hennig F, Potapov E. Temporary mechanical circulatory support: devices, outcomes, and future directions. J Heart Lung Transplant. 2022;41:678–91.
13. Miller PE, Bromfield SG, Ma Q, et al. Clinical outcomes and cost associated with an intravascular microaxial left ventricular assist device vs intra-aortic balloon pump in patients presenting with acute myocardial infarction complicated by cardiogenic shock. JAMA Intern Med. 2022;182:926–33.
14. Dhruva SS, Ross JS, Mortazavi BJ, et al. Association of use of an intravascular microaxial left ventricular assist device vs intra-aortic balloon pump with in-hospital mortality and major bleeding among patients with acute myocardial infarction complicated by cardiogenic shock. JAMA. 2020;323:734–45.
15. Udesen NJ, Møller JE, Lindholm MG, et al. Rationale and design of DanGer shock: Danish-German cardiogenic shock trial. Am Heart J. 2019;214:60–8.
16. Salna M, Garan AR, Kirtane AJ, et al. Novel percutaneous dual-lumen cannula-based right ventricular assist device provides effective support for refractory right ventricular failure after left ventricular assist device implantation. Interact Cardiovasc Thorac Surg. 2020;30:499–506.
17. Atiemo AD, Conte JV, Heldman AW. Resuscitation and recovery from acute right ventricular failure using a percutaneous right ventricular assist device. Catheter Cardiovasc Interv. 2006;68:78–82.
18. Eckman PM, Katz JN, El Banayosy A, Bohula EA, Sun B, van Diepen S. Veno-arterial extracorporeal membrane oxygenation for cardiogenic shock: an introduction for the busy clinician. Circulation. 2019;140:2019–37.
19. Keebler ME, Haddad EV, Choi CW, et al. Venoarterial extracorporeal membrane oxygenation in cardiogenic shock. JACC Heart Fail. 2018;6:503–16.
20. Yannopoulos D, Bartos J, Raveendran G, et al. Advanced reperfusion strategies for patients with out-of-hospital cardiac arrest and refractory ventricular fibrillation (ARREST): a phase 2, single centre, open-label, randomised controlled trial. Lancet. 2020;396:1807–16.
21. Grandin EW, Nunez JI, Willar B, et al. Mechanical left ventricular unloading in patients undergoing venoarterial extracorporeal membrane oxygenation. J Am Coll Cardiol. 2022;79:1239–50.
22. Takeda K, Garan AR, Ando M, et al. Minimally invasive CentriMag ventricular assist device support integrated with extracorporeal membrane oxygenation in cardiogenic shock patients: a comparison with conventional CentriMag biventricular support configuration. Eur J Cardiothorac Surg. 2017;52:1055–61.
23. Geller BJ, Sinha SS, Kapur NK, et al. Escalating and de-escalating temporary mechanical circulatory support in cardiogenic shock: a scientific statement from the American Heart Association. Circulation. 2022;146:e50–68.
24. Randhawa VK, Al-Fares A, Tong MZY, et al. A pragmatic approach to weaning temporary mechanical circulatory support: a state-of-the-art review. JACC Heart Fail. 2021;9:664–73.
25. Kennel PJ, Lumish H, Kaku Y, et al. A case series analysis on the clinical experience of Impella 5.5® at a large tertiary care centre. ESC Heart Fail. 2021;8:3720–5.
26. Slaughter MS, Rogers JG, Milano CA, et al. Advanced heart failure treated with continuous-flow left ventricular assist device. N Engl J Med. 2009;361:2241–51.
27. Milano CA, Rogers JG, Tatooles AJ, et al. HVAD: The ENDURANCE Supplemental Trial. JACC Heart Fail. 2018;6:792–802.
28. Mehra MR, Cleveland JC, Uriel N, et al. Primary results of long-term outcomes in the MOMENTUM 3 pivotal trial and continued access protocol study phase: a study of 2200 HeartMate 3 left ventricular assist device implants. Eur J Heart Fail. 2021;23:1392–400.

29. Kapelios CJ, Lund LH, Wever-Pinzon O, et al. Right heart failure following left ventricular device implantation: natural history, risk factors, and outcomes: An analysis of the STS INTERMACS Database. Circ Heart Fail. 2022;15:e008706.
30. Mehra MR. The burden of haemocompatibility with left ventricular assist systems: a complex weave. Eur Heart J. 2019;40:673–7.
31. Willey JZ, Demmer RT, Takayama H, Colombo PC, Lazar RM. Cerebrovascular disease in the era of left ventricular assist devices with continuous flow: risk factors, diagnosis, and treatment. J Heart Lung Transplant. 2014;33:878–87.
32. Han JJ, Acker MA, Atluri P. Left ventricular assist devices. Circulation. 2018;138:2841–51.
33. Pinsino A, Castagna F, Zuver AM, et al. Prognostic implications of serial outpatient blood pressure measurements in patients with an axial continuous-flow left ventricular assist device. J Heart Lung Transplant. 2019;38:396–405.
34. Colombo PC, Mehra MR, Goldstein DJ, et al. Comprehensive analysis of stroke in the long-term cohort of the MOMENTUM 3 study. Circulation. 2019;139:155–68.
35. Cho SM, Mehaffey JH, Meyers SL, et al. Cerebrovascular events in patients with centrifugal-flow left ventricular assist devices: propensity score-matched analysis from the Intermacs Registry. Circulation. 2021;144:763–72.
36. Mehra MR, Crandall DL, Gustafsson F, et al. Aspirin and left ventricular assist devices: rationale and design for the international randomized, placebo-controlled, non-inferiority ARIES HM3 trial. Eur J Heart Fail. 2021;23:1226–37.
37. Schlöglhofer T, Michalovics P, Riebandt J, et al. Left ventricular assist device driveline infections in three contemporary devices. Artif Organs. 2021;45:464–72.
38. Lumish HS, Cagliostro B, Braghieri L, et al. Driveline infection in left ventricular assist device patients: effect of standardized protocols, pathogen type, and treatment strategy. ASAIO J. 2022;68:1450–8.
39. Zaidi SH, Minhas AMK, Sagheer S, et al. Clinical outcomes of transcatheter aortic valve replacement (TAVR) vs. surgical aortic valve replacement (SAVR) in patients with durable left ventricular assist device (LVAD). Curr Probl Cardiol. 2022;47:101313.
40. Jimenez Contreras F, Mendiola Pla M, Schroder J, et al. Progression of aortic valve insufficiency during centrifugal versus axial flow left ventricular assist device support. Eur J Cardiothorac Surg. 2022;61:1188–96.
41. Burrell AJC, Pellegrino VA, Sheldrake J, Pilcher DV. Percutaneous cannulation in predominantly venoarterial extracorporeal membrane oxygenation by intensivists. Crit Care Med. 2015;43:e595.
42. Condello I. Percutaneous right ventricular assist device, rapid employment in right ventricular failure during septic shock. Crit Care. 2020;24:674.
43. Chang HH, Chen YC, Huang CJ, Kuo CC, Wang YM, Sun CW. Optimization of extracorporeal membrane oxygenation therapy using near-infrared spectroscopy to assess changes in peripheral circulation: a pilot study. J Biophotonics. 2020;13:e202000116.

# Part VI

# Fluids and Transfusion

# Venous Congestion: Why Examine the Abdomen with Ultrasound in Critically Ill Patients?

24

A. Y. Denault, P. Rola, and W. Beaubien-Souligny

## 24.1 Introduction

Signs of venous congestion can be present in critically ill patients and their prompt recognition is essential for several key clinical elements: (a) prognostication, (b) fluid management, and (c) identifying the pathological cause. In this chapter, we will briefly review the importance of fluid overload and discuss the bedside ultrasound examination allowing detection of venous congestion using Doppler technology. We will start with a case illustrating the role of those indices in the operating room and intensive care unit (ICU).

## 24.2 Case Study

May 10th 2017 Montreal: an 84-year-old woman is scheduled for aortic, mitral valve, and tricuspid valve replacement. She has hypertension, non-insulin dependent diabetes, and chronic renal failure with an estimated glomerular filtration

A. Y. Denault (✉)
Department of Anesthesiology, Montreal Heart Institute, Université de Montréal, Montreal, QC, Canada
e-mail: andre.denault@umontreal.ca

P. Rola
Intensive Care Unit, Chief of Service, Santa Cabrini Hospital, Montreal, QC, Canada

W. Beaubien-Souligny
Division of Nephrology, Centre Hospitalier de l'Université de Montréal (CHUM), Montreal, QC, Canada

Innovation Hub, Centre de recherche du CHUM, Montreal, QC, Canada



J.-L. Vincent (ed.), *Annual Update in Intensive Care and Emergency Medicine 2023*, Annual Update in Intensive Care and Emergency Medicine,
https://doi.org/10.1007/978-3-031-23005-9_24

rate of 50 ml/min. She also has a systolic pulmonary artery pressure of 59 mmHg. Her European System for Cardiac Operative Risk Evaluation (EuroSCORE II) is 13%. The cardiopulmonary bypass (CPB) lasts 121 min. Blood losses were approximately 400 ml and she had fluid removal performed through ultrafiltration for a total of 2.2 l. Her urine output was 365 ml intraoperatively. Her final fluid balance was −166 ml (intake of 2849 ml in and output of 3015 ml). She arrived in the ICU without any vasoactive agents, receiving only insulin and propofol. She was extubated 4.7 h after admission. She did not develop any ICU delirium or atrial fibrillation and did not receive pacemaker support, blood transfusion, or intravenous albumin. She was discharged on day 2 after 50 h in the ICU. Multiple decisions during perioperative care were guided by the assessment of venous congestion indices as will be presented in the closing section of this chapter.

## 24.3 Importance of Fluid Overload

Fluid overload is epidemiologically associated with adverse outcomes in multiple settings. A systematic review and meta-analysis including 34 studies and 31,076 patients confirmed the association between fluid overload and mortality in critically ill patients [1]. Congestive organ injury may be the consequence of multiple factors including increased interstitial pressure, creating a compartment syndrome phenomenon, an increase in the diffusion distance from the blood to the tissue, as well as a reduction in the arterio-venous pressure gradient, otherwise named perfusion pressure. This can affect several organs including the brain, heart, lung, kidney, and abdomen. This relationship between fluid balance and morbidity/mortality is not linear but most likely curvilinear [2] indicating that excessive fluid restriction and excessive fluid administration will be associated with adverse outcomes. This U-shaped relationship has been observed in patients undergoing aortic valve replacement [3], as a risk factor for acute kidney injury [4] and post-op atrial arrhythmias [5]. This U-shaped relationship represents the balance between congestive organ injury and insufficient cardiac preload. It appears therefore important to identify at the bedside not only signs of hypoperfusion but also signs of venous congestion.

## 24.4 Diagnosis of Venous Congestion

The diagnosis of venous congestion can be obtained at the bedside using ultrasound. Combining two-dimensional and Doppler ultrasound, there are several portions of the venous system that can be examined in order to detect venous congestion. Those include the inferior vena cava (IVC) and venous Doppler assessment of the hepatic vein, portal, splenic, renal, and femoral veins.

### 24.4.1 Inferior Vena Cava

The IVC is relatively easy to image with ultrasound. Two-dimensional IVC characteristics, such as size and respiratory variation, have been used to estimate filling pressure and to predict intraoperative hypotension after induction [6]. However its predictive ability for fluid responsiveness is inferior to the measurement of the maximal aortic velocity in the left ventricular (LV) outflow tract [7]. Measurement of IVC characteristics in spontaneously breathing patients and those receiving mechanical ventilation also differs. There are several pitfalls [8] in the measurement of IVC, one being the effect of abdominal pressure, which reduces the dimension of the IVC and the site of measurement for the collapsibility index [9]. The cut-off for IVC size is 2.1 cm [10]. If the IVC diameter is less than 2.1 cm and collapses >50% with a sniff, this suggests a normal central venous pressure (CVP) of about 3 mmHg (range 0–5 mmHg), whereas an IVC diameter >2.1 cm that collapses <50% with a sniff suggests elevated CVP of 15 mmHg (range 10–20 mmHg). Measurement of the IVC alone is insufficient to diagnose venous congestion but dilatation and reduced respiratory variation correlate with portal vein pulsatility [11].

Some of the limitations with IVC imaging found in the current literature relate to two factors, one geometrical and one pathophysiological. The first, the traditional long axis, single diameter method of measurement unfortunately ignores the anatomical detail that the IVC, in almost all cases, does not behave in a cylindrical fashion, but rather has an elliptoid shape, with an oblique axis. Hence the antero-posterior diameter, particularly in non-plethoric IVCs, may misrepresent distension, particularly if the long axis of the ellipse is vertical (from a sonographic standpoint). In plethoric IVCs, which approach spherical proportions, this becomes less of a concern. The second issue is that the IVC is distensible, such that, chronically exposed to elevated right atrial pressures, it may reach much larger sizes (diameters up to 4.0 cm or more), and thus, in such cases, a 2.1 cm IVC may represent a lower CVP than one that had not been exposed to chronically elevated right atrial pressures. Hence, we suggest that in future studies the IVC should also be examined in the short axis to assess sphericity index and variation. This is why biplane measurement might be more precise in estimating CVP [12].

### 24.4.2 Hepatic Veins

The hepatic vein Doppler signal will be influenced by the CVP but also by the severity of pulmonary hypertension [13]. Several studies have reported on hepatic vein significance in normal adults [14] and children [15], in tricuspid regurgitation [16], in right heart dysfunction [11, 17], in the estimation of right atrial filling pressure [18], and in the ability to predict renal failure [19].

The triphasic hepatic vein Doppler signal corresponds to the CVP pressure waveform (Fig. 24.1). There is a predominant systolic velocity, a lower diastolic velocity, and an atrial reversal velocity that should be less than 50% of the systolic velocity (Fig. 24.1g). The hepatic vein Doppler signal is a very sensitive marker of right ventricular (RV) diastolic function [10]. As CVP increases and RV function deteriorates, the systolic velocity becomes smaller and reversed (Fig. 24.1h, i).

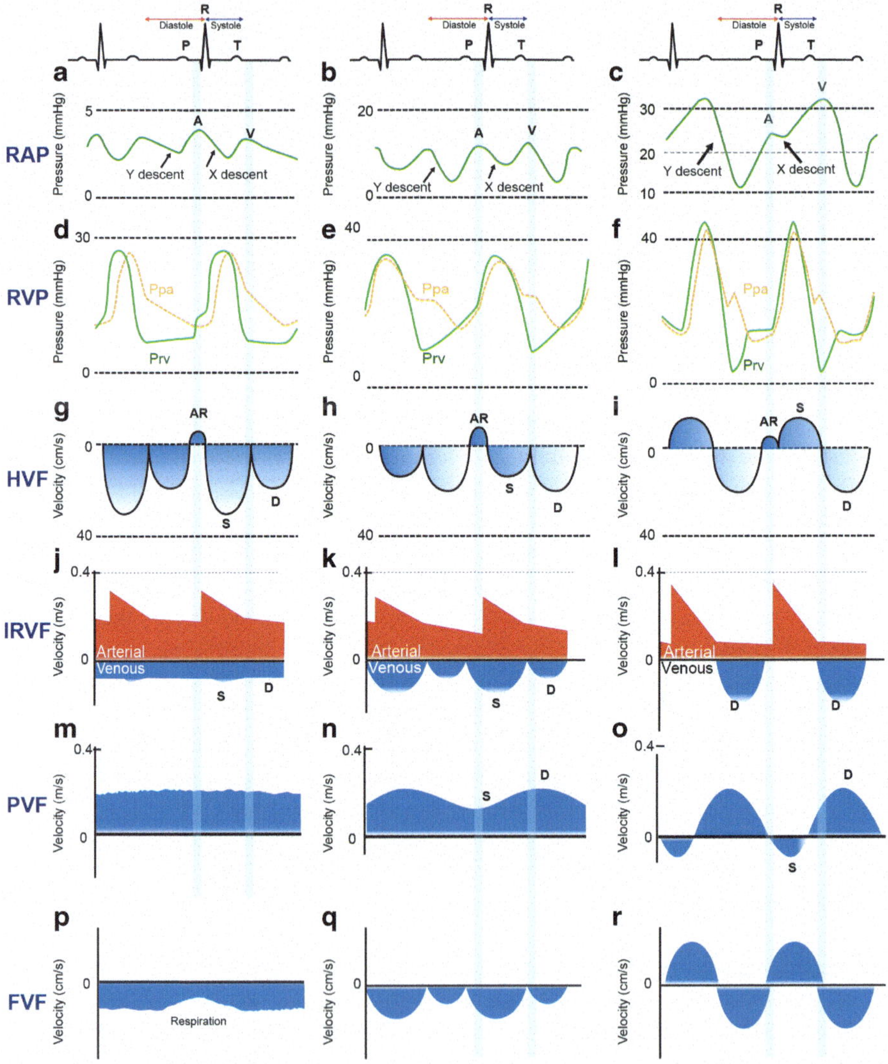


**Fig. 24.1** Correlation between right atrial pressure waveform (RAP), right ventricular pressure waveform (RVP), hepatic venous flow (HVF), interlobar renal venous flow (IRVF), portal venous flow (PVF) and femoral venous flow (FVF) with progressive right ventricular (RV) dysfunction and venous congestion in normal patients (**a**, **d**, **g**, **j**, **m**, **p**). Typical patterns are commonly observed in patients with mild (**b**, **e**, **h**, **k**, **n**, **q**) and severe (**c**, **f**, **i**, **l**, **o**, **r**) RV dysfunction. *AR* atrial reversal Doppler flow velocity, *D* diastolic Doppler flow velocity, *Ppa* pulmonary artery pressure, *Prv* right ventricular pressure, *S* systolic Doppler flow velocity. (Adapted from [20] with permission)

The aspect of the hepatic veins can also orient toward the mechanisms of hemodynamic instability. Normal or elevated hepatic vein Doppler velocities are suggestive of non-cardiac etiology such as hemorrhagic or vasodilatory shock [21]. Abnormal velocities with a reduced or reversed systolic component are suggestive of RV dysfunction. In a shock state, the absence of a velocity or a blunted signal may indicate an obstruction to venous return, such as IVC stenosis [22]. Abnormal hepatic vein velocities after cardiac surgery are very frequent due to the presence of abnormal RV diastolic function in up to 48% of cases [23]. However, the use of hepatic vein Doppler as an indicator of venous congestion is not as specific as the detection of abnormal portal vein pulsatility [11]. The reported interobserver agreement for hepatic vein grading as normal or abnormal is high, yielding a Kappa value of 0.95 [24].

### 24.4.3 Renal Veins

Renal venous Doppler was originally described for its diagnostic role in obstructive uropathy and in diabetes. An article by Iida et al in 2016 brought attention to the role of venous Doppler interrogation in heart failure [25]. In this cohort study, which included 217 patients with heart failure, abnormal renal venous Doppler signals were independently associated with endpoints that included death from cardiovascular disease and unplanned hospitalization for heart failure. Subsequently, those Doppler signals were demonstrated to be very sensitive in detecting venous congestion and resistance to diuretics [26]. Beaubien-Souligny et al. performed a retrospective and a prospective study in cardiac surgical patients [17]. They demonstrated that abnormal renal venous patterns were associated with the development of acute kidney injury in cardiac surgery. Several other authors made similar observations in various perioperative and ICU populations [27, 28].

A normal renal venous Doppler signal is continuous. An abnormal signal will become pulsatile. The very severe pattern will show a signal only present in diastole [29] (Fig. 24.1j–l). The success rate for obtaining a signal is 94.8% for the right kidney, and 85.4% for the left kidney in cardiac surgery patients [17], but may be less in general ICU patients [19]. The interobserver agreement was reported to be 87–94% in one study [17].

### 24.4.4 Portal Veins

The association between abnormal portal pulsatility and RV dysfunction was reported in 1990 by Abu-Yousef et al. [30]. Subsequently several authors reported abnormal portal vein patterns in congestive heart failure, tricuspid regurgitation, RV dysfunction [11], cardiac surgery [31], ICU patients [19], patients with elevated liver enzymes [32], pericarditis, [33] hyponatremia [34], renal failure [17], and post-cardiac surgical delirium [35]. Assessment of fluid responsiveness using portal pulsatility was recently reported using magnetic resonance imaging (MRI) [36]. Fluid unresponsiveness is associated with the appearance of portal pulsatility.

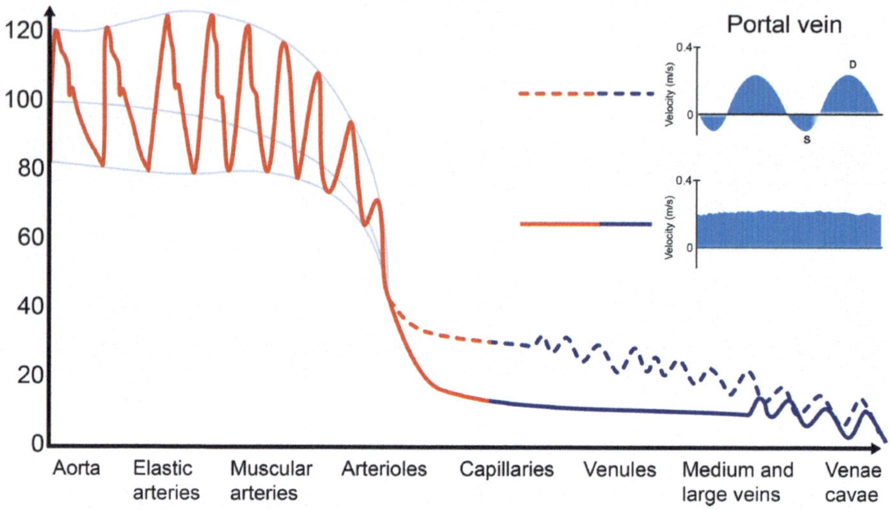


**Fig. 24.2** Doppler assessment of the circulatory system. Normal right-sided filling pressure (continuous line) and elevated right-sided filling pressure (dotted line). In the latter, venous pulsatility will be present in venules and in medium and large veins. This explains why a normal continuous portal vein Doppler signal becomes pulsatile when right-sided filling pressure is elevated

At a normal or low CVP, the waveform pattern of venous flow is not visible far from the right atrium, as venous wall compliance buffers any pulsatility. As CVP increases and the venous reservoir compliance is reduced, the pulsatility of the waveform is transferred to the periphery (Fig. 24.2). Therefore, the presence of portal pulsatility indicates significant CVP elevation, and RV dysfunction with its potential consequence not only on the liver but also on the gut leading to a cardio-intestinal syndrome with bowel edema and bacterial translocation [37]. Indeed, reduction of endotoxemia with diuretics in heart failure patients has been reported [38]. The elevated CVP will be transmitted to the kidney leading to a cardiorenal syndrome in association with portal pulsatility [39]. In addition elevated filling pressure will reach the brain leading to a cardio-cerebral syndrome [35] (Fig. 24.3). Major complications after cardiac surgery have been reported in patients with intra-operative portal pulsatility in single-center studies [11, 40] and in an international multicenter cohort study [41]. The success rate to obtain a portal vein signal with surface ultrasound is close to 99% [11].

A normal portal venous Doppler signal is monophasic (Fig. 24.1m). As the CVP increases, pulsatility appears (Fig. 24.1n, o). A portal pulsatility (maximal velocity – minimal velocity) fraction of 50% or more (PPF50) is considered pathologic and has been used as a threshold in several studies [11, 41]. Interobserver agreement and variability for renal venous flow patterns were reported [17]. The agreement ranges from 91.3 to 100% with a Kappa from 0.738 to 0.868.

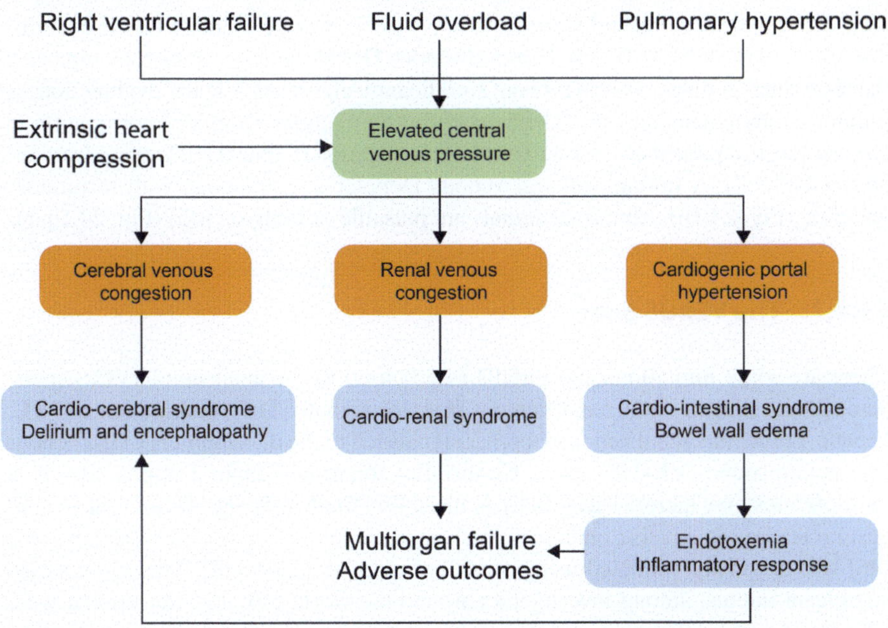


**Fig. 24.3** The combination of right ventricular failure, fluid overload, and pulmonary hypertension will lead to elevated central venous pressure (CVP). Extrinsic cardiac compression, such as tension pneumothorax, pericardial tamponade, or abdominal compartment syndrome, can also increase CVP. The consequence will be cerebral, renal, and cardiogenic portal venous congestion. The latter will lead to gut edema, bacterial translocation, and an inflammatory reaction through the release of cytokines that will cross the blood-brain barrier leading to delirium and encephalopathy. If portal hypertension and renal venous congestion are uncorrected, adverse outcomes and multisystem organ failure will occur. Portal pulsatility, renal venous pulsatility, and asterixis [35] are ultrasound and clinical signs of venous congestion

### 24.4.5 Splenic Veins

Only a few studies have explored the role of splenic vein Doppler interrogation [31], however, in our experience splenic veins behave similarly to the portal vein. They represent an alternative to the portal vein, particularly in very obese patients with liver steatosis. The aspect of the splenic venous Doppler is similar to that of the portal vein.

### 24.4.6 Femoral Veins

Pulsatile venous Doppler signals in the lower extremity or the femoral vein were reported in 1996 [42]. Their presence indicates elevated CVP. The mechanism is the same as for the other venous signals, such as the pulsatile varicose veins described in

1962 [43] and, more recently, pulsatile popliteal veins in patients with coronavirus disease 2019 (COVID-19) [44]. Femoral venous Doppler interrogation may represent the fastest and simplest way to rule out significantly elevated CVP, RV dysfunction, or pulmonary hypertension [45]. The role of femoral venous Doppler interrogation in cardiac surgical patients is currently under investigation (ClinicalTrials.gov Identifier: NCT05038267). A normal femoral venous Doppler is continuous with respiratory variation (Fig. 24.1p). Abnormal signals are pulsatile or biphasic [45] (Fig. 24.1q, r).

### 24.4.7 The VExUS Score

There are some limitations and pitfalls (see below) in the analysis of IVC, hepatic vein, portal, splenic, and renal venous Doppler signals. The combination of IVC, hepatic, portal, and renal venous Doppler signals led to the development of the venous excess ultrasound (VExUS) score. Confirming abnormal venous Doppler signals at multiple sites may increase specificity in the ability to identify significant venous congestion leading to adverse outcomes, such as acute kidney injury. The VExUS score [46] was originally validated using a cardiac surgical cohort [17]. This score raised significant interest among investigators around the world [46] and educational websites have been developed in order to teach how to use it [47]. In a patient with a severe VExUS grade, the IVC diameter will be more than 2 cm, and there will be at least two of the following: an hepatic vein with systolic reversal, a pulsatile portal vein with a PPF ≥50%, and the intrarenal venous Doppler signal only present in diastole. In this derivation cohort, this combination, when detected at ICU admission, had high specificity (96%) for the subsequent development of acute kidney injury [46].

### 24.4.8 Surface Ultrasound or Transesophageal Echocardiography

The acquisition of venous Doppler signals can be obtained with transthoracic and curvilinear probes. We use linear probes for femoral venous Doppler interrogation [45]. Venous Doppler signals can also be obtained using abdominal transesophageal echocardiography (TEE) or transgastric abdominal ultrasound (TGAUS). The success rates for portal venous Doppler interrogation using TGAUS are 94.0% and 95.7% before and after CPB [11, 31]. Interrogation of the retropancreatic and intrasplenic vein increased the success rate up to 99.2% before CPB and 94.9% after CPB in a multicenter cohort study [41]. Interrogation of the left renal vein using TGAUS can also be obtained [48]. Therefore hepatic, renal, portal, and splenic signals can be obtained intraoperatively with TGAUS.

## 24.5 Venous Congestion and RV Dysfunction

As RV dysfunction develops, signs of venous congestion will appear. Using RV and CVP pressure waveform (Fig. 24.1a–f), we and others have previously established the relationship between RV function and all the venous patterns that have been presented [29].

## 24.6 The Importance of Examining the Abdomen of Critically Ill Patients

Bedside ultrasound in the ICU initially focused on cardiac ultrasound and then lung ultrasound. However, there is significant interest in the routine examination of the abdomen not only to assess the degree of venous congestion but to diagnose other critical conditions such as free fluid, abdominal aortic aneurysm, air in the liver or bowel wall, and distended or full stomach to name a few. In order, however, to teach abdominal ultrasound, new techniques have been developed using augmented reality which facilitates the understanding of abdominal anatomy.

## 24.7 Limitations and Pitfalls of Venous Congestion Indices

Every element used in the evaluation of venous congestion has its own limitations. For example, the IVC will be enlarged in normal athletes [49], portal pulsatility can be observed in thin and young individuals [50], renal venous Doppler may be abnormal in pregnant women, and all venous Doppler measures will be altered in patients with abdominal compartment syndrome. It is therefore important not to treat an ultrasound image but a patient, considering other important data such as the history, physical examination, laboratory data, and other imaging modalities. Abnormal signs of venous congestion indicate elevated CVP, however they do not provide the etiology of this abnormal elevation of the right-sided structure. For example, pre or post-capillary hypertension will be treated differently but can lead to the same abnormal venous Doppler signals. Cardiac and lung ultrasound will be required in such cases to precisely determine the mechanism and subsequently the treatment. Finally, the association between abnormal venous Doppler signal and outcome is supported by an increasing number of studies [11, 17, 27, 41]. The impact and outcome of correcting those signals are currently being evaluated but their value and benefit remain to be determined.

## 24.8 Back to the Case Study

The elderly lady was monitored using a dual radial and femoral artery catheter [51], pulmonary artery catheter, brain monitoring using a processed electroencephalogram, brain oximetry, and TEE. TGAUS was performed which showed a PPF50. At this point, the patient was given inhaled prostacyclin and inhaled milrinone before

CPB. Weaning from CPB was easy and required no vasoactive agents. Upon arrival on the ICU, the intensivist examined the patient and observed PPF50 for which diuretics were initiated immediately. The next day, the creatinine increased but there was still a PPF50. The intensivist doubled the diuretic dosage and the creatinine returned to normal the following day. No intravenous fluids or blood were administered in the ICU. This case of a very high-risk patient illustrates the intra- and post-operative values of venous congestion indices, the impact on management, and the importance of abdominal examination of the critically ill patient at the bedside by the intensivist.

## 24.9 Conclusion

Venous congestion indices are an essential part of the evaluation of the critically ill patient, as it is necessary for the physicians managing such patients to have a hemodynamic approach that is not based solely on forward flow. It has been established that elevated levels of venous congestion are associated with organ dysfunction. As part of a holistic point-of-care ultrasound (POCUS) approach, this highlights the importance of bedside ultrasound examination of the abdomen in critically ill patients.

## References

1. Messmer AS, Zingg C, Muller M, Gerber JL, Schefold JC, Pfortmueller CA. Fluid overload and mortality in adult critical care patients—a systematic review and meta-analysis of observational studies. Crit Care Med. 2020;48:1862–70.
2. Shin CH, Long DR, McLean D, et al. Effects of intraoperative fluid management on postoperative outcomes: a hospital registry study. Ann Surg. 2018;267:1084–92.
3. Smith BB, Mauermann WJ, Yalamuri SM, et al. Intraoperative fluid balance and perioperative outcomes after aortic valve surgery. Ann Thorac Surg. 2020;110:1286–93.
4. Chen X, Xu J, Li Y, et al. The effect of postoperative fluid balance on the occurrence and progression of acute kidney injury after cardiac surgery. J Cardiothorac Vasc Anesth. 2021;35:2700–6.
5. Minami K, Kabata D, Kakuta T, et al. U-shaped association between intraoperative net fluid balance and risk of postoperative recurrent atrial tachyarrhythmia among patients undergoing the cryo-maze procedure: an observational study. J Cardiothorac Vasc Anesth. 2021;35:2392–6.
6. Zhang J, Critchley LA. Inferior vena cava ultrasonography before general anesthesia can predict hypotension after induction. Anesthesiology. 2016;124:580–9.
7. Vignon P, Repesse X, Begot EL, et al. Comparison of echocardiographic indices used to predict fluid responsiveness in ventilated patients. Am J Respir Crit Care Med. 2017;195:1022–32.
8. Via G, Tavazzi G, Price S. Ten situations where inferior vena cava ultrasound may fail to accurately predict fluid responsiveness: a physiologically based point of view. Intensive Care Med. 2016;42:1164–7.
9. Caplan M, Durand A, Bortolotti P, et al. Measurement site of inferior vena cava diameter affects the accuracy with which fluid responsiveness can be predicted in spontaneously breathing patients: a post hoc analysis of two prospective cohorts. Ann Intensive Care. 2020;10:168.
10. Rudski LG, Lai WW, Afilalo J, et al. Guidelines for the echocardiographic assessment of the right heart in adults: a report from the American Society of Echocardiography endorsed by the European Association of Echocardiography, a registered branch of the European Society of Cardiology, and the Canadian Society of Echocardiography. J Am Soc Echocardiogr. 2010;23:685–713; quiz 786–8.

11. Eljaiek R, Cavayas YA, Rodrigue E, et al. High postoperative portal venous flow pulsatility indicates right ventricular dysfunction and predicts complications in cardiac surgery patients. Br J Anaesth. 2019;122:206–14.
12. Huguet R, Fard D, d'Humieres T, et al. Three-dimensional inferior vena cava for assessing central venous pressure in patients with cardiogenic shock. J Am Soc Echocardiogr. 2018;31:1034–43.
13. Zhang A, Himura Y, Kumada T, et al. The characteristics of hepatic venous flow velocity pattern in patients with pulmonary hypertension by pulsed Doppler echocardiography. Jpn Circ J. 1992;56:317–24.
14. Abu-Yousef MM. Normal and respiratory variations of the hepatic and portal venous duplex Doppler waveforms with simultaneous electrocardiographic correlation. J Ultrasound Med. 1992;11:263–8.
15. Patel SG, Woolman P, Li L, Craft M, Danford DA, Kutty S. Relation of right atrial volume, systemic venous dimensions, and flow patterns to right atrial pressure in infants and children. Am J Cardiol. 2017;119:1473–8.
16. Sakai K, Nakamura K, Satomi G, Kondo M, Hirosawa K. Evaluation of tricuspid regurgitation by blood flow pattern in the hepatic vein using pulsed Doppler technique. Am Heart J. 1984;108:516–23.
17. Beaubien-Souligny W, Benkreira A, Robillard P, et al. Alterations in portal vein flow and intrarenal venous flow are associated with acute kidney injury after cardiac surgery: a prospective observational cohort study. J Am Heart Assoc. 2018;7:e009961.
18. Nagueh SF, Kopelen HA, Zoghbi WA. Relation of mean right atrial pressure to echocardiographic and Doppler parameters of right atrial and right ventricular function. Circulation. 1996;93:1160–9.
19. Spiegel R, Teeter W, Sullivan S, et al. The use of venous Doppler to predict adverse kidney events in a general ICU cohort. Crit Care. 2020;24:615.
20. Couture EJ, Gronlykke L, Denault AY. New developments in the understanding of right ventricular function in acute care. Curr Opin Crit Care. 2022;28:331–9.
21. Vegas A, Denault A, Royse C. A bedside clinical and ultrasound-based approach to hemodynamic instability—part II: bedside ultrasound in hemodynamic shock: continuing professional development. Can J Anesth. 2014;61:1008–27.
22. Hulin J, Aslanian P, Desjardins G, Belaidi M, Denault A. The critical importance of hepatic venous blood flow Doppler assessment for patients in shock. A A Case Rep. 2016;6:114–20.
23. Gronlykke L, Couture EJ, Haddad F, et al. Preliminary experience using diastolic right ventricular pressure gradient monitoring in cardiac surgery. J Cardiothorac Vasc Anesth. 2020;34:2116–25.
24. Carricart M, Denault AY, Couture P, et al. Incidence and significance of abnormal hepatic venous Doppler flow velocities before cardiac surgery. J Cardiothorac Vasc Anesth. 2005;19:751–8.
25. Iida N, Seo Y, Sai S, et al. Clinical implications of intrarenal hemodynamic evaluation by Doppler ultrasonography in heart failure. JACC Heart Fail. 2016;4:674–82.
26. Nijst P, Martens P, Dupont M, Tang WHW, Mullens W. Intrarenal flow alterations during transition from euvolemia to intravascular volume expansion in heart failure patients. JACC Heart Fail. 2017;5:672–81.
27. Husain-Syed F, Birk HW, Ronco C, et al. Doppler-derived renal venous stasis index in the prognosis of right heart failure. J Am Heart Assoc. 2019;8:e013584.
28. Yoshihisa A, Watanabe K, Sato Y, et al. Intrarenal Doppler ultrasonography reflects hemodynamics and predicts prognosis in patients with heart failure. Sci Rep. 2020;10:22257.
29. Tang WH, Kitai T. Intrarenal venous flow: a window into the congestive kidney failure phenotype of heart failure? JACC Heart Fail. 2016;4:683–6.
30. Abu-Yousef MM, Milam SG, Farner RM. Pulsatile portal vein flow: a sign of tricuspid regurgitation on duplex Doppler sonography. Am J Roentgenol. 1990;155:785–8.
31. Denault AY, Beaubien-Souligny W, Elmi-Sarabi M, et al. Clinical significance of portal hypertension diagnosed with bedside ultrasound after cardiac surgery. Anesth Analg. 2017;124:1109–15.

32. Styczynski G, Milewska A, Marczewska M, et al. Echocardiographic correlates of abnormal liver tests in patients with exacerbation of chronic heart failure. J Am Soc Echocardiogr. 2016;29:132–9.
33. Gonzalez C, Chamberland ME, Aldred MP, et al. Constrictive pericarditis: portal, splenic, and femoral venous Doppler pulsatility: a case series. Can J Anesth. 2022;69:119–28.
34. Singh G, Rachoin JS, Chien C, Patel S. The use of portal vein pulsatility to differentiate hypervolemic and hypovolemic hyponatremia. Case Rep Crit Care. 2019;2019:9591823.
35. Benkreira A, Beaubien-Souligny W, Mailhot T, et al. Portal hypertension is associated with congestive encephalopathy and delirium after cardiac surgery. Can J Cardiol. 2019;35:1134–41.
36. Abou-Arab O, Beyls C, Moussa MD, et al. Portal vein pulsatility index as a potential risk of venous congestion assessed by magnetic resonance imaging: a prospective study on healthy volunteers. Front Physiol. 2022;13:811286.
37. Sundaram V, Fang JC. Gastrointestinal and liver issues in heart failure. Circulation. 2016;133:1696–703.
38. Niebauer J, Volk HD, Kemp M, et al. Endotoxin and immune activation in chronic heart failure: a prospective cohort study. Lancet. 1999;353:1838–42.
39. Beaubien-Souligny W, Denault A, Robillard P, Desjardins G. The role of point-of-care ultrasound monitoring in cardiac surgical patients with acute kidney injury. J Cardiothorac Vasc Anesth. 2019;33:2781–96.
40. Singh NG, Kumar KN, Nagaraja PS, Manjunatha N. Portal venous pulsatility fraction, a novel transesophageal echocardiographic marker for right ventricular dysfunction in cardiac surgical patients. Ann Card Anaesth. 2020;23:39–42.
41. Denault A, Couture EJ, De Medicis É, et al. Portal vein Doppler in high-risk cardiac surgery patients: a multicenter prospective cohort study. Crit Care. 2022;26:P025. (abst)
42. Abu-Yousef MM, Kakish ME, Mufid M. Pulsatile venous Doppler flow in lower limbs: highly indicative of elevated right atrium pressure. AJR Am J Roentgenol. 1996;167:977–80.
43. Brickner PW, Scudder WT, Weinrib M. Pulsating varicose veins in functional tricuspid insufficiency. Case report and venous pressure tracing. Circulation. 1962;25:126–9.
44. Malinovska A, Arslani K, Zellweger N, et al. Femoral and popliteal venous Doppler during prone and supine position in COVID-19 patients: a potential diagnostic tool to detect abnormal right ventricular function. Can J Anesth. 2021;68:737–9.
45. Denault AY, Aldred MP, Hammoud A, et al. Doppler interrogation of the femoral vein in the critically ill patient: the fastest potential acoustic window to diagnose right ventricular dysfunction? Crit Care Explor. 2020;2:e0209.
46. Beaubien-Souligny W, Rola P, Haycock K, et al. Quantifying systemic congestion with Point-Of-Care ultrasound: development of the venous excess ultrasound grading system. Ultrasound J. 2020;12:16.
47. Pocus 101. VExUS ultrasound score—fluid overload and venous congestion assessment. Available at: https://www.pocus101.com/vexus-ultrasound-score-fluid-overload-and-venous-congestion-assessment/. Accessed 3 Nov 2022
48. Denault AY, Roberts M, Cios T, et al. Transgastric abdominal ultrasonography in anesthesia and critical care: review and proposed approach. Anesth Analg. 2021;133:630–47.
49. Hedman K, Nylander E, Henriksson J, Bjarnegard N, Brudin L, Tamas E. Echocardiographic characterization of the inferior vena cava in trained and untrained females. Ultrasound Med Biol. 2016;42:2794–802.
50. Gallix BP, Taourel P, Dauzat M, Bruel JM, Lafortune M. Flow pulsatility in the portal venous system: a study of Doppler sonography in healthy adults. AJR Am J Roentgenol. 1997;169:141–4.
51. Bouchard-Dechene V, Kontar L, Couture P, et al. Radial-to-femoral pressure gradient quantification in cardiac surgery. JTCVS Open. 2021;8:446–60.

# The Most Important Questions in the Current Practice of Transfusion of Critically Bleeding Patients

25

A. W. Flint, J. Winearls, and M. C. Reade

## 25.1 Introduction

Bleeding in the context of critical illness must be distinguished from critical (or major) bleeding, although the two circumstances are often conflated. Recent comprehensive guidelines exist for both circumstances. This narrative review

A. W. Flint
Department of Intensive Care Medicine, Royal Brisbane and Women's Hospital, Herston, QLD, Australia

Medical School, University of Queensland, Brisbane, QLD, Australia

Royal Australian Navy, Canberra, ACT, Australia

Transfusion Research Unit, Department of Epidemiology and Preventive Medicine, Monash University, Melbourne, VIC, Australia

The Australian and New Zealand Intensive Care Research Centre (ANZIC-RC), School of Public Health and Preventive Medicine, Monash University, Melbourne, VIC, Australia

J. Winearls
Medical School, University of Queensland, Brisbane, QLD, Australia

Intensive Care Unit, Gold Coast University Hospital, Southport, QLD, Australia

M. C. Reade (✉)
Department of Intensive Care Medicine, Royal Brisbane and Women's Hospital, Herston, QLD, Australia

Medical School, University of Queensland, Brisbane, QLD, Australia

Transfusion Research Unit, Department of Epidemiology and Preventive Medicine, Monash University, Melbourne, VIC, Australia

The Australian and New Zealand Intensive Care Research Centre (ANZIC-RC), School of Public Health and Preventive Medicine, Monash University, Melbourne, VIC, Australia

Joint Health Command, Australian Defence Force, Canberra, ACT, Australia
e-mail: m.reade@uq.edu.au



J.-L. Vincent (ed.), *Annual Update in Intensive Care and Emergency Medicine 2023*, Annual Update in Intensive Care and Emergency Medicine,
https://doi.org/10.1007/978-3-031-23005-9_25

will concentrate exclusively on major bleeding. Research programs ranging from preclinical studies to multicenter randomized trials with patient-centered outcomes are underway to address identified knowledge gaps. However, some questions that are highly relevant to clinicians—e.g. identifying when the benefit of transfusion (of red blood cells [RBCs], clotting factors, or platelets) outweighs the risk, or when to change from a pro- to an anti-thrombotic strategy, are unlikely to be answered using currently available technology. Such questions are likely to require cost-effective, rapid and repeatable diagnostic tests for individual patients, validated in studies that pair testing with interventions. Further, many current trial designs, which aim to observe the effect of an intervention applied in the first few hours of a patient's treatment through the subsequent 'noise' of the next 90 days or 6 months when all-cause mortality is assessed, seem unlikely to succeed. Personalizing interventions and seeking meaningful outcomes plausibly amenable to improvement are the two major challenges in this field. Rather than explore many promising experimental tests and therapies, in this chapter we examine six questions that clinicians must answer in current routine practice. What evidence exists will be presented, highlighting reasons for uncertainty. Trials currently underway will be critiqued, followed by discussion of what innovations in study design might lead to even better guidance for clinicians.

## 25.2 Therapeutic Goals in Treating Major Hemorrhage

Goals in the treatment of major hemorrhage include:

- Maintaining or restoring sufficient circulating blood volume to prevent organ failure and preserve life. A 1994 trial [1] of 598 adults with penetrating torso trauma that found an 8% absolute risk reduction in hospital mortality associated with giving no pre-hospital fluid compared to standard crystalloid resuscitation demonstrated that, at least briefly, even substantial hypovolemia can be tolerated. However, the optimal duration of hypovolemia is increasingly questioned, as shown in the elegant preclinical "hybrid resuscitation" experiments of Doran et al. [2] that found fluid resuscitation to normotension after 60 min superior to ongoing hypovolemic hypotension.
- Maintaining or restoring the integrity of the endothelial glycocalyx, which in health regulates vascular permeability and prevents thrombomodulin exposure to the circulation. In trauma and perhaps other forms of major hemorrhage the glycocalyx degrades, most likely accentuated by the choice of crystalloid over plasma as a resuscitation fluid [3].
- Avoiding thrombomodulin/activated protein C-modulated acute traumatic coagulopathy [4].

Achieving these goals requires intravenous fluid—but clinicians must decide how much of what type.

## 25.3 Question 1: Fibrinogen Concentrate vs. Cryoprecipitate?

Fibrinogen plays a critical role in maintaining effective hemostasis in major hemorrhage. Hypofibrinogenemia is associated with increased morbidity and mortality [5], and early fibrinogen replacement may assist in hemorrhage control, improve coagulopathy, and reduce transfusion requirements. Published guidelines suggest fibrinogen replacement should occur when plasma fibrinogen levels fall to <1.5–2 g/l or there are thromboelastometric signs of fibrinogen deficiency [6].

Fibrinogen can be replaced with cryoprecipitate or fibrinogen concentrate, each with advantages and disadvantages. The use of cryoprecipitate or fibrinogen concentrate for fibrinogen replacement remains one of the most hotly debated topics in major hemorrhage resuscitation with no Level 1 evidence to support one above the other.

Fibrinogen concentrate has several theoretical advantages, including standardized dose, viral inactivation, no requirement for ABO compatibility matching, long shelf-life, ease of transport, and rapidity of reconstitution and administration. These advantages are particularly attractive for use in austere medical environments and in countries with dispersed populations where maintaining stocks of allogenic blood products is difficult.

Several pilot trials have investigated the feasibility of rapidly administering fibrinogen concentrate in the trauma patient with major hemorrhage. The Canadian Fibrinogen In the Initial Resuscitation of Severe Trauma (FiiRST) trial reported early fibrinogen concentrate administration was feasible and increased plasma fibrinogen levels during traumatic hemorrhage compared to placebo [7]. The Efficacy of pre-hospital administration of Fibrinogen concentrate In Trauma patients bleeding or presumed to bleed (FlinTIC) trial demonstrated the feasibility of pre-hospital administration of fibrinogen concentrate and increased clot stability compared to placebo in trauma patients [8]. In contrast, the UK Early Fibrinogen concentrate therapy for major hemorrhage In Trauma (E-FIT) 1 trial reported that the administration of fibrinogen concentrate within 45 min of hospital admission was not feasible [9]. The Fibrinogen Early In Severe Trauma (FEISTY) compared time to administration of fibrinogen concentrate and cryoprecipitate in bleeding trauma patients with hypofibrinogenaemia, demonstrating fibrinogen concentrate could be administered significantly more quickly than cryoprecipitate and that both products resulted in appropriate increments in fibrinogen levels [10]. The CRYOSTAT 1 trial reported that it was feasible to use cryoprecipitate empirically as part of a fixed ratio major hemorrhage protocol in traumatic hemorrhage and maintain normal fibrinogen levels [11]. The results of CRYOSTAT 2 (ISRCTN 4998314) are eagerly awaited. The only large scale randomized controlled trial (RCT) comparing cryoprecipitate to fibrinogen concentrate is the Effect of Fibrinogen Concentrate vs. Cryoprecipitate on Blood Component Transfusion After Cardiac Surgery (FIBRES) trial in bleeding post-cardiac surgical patients with hypofibrinogenemia, which found fibrinogen concentrate was non-inferior to cryoprecipitate in terms of number of blood components transfused [12]. FEISTY II (ClinicalTrials.gov Identifier: NCT05449834), a phase III, multicenter RCT comparing fibrinogen concentrate to cryoprecipitate in bleeding trauma patients, started recruiting at the end of 2022.

Although time to administration of fibrinogen replacement in major hemorrhage may be important, it may be just as crucial to form a robust clot. The time to administration advantage of fibrinogen concentrate compared to cryoprecipitate may be offset by the additional coagulation factors present in cryoprecipitate (factor VIII, von Willebrand factor, factor XIII, fibronectin, antithrombin, and alpha-2 antiplasmin). These additional factors might play a significant role in balancing hemostasis and potentially mitigating hyperfibrinolysis: cryoprecipitate achieves a more rapid and greater thrombin-generating capacity, forms a different fibrinogen clot structure to fibrinogen concentrate, and has greater resistance to clot lysis (Fig. 25.1) [13]. Whether these hemostatic effects translate to differences in clinical outcomes is unknown.

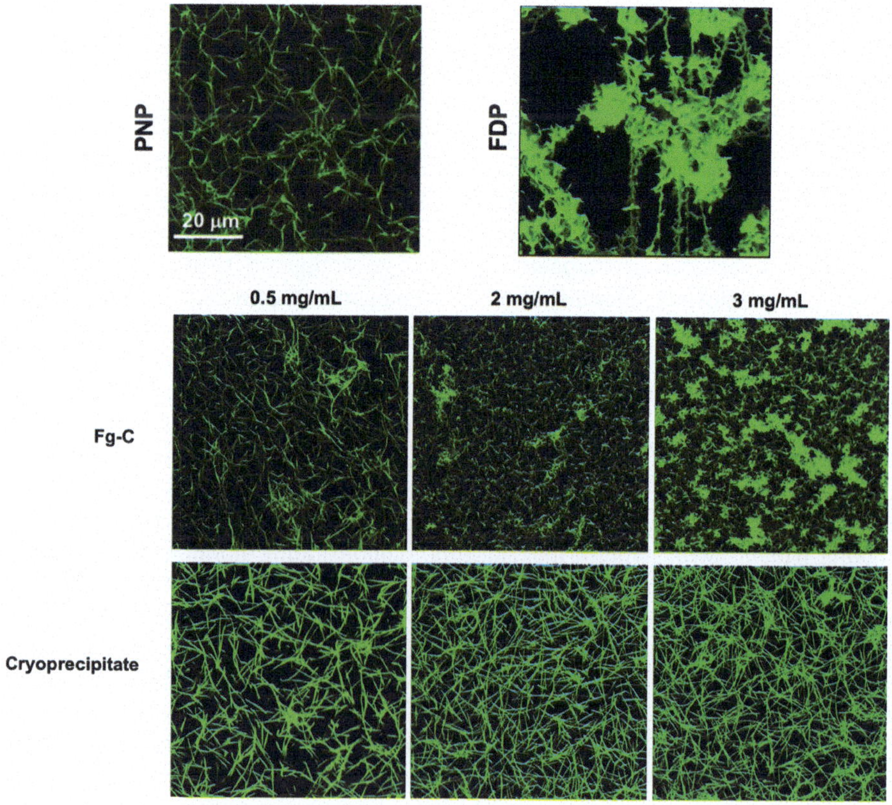


**Fig. 25.1** The fibrin networks of thrombi formed from cryoprecipitate are more homogeneous than those formed from fibrinogen concentrate. Clots were formed from 30% pooled normal plasma (PNP) or freeze-dried plasma (FDP) and spiked with 0.5, 2, or 3 mg/ml cryoprecipitate or fibrinogen concentrate (Fg-C). Clots were imaged using a ×63 1.4 oil immersion objective and Zeiss 710 laser scanning confocal microscope. Representative image of $n = 3$. (Reproduced from [13] using a Creative Commons Attribution (CC BY) license)

In addition to the coagulation factor differences between cryoprecipitate and fibrinogen concentrate it is also worth highlighting that fibrinogen concentrates from different manufacturing processes differ in composition [14]. In addition to fibrinogen, the various fibrinogen concentrates contain differing quantities of other coagulation factors. Whether this results in differing hemostatic effects between the products is unknown.

Large scale trials with patient-centered outcomes performed in conjunction with quality mechanistic studies are urgently required to elucidate the optimum form of fibrinogen replacement in patients with major hemorrhage.

## 25.4 Question 2: Early Empiric Fibrinogen, Prothrombin Complex Concentrate, and Other Coagulation Factors (Usually in Combination with Crystalloid for Volume) vs. Fresh-Frozen Plasma?

There is ongoing debate regarding the use of a predominantly factor-based resuscitation strategy (often guided by viscoelastic hemostatic assays) vs. an empiric fixed ratio blood component strategy. There are staunch proponents for each but no Level 1 evidence to support one over the other.

A number of studies in trauma, obstetrics, and cardiac surgery have reported positive outcomes with a factor-based strategy but these have not been replicated in well-designed large scale RCTs.

In two RCTs in obstetric patients, neither empiric nor guided fibrinogen concentrate administration improved patient outcomes [15, 16]. In cardiac surgery, two RCTs failed to demonstrate patient benefit with an early fibrinogen concentrate resuscitation strategy [17, 18]. A recently published RCT reported reduced transfusion requirements in cardiac surgical patients receiving prothrombin complex concentrate (PCC) compared to plasma [19]. Trauma patients are the most extensively studied. Observational studies report improved patient outcomes with a factor-based resuscitation strategy [20]. A small single-center RCT that was terminated early reported superiority of a factor-based strategy compared to plasma in terms of transfusion requirements [21]. There is increasing interest in empiric PCC in trauma hemorrhage, but this is not supported by quality evidence. The currently recruiting FiiRST-2 trial is a large multicenter RCT comparing empiric fibrinogen concentrate and PCC to a standard plasma-based major hemorrhage protocol in bleeding trauma patients [22]. Although the primary outcome of cumulative blood product transfusion volumes is not truly patient centered, this trial will certainly further the evidence base.

In the absence of high-quality evidence supporting a factor-based strategy it could be argued that 'deconstructing' blood components to factor concentrates is not warranted. However, it could also be argued that an initial factor-based strategy should be utilized when the rapid availability of blood components is not feasible—for example in the austere pre-hospital environment or when rapid replacement of coagulation factors is required.

As is the case for fibrinogen replacement, large scale RCTs with patient-centered outcomes will be required to define the optimum strategy for coagulation factor replacement in patients with major hemorrhage. It might be that one strategy more than another is amenable to a personalized medicine approach. Demonstrating this will require trials simultaneously testing a diagnostic modality and the treatment it suggests is indicated.

## 25.5 Question 3: Whole Blood vs. Fractionated Blood Components?

Whole blood can be transfused in two forms:

- Fresh, meaning blood from a donor that has not been fractionated or cooled, and which is administered within 24 h of donation. There is no evidence that whole blood transfused sooner within this 24-h period confers any different clinical effect;
- After storage at 4 °C (to reduce the risk of bacterial contamination) for up to 14 days, although up to 35 days has been explored [23].

While fresh whole blood has long been assumed to be the superior product to facilitate hemostasis, there is no evidence stored whole blood is substantially inferior. For example, in whole blood stored at 4 °C [23], platelets declined as aggregation occurred over time, but aggregation activity in the remaining platelets was normal. Thrombin generation increased over time. Functional fibrinogen responses remained consistent regardless of length of storage.

Whole blood in one or both of these forms is used extensively throughout the developing world, and by many armed forces, due to lower technological requirements compared to fractionation. Anecdotal military experience during the 2001+ wars in Iraq and Afghanistan, compelling civilian case reports [24], and retrospective military cohort studies [25], have led many to advocate whole blood transfusion over component therapy, particularly in trauma. Some pre-hospital services have introduced this practice [26], as have an increasing number of civilian hospitals [27].

The most often quoted military study of whole blood transfusion is that of Spinella et al. [25]. This retrospective study reported on 354 United States (US) military trauma patients treated at Role II or III (small or large surgical) facilities in Iraq and Afghanistan, 100 of whom were transfused at least one unit of fresh whole blood. There was a survival benefit both at 24 h (96% vs. 88%, $p = 0.018$) and at 30 days (95% vs. 82%, $p = 0.02$) that translated to an odds ratio of survival (adjusted for Injury Severity Score, Glasgow Coma Scale (GCS) score (eye component) and base deficit) of 12.4 (95% CI 1.8–80, $p = 0.01$). However, there is a substantial risk of residual confounding. Patients receiving fresh whole blood had to survive long enough for the blood to be requested, collected, processed, and released for transfusion.

The military observational study of Perkins et al. [28] receives comparatively less attention. In contrast to most of the patients included in the Spinella study, all of the component-therapy patients in this analysis also received platelets. When survival of 85 patients transfused fresh whole blood was compared to that of 284 who received component therapy, the dramatic mortality difference observed by Spinella was not apparent. Indeed, the incidence of acute respiratory distress syndrome (ARDS) was higher in the fresh whole blood group (7.4% vs. 18.8%, $p = 0.002$), and there were no other differences in patient outcomes.

The first RCT of whole blood in trauma [29] was performed in a single US civilian trauma hospital. Adult patients who met trauma activation criteria and had evidence of active bleeding requiring un-crossmatched blood while in the emergency department received up to 6 units of whole blood (stored at 4 °C for up to 5 days) or 6 units of RBCs and 6 units of plasma. Both groups could receive 1 unit of apheresis platelets, as the whole blood was passed through a leukoreduction filter that removed the platelets. Outcomes were similar between the groups, but there was a trend to higher 30-day mortality (27% vs. 15%, $p = 0.16$) associated with whole blood. The authors noted several limitations: they initially failed to exclude patients with severe traumatic brain injury (TBI), leading to an imbalance in TBI patients that might have been the cause of the trend to higher mortality in the whole blood group. Moreover, many patients did not ultimately require a massive transfusion, perhaps reducing the opportunity for whole blood to be of benefit. Their protocol required blood typing in the whole blood group, introducing a 5–10 min delay compared to universal donor component therapy. Finally, the leukoreduction filter, which retained platelets, necessitated a separate platelet transfusion, arguably meaning they were in fact not transfusing 'whole blood'. The only other trial was published in 2022: the Pragmatic Pre-hospital Group O Whole Blood Early Resuscitation (PPOWER) study [30] randomized 86 trauma patients transported by air ambulance with hypotension to either 2 units of low titer leukocyte-reduced whole blood pre-hospital and up to a further 6 units in hospital, or standard pre-hospital care (up to 2 units RBC) with 1:1:1 component therapy in hospital. The primary outcome of this pilot study, 28-day mortality, was no different between trial groups.

Three systematic reviews have addressed this topic [31–33], all of which identified the poor quality of the published studies, concluding there is currently no evidence showing benefit of whole blood over component therapy. At least two more RCTs are planned or underway: (1) the Evaluation of a Transfusion Therapy using Whole Blood in the Management of Coagulopathy in Patients with Acute Traumatic Hemorrhage (T-STORHM) trial (ClinicalTrials.gov Identifier: NCT04431999), comparing up to 3 units of whole blood with the same number of component packs, with non-inferiority of the correction of coagulopathy as the primary outcome in 200 patients; and (2) the 848-patient pre-hospital Study of Whole Blood in Frontline Trauma (SWiFT) trial [34] (isrctn.com Identifier: ISRCTN23657907). Hopefully these trials will answer definitively the question of whole blood, including its cost effectiveness and impact on other aspects of blood supply. Wastage has been identified as a particularly important consideration: in its 12-month experience of a low-titer O whole blood program, a major USA trauma center reported a 42% wastage rate of whole blood units, without any demonstrable improvement in patient outcomes [35]. For now, it only seems certain that whole blood is not clinically inferior to appropriately titrated component therapy, and so logically has a role only in resource-limited environments such as pre-hospital or in hospitals with minimal laboratory facilities.

## 25.6 Question 4: Lyophilized Plasma vs. FFP?

Historically developed and used for military purposes, lyophilized or freeze-dried plasma (FDP) contains plasma components in powder form for reconstitution with sterile water. Compared to fresh-frozen plasma (FFP), which is stored at −20 °C and must be thawed prior to transfusion, FDP has the potential benefits of faster administration (within 10 min) and therefore correction of coagulopathy. FDP is stored over a range of temperatures up to 25 °C, making its use suitable for pre-hospital, remote, and military settings.

The only in-hospital trial of FDP has been the French lyophilized plasma versus FFP for the initial management of trauma-induced coagulopathy (TRAUCC) trial of 48 severe trauma patients at a single center randomized to either 4 units of FDP or 4 units of FFP [36], which found shorter time to transfusion of the first plasma unit for FDP compared to FFP (median 14 vs. 77 min). By 45 min there was also significant improvement in indicators of hemostatic activity in the FDP group (increased fibrinogen concentration, factor V and thrombin levels, and lower prothrombin time ratios), unsurprising given the measurement time (45 min) was before the median time for FFP administration. These benefits of FDP over FFP did not result in a significant reduction in all-cause in-hospital mortality (22% for FDP vs. 29% for FFP, $p = 0.56$), although the small sample size was not powered to detect mortality difference.

There have been two randomized trials of FDP in the pre-hospital setting. In the Pre-hospital Lyophilized Plasma (PREHO-PLYO) trial of FDP vs. FFP involving 134 trauma patients at risk of hemorrhagic shock and coagulopathy, the primary outcome of reduced trauma-induced coagulopathy (as indicated by international normalized ratio) did not differ between trial groups (mean difference −0.01, $p = 0.88$) [37]. While the small sample size limited subgroup analysis, there was also no difference in the incidence of massive transfusion or 30-day survival. In a larger study of 432 trauma patients with hemorrhagic shock and hypotension, the RePHILL (Resuscitation with blood products in patients with trauma-related hemorrhagic shock receiving pre-hospital care) study [38] did not find superiority of combined RBCs and FDP (1:1 FFP to RBC ratio) vs. standard care (crystalloid) for the primary composite outcome of mortality or impaired lactate clearance (64% versus 65%, adjusted risk difference 0.025%, $p = 0.996$), but intervention did lead to more RBCs (adjusted average difference 1.8, $p = 0.004$) and plasma (adjusted average difference 1.54, $p = 0.002$) being transfused.

Inability to observe benefit from pre-hospital FDP is not surprising given the conflicting evidence from the two recent trials of pre-hospital plasma transfusion in trauma. However, a *post hoc* combined analysis of these two trials found higher survival with pre-hospital plasma (hazard ratio (HR) 0.65, $p = 0.01$) after adjusting for injury severity, age, and trial cohort [39]—and pre-hospital transport time was a significant interaction term, with greater mortality in the standard care (crystalloid) group beyond 20 min (HR 2.12, p = 0.04), but not in the pre-hospital plasma group (HR 0.78, p = 0.46). This 20-min minimum threshold for potential benefit of pre-hospital plasma was not found in the RePHILL study [38], where mean time from randomization to hospital was longer than 20 min for both groups (FDP 37 vs. crystalloid 35 min), leading to further uncertainty on the benefit of FDP in pre-hospital urban settings.

Accordingly, trial evidence supporting FDP use in trauma is lacking. To justify the additional cost of FDP over FFP or standard care, future trials and economic evaluations are required to determine the settings and patients where FDP administration is beneficial.

## 25.7 Question 5: The Value of Viscoelastic Testing

The incorporation of viscoelastic hemostatic assays into the major hemorrhage protocol has gained popularity in the last few years. Despite increasing adoption of viscoelastic hemostatic assays there remains a paucity of evidence to support their routine use. The concept of thromboelastometric methods to define coagulopathy is not new and was first described in the 1950s. Two devices performing viscoelastic hemostatic assays are widely and commercially available: TEG® (Haemonetics, Braintree, MA, USA) and ROTEM® (Werfen, Barcelona, Spain); neither device is superior and market share differs geographically.

Viscoelastic hemostatic assays have potential advantages over standard laboratory tests in the management of patients with major hemorrhage in terms of detecting coagulopathy and guiding therapy. Viscoelastic hemostatic assays provide dynamic information regarding clot formation, clot strength, and clot lysis, and have a higher sensitivity for the rapid detection of coagulopathy compared to standard laboratory tests.

A number of observational studies (the majority in the cardiac surgical and trauma patient populations) have reported improved patient outcomes with the incorporation of viscoelastic hemostatic assays in the management of major hemorrhage. However, these findings have not been replicated in well-designed RCTs. The most recent systematic review only conditionally recommends the use of viscoelastic hemostatic assays to guide blood component transfusion in major hemorrhage [40].

In the trauma patient population, a single-center RCT reported significant reductions in blood component transfusion and improved survival with a viscoelastic hemostatic assay-guided major hemorrhage protocol [41]. Several trauma centers have established evidence-based viscoelastic-guided trauma major hemorrhage protocols, specifically using early parameters of clot strength, and the use of viscoelastic hemostatic assays is supported by the European Trauma Guidelines. However, the recently published Viscoelastic hemostatic assay augmented protocols for major trauma haemorrhage (ITACTIC) trial did not demonstrate a statistically significant difference in patient outcomes between a viscoelastic hemostatic assay and a standard laboratory test augmented major hemorrhage protocol [42].

Whilst evidence of impact on mortality is currently equivocal, it is apparent that viscoelastic hemostatic assays can be used to rapidly and reliably identify coagulopathic bleeding patients [40]. To what extent abnormalities in the coagulation system detected by viscoelastic hemostatic assays can be used to guide coagulation therapy as part of a major hemorrhage protocol remains to be elucidated. However, it would seem logical to only treat patients in whom coagulopathy is contributing to ongoing hemorrhage.

Viscoelastic hemostatic assays are extremely sensitive at identifying fibrinogen deficiency and potentially have significant value in guiding fibrinogen replacement [10]. However, commonly-used viscoelastic hemostatic assays are not as sensitive in identifying platelet deficit or dysfunction and there is limited evidence to support the use of these assays to guide platelet transfusion [43].

Several trials have evaluated unguided coagulation factor replacement and failed to demonstrate benefit. This suggests it is difficult to predict those patients who will benefit from coagulation factor replacement based on clinical features alone, and there is likely to be no benefit in treating those who are not coagulopathic [16, 18]. It is imperative that future trials specifically investigate the cohort of patients with major hemorrhage and coagulopathy, utilizing standardized intervention triggers and endpoints with patient-centered outcomes.

## 25.8 Question 6: The Value of Platelets (Including Cold Stored and Cryopreserved)

Platelets are vital components of hemostasis, and thrombocytopenia has been shown to be associated with poor outcomes in some trauma and massively transfused patient cohorts [6]. The timing and threshold for platelet transfusion, and in which form—liquid-stored, cryopreserved, or cold-stored—is however uncertain.

Evidence for platelet transfusion in major bleeding patients is primarily observational. In a multicenter retrospective US study of 466 trauma patients who received massive transfusions, higher ratios of platelets to RBCs were associated with decreased 6-h and in-hospital mortality [44]. This was supported by the PROMMTT (Prospective, Observational, Multicenter, Major Trauma Transfusion) study [45], a prospective study of 905 trauma patients who received at least 3 units of blood products: higher ratios of platelets to RBCs were associated with a decreased mortality within the first 6 h, however the mortality benefit was not significant beyond 6 h. These results support early administration of platelets in trauma, but may be confounded by survival bias, where patients in the higher ratio groups were those who survived long enough to receive higher ratios of transfusions.

These observational findings were not found in the subsequent PROPPR (Pragmatic, Randomized Optimal Platelet and Plasma Ratios) trial of 680 severe trauma and major bleeding patients across 12 trauma centers in the USA, investigating higher ratios of FFP *and* platelets to RBCs. In this study, there was no difference in mortality at 24 h or 30 days for early administration of higher ratios of plasma and platelets to RBCs (1:1:1 ratio compared with 1:1:2). However, in a *post hoc* analysis of the subset of 261 patients who received, or did not receive, platelets as part of their first transfusion pack, patients who received platelets had significantly lower mortality at 24 h (5.8% vs. 16.9%, $p < 0.05$) and 30 days (9.5% vs. 20.2%, $p < 0.01$), and were more likely to achieve hemostasis and less likely to die of exsanguination [46].

While maintaining platelet counts of $>50 \times 10^9$/l for severe bleeding and $>100 \times 10^9$/l in some trauma situations has been recommended [6], there is a lack of high-quality evidence to guide triggers for platelet transfusions. Adding to uncertainty, in one study of trauma patients, platelet transfusion was not shown to increase platelet counts [47] and in the previously mentioned *post hoc* analysis of the PROPPR data, mortality reduction was found despite platelet counts of $>100 \times 10^9$/l for all patients [46]. This suggests a potential benefit of platelet transfusion independent of platelet count in a patients with major hemorrhage.

Platelets are normally stored in liquid form at 20–24 °C with a shelf-life of only 5–7 days due to development of a storage lesion and risk of bacterial proliferation with prolonged storage. With their short shelf-life and difficult to predict demand for major bleeding, supply of liquid-stored platelets is challenging and results in significant wastage. Cryopreserved platelets are stored for more than 2 years and overcome the logistical issues of liquid-stored platelets but have reduced circulation times *in vivo*. Despite this, cryopreserved platelets have potentially greater hemostatic properties when compared to liquid-stored platelets, and the issue of reduced circulation times is less relevant to major bleeding patients. Three trials of cryopreserved platelets in cardiac surgery patients are underway—the Cryopreserved vs. Liquid Platelets (CLIP) II study (ClinicalTrials.gov Identifier: NCT03991481), the CLIPNZ-II study, and the Cryopreserved Platelets in Cardiopulmonary Bypass Surgery (CRYPTICS) study (ClinicalTrials.gov Identifier: NCT04709705). Cold-stored platelets stored at 2–6 °C for 14–21 days have also demonstrated superior hemostatic activity in bleeding patients compared to liquid-stored platelets [48]. The CHIlled Platelet Study (CHIPS) (ClinicalTrials.gov Identifier: NCT04834414) is investigating hemostatic efficacy of cold-stored platelets, also in cardiac surgery patients. While optimal triggers and timing of platelet transfusions remain controversial, these trials of cryopreserved and cold-stored platelets will offer insight into which form of platelet should be transfused to major bleeding patients.

## 25.9 Conclusion

Despite many attempts, only one trial [49] has ever demonstrated benefit of a transfusion intervention for major hemorrhage in trauma. However, it seems biologically implausible that transfusion would not help at least some patients. Therefore, the many trials that have failed to show benefits must logically have (1) been too small (the least likely explanation, as effect sizes based on biological understandings should have been sufficiently large); (2) enrolled a mixture of patients who were both helped and harmed (suggesting a better method of personalizing interventions

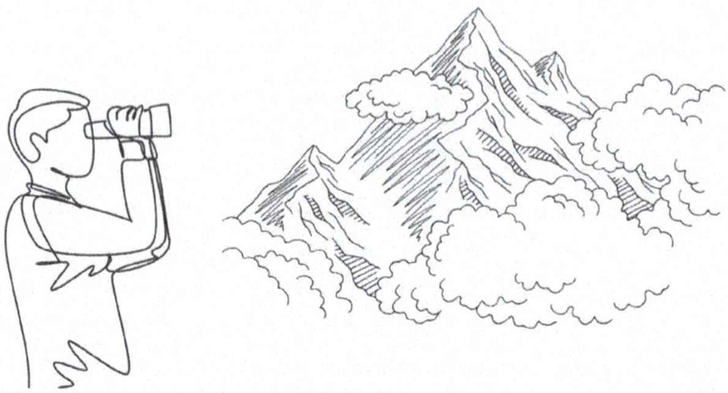

**Fig. 25.2** Observing the effect of a brief intervention applied early in a disease course several months later in any randomized controlled trial is analogous to attempting to define the shape of a mountain from a distance through the "noise" of cloud cover. This requires at least one of (1) a very large mountain (analogous to a large intervention effect size); (2) watching for a long time (analogous to a large study sample size); (3) accepting the validity of effects of the mountain (e.g. the way it affects wind patterns) as surrogates for its actual shape (analogous to biological surrogate outcomes); (4) extrapolating from brief glimpses (analogous to measuring only very early outcomes); or (5) incorporating prior knowledge to guide a constantly updating picture (Bayesian rather than frequentist statistical analysis)

is required); or (3) measured outcomes that could not have been plausibly affected by the intervention. Expecting that all-cause 6-month mortality will be significantly affected by an intervention lasting minutes when so many other factors influence mortality in the following months is analogous to listening for a faint noise in a snowstorm. Considerations in clinical trial design are shown in Fig. 25.2. A USA National Institutes of Health/Department of Defense working group [50] recently recommended 3 to 6-h all-cause mortality as the primary outcome for these types of study—a major departure from the more general trend in critical care to favor longer-term functional outcomes. Statistical approaches to account for the competing effect of short-term mortality and later outcomes of interest were suggested by some of the same authors. Whatever approach to better trial design is chosen, what should be clear is that persisting with studies in which heterogenous patient groups receive brief non-titrated interventions and expecting to observe effects 6 months later is likely to remain unsuccessful.

## References

1. Bickell WH, Wall MJ Jr, Pepe PE, et al. Immediate versus delayed fluid resuscitation for hypotensive patients with penetrating torso injuries. N Engl J Med. 1994;331:1105–9.
2. Doran CM, Doran CA, Woolley T, et al. Targeted resuscitation improves coagulation and outcome. J Trauma Acute Care Surg. 2012;72:835–43.
3. Milford EM, Reade MC. Resuscitation fluid choices to preserve the endothelial glycocalyx. Crit Care. 2019;23:77.
4. Brohi K, Cohen MJ, Ganter MT, Matthay MA, Mackersie RC, Pittet JF. Acute traumatic coagulopathy: initiated by hypoperfusion: modulated through the protein C pathway? Ann Surg. 2007;245:812–8.

5. McQuilten ZK, Bailey M, Cameron PA, et al. Fibrinogen concentration and use of fibrinogen supplementation with cryoprecipitate in patients with critical bleeding receiving massive transfusion: a bi-national cohort study. Br J Haematol. 2017;179:131–41.
6. Spahn DR, Bouillon B, Cerny V, et al. The European guideline on management of major bleeding and coagulopathy following trauma: fifth edition. Crit Care. 2019;23:98.
7. Nascimento B, Callum J, Tien H, et al. Fibrinogen in the initial resuscitation of severe trauma (FiiRST): a randomized feasibility trial. Br J Anaesth. 2016;117:775–82.
8. Ziegler B, Bachler M, Haberfellner H, et al. Efficacy of prehospital administration of fibrinogen concentrate in trauma patients bleeding or presumed to bleed (FIinTIC): a multicentre, double-blind, placebo-controlled, randomised pilot study. Eur J Anaesthesiol. 2021;38:348–57.
9. Curry N, Foley C, Wong H, et al. Early fibrinogen concentrate therapy for major haemorrhage in trauma (E-FIT 1): results from a UK multi-centre, randomised, double blind, placebo-controlled pilot trial. Crit Care. 2018;22:164.
10. Winearls J. Fibrinogen Early In Severe Trauma studY (FEISTY): results from an Australian multicentre randomised controlled pilot trial. Crit Care Resusc. 2021;23:32–46.
11. Curry N, Rourke C, Davenport R, et al. Early cryoprecipitate for major haemorrhage in trauma: a randomised controlled feasibility trial. Br J Anaesth. 2015;115:76–83.
12. Callum J, Farkouh ME, Scales DC, et al. Effect of fibrinogen concentrate vs cryoprecipitate on blood component transfusion after cardiac surgery: The FIBRES randomized clinical trial. JAMA. 2019;322:1966–76.
13. Morrow GB, Carlier MSA, Dasgupta S, Craigen FB, Mutch NJ, Curry N. Fibrinogen replacement therapy for traumatic coagulopathy: does the fibrinogen source matter? Int J Mol Sci. 2021;22:2185.
14. Neisser-Svae A, Hegener O. Gorlinger K Differences in the biochemical composition of three plasma derived human fibrinogen concentrates. Thromb Res. 2021;205:44–6.
15. Wikkelso AJ, Edwards HM, Afshari A, et al. Pre-emptive treatment with fibrinogen concentrate for postpartum haemorrhage: randomized controlled trial. Br J Anaesth. 2015;114:623–33.
16. Collins PW, Cannings-John R, Bruynseels D, et al. Viscoelastometric-guided early fibrinogen concentrate replacement during postpartum haemorrhage: OBS2, a double-blind randomized controlled trial. Br J Anaesth. 2017;119:411–21.
17. Ranucci M, Baryshnikova E, Crapelli GB, Rahe-Meyer N, Menicanti L, Frigiola A. Randomized, double-blinded, placebo-controlled trial of fibrinogen concentrate supplementation after complex cardiac surgery. J Am Heart Assoc. 2015;4:e002066.
18. Rahe-Meyer N, Levy JH, Mazer CD, et al. Randomized evaluation of fibrinogen vs placebo in complex cardiovascular surgery (REPLACE): a double-blind phase III study of haemostatic therapy. Br J Anaesth. 2016;117:41–51.
19. Smith MM, Schroeder DR, Nelson JA, et al. Prothrombin complex concentrate vs plasma for post-cardiopulmonary bypass coagulopathy and bleeding: a randomized clinical trial. JAMA Surg. 2022;157:757–64.
20. Innerhofer P, Westermann I, Tauber H, et al. The exclusive use of coagulation factor concentrates enables reversal of coagulopathy and decreases transfusion rates in patients with major blunt trauma. Injury. 2013;44:209–16.
21. Innerhofer P, Fries D, Mittermayr M, et al. Reversal of trauma-induced coagulopathy using first-line coagulation factor concentrates or fresh frozen plasma (RETIC): a single-centre, parallel-group, open-label, randomised trial. Lancet Haematol. 2017;4:e258–71.
22. da Luz LT, Callum J, Beckett A, et al. Protocol for a multicentre, randomised, parallel-control, superiority trial comparing administration of clotting factor concentrates with a standard massive haemorrhage protocol in severely bleeding trauma patients: the FiiRST 2 trial (a 2020 EAST multicentre trial). BMJ Open. 2021;11:e051003.
23. Meledeo MA, Peltier GC, McIntosh CS, Bynum JA, Cap AP. Optimizing whole blood storage: hemostatic function of 35-day stored product in CPD, CP2D, and CPDA-1 anticoagulants. Transfusion. 2019;59:1549–59.
24. Condron M, Scanlan M, Schreiber M. Massive transfusion of low-titer cold-stored O-positive whole blood in a civilian trauma setting. Transfusion. 2019;59:927–30.

25. Spinella PC, Perkins JG, Grathwohl KW, Beekley AC, Holcomb JB. Warm fresh whole blood is independently associated with improved survival for patients with combat-related traumatic injuries. J Trauma. 2009;66:S69–76.
26. McGinity AC, Zhu CS, Greebon L, et al. Prehospital low-titer cold-stored whole blood: philosophy for ubiquitous utilization of O-positive product for emergency use in hemorrhage due to injury. J Trauma Acute Care Surg. 2018;84:S115–S9.
27. Hashmi ZG, Chehab M, Nathens AB, et al. Whole truths but half the blood: addressing the gap between the evidence and practice of pre-hospital and in-hospital blood product use for trauma resuscitation. Transfusion. 2021;61(Suppl 1):S348–53.
28. Perkins JG, Cap AP, Spinella PC, et al. Comparison of platelet transfusion as fresh whole blood versus apheresis platelets for massively transfused combat trauma patients (CME). Transfusion. 2011;51:242–52.
29. Cotton BA, Podbielski J, Camp E, et al. A randomized controlled pilot trial of modified whole blood versus component therapy in severely injured patients requiring large volume transfusions. Ann Surg. 2013;258:527–32.
30. Guyette FX, Zenati M, Triulzi DJ, et al. Prehospital low titer group O whole blood is feasible and safe: results of a prospective randomized pilot trial. J Trauma Acute Care Surg. 2022;92:839–47.
31. Avery P, Morton S, Tucker H, Green L, Weaver A, Davenport R. Whole blood transfusion versus component therapy in adult trauma patients with acute major haemorrhage. Emerg Med J. 2020;37:370–8.
32. Crowe E, DeSantis SM, Bonnette A, et al. Whole blood transfusion versus component therapy in trauma resuscitation: a systematic review and meta-analysis. J Am Coll Emerg Physicians Open. 2020;1:633–41.
33. Naumann DN, Boulton AJ, Sandhu A, et al. Fresh whole blood from walking blood banks for patients with traumatic hemorrhagic shock: a systematic review and meta-analysis. J Trauma Acute Care Surg. 2020;89:792–800.
34. NHS Clinical Trials Unit. SWIFT study of whole blood in frontline trauma. Available at: https://www.nhsbt.nhs.uk/clinical-trials-unit/current-trials-and-studies/swift/. Accessed 3 Nov 2022
35. Barmparas G, Huang R, Hayes C, et al. Implementation of a low-titer stored whole blood transfusion program for civilian trauma patients: early experience and logistical challenges. Injury. 2022;53:1576–80.
36. Garrigue D, Godier A, Glacet A, et al. French lyophilized plasma versus fresh frozen plasma for the initial management of trauma-induced coagulopathy: a randomized open-label trial. J Thromb Haemost. 2018;16:481–9.
37. Jost D, Lemoine S, Lemoine F, et al. Prehospital lyophilized plasma transfusion for trauma-induced coagulopathy in patients at risk for hemorrhagic shock: a randomized clinical trial. JAMA Netw Open. 2022;5:e2223619.
38. Crombie N, Doughty HA, Bishop JRB, et al. Resuscitation with blood products in patients with trauma-related haemorrhagic shock receiving prehospital care (RePHILL): a multicentre, open-label, randomised, controlled, phase 3 trial. Lancet Haematol. 2022;9:e250–61.
39. Pusateri AE, Moore EE, Moore HB, et al. Association of prehospital plasma transfusion with survival in trauma patients with hemorrhagic shock when transport times are longer than 20 minutes: a post hoc analysis of the PAMPer and COMBAT clinical trials. JAMA Surg. 2020;155:e195085.
40. Bugaev N, Como JJ, Golani G, et al. Thromboelastography and rotational thromboelastometry in bleeding patients with coagulopathy: practice management guideline from the Eastern Association for the Surgery of Trauma. J Trauma Acute Care Surg. 2020;89:999–1017.
41. Gonzalez E, Moore EE, Moore HB, et al. Goal-directed hemostatic resuscitation of trauma-induced coagulopathy: a pragmatic randomized clinical trial comparing a viscoelastic assay to conventional coagulation assays. Ann Surg. 2016;263:1051–9.

42. Baksaas-Aasen K, Gall LS, Stensballe J, et al. Viscoelastic haemostatic assay augmented protocols for major trauma haemorrhage (ITACTIC): a randomized, controlled trial. Intensive Care Med. 2021;47:49–59.
43. Curry NS, Davenport R, Pavord S, et al. The use of viscoelastic haemostatic assays in the management of major bleeding: a British Society for Haematology Guideline. Br J Haematol. 2018;182:789–806.
44. Zink KA, Sambasivan CN, Holcomb JB, Chisholm G, Schreiber MA. A high ratio of plasma and platelets to packed red blood cells in the first 6 hours of massive transfusion improves outcomes in a large multicenter study. Am J Surg. 2009;197:565–70.
45. Holcomb JB, del Junco DJ, Fox EE, et al. The prospective, observational, multicenter, major trauma transfusion (PROMMTT) study: comparative effectiveness of a time-varying treatment with competing risks. JAMA Surg. 2013;148:127–36.
46. Cardenas JC, Zhang X, Fox EE, et al. Platelet transfusions improve hemostasis and survival in a substudy of the prospective, randomized PROPPR trial. Blood Adv. 2018;2:1696–704.
47. Vulliamy P, Gillespie S, Gall LS, Green L, Brohi K, Davenport RA. Platelet transfusions reduce fibrinolysis but do not restore platelet function during trauma hemorrhage. J Trauma Acute Care Surg. 2017;83:388–97.
48. Strandenes G, Sivertsen J, Bjerkvig CK, et al. A pilot trial of platelets stored cold versus at room temperature for complex cardiothoracic surgery. Anesthesiology. 2020;133:1173–83.
49. Sperry JL, Guyette FX, Brown JB, et al. Prehospital plasma during air medical transport in trauma patients at risk for hemorrhagic shock. N Engl J Med. 2018;379:315–26.
50. Spinella PC, El Kassar N, Cap AP, et al. Recommended primary outcomes for clinical trials evaluating hemostatic blood products and agents in patients with bleeding: proceedings of a National Heart Lung and Blood Institute and US Department of Defense Consensus Conference. J Trauma Acute Care Surg. 2021;91:S19–25.

# Part VII

# Acute Renal Failure

# Fluid Management and Acute Kidney Injury

# 26

N. Lumlertgul, N. Z. Nordin, and M. Ostermann

## 26.1 Introduction

Acute kidney injury (AKI) is common in critical illness and is associated with increased short- and long-term complications. Both hypovolemia and fluid accumulation affect renal blood flow, can lead to worsening kidney function, and impact outcomes. When prescribing fluids for patients at risk of AKI or with AKI, clinicians should focus on the four Ds (drug, dose, duration, and de-escalation), four questions (when to initiate and when to discontinue fluid therapy, and when to initiate and when to discontinue fluid removal), four indications (resuscitation, maintenance, replacement, and nutrition), and the conceptual SOSD or ROSE model describing four fluid phases (salvage/resuscitation, optimization, stabilization, and de-escalation/evacuation) [1, 2] (Fig. 26.1).

N. Lumlertgul
Department of Critical Care, King's College London, Guy's & St Thomas' NHS Foundation Trust, London, UK

Division of Nephrology, Department of Internal Medicine and Excellence Center in Critical Care Nephrology, King Chulalongkorn Memorial Hospital, Bangkok, Thailand

Faculty of Medicine, Center of Excellence in Critical Care Nephrology, Chulalongkorn University, Bangkok, Thailand

N. Z. Nordin
Department of Critical Care, King's College London, Guy's & St Thomas' NHS Foundation Trust, London, UK

Nephrology Department, Hospital Kuala Lumpur, Ministry of Health, Kuala Lumpur, Malaysia

M. Ostermann (✉)
Department of Critical Care, King's College London, Guy's & St Thomas' NHS Foundation Trust, London, UK
e-mail: Marlies.Ostermann@gstt.nhs.uk



J.-L. Vincent (ed.), *Annual Update in Intensive Care and Emergency Medicine 2023*, Annual Update in Intensive Care and Emergency Medicine,
https://doi.org/10.1007/978-3-031-23005-9_26

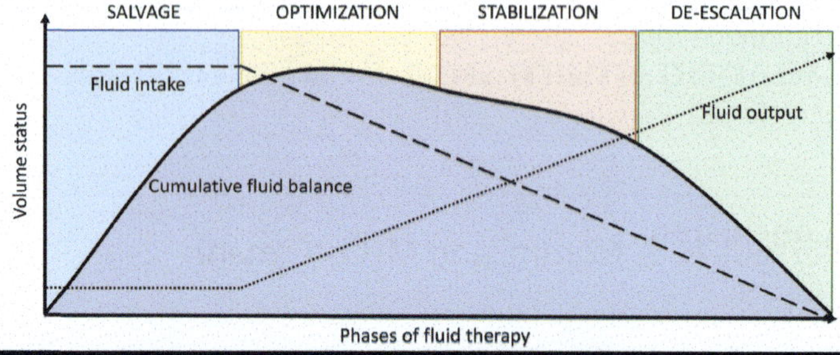


| Triggers | Fluid administration | | Fluid removal | |
|---|---|---|---|---|
| | Initiation | Discontinuation | Initiation | Discontinuation |
| Perfusion | Decreased | Improved | Maintained | Decreased |
| Fluid responsiveness | Yes | No | No | Yes |
| Fluid accumulation | No | Variable | Yes | Variable |

**Fig. 26.1** Schematic presentation of the relationship between phases of fluid therapy, fluid intake **(dashed line)**, fluid output (dotted line), and cumulative fluid balance **(solid line)** in critically ill patients. The table outlines triggers to start and stop fluid therapy and triggers to start and stop fluid removal

## 26.2 Fluid Status and Kidney Function

In normal physiology, renal blood flow (RBF) is determined by the difference between inflow and outflow pressures (transrenal pressure gradient). Interestingly, compared to all other vital organs, the kidneys have a complicated glomerular autoregulation, which keeps this gradient between 50 and 150 mmHg in a normotensive patient, therefore protecting them against vascular injury under various physiologic and pathophysiologic conditions. Nevertheless, this autoregulation is deranged when the systolic blood pressure falls below 80 mmHg. The kidney is a highly perfused organ; therefore, any significant reduction in systolic blood pressure will lead to poor kidney perfusion. Fluid therapy may increase RBF and glomerular filtration but will also increase workload to the kidneys from increased resorption of sodium chloride, thus increasing oxygen consumption. Stressed tubular cells also consume oxygen at twice the rate of healthy kidneys. Furthermore, hemodilution from fluid therapy will decrease renal oxygen delivery. Therefore, restoration of cardiac output by fluid might not always improve renal oxygenation due to the supply-demand mismatch [3].

Whilst it is important to restore adequate volume to maintain cardiac output and forward flow, there is growing evidence that overzealous fluid administration and positive net body balance also lead to the development of AKI. There are several potential mechanisms. First, high central venous pressure (CVP) leads to renal congestion, subsequently causing a reduction in net glomerular filtration. An increase in CVP has been linked to worsening kidney function independent of mean arterial pressure (MAP) or cardiac output [4]. Second, raised intra-abdominal pressure (IAP) due to fluid accumulation also aggravates renal interstitial edema by

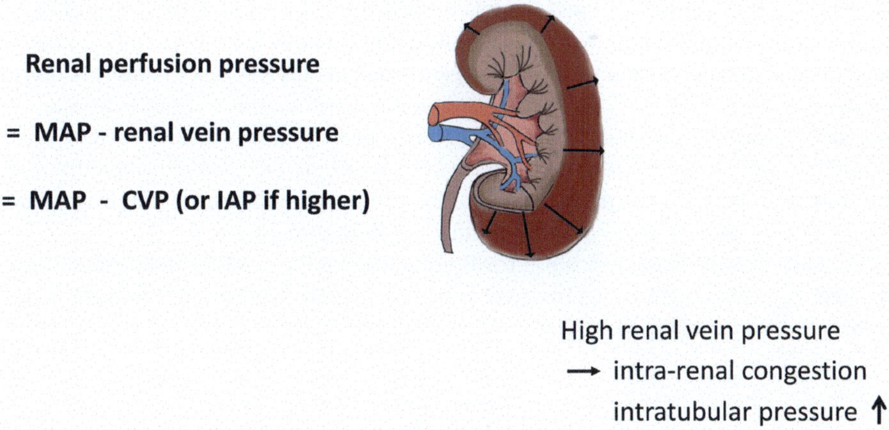


**Fig. 26.2** Relationship between fluid accumulation, high renal vein pressure, and renal perfusion pressure. *MAP* mean arterial pressure, *CVP* central venous pressure, *IAP* intra-abdominal pressure

externally compressing the encapsulated kidneys [5]. Finally, septic patients also suffer from increased capillary permeability leading to extravasation of protein and large molecules into the interstitial spaces. The high oncotic shift will lead to further extravasation of fluids, leaving the intravascular columns depleted, which may aggravate existing hypotension further. In this scenario, giving more fluids to achieve a target MAP may worsen fluid accumulation. In severe cases, this could lead to renal compartment syndrome. All these factors will further impair renal perfusion pressure and venous return, leading to AKI. It is becoming increasingly evident that liberal use of fluids in this group of patients increases morbidity and mortality, including the risk of AKI progression, AKI non-recovery, and renal replacement therapy (RRT) [6].

Systemic blood pressure is often used to evaluate renal perfusion. However, there is increasing recognition that renal perfusion pressure (RPP), the difference between in- and outflow, is a better indicator [7]. RPP is estimated as MAP – CVP (or IAP, whichever is higher) (Fig. 26.2).

## 26.3 Why Prescribe Fluids?

The physiological goals for fluid administration in AKI are to optimize intravascular circulating volume, increase cardiac output, and maintain perfusion pressure in order to improve RBF and glomerular filtration. Intravenous fluid can be given as a bolus during resuscitation, as maintenance fluid during the optimization phase, as an infusion to replace water and electrolytes lost during critical illness, or as a route for nutrition.

Hypotension and oliguria are the most common indications for fluid therapy in patients at risk of AKI or with AKI. In absolute hypovolemia, renal hypoperfusion may result from decreased cardiac output. Giving fluid seems logical in order to increase stroke volume (SV) and cardiac output, thus increasing RBF and glomerular filtration rate (GFR). However, RBF and GFR correlate poorly in AKI. In addition, RBF might be normal or high in sepsis-associated AKI [3]. Administration of fluids to increase RBF may in fact not augment GFR if cardiac output is normal or increased. Recent studies have shown that a rise in MAP after the administration of a fluid bolus did not necessarily produce a corresponding increase in urine output or an improvement in renal perfusion [8]. Therefore, hypotension or oliguria alone should not be viewed as triggers for immediate fluid therapy.

In summary, the only indication for fluid resuscitation in AKI is to correct intravascular hypovolemia and to improve renal perfusion. This should be done judiciously without causing fluid accumulation (Fig. 26.3).

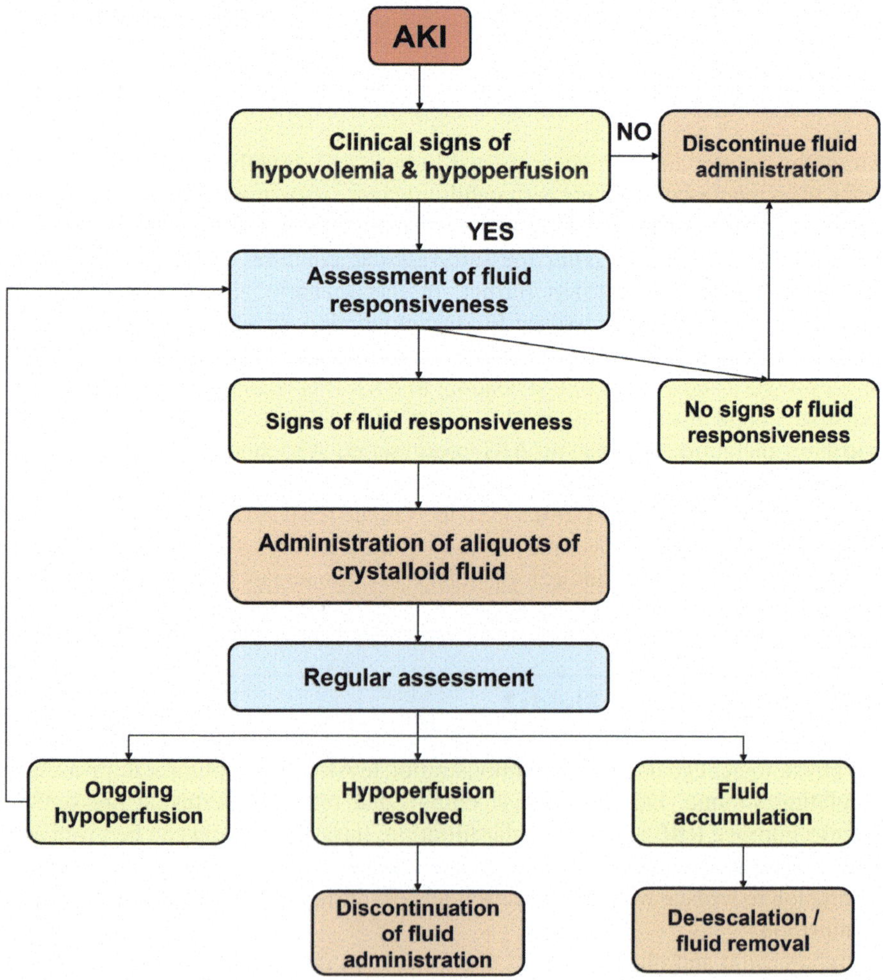


**Fig. 26.3** Algorithm to guide fluid management in acute kidney injury (AKI)

## 26.4 What to Prescribe: Types of Fluids

Intravenous (i.v.) fluids are broadly categorized as colloids and crystalloids and vary in electrolyte composition, osmolarity, pH, and clinical effect [9]. The choice of fluid is one of the most controversial issues, and there is growing evidence that certain types of fluids are nephrotoxic.

### 26.4.1 Colloids

Colloids are solutions that contain macrooncotic molecules. They are proposed as an alternative to crystalloids to expand intravascular volume quicker and maintain intravascular oncotic pressure for longer. The volume-sparing effect (the ratio of administered colloids:crystalloids needed to achieve hemodynamic targets) is 1:1.1 to 1:1.4 and the duration of intravascular volume expansion of colloids (4–6 h) is longer than that of crystalloids (1–4 h) [3].

Several randomized controlled trials (RCTs) have confirmed that hydroxyethyl starch (HES) is associated with increased rates of AKI and RRT, and increased mortality in sepsis patients [10]. Consequently, the Food and Drug Administration (FDA) and European Medicines Agency (EMA) issued recommendations against the use of HES.

Gelatin is another commonly used synthetic colloid. Various observational studies have reported an increased risk of osmosis nephrosis-induced AKI with gelatin [11], but a meta-analysis including 212 patients from three RCTs comparing gelatin with crystalloid/albumin showed no significant difference in the risk of AKI (RR 1.35, 95% CI 0.58–3.14) [12]. Although the quality of the evidence is low, potential harms outweigh its benefits. Hence, gelatin-based colloids should be avoided in patients at risk of AKI or with AKI.

Albumin is a natural colloid. There are various preparations of albumin including iso-oncotic (4–5%) and hyper-oncotic (20–25%) solutions, which contain lower sodium concentrations than do iso-oncotic solutions. Albumin appears to be safe in patients at risk of AKI or with AKI, although it has not been shown in large RCTs to reduce the rate of RRT or improve survival in critically ill patients [13, 14]. The 2021 Surviving Sepsis Campaign (SSC) Guidelines suggest, "In situations when further crystalloid use would result in fluid accumulation, albumin administration is an alternative" [15]. However, the modest volume-sparing effect and higher cost warrant for judicious albumin use. Exceptions are patients with cirrhosis and massive ascites requiring large-volume paracentesis or those with spontaneous bacterial peritonitis where albumin administration appears to protect kidney function [16]. Albumin is also recommended by the European Association for the Study of the Liver (EASL) in hepatorenal syndrome in combination with vasopressors [17].

Other possible roles of albumin include cardiac surgery, diuretic resistance, and patients receiving RRT with hypoalbuminemia. A single-center RCT in patients undergoing off-pump cardiac surgery showed that correction of hypoalbuminemia

(<4 g/dl) by administering 20% albumin reduced the risk of postoperative AKI [18]. The co-administration of albumin with diuretics was shown to increase urine output in diuretic-resistant cases. The effect was more pronounced in patients with serum albumin <2.5 g/dl and when using higher albumin doses (30 g) [19]. In AKI and end-stage kidney disease patients with hypoalbuminemia (<3 g/dl) receiving RRT, albumin administration helped to achieve more negative fluid balance and prevented episodes of intradialytic hypotension compared with usual care [20].

### 26.4.2 Crystalloids

The compositions of commonly used crystalloid solutions are shown in Table 26.1. Saline (0.9% sodium chloride solution) is the most frequently administered crystalloid globally. However, its unphysiological sodium and chloride concentrations and the absence of buffer can result in hyperchloremic acidosis. Preclinical studies have demonstrated that hyperchloremia induces afferent arteriolar vasoconstriction and possibly reduces glomerular filtration via tubulo-glomerular feedback [21]. The infusion of 2 l of 0.9% saline in healthy human adult volunteers has been shown to decrease the velocity of renal arterial flow, the perfusion of renal cortical tissue, and urinary excretion of water and sodium [22].

Balanced or buffered crystalloid solutions, in which chloride ions are replaced by bicarbonate or buffer to reduce acid-base perturbations, contain similar electrolyte concentrations to human plasma. Examples of buffers include lactate, acetate, and gluconate, which are rapidly metabolized and excreted. Although balanced solutions contain potassium, the risk of aggravating hyperkalemia is high only in those with markedly raised serum potassium levels [23]. Of note, a study in post kidney transplant recipients comparing 0.9% saline versus balanced crystalloids reported a higher risk of hyperkalemia in the saline group, possibly explained by the potassium efflux from metabolic acidosis [24]. Additionally, the use of balanced crystalloids was associated with lower concentrations of urinary neutrophil gelatinase-associated lipocalin (NGAL), a biomarker of tubular cell damage, compared with saline [25].

However, despite the lower risk of AKI, RRT, and death with balanced crystalloids in animal studies, healthy volunteers, and observational studies, the results from RCTs are more conflicting (Table 26.2). The Saline vs. Plasma-Lyte 148 for ICU Fluid Therapy (SPLIT) trial was a double-blind, cluster-randomized, double-crossover trial conducted in four intensive care units (ICUs) in New Zealand and included 2278 patients. Compared with saline, Plasma-Lyte did not result in a difference in the AKI incidence, use of RRT, and in-hospital mortality. However, it was a feasibility trial, and the cohort was less acutely ill, being predominantly surgical patients [26].

The Isotonic Solutions and Major Adverse Renal Events Trial (SMART) trial was an open-label, pragmatic, cluster-crossover, single-center trial conducted in five ICUs in the United States [27]. A total of 15,802 critically ill participants were recruited. The primary outcome was major adverse kidney events at 30 days (MAKE30), which is a composite endpoint comprising death, new RRT, and

**Table 26.1** Composition of commonly used crystalloid fluids compared with human plasma

| Components | pH | $Na^+$, [mmol/l] | $Cl^-$, [mmol/l] | $K^+$, [mmol/l] | $Ca^{2+}$, [mmol/l] | $Mg^{2+}$, [mmol/l] | Phosphate, [mmol/l] | Buffer, [mmol/l] | Glucose, [mmol/l] | Osmolarity, [mOsm/l] |
|---|---|---|---|---|---|---|---|---|---|---|
| Human plasma | 7.35–7.45 | 135–145 | 100–110 | 3.5–5.0 | 2.2–2.6 | 0.8–1.2 | 0.8–1.2 | $HCO_3^-$ 22–26 | 4–7 | 275–295 |
| 0.9% NaCl | 5.5 | 154 | 154 | – | – | | | – | – | 308 |
| Hartmann's solution | 5.0–7.0 | 131 | 111 | 5 | 2 | | | Lactate 29 | – | 278 |
| Plasma-Lyte A | 7.4 | 140 | 98 | 5 | – | 3 | – | Acetate 27/ Gluconate 23 | – | 294 |
| Plasma-Lyte 148 | 5.5 | 140 | 98 | 5 | – | 3 | – | Acetate 27/ Gluconate 23 | – | 294 |
| Ringer lactate | 6.0–7.5 | 130 | 109 | 4 | 1.5 | – | | Lactate 28 | – | 273 |
| Ringer acetate | 6–8 | 130 | 112 | 5 | 1 | 1 | | Acetate 27 | – | 277 |
| Sterofundin | 5.1–5.9 | 145 | 127 | 4 | 2.5 | 1 | – | Acetate 24/ Malate 5 | – | 309 |
| Isolyte S | 6.3–7.3 | 141 | 98 | 5 | – | 3 | 1 | Acetate 27/ Gluconate 23 | – | 295 |
| 0.45% NaCl/4% glucose | 3.5–6.5 | 77 | 77 | – | – | – | – | – | 278 | 406 |
| 5% glucose | 3.5–5.5 | – | – | – | – | – | – | – | 252 | 278 |
| 1.26% $NaHCO_3$ | 7.0–8.5 | 150 | – | – | – | – | – | $HCO_3^-$ 150 | – | 301 |
| 1.4% $NaHCO_3$ | 7.0–8.5 | 167 | – | – | – | – | – | $HCO_3^-$ 167 | – | 333 |
| 8.4% $NaHCO_3$ | 7.0–8.5 | 1000 | – | – | – | – | – | $HCO_3^-$ 1000 | – | 2000 |

*Ca* calcium, *Cl* chloride, $HCO_3$ bicarbonate, *K* potassium, *Mg* magnesium, *Na* sodium

**Table 26.2** Randomized controlled trials comparing balanced crystalloids with 0.9% saline in acutely ill or critically ill patients

| Study [Ref] | SPLIT [26] | SALT-ED [28] | SMART [27] | BaSICS [29] | PLUS [30] |
|---|---|---|---|---|---|
| Setting and design | New Zealand | USA | USA | Brazil | Australia and New Zealand |
| | Double-blind, cluster-crossover, multicenter (4 ICUs) | Open-label, cluster-crossover, single-center | Open-label, cluster-crossover, single-center | Double-blind, parallel-group, multicenter (75 ICUs) | Double-blind, parallel-group, multicenter (53 ICUs) |
| Number | 2278 | 13,347 | 15,802 | 11,052 | 5037 |
| Population | Critically ill (57% elective surgical) | ER (81% medical) | Critically ill (71% medical) | Critically ill (48% elective surgical) | Critically ill (42% elective surgical) |
| Intervention | Plasma-Lyte 148 | RL/Plasma-Lyte A | RL/Plasma-Lyte A | Plasma-Lyte 148 | Plasma-Lyte 148 |
| Control | 0.9% NaCl | 0.9% NaCl | 0.9% NaCl | 0.9% NaCl | 0.9% NaCl |
| Median volume of administered fluids | ~2 l | ~1 l | ~1 l | ~3 l | ~4 l |
| Primary outcome | AKI (RR 1.04, 95% CI 0.80–1.36) | Hospital-free days (OR 0.98, 95% CI 0.92–1.04) | MAKE30 (OR 0.90, 95% CI 0.82–0.99, p = 0.04) | 90-day mortality (HR 0.97, 95% CI 0.90–1.05) | 90-day mortality (OR 0.99, 95% CI 0.86–1.14) |
| Secondary outcomes | No difference in RRT, in-hospital mortality | MAKE30 (OR 0.82, 95% CI 0.70–0.95, p = 0.01) | In-hospital mortality (OR 0.90, 95% CI 0.80–1.01, p = 0.06) | Neurological SOFA > 2 (OR 1.40, 95% CI 1.18–1.66) | No difference in RRT, maximum SCr levels, maximum increase in SCr levels, ICU stay, MV-free days |
| | | No difference in AKI stage ≥2 and in-hospital mortality | RRT (OR 0.84, 95% CI 0.68-1.02, p = 0.08) | No difference in AKI, RRT incidence, ICU stay | |
| | | | No difference in persistent kidney dysfunction, ICU- and MV-free days | | |

*AKI* acute kidney injury, *CI* confidence interval, *HR* hazard ratio, *ICU* intensive care unit, *MAKE30* 30-day major adverse kidney events, *MV* mechanical ventilation, *OR* odds ratio, *RR* relative risk, *RRT* renal replacement therapy, *SCr* serum creatinine, *SOFA* Sequential Organ Failure Assessment, *RL* Ringer's lactate solution persistent kidney dysfunction, defined as doubling in serum creatinine compared to baseline. Balanced crystalloids (Plasma-Lyte or Ringer's lactate solution) were associated with a significantly lower incidence of MAKE30 compared with saline (14.3% vs. 15.4%, p = 0.04), driven mainly by marginal reduction in RRT rates and in-hospital mortality. The effect was more pronounced in the sepsis group. Similarly, the Saline against Lactated Ringer's or Plasma-Lyte in the Emergency Department (SALT-ED) trial including 13,347 non-critically ill patients demonstrated a lower incidence of MAKE30 in the balanced crystalloid group (4.7% vs. 5.6%, p = 0.01) [28]. However, it is argued that the use of a composite endpoint assumed the equivalency of all three components. In this regard, it should be acknowledged that the initiation of RRT is clinician dependent. Further, the availability of baseline creatinine concentrations and potential confounding by various factors, including muscle wasting and liver disease during and after the acute illness, could affect the ascertainment of kidney dysfunction.

The Balanced Solutions in Intensive Care Study (BaSICS) was a multicenter, double-blind, factorial design RCT in 75 ICUs in Brazil [29]. A total of 11,052 critically ill patients (48% elective surgery) requiring fluid resuscitation with at least one risk factor for AKI were randomized to Plasma-Lyte or saline. Contrary to the SMART and SALT-ED trials, Plasma-Lyte did not result in a reduction in 90-day mortality and RRT receipt compared with saline. The results were consistent in the pre-specified subgroup analyses, in particular in patients with sepsis or moderate to severe AKI.

The Plasma-Lyte 148 versus Saline (PLUS) study was a double-blinded RCT undertaken in 53 ICUs in Australia and New Zealand and recruited 5037 critically ill patients (42% elective surgery) [30]. The median volume of received fluid was 4 l in 6 days, which is larger compared with previous studies (2.9 l in the BaSICS trial, 2 l in the SPLIT trial, and 1 l in the SMART and SALT-ED trials). Similar to the BaSICS trial, administration of balanced solution did not result in a reduction in 90-day mortality compared with saline. Despite a clear separation in serum chloride levels (~2 mmol/l) and pH values between the groups, the incidence of RRT and maximum increase in serum creatinine concentrations did not differ. The results were also consistent when adjusted by the amount of fluids received before randomization. There were no differences in subgroup analyses, including those with sepsis. Notably, the sample size was revised from 8800 to 5000 during the coronavirus disease 2019 (COVID-19) pandemic. However, the futility analysis suggests that it is highly unlikely that the results would have changed had the trial been continued.

The discordance of these findings could be explained by several factors, such as the difference in trial design (cluster-crossover vs. parallel group), the heterogeneity and acuity of the patients, the electrolyte compositions of each fluid, the volume of administered fluids pre- and post-randomization, clinician blinding to the study fluids, the amount of non-study fluids, infusion rates, or concomitant therapies, e.g., vasopressors. It is also postulated that the adverse effects of saline might be dose dependent. However, a study in ICU patients receiving large volumes of fluid resuscitation (>60 ml/kg body weight) did not show any association between chloride load and risk of AKI after adjusting for illness severity [31]. An updated meta-analysis comprising 35,884 patients concluded that the effect of balanced crystalloid fluids, as compared with saline, ranged from a 9% relative reduction to a 1% relative increase in risk of AKI. The effect on mortality was similar [32].

There may be subgroups of patients in which the use of one type of fluid is preferred. For example, saline is the fluid of choice in patients with traumatic brain injury (TBI) and those with hypovolemia and hypochloremia, e.g., from upper gastrointestinal losses. In diabetic ketoacidosis patients, the use of balanced crystalloids was associated with faster resolution of acidosis [33]. *Post hoc* analyses of previous RCTs also showed potential benefits of balanced crystalloids in patients who had exclusively received balanced solutions before randomization [34], patients with severe hyperkalemia (potassium ≥6.5 mmol/l) [23], and patients with AKI at least stage 2 [23].

In conclusion, the current evidence does not show clear superiority of balanced crystalloids over saline for protection of kidney function. Instead, individual patient cohorts may benefit more from one type of crystalloid over the other. If saline is given, it is important that biochemical parameters are appropriately monitored.

### 26.4.3 Bicarbonate Infusion and Acute Kidney Injury

In the 'Sodium bicarbonate therapy for patients with severe metabolic acidemia in the intensive care unit' (BICAR-ICU) multicenter, open-label RCT (n = 389), administration of bicarbonate to raise blood pH to a target of ≥7.3 had no effect on the primary composite outcome of death and organ failure at day 7. However, in the prespecified subgroup of patients with AKI stage 2 or 3, there were statistically significant fewer composite outcomes, 28-day mortality, and occurrence of organ failure with the infusion of bicarbonate compared with placebo [35]. Further studies exploring the role of bicarbonate in AKI are in progress.

## 26.5 How to Prescribe: Volume of Fluids

There is no consensus on how much fluid to prescribe in critically ill patients at risk of AKI or with AKI. However, the clinical phase, degree of hypovolemia, and response to fluid administration should be considered. During the salvage/resuscitation phase, it is suggested that fluid administration be individualized with regular assessment guided by dynamic variables rather than static measurements. Importantly, fluid responsiveness is not equal to intravascular hypovolemia. It should also be noted that fluid responsiveness is short-lived and diminishes over time.

Several studies have investigated different fluid management strategies in critically ill patients. The 2006 multicenter Fluids and Catheters Treatment Trial (FACTT) randomized 1000 patients with ARDS to liberal or conservative fluid strategy guided by CVP or pulmonary artery occlusion pressure (PAOP). Compared with a liberal fluid strategy, the conservative strategy resulted in a lower cumulative fluid balance, increased $PaO_2/FiO_2$ ratio, and increased mechanical ventilator-free days and ICU-free days but there was no difference in the use of RRT [36]. In contrast, perioperative fluid restriction in patients undergoing major abdominal surgery (RELIEF trial) increased the risks of AKI and RRT [37].

Three RCTs comparing three resuscitation approaches in sepsis/septic shock including (1) protocolized resuscitation guided by CVP and oxygen monitoring, (2) protocolized resuscitation without the use of CVP, and (3) usual care by the treating physician concluded no difference in outcomes [38]. The Conservative versus Liberal Approach to Fluid Therapy of Septic Shock in Intensive care (CLASSIC) study was a multinational, multicenter RCT aiming to evaluate two fluid management strategies in early septic shock after the initial resuscitation phase [39]. In the restrictive fluid group, fluid boluses were allowed only if signs of hypoperfusion were present. In the standard group, i.v. fluid therapy was entirely directed by the clinical teams. There was no between-group difference in 90-day mortality, severe AKI incidence, or days alive without organ support. Of note, the between-group difference in the median volume of administered i.v. fluids and cumulative fluid balance at day 5 were 2 l and ~800 ml, respectively, which may point towards a cautious approach to fluid administration in modern European ICU practice.

Among patients with established AKI, the effect of fluid restriction on AKI progression and RRT requirement remains uncertain and is likely affected by volume status. The Restrictive Fluid Management versus Usual Care in Acute Kidney Injury (REVERSE-AKI) study was a pilot multinational, multicenter RCT aiming to investigate the feasibility of a restrictive fluid management regimen versus usual care in patients with AKI who were not hypovolemic. The restrictive fluid management bundle consisted of limiting fluid input as well as targeting output by diuretics with or without extracorporeal fluid removal with the overall aim to prevent an increase in cumulative fluid balance. Patients randomized to the restrictive fluid regimen had a lower cumulative fluid balance at 72 h post-randomization, as well as less need for RRT, a shorter duration of AKI, and fewer adverse events compared with usual care [40]. An adequately powered RCT is needed to confirm these findings.

Based on current evidence, fluid restriction in patients at risk of AKI or with AKI who are considered not to be hypovolemic appears to be safe except in those undergoing major abdominal surgery. When required, fluids should be given in small aliquots with frequent monitoring of hemodynamic indices and clinical response and should be individualized rather than employing a 'one-size-fits-all' approach. Regular adjustments based on the phase of resuscitation and clinical response are needed (Fig. 26.3) using basic and advanced assessment tools (Table 26.3).

**Table 26.3** Hemodynamic parameters to assess fluid status

| Parameters | Techniques/devices | Advantages | Limitations |
|---|---|---|---|
| *Static parameters* | | | |
| Capillary refill time | Clinical examination | Non-invasive | Operator dependent |
| Skin temperature | | Low cost | Lag time following resuscitation |
| Mottling | | Not dependent on resources | |
| Central venous pressure (CVP) | Central venous catheter insertion through internal jugular or subclavian vein | Useful to assess volume tolerance—an increase in CVP without improvement in CO indicates fluid non-tolerance | Invasive<br>Complications of central line<br>Not reliable in predicting CO in response to fluid challenge<br>Limited role in right sided heart failure<br>Median values (7–15 mmHg) are less informative |
| PA catheter | PA catheter insertion through pulmonary artery | Evaluation of volume status and hemodynamic parameters in patients with hemodynamic compromise | Invasive<br>More costly<br>Risk of mechanical and infectious complications |
| Evaluation of IVC | Ultrasound | Non-invasive | Operator dependent |
| – Diameter | | Estimates of CVP and caval index | Affected by changes in intrathoracic pressure/respiration/increased intra-abdominal pressure |
| – Collapsibility and distensibility | | Can be used in ventilated or spontaneously breathing patients | A negative test cannot rule out fluid responsiveness.<br>Challenges in obesity |
| Left ventricular end-diastolic volume | Trans thoracic echocardiography | Non-invasive | Operator dependent |
| | 2D Doppler | Assessment of cardiac anatomy and ejection fraction<br>Bedside availability | Poor echo window in obesity and ventilated patients<br>Real-time but non-continuous monitoring |
| Electrical bioimpedance | Constant electrical current stimulation for identification of thoracic or body impedance variations induced by vascular blood flow | Non-invasive | Inconsistent outcomes in case reports<br>Reliability in critically ill patients not clear |

| | | | |
|---|---|---|---|
| *Dynamic parameters* | | | |
| Pulse contour analysis | Pulse pressure variation (PPV) | Advanced hemodynamic and volumetric management | Invasive |
| | Stroke volume variation (SVV) | Allows continuous CO/CI measurements | Unreliable in patients with cardiac arrhythmias/IABP |
| Plethysmographic variability index (PVI) | Modified pulse oximeter to measure respiratory cycle-induced variation in the plethysmograph waveform | Non-invasive<br>Can be used in ED setting | |
| End-expiratory occlusion test | A 15-s end-expiratory occlusion to augment cardiac preload; an increase in cardiac output by >5% predicts fluid responsiveness, regardless of PEEP reading | Detection of preload responsiveness in mechanically ventilated patients | Ineffective if the spontaneous breathing activity is too high for sustaining the 15-s end-expiratory occlusion<br>Not suitable for non-intubated patients |
| Passive leg raising (PLR) test | A 45° PLR maneuver is performed in a recumbent patient | Most reliable to predict fluid responsiveness in both spontaneously breathing and intubated patient | Sensitivity depends on timing—hemodynamic effects reach their maximum within 1 min and diminish thereafter |
| | PLR mobilizes approximately 300 ml (4 ml/kg) from the lower extremities and transiently increases venous return as an internal fluid bolus | Reliable in cardiac arrhythmias and with low tidal ventilation, low lung compliance | Use in patients with high intra-abdominal pressure is not validated |
| | More reliable when coupled with SV monitoring; an increase in >10% in SV is considered fluid responsive | Good specificity | |
| Mini fluid bolus (100–200 ml) | A mini fluid bolus is given fast, followed by assessment of SVV and PPV | Use as an alternative in patients on low tidal volume ventilation | Effects are often short-lived.<br>Repeated mini boluses contribute to fluid accumulation |

*CI* cardiac index, *CO* cardiac output, *CVP* central venous pressure, *ER* emergency department, *IABP* intra-arterial balloon pump, *IVC* inferior vena cava, *PA* pulmonary artery, *PEEP* positive end-expiratory pressure, *SV* stroke volume

## 26.6 When to Stop Fluid Therapy?

The duration of fluid therapy should be as short as possible but as long as needed to correct hypovolemia. Fluids should be stopped once circulatory failure has resolved, patients are no longer preload responsive, or there are signs of fluid accumulation [10]. Prevention of further fluid accumulation and maintaining a neutral fluid balance should be the targets during the optimization phase. There is increasing recognition that hidden "fluid creep" from maintenance fluids and drug administration poses a risk during this period [41]. Excessive fluid administration after the onset of AKI is an independent risk factor for progression to severe AKI and non-recovery of kidney function [42].

Fluid accumulation syndrome is described as the presence of fluid accumulation with a negative impact on end-organ function, including kidney function. Indicators of fluid accumulation include clinical signs (daily weight change, positive cumulative fluid balance, raised CVP, raised IAP), laboratory parameters (hemodilution), radiographic signs (pulmonary edema on chest radiography, B-lines on lung ultrasonography, pleural effusion), or changes on echocardiography (raised filling pressure, increased extracellular lung water [ECLW] or global end-diastolic volume index [GEDVI]). The role of ultrasound to diagnose renal congestion in patients with AKI remains unclear. Fluid balance charting and daily weight measurement are easily acquired at the bedside. However, they do not specify the location of fluids or account for insensible losses and should be interpreted accordingly [1].

Various novel techniques are available to assess fluid accumulation. Bioelectrical impedance analysis (BIA) is a non-invasive method for estimating body fluid composition i.e., total, intracellular, and extracellular body water. This technique can quantify the degree of fluid excess and monitor intercompartmental changes after fluid removal but its role in critically ill patients receiving mechanical ventilation is unclear. Serum N-terminal pro-B-type natriuretic peptide (BNP) is associated with circulatory overfilling but does not provide any specific information about kidney function. The venous excess ultrasound score (VExUS) is derived from using point-of-care ultrasound to examine the inferior vena cava (IVC), hepatic vein, portal vein, and ideally intrarenal venous plexi. Venous congestion in these vessels may cause a change in blood flow velocities and directions. Whether there is a role of VExUS to guide fluid removal in patients receiving RRT or in patients with cardio-renal syndrome is under investigation .

## 26.7 De-escalation of Fluid Therapy

Fluid accumulation is common following initial resuscitation, in particular in patients with AKI. To date, there is no single parameter that indicates when fluid removal should begin. In fact, need for de-escalation, defined as rationalization of fluid intake, use of diuretic agents, and/or extracorporeal therapies, should be regularly considered during all phases of critical illness. Current practice of fluid removal is varied [43]. Small RCTs have shown that protocolized de-escalation/fluid removal is feasible, well-tolerated, and associated with improved outcomes and a more negative balance [44, 45]. The results of larger trials are awaited (ClinicalTrials.gov Identifiers: NCT04180397, NCT02765009).

To avoid harm from removing fluid ‘too fast’ but also ‘not fast enough’, it is important to determine fluid removal targets and fluid removal tolerance. The rate of fluid removal should not exceed the refilling capacity of fluid movement from the extravascular compartments back into the vascular space. The maximal refill rate is around 5 ml/kg/h in health but lower during critical illness. At present, there is no single factor that determines the optimal fluid removal rate. Parameters of fluid responsiveness can be used to indicate fluid removal tolerance. Fluid responsiveness during passive straight leg raising has been shown to predict inability to tolerate fluid removal during RRT [46]. Fluid removal should be stopped once the goal is achieved and/or signs of hypoperfusion occur.

The choice between diuretics and RRT depends on kidney function, urine output, electrolyte abnormalities, diuretic responsiveness, and degree of fluid accumulation. Diuretics have not been shown to prevent or reverse AKI, and oliguria alone should not trigger diuretic prescription without an assessment of volume status. Meta-analyses comparing intermittent bolus strategy over a bolus followed by a continuous infusion of furosemide in critically ill patients showed higher urine output achieved with the latter arm. However, there was no significant difference in mortality or ventilator days between the arms [47]. Diuretic non-responsiveness is defined as a furosemide dose equivalent to 1 mg/ml of daily urine output (e.g., 200 ml urine output in response to 200 mg of furosemide equates to an equivalent dose ratio of 1 mg/ml). Furosemide-nonresponsiveness has been shown to identify those at risk for RRT [48]. Further attempt to continue diuretics when target urine output is not achieved is not justified bearing the risks of side effects.

## 26.8 Fluid Management During RRT

In patients receiving RRT, the general principles of fluid management apply: in case of hypovolemia or reduced cardiac preload, fluid administration may be necessary. If fluid has accumulated and is contributing to organ dysfunction, including AKI, fluid should be removed. In this case, fluid removal may not only improve cardiac output but also decongest the kidneys and improve the chances of renal recovery. Adjustment of the fluid removal rate is essential to minimize the risks of hemodynamic instability and compromised renal perfusion. Data from an observational study indicate that the relationship between net removal rate and mortality has a U-shaped curve, with the lowest mortality associated with net ultrafiltration rates of 1.0–1.75 ml/kg/h [49]. Further sub-analysis from the same observational cohort also concluded that every 1.0 ml/kg/h increase in ultrafiltration rate is associated with a faster decline in renal function and a delay in renal recovery [50].

## 26.9 Areas for Further Research

Sparse data exist to guide fluid management in patients with AKI. Several biomarkers of renal damage have emerged over the past decade e.g., NGAL, cell cycle arrest biomarkers, etc. However, their clinical relevance as surrogates for patient-centered outcomes in fluid therapy are uncertain. Larger trials are required to determine the effects of a restrictive fluid regimen versus a conservative fluid regimen and the effects of de-escalation strategies on AKI progression. During RRT, the determination of optimal fluid removal rates, either by weight-based or physiologic parameters-based, needs to be investigated. Finally, the role of adjunctive techniques, such as machine learning to assess volume status and to assist fluid management in patients at risk of AKI or with AKI, requires further studies.

## 26.10 Conclusion

Fluids are drugs and should be administered to patients at risk or with AKI to correct intravascular hypovolemia and to improve cardiac preload. Various techniques are available to guide the assessment of volume status although preload responsiveness does not equate to 'need for fluids'. Current evidence does not suggest clear benefits of balanced crystalloids over saline to protect kidney function, but a signal in favour of balanced solutions. Saline has a role in correcting hypovolemia in patients with hypochloremia, and HES and gelatin should be avoided. There is a weak recommendation supporting albumin as an alternative to crystalloids during resuscitation, and for specific patient cohorts. After the initial resuscitation and correction of hypovolemia, conservative fluid management is safe in patients with AKI. De-escalation of fluid therapy includes minimizing fluid input and optimizing output by using diuretics and/or RRT. In patients treated with RRT, adjustment of the fluid removal prescription and monitoring of complications are essential to improve the chances of renal recovery.

## References

1. Malbrain MLNG, Martin G, Ostermann M. Everything you need to know about deresuscitation. Intensive Care Med. 2022;48:1781–6.
2. Vincent JL. Fluid management in the critically ill. Kidney Int. 2019;96:52–7.
3. Perner A, Prowle J, Joannidis M, Young P, Hjortrup PB, Pettilä V. Fluid management in acute kidney injury. Intensive Care Med. 2017;43:807–15.
4. Legrand M, Dupuis C, Simon C, et al. Association between systemic hemodynamics and septic acute kidney injury in critically ill patients: a retrospective observational study. Crit Care. 2013;17:R278.
5. de Laet IE, Malbrain M. Current insights in intra-abdominal hypertension and abdominal compartment syndrome. Med Intensiva. 2007;31:88–99.

6. Messmer AS, Zingg C, Müller M, Gerber JL, Schefold JC, Pfortmueller CA. Fluid overload and mortality in adult critical care patients—a systematic review and meta-analysis of observational studies. Crit Care Med. 2020;48:1862–70.
7. Ostermann M, Hall A, Crichton S. Low mean perfusion pressure is a risk factor for progression of acute kidney injury in critically ill patients—a retrospective analysis. BMC Nephrol. 2017;18:151.
8. Hjortrup PB, Haase N, Bundgaard H, et al. Restricting volumes of resuscitation fluid in adults with septic shock after initial management: the CLASSIC randomised, parallel-group, multicentre feasibility trial. Intensive Care Med. 2016;42:1695–705.
9. Varrier M, Ostermann M. Fluid composition and clinical effects. Crit Care Clin. 2015;31:823–37.
10. Ostermann M, Liu K, Kashani K. Fluid management in acute kidney injury. Chest. 2019;156:594–603.
11. Heringlake M, Berggreen AE, Reemts E, et al. Fluid therapy with gelatin may have deleterious effects on kidney function: an observational trial. J Cardiothorac Vasc Anesth. 2020;34:2674–81.
12. Moeller C, Fleischmann C, Thomas-Rueddel D, et al. How safe is gelatin? A systematic review and meta-analysis of gelatin-containing plasma expanders vs crystalloids and albumin. J Crit Care. 2016;35:75–83.
13. Finfer S, Bellomo R, Boyce N, French J, Myburgh J, Norton R. A comparison of albumin and saline for fluid resuscitation in the intensive care unit. N Engl J Med. 2004;350:2247–56.
14. Caironi P, Tognoni G, Masson S, Fumagalli R, Pesenti A, Romero M, et al. Albumin replacement in patients with severe sepsis or septic shock. N Engl J Med. 2014;370:1412–21.
15. Evans L, Rhodes A, Alhazzani W, et al. Surviving sepsis campaign: international guidelines for management of sepsis and septic shock 2021. Crit Care Med. 2021;49:e1063–143.
16. Joannidis M, Wiedermann CJ, Ostermann M. Ten myths about albumin. Intensive Care Med. 2022;48:602–5.
17. EASL clinical practice guidelines on the management of ascites, spontaneous bacterial peritonitis, and hepatorenal syndrome in cirrhosis. J Hepatol. 2010;53:397–417.
18. Lee EH, Kim WJ, Kim JY, Chin JH, Choi DK, Sim JY, et al. Effect of exogenous albumin on the incidence of postoperative acute kidney injury in patients undergoing off-pump coronary artery bypass surgery with a preoperative albumin level of less than 4.0 g/dl. Anesthesiology. 2016;124:1001–11.
19. Lee TH, Kuo G, Chang CH, et al. Diuretic effect of co-administration of furosemide and albumin in comparison to furosemide therapy alone: an updated systematic review and meta-analysis. PLoS One. 2021;16:e0260312.
20. Macedo E, Karl B, Lee E, Mehta RL. A randomized trial of albumin infusion to prevent intradialytic hypotension in hospitalized hypoalbuminemic patients. Crit Care. 2021;25:18.
21. Wilcox CS. Regulation of renal blood flow by plasma chloride. J Clin Invest. 1983;71:726–35.
22. Chowdhury AH, Cox EF, Francis ST, Lobo DN. A randomized, controlled, double-blind crossover study on the effects of 2-L infusions of 0.9% saline and plasma-lyte® 148 on renal blood flow velocity and renal cortical tissue perfusion in healthy volunteers. Ann Surg. 2012;256:18–24.
23. Toporek AH, Semler MW, Self WH, Bernard GR, Wang L, Siew ED, et al. Balanced crystalloids versus saline in critically ill adults with hyperkalemia or acute kidney injury: secondary analysis of a clinical trial. Am J Respir Crit Care Med. 2021;203:1322–5.
24. Khajavi MR, Etezadi F, Moharari RS, et al. Effects of normal saline vs. lactated ringer's during renal transplantation. Ren Fail. 2008;30:535–9.
25. Funke BE, Jackson KE, Self WH, et al. Effect of balanced crystalloids versus saline on urinary biomarkers of acute kidney injury in critically ill adults. BMC Nephrol. 2021;22:54.
26. Young P, Bailey M, Beasley R, et al. Effect of a buffered crystalloid solution vs saline on acute kidney injury among patients in the intensive care unit: the SPLIT Randomized Clinical Trial. JAMA. 2015;314:1701–10.

27. Semler MW, Self WH, Wanderer JP, et al. Balanced crystalloids versus saline in critically ill adults. N Engl J Med. 2018;378:829–39.
28. Self WH, Semler MW, Wanderer JP, et al. Balanced crystalloids versus saline in noncritically ill adults. N Engl J Med. 2018;378:819–28.
29. Zampieri FG, Machado FR, Biondi RS, et al. Effect of intravenous fluid treatment with a balanced solution vs 0.9% saline solution on mortality in critically ill patients: the BaSICS randomized clinical trial. JAMA. 2021;326(9):1–12.
30. Finfer S, Micallef S, Hammond N, et al. Balanced multielectrolyte solution versus saline in critically ill adults. N Engl J Med. 2022;386:815–26.
31. Sen A, Keener CM, Sileanu FE, et al. Chloride content of fluids used for large-volume resuscitation is associated with reduced survival. Crit Care Med. 2017;45:e146–53.
32. Hammond Naomi E, Zampieri Fernando G, Di Tanna GL, et al. Balanced crystalloids versus saline in critically ill adults—a systematic review with meta-analysis. NEJM Evid. 2022;1:EVIDoa2100010.
33. Ramanan M, Attokaran A, Murray L, et al. Sodium chloride or Plasmalyte-148 evaluation in severe diabetic ketoacidosis (SCOPE-DKA): a cluster, crossover, randomized, controlled trial. Intensive Care Med. 2021;47:1248–57.
34. Zampieri FG, Machado FR, Biondi RS, et al. Association between type of fluid received prior to enrollment, type of admission, and effect of balanced crystalloid in critically ill adults: a secondary exploratory analysis of the BaSICS clinical trial. Am J Respir Crit Care Med. 2022;205:1419–28.
35. Jaber S, Paugam C, Futier E, et al. Sodium bicarbonate therapy for patients with severe metabolic acidaemia in the intensive care unit (BICAR-ICU): a multicentre, open-label, randomised controlled, phase 3 trial. Lancet. 2018;392:31–40.
36. Wiedemann HP, Wheeler AP, Bernard GR, et al. Comparison of two fluid-management strategies in acute lung injury. 2006;354:2564–75.
37. Myles PS, Bellomo R, Corcoran T, et al. Restrictive versus liberal fluid therapy for major abdominal surgery. N Engl J Med. 2018;378:2263–74.
38. Rowan KM, Angus DC, Bailey M, et al. Early, goal-directed therapy for septic shock—a patient-level meta-analysis. N Engl J Med. 2017;376:2223–34.
39. Meyhoff TS, Hjortrup PB, Wetterslev J, et al. Restriction of intravenous fluid in ICU patients with septic shock. N Engl J Med. 2022;386:2459–70.
40. Vaara ST, Ostermann M, Bitker L, et al. Restrictive fluid management versus usual care in acute kidney injury (REVERSE-AKI): a pilot randomized controlled feasibility trial. Intensive Care Med. 2021;47:665–73.
41. Van Regenmortel N, Verbrugghe W, Roelant E, Van den Wyngaert T, Jorens PG. Maintenance fluid therapy and fluid creep impose more significant fluid, sodium, and chloride burdens than resuscitation fluids in critically ill patients: a retrospective study in a tertiary mixed ICU population. Intensive Care Med. 2018;44:409–17.
42. Zhang J, Crichton S, Dixon A, Seylanova N, Peng ZY, Ostermann M. Cumulative fluid accumulation is associated with the development of acute kidney injury and non-recovery of renal function: a retrospective analysis. Crit Care. 2019;23:392.
43. Murugan R, Ostermann M, Peng Z, et al. Net ultrafiltration prescription and practice among critically ill patients receiving renal replacement therapy: a multinational survey of critical care practitioners. Crit Care Med. 2020;48:e87–97.
44. Silversides JA, McMullan R, Emerson LM, et al. Feasibility of conservative fluid administration and deresuscitation compared with usual care in critical illness: the Role of Active Deresuscitation After Resuscitation-2 (RADAR-2) randomised clinical trial. Intensive Care Med. 2022;48:190–200.

45. Bissell BD, Laine ME, Thompson Bastin ML, et al. Impact of protocolized diuresis for de-resuscitation in the intensive care unit. Crit Care. 2020;24:70.
46. Monnet X, Cipriani F, Camous L, et al. The passive leg raising test to guide fluid removal in critically ill patients. Ann Intensive Care. 2016;6:46.
47. Ng KT, Yap JLL. Continuous infusion vs. intermittent bolus injection of furosemide in acute decompensated heart failure: systematic review and meta-analysis of randomised controlled trials. Anaesthesia. 2018;73:238–47.
48. Chawla LS, Davison DL, Brasha-Mitchell E, et al. Development and standardization of a furosemide stress test to predict the severity of acute kidney injury. Crit Care. 2013;17:R207.
49. Murugan R, Kerti SJ, Chang CH, et al. Association of net ultrafiltration rate with mortality among critically ill adults with acute kidney injury receiving continuous venovenous hemodiafiltration: a secondary analysis of the randomized evaluation of normal vs augmented level (RENAL) of renal replacement therapy trial. JAMA Netw Open. 2019;2:e195418.
50. Murugan R, Kerti SJ, Chang CH, et al. Association between net ultrafiltration rate and renal recovery among critically ill adults with acute kidney injury receiving continuous renal replacement therapy: an observational cohort study. Blood Purif. 2022;51:397–409.

# Cardiorenal Syndrome 1: What's in a Name?

27

H. A. I. Schaubroeck, W. Vandenberghe, and E. A. J. Hoste

## 27.1 Introduction

Cardiorenal syndrome (CRS) is defined as the pathophysiologic disorder of the heart and the kidneys whereby acute or chronic dysfunction in one organ induces acute or chronic dysfunction in the other organ, and consists of five subtypes. Any acute cardiac event leading to acute kidney injury (AKI) is called CRS type 1 or acute CRS (CRS-1) [1]. The kidneys are responsible for maintaining volume and electrolyte homeostasis and act as neurohormonal regulators [2]. As a consequence, the functions of the kidneys and the heart are heavily intertwined. Kidney impairment complicates the course of patients with cardiac disease and could in turn contribute to the progression of the acute cardiac disorder.

Depending on the underlying cardiac disorder (e.g., arrhythmia, acute coronary syndrome, acute heart failure, etc.), the pathophysiology and hence management of CRS-1 can be different. In this chapter, we focus on the definition of AKI and the specific issues of this definition regarding CRS-1 in the settings of acute heart failure and cardiac surgery. In addition, we briefly discuss management of these entities within CRS-1.

H. A. I. Schaubroeck (✉) · W. Vandenberghe
Intensive Care Unit, Ghent University Hospital, Ghent University, Gent, Belgium
e-mail: Hannah.Schaubroeck@Uzgent.be

E. A. J. Hoste
Intensive Care Unit, Ghent University Hospital, Ghent University, Gent, Belgium

Research Foundation-Flanders (FWO), Brussels, Belgium



J.-L. Vincent (ed.), *Annual Update in Intensive Care and Emergency Medicine 2023*,
Annual Update in Intensive Care and Emergency Medicine,
https://doi.org/10.1007/978-3-031-23005-9_27

## 27.2 Epidemiology

CRS-1 is a frequent condition, occurring in 47% of patients with acute heart failure, in 15% of patients suffering from an acute coronary syndrome, and in 22% of post-cardiac surgery patients [3]. Renal replacement therapy (RRT) is used in 4.3% of patients with acute heart failure and in 3.1% postoperatively after cardiac surgery [3]. In cardiogenic shock due to acute myocardial infarction, AKI occurs in 50% of patients, with up to 25% receiving RRT [4].

The occurrence of CRS-1 influences the prognosis of patients with acute heart failure or following cardiac surgery, even after correction for confounders, resulting in a longer hospital stay and increased mortality [3].

## 27.3 Pathophysiology

Similar to other types of AKI, CRS-1 is a syndrome with many causes leading to the same phenotype, i.e., AKI. In severely ill patients, the etiology is mostly multifactorial and several 'hits' may occur over a certain period of time. In addition to the impact of altered hemodynamics, other mechanisms may play a role, such as inflammation or toxicity by free hemoglobin [5]. Two hemodynamic concepts in the patient with cardiac disease are important for kidney function: perfusion and congestion [6]. A generally accepted mechanism of acute CRS in acute heart failure and following cardiac surgery is a low cardiac output, leading to increased sympathetic tone and renin-angiotensin-aldosterone-system (RAAS) activation, which causes sodium and water retention precipitating a vicious circle of progressive heart failure [2, 7]. Venous congestion plays a major role in the pathophysiology of acute CRS. Elevated central venous pressure (CVP) increases 'kidney afterload', which is even worse in the presence of increased intra-abdominal pressure (IAP) due to intra-abdominal fluid accumulation [8–10]. A low mean perfusion pressure (mean arterial pressure [MAP] minus CVP) causes decreased renal perfusion and possible renal ischemia despite the protective mechanism of renal blood flow autoregulation [10]. Additional contributing factors are activation of other neurohormonal pathways and induction of inflammatory cascades [2, 11].

Acute heart failure encompasses a heterogeneous syndrome which can be classified into several subtypes, depending on the predominant clinical feature (Table 27.1) [6]. The majority of patients with acute heart failure present with congestion and normal perfusion, and approximately 4% of patients with acute heart failure develop cardiogenic shock with predominantly left ventricular (LV) failure and marked hypoperfusion which can induce CRS-1 [12]. In patients with predominantly right ventricular (RV) failure and/or tricuspid regurgitation, congestion is the main driver for CRS-1 and can even induce liver failure or a cardiohepatic syndrome. These

**Table 27.1** Subtypes of acute heart failure according to mechanism, according to the 2021 European Society of Cardiology (ESC) heart failure guidelines [6]

| Acute heart failure phenotypes | Main mechanism |
|---|---|
| 1. Acute decompensated heart failure | LV dysfunction |
| | Sodium and water retention |
| 2. Acute pulmonary edema | Increased afterload and/or predominant LV diastolic dysfunction or valvular heart disease |
| 3. Isolated right ventricular failure | RV dysfunction and/or precapillary pulmonary hypertension |
| 4. Cardiogenic shock | Decreased cardiac output with hypoperfusion |

*LV* left ventricular, *RV* right ventricular

subtypes can also be observed following cardiac surgery, depending on the type of surgery and the pre-existent cardiac disease. Other important pathophysiologic pathways include inflammation caused by the surgical procedure and exposure to extracorporeal cardiopulmonary bypass, thromboembolic events, and altered hemodynamics during and following the operation [10].

Therefore, different phenotypes of acute heart failure have a specific trajectory and specific factors contributing to the occurrence of CRS-1.

## 27.4 Definitions

Since 2012, the Kidney Disease: Improving Global Outcomes (KDIGO) consensus group has standardized the definition and classification of AKI according to change in serum creatinine and/or urinary output (Tables 27.2 and 27.3), replacing previous AKI classifications (RIFLE, AKIN) [13]. Recently, KDIGO updated this definition and specified the concept of acute kidney disease (AKD) in order to harmonize the existing definitions of AKI and chronic kidney disease (CKD) [14]. AKD is used for patients with structural or functional abnormalities of the kidneys who do not fulfill the definitions of AKI or CKD. CKD requires at least a 3-month period of kidney impairment, AKI specifies a 7-day period of kidney impairment, while AKD is for episodes with a duration of less than 3 months (Table 27.2). In practical terms, AKD includes patients meeting AKI criteria but also patients with a more gradual decline in kidney function, such as a 50% increase of serum creatinine occurring over a period lasting more than 7 days (as opposed to AKI where the time-window is 7 days or less). Patients with an estimated glomerular filtration rate (eGFR) <60 ml/min/1.73 $m^2$, patients with a decrease in eGFR of 35%, and patients with markers of glomerular or tubular damage (e.g., hematuria, albuminuria, or pyuria) are also classified as AKD [14].

In the setting of CRS-1 caused by acute heart failure and following cardiac surgery, there are some important issues concerning the definition of AKI.

**Table 27.2** Definitions of acute kidney injury (AKI), acute kidney disease (AKD), and chronic kidney disease (CKD) according to the 2012 Kidney Disease: Improving Global Outcomes (KDIGO) guidelines and the updated guideline in 2021 [13, 14]

| | AKI | AKD | CKD |
|---|---|---|---|
| Duration | Within 7 days | ≤3 months | >3 months |
| Functional criteria | sCr ↑ 0.3 mg/dl over 48 h or >50% within 7 days or UO <0.5 ml/kg/h >6 h | AKI or GFR <60 ml/min/1.73 m$^2$ or ↓ GFR by ≥35% or ↑ sCr by >50% | GFR <60 ml/min/1.73 m$^2$ |
| Structural criteria | Not defined | Marker of kidney damage | Marker of kidney damage |

*sCr* serum creatinine, *UO* urine output, *GFR* glomerular filtration rate

**Table 27.3** Acute kidney injury (AKI) stages according to the 2012 Kidney Disease: Improving Global Outcomes (KDIGO) guidelines [13]

| AKI stage | Serum creatinine criteria | Urine output criteria |
|---|---|---|
| 1 | ≥1.5–1.9 × baseline or >0.3 mg/dl | <0.5 ml/kg/h for 6–12 h |
| 2 | ≥2.0–2.9 × baseline | <0.5 ml/kg/h for ≥12 h |
| 3 | ≥3 × baseline or ≥4 mg/dl or RRT | <0.3 ml/kg/h for ≥24 h or anuria for ≥12 h |

*RRT* renal replacement therapy

### 27.4.1 Urine Output Criteria

To meet the urine output criteria for AKI, a patient needs to have decreased urine output every hour for a period of at least 6 h. Staging of AKI using urine output translates to a less severe impact on outcomes compared to the same staging when using serum creatinine criteria [15–17].

As a first limitation, use of urine output criteria is only feasible in a patient with a urinary catheter in place and with staffing available for hourly recording of urine output. This requirement is difficult to meet outside the intensive care or cardiac care unit. Second, almost all these patients receive diuretics, which is not mentioned when defining AKI according to the KDIGO criteria. A more important concept in the setting of acute heart failure is the presence of diuretic resistance, caused by several factors, such as enteral malabsorption due to congestion, decreased renal blood flow, tubular injury, and low albumin. Diuretic resistance causes residual congestion and leads to increased rehospitalization and mortality rates [18]. Unfortunately, the definition of diuretic resistance, which could contain urine volume or natriuresis at a certain time interval following a fixed dose of diuretics, is not yet universal and needs validation in future research [18]. A furosemide stress test (bolus of 1 mg/kg furosemide in diuretic naïve patients and 1.5 mg/kg in previously exposed patients) has been used in critically ill patients with AKI to predict the severity of AKI [19]. The use of a furosemide stress test to predict development of AKI or even to guide treatment of acute heart failure is still under investigation (ClinicalTrials.gov Identifiers: NCT04464811 [ENACT-HF] and NCT04606927 [PUSH-AHF]).

### 27.4.2 Baseline Serum Creatinine

Establishing a baseline or reference value of serum creatinine may be particularly challenging in patients with heart failure. This baseline serum creatinine value is necessary to use as a reference for establishing a 50% increase of serum creatinine. KDIGO states that this value is "known or presumed to have occurred within the prior 7 days". A value that is representative for baseline kidney function may be determined from previous laboratory results up to 1 year prior to current diagnosis [13]. This implicates clinical judgement as blood draws are often triggered by clinical deterioration of the patient. In other words, creatinine values obtained, e.g., at admission for worsening heart failure do not reflect true baseline kidney function. This is especially relevant in heart failure patients in whom serum creatinine values are known to fluctuate over time [20].

If there are no serum creatinine values from the preceding year, several methods have been used in the literature. First, an estimated baseline serum creatinine can be calculated. This is based on "back-calculation" with the Modifying Diet in Renal Disease (MDRD) equation for eGFR and a conservative baseline eGFR of 75 ml/min/1.73 $m^2$ [21]. Alternatively, the nadir of serum creatinine during hospital stay, and the admission serum creatinine value have been used [22].

### 27.4.3 Serum Creatinine Criteria

Increases in serum creatinine are frequently seen in the course of acute cardiac disease, especially in acute heart failure and following cardiac surgery.

#### 27.4.3.1 Worsening Renal Function

The term 'worsening renal function' is frequently used to indicate these changes. An important constraint to the use of 'worsening renal function' is a lack of a consistent definition. Worsening renal function is often defined as an increase in serum creatinine of 0.3 mg/dl (26.5 μmol/l) or greater, which is similar to the KDIGO criteria for AKI, except for the fact that in worsening renal function there is no 48-h time window for changes in serum creatinine. However, other definitions of worsening renal function can be encountered such as an increase in serum creatinine of 0.5 mg/dl (44.2 μmol/l) or 25%, or a 20% decrease in eGFR [11]. In the past, worsening renal function has been associated with worse prognosis in patients with acute heart failure [3]. This observation has been challenged in more recent studies demonstrating that hemoconcentration is associated with a better prognosis despite occurrence of worsening renal function [23]. Similarly, when worsening renal function is associated with significant brain natriuretic peptide (BNP) reduction (>40%), patients are adequately decongested at discharge with favorable outcomes [24]. However, in the presence of congestion, worsening renal function is an independent predictor of death and death or rehospitalization [25]. These findings are consistent with the observation that worsening renal function in the context of aggressive forced diuresis by loop diuretics in patients with acute heart failure is not associated with acute kidney tubular injury as shown by kidney biomarkers [26]. In addition to diuretic treatment, there are several disease-modifying therapies for patients with acute heart failure, with proven benefit on hard outcomes that are associated with an increased risk for elevation in serum creatinine levels, such as angiotensin converting enzyme (ACE) inhibitors, angiotensin II receptor blockers or angiotensin receptor neprilysin inhibitors, and sodium glucose transport protein 2 (SGLT2) inhibitors. By contrast, over the long term, these drugs have proven to slow down deterioration of kidney function [27, 28].

#### 27.4.3.2 Pseudo-AKI, Functional AKI, and Subclinical AKI

To counter these discrepancies, Damman et al. introduced the concept of pseudo-worsening renal function and pseudo-AKI which indicate functional changes without structural damage to the kidneys ('functional AKI') [29, 30]. In patients with acute heart failure or following cardiac surgery, a change in kidney function is often due to either hypoperfusion or congestion and can be rapidly reversed after hemodynamic optimization. If AKI persists despite correction of congestion and perfusion, there might be structural kidney damage or 'true AKI' [29, 30]. Functional AKI has been observed in several prospective studies conducted in the immediate postoperative phase after cardiac surgery [31]. These patients have better kidney and overall outcomes compared to patients with AKI with evidence of tubular damage [31–33]. When kidney biomarkers are positive, but the patient does not meet the serum creatinine criteria for AKI, the term 'subclinical AKI' is used. Several studies have found an association of subclinical AKI and worse prognosis [34, 35] (Fig. 27.1).

Novel kidney stress or damage biomarkers measured in urine, such as neutrophil gelatinase-associated lipocalin (NGAL) and the NephroCheck® (Astute Medical, Inc., San Diego, CA, USA), which measures presence of insulin-like growth factor binding protein 7 (IGFBP7) and tissue inhibitor of metalloproteinases 2 (TIMP-2), have the potential to illustrate whether stress or damage to the kidneys is present. As such, the Acute Disease Quality Initiative (ADQI) envisions the use of these biomarkers in conjunction with the existing KDIGO AKI criteria in the future [36] (Fig. 27.2).

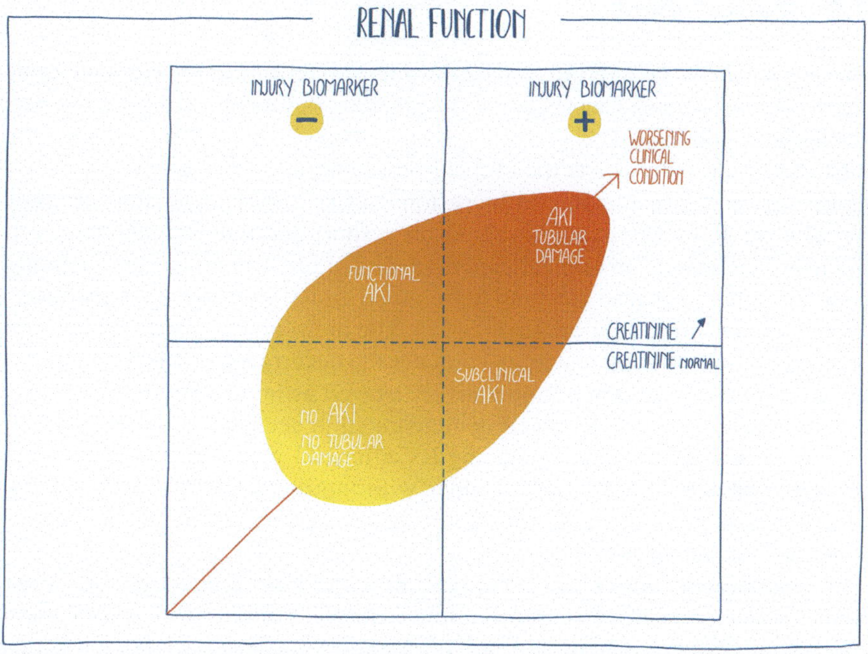


**Fig. 27.1** Spectrum of acute kidney injury (AKI) in patients with underling cardiac disease defined by injury biomarkers and serum creatinine values. Depending on these biomarkers, AKI can be divided into functional, subclinical, and 'true' AKI. Yellow indicates a good prognosis, orange a worse prognosis

| Functional criteria | Stage | Damage criteria |
|---|---|---|
| No change or sCr level increase <0.3 mg/dl and no UO criteria | 1S | Biomarker positive |
| Increase of sCr level by ≥0.3 mg/dl for ≤48 h or ≥150% for ≤7 days and/or UO <0.5 ml/kg/h for >6 h | 1A | Biomarker negative |
| | 1B | Biomarker positive |
| Increase of sCr level by > 200% and/or UO <0.5 ml/kg/h for >12 h | 2A | Biomarker negative |
| | 2B | Biomarker positive |
| Increase of sCr level by> 300% (≥4.0 mg/dl with an acute increase of ≥0.5 mg/dl) and/or UO <0.3 ml/kg/h for >24 h or anuria for >12 h and/or acute RRT | 3A | Biomarker negative |
| | 3B | Biomarker positive |

**Fig. 27.2** Proposed new definition of acute kidney injury: functional markers include serum creatinine (sCr) and urine output (UO) but new functional markers may be included. (Reproduced from [36] under the terms of a CC-BY license)

## 27.5 Management

To treat CRS-1, the underlying cardiac disorder should be tackled considering the underlying mechanism of acute cardiac dysfunction. Reversible cardiac causes need to be detected and treated.

The first step is to assess the clinical presentation of the patient. In case of hypoperfusion, perfusion should be restored using inotropes and/or vasopressors with the lowest possible dose and for a short duration [6]. The choice of drug heavily depends on clinical expertise taking into account several hemodynamic variables, because randomized clinical trials have not demonstrated a benefit from one drug over another [6, 37]. The inotrope levosimendan has beneficial effects on renal perfusion and reduces the occurrence of CRS-1 following cardiac surgery when used perioperatively as well as in the setting of advanced heart failure. Its effect is less well demonstrated in acute heart failure [38, 39]. If RV failure is predominant, reducing RV afterload with pulmonary vasodilators and/or inhaled nitric oxide together with inotropes and vasopressors may stabilize the patient. If drugs fail, short-term mechanical circulatory support should be considered [6].

In most patients with CRS-1, congestion is the main clinical feature. First-line treatment consists of loop diuretics, with early addition of add-ons with acetazolamide and/or thiazides in case of diuretic resistance [40]. For a practical approach to decongestion, we refer to a position paper by the European Heart Failure association [41]. An interesting and promising therapy is the RenalGuard® system (RenalGuard Solutions, Milford, MA, USA). This device combines furosemide-induced forced diuresis with real-time urine output measurement and closed loop fluid administration to prevent volume depletion. Several studies showed a lower incidence of AKI in RenalGuard® treated patients after percutaneous coronary intervention (PCI), transcatheter aortic valve implantation, and on-pump cardiac surgery [42].

In acute decompensated heart failure, maldistribution rather than overt fluid overload might be the main cause of congestion, and venodilatation (e.g., nitrates) is indicated [43].

In addition to targeting the underlying cardiac disease, further harm to the kidneys needs to be minimized. The potential risk of iodinated radiocontrast agents, nephrotoxic drugs, e.g., non-steroidal anti-inflammatory drugs (NSAIDs) and certain antibiotics, should be balanced against the potential benefit. Moreover, obstructive causes should be considered and treated accordingly. In view of toxicity, the dose of drugs cleared by the kidneys should be adapted to the GFR [13]. Whenever possible, up-titration of heart failure treatment should be performed to improve outcomes in patients with CRS-1. Studies are needed to explore continuation of these drugs in AKI KDIGO stage 3. SGLT2-inhibition has renoprotective effects and its early introduction in acute heart failure is safe [44]. Further research is warranted to explore the potential benefit of this class in CRS-1.

### 27.5.1 Renal Replacement Therapy

RRT is used in only a minority of patients with CRS-1 in acute heart failure and following cardiac surgery. In the last decade, several important randomized studies have been published regarding the indications and timing for initiation of RRT in cohorts of critically ill patients [45–47]. While a decade ago, early initiation of RRT was thought to lead to better patient outcomes, several large prospective studies have demonstrated that delayed initiation is associated with better patient outcomes as well as with a decreased use of resources as a sizeable number of patients was not treated with RRT at all. These studies demonstrate that RRT should be initiated when potentially life-threatening complications of AKI are present. These include severe hyperkalemia (>6.5 mmol/l, rapidly increasing, or with electrocardiogram [EKG] changes) and severe metabolic acidosis (pH <7.15). The threshold of azotemia to start RRT is less well defined [13]. The main indication for RRT in CRS-1 is fluid overload due to failure to decongest in the presence of diuretic resistance or anuria [13]. Ultrafiltration has been used as an alternative to loop diuretics for treating venous congestion, even in the absence of AKI. At present, data are inconclusive for the use of ultrafiltration compared to diuretics alone in CRS-1 [48]. Importantly, if initiation is delayed too long (oliguria for >72 h or blood urea nitrogen >112 mg/day), this is associated with worse outcomes [45].

In acute heart failure not related to cardiac surgery, evidence about the timing of RRT initiation is lacking. When looking at the evidence in patients following cardiac surgery, some small trials argue in favor of early initiation. This was consistent with the ELAIN trial, in which 40% of the included population had AKI following cardiac surgery. These patients had a survival benefit with early (defined as initiation within 8 h when criteria for AKI KDIGO stage 2 were fulfilled) compared to later RRT initiation [49].

Modalities of RRT in CRS-1 (intermittent, continuous, and hybrid techniques) have been reviewed elsewhere [47, 50].

## 27.6 Conclusion

The function of the kidneys and the heart are heavily intertwined. CRS-1 is frequent in patients with acute heart failure and following cardiac surgery and has a negative impact on prognosis. Defining CRS-1 in this specific population is challenging due to several limitations. Differentiation between functional AKI, subclinical AKI, and true AKI, based on biomarker assessment, should be targeted in future research. Management of CRS-1 in acute heart failure and after cardiac surgery primarily focuses on hemodynamic optimization, which should be tailored to the main mechanism of cardiac dysfunction. Effective and complete decongestion improves outcomes of these patients despite CRS-1. RRT is seldom needed. Interruptions in goal-directed medical heart failure treatment should be minimized. Other causes of AKI in this patient population should be excluded and treated.

## References

1. Ronco C, Haapio M, House AA, Anavekar N, Bellomo R. Cardiorenal syndrome. J Am Coll Cardiol. 2008;52:1527–39.
2. Harjola VP, Mullens W, Banaszewski M, et al. Organ dysfunction, injury and failure in acute heart failure: from pathophysiology to diagnosis and management. A review on behalf of the Acute Heart Failure Committee of the Heart Failure Association (HFA) of the European Society of Cardiology (ESC). Eur J Heart Fail. 2017;19:821–36.
3. Vandenberghe W, Gevaert S, Kellum JA, et al. Acute kidney injury in cardiorenal syndrome type 1 patients: a systematic review and meta-analysis. Cardiorenal Med. 2016;6:116–28.
4. Marenzi G, Assanelli E, Campodonico J, et al. Acute kidney injury in ST-segment elevation acute myocardial infarction complicated by cardiogenic shock at admission. Crit Care Med. 2010;38:438–44.
5. Wang Y, Bellomo R. Cardiac surgery-associated acute kidney injury: risk factors, pathophysiology and treatment. Nat Rev Nephrol. 2017;13:697–711.
6. McDonagh TA, Metra M, Adamo M, et al. 2021 ESC Guidelines for the diagnosis and treatment of acute and chronic heart failure. Eur Heart J. 2021;42:3599–726.
7. Rangaswami J, Bhalla V, Blair JEA, et al. Cardiorenal syndrome: classification, pathophysiology, diagnosis, and treatment strategies: a Scientific Statement From the American Heart Association. Circulation. 2019;139:e840–78.
8. Damman K, Navis G, Smilde TD, et al. Decreased cardiac output, venous congestion and the association with renal impairment in patients with cardiac dysfunction. Eur J Heart Fail. 2007;9:872–8.
9. Mullens W, Abrahams Z, Francis GS, et al. Importance of venous congestion for worsening of renal function in advanced decompensated heart failure. J Am Coll Cardiol. 2009;53:589–96.
10. Vandenberghe W, Bove T, De Somer F, et al. Impact of mean perfusion pressure and vasoactive drugs on occurrence and reversal of cardiac surgery-associate acute kidney injury: a cohort study. J Crit Care. 2022;71:154101.
11. Haase M, Muller C, Damman K, et al. Pathogenesis of cardiorenal syndrome type 1 in acute decompensated heart failure: workgroup statements from the eleventh consensus conference of the Acute Dialysis Quality Initiative (ADQI). Contrib Nephrol. 2013;182:99–116.
12. Crespo-Leiro MG, Anker SD, Maggioni AP, et al. European Society of Cardiology Heart Failure Long-Term Registry (ESC-HF-LT): 1-year follow-up outcomes and differences across regions. Eur J Heart Fail. 2016;18:613–25.
13. KDIGO working group. KDIGO clinical practice guideline for acute kidney injury. Kidney Int Suppl. 2012;2:1–138.
14. Lameire NH, Levin A, Kellum JA, et al. Harmonizing acute and chronic kidney disease definition and classification: report of a Kidney Disease: Improving Global Outcomes (KDIGO) Consensus Conference. Kidney Int. 2021;100:516–26.
15. Kellum JA, Sileanu FE, Murugan R, Lucko N, Shaw AD, Clermont G. Classifying AKI by urine output versus serum creatinine level. J Am Soc Nephrol. 2015;26:2231–8.
16. Priyanka P, Zarbock A, Izawa J, Gleason TG, Renfurm RW, Kellum JA. The impact of acute kidney injury by serum creatinine or urine output criteria on major adverse kidney events in cardiac surgery patients. J Thorac Cardiovasc Surg. 2021;162:143–51.e7.
17. Schaubroeck H, Vandenberghe W, Boer W, et al. Acute kidney injury in critical COVID-19: a multicenter cohort analysis in seven large hospitals in Belgium. Crit Care. 2022;26:225.
18. ter Maaten JM, Valente MA, Damman K, Hillege HL, Navis G, Voors AA. Diuretic response in acute heart failure-pathophysiology, evaluation, and therapy. Nat Rev Cardiol. 2015;12:184–92.
19. Koyner JL, Davison DL, Brasha-Mitchell E, et al. Furosemide stress test and biomarkers for the prediction of AKI severity. J Am Soc Nephrol. 2015;26:2023–31.
20. Mullens W, Damman K, Testani JM, et al. Evaluation of kidney function throughout the heart failure trajectory—a position statement from the Heart Failure Association of the European Society of Cardiology. Eur J Heart Fail. 2020;22:584–603.

21. Bellomo R, Ronco C, Kellum JA, Mehta RL, Palevsky P, Acute Dialysis Quality Initiative workgroup. Acute renal failure—definition, outcome measures, animal models, fluid therapy and information technology needs: the Second International Consensus Conference of the Acute Dialysis Quality Initiative (ADQI) Group. Crit Care. 2004;8:R204–12.
22. Hoste EA, Clermont G, Kersten A, et al. RIFLE criteria for acute kidney injury are associated with hospital mortality in critically ill patients: a cohort analysis. Crit Care. 2006;10:R73.
23. Breidthardt T, Weidmann ZM, Twerenbold R, et al. Impact of haemoconcentration during acute heart failure therapy on mortality and its relationship with worsening renal function. Eur J Heart Fail. 2017;19:226–36.
24. Stolfo D, Stenner E, Merlo M, et al. Prognostic impact of BNP variations in patients admitted for acute decompensated heart failure with in-hospital worsening renal function. Heart Lung Circ. 2017;26:226–34.
25. Metra M, Davison B, Bettari L, et al. Is worsening renal function an ominous prognostic sign in patients with acute heart failure? The role of congestion and its interaction with renal function. Circ Heart Fail. 2012;5:54–62.
26. Ahmad T, Jackson K, Rao VS, et al. Worsening renal function in patients with acute heart failure undergoing aggressive diuresis is not associated with tubular injury. Circulation. 2018;137:2016–28.
27. Wanner C, Heerspink HJL, Zinman B, et al. Empagliflozin and kidney function decline in patients with type 2 diabetes: a slope analysis from the EMPA-REG OUTCOME Trial. J Am Soc Nephrol. 2018;29:2755–69.
28. Fu EL, Trevisan M, Clase CM, et al. Association of acute increases in plasma creatinine after renin-angiotensin blockade with subsequent outcomes. Clin J Am Soc Nephrol. 2019;14:1336–45.
29. Damman K, Tang WH, Testani JM, McMurray JJ. Terminology and definition of changes renal function in heart failure. Eur Heart J. 2014;35:3413–6.
30. Damman K, Testani JM. The kidney in heart failure: an update. Eur Heart J. 2015;36:1437–44.
31. De Loor J, Herck I, Francois K, et al. Diagnosis of cardiac surgery-associated acute kidney injury: differential roles of creatinine, chitinase 3-like protein 1 and neutrophil gelatinase-associated lipocalin: a prospective cohort study. Ann Intensive Care. 2017;7:24.
32. de Geus HR, Ronco C, Haase M, Jacob L, Lewington A, Vincent JL. The cardiac surgery-associated neutrophil gelatinase-associated lipocalin (CSA-NGAL) score: a potential tool to monitor acute tubular damage. J Thorac Cardiovasc Surg. 2016;151:1476–81.
33. McCullough PA, Shaw AD, Haase M, et al. Diagnosis of acute kidney injury using functional and injury biomarkers: workgroup statements from the tenth Acute Dialysis Quality Initiative Consensus Conference. Contrib Nephrol. 2013;182:13–29.
34. Haase M, Devarajan P, Haase-Fielitz A, et al. The outcome of neutrophil gelatinase-associated lipocalin-positive subclinical acute kidney injury: a multicenter pooled analysis of prospective studies. J Am Coll Cardiol. 2011;57:1752–61.
35. Albert C, Albert A, Kube J, et al. Urinary biomarkers may provide prognostic information for subclinical acute kidney injury after cardiac surgery. J Thorac Cardiovasc Surg. 2018;155:2441–52.e13.
36. Ostermann M, Zarbock A, Goldstein S, et al. Recommendations on acute kidney injury biomarkers from the Acute Disease Quality Initiative Consensus Conference: a consensus statement. JAMA Netw Open. 2020;3:e2019209.
37. Mathew R, Di Santo P, Jung RG, et al. Milrinone as compared with dobutamine in the treatment of cardiogenic shock. N Engl J Med. 2021;385:516–25.
38. Zhou C, Gong J, Chen D, Wang W, Liu M, Liu B. Levosimendan for prevention of acute kidney injury after cardiac surgery: a meta-analysis of randomized controlled trials. Am J Kidney Dis. 2016;67:408–16.
39. Tholen M, Ricksten SE, Lannemyr L. Effects of levosimendan on renal blood flow and glomerular filtration in patients with acute kidney injury after cardiac surgery: a double blind, randomized placebo-controlled study. Crit Care. 2021;25:207.

40. Mullens W, Dauw J, Martens P, et al. Acetazolamide in acute decompensated heart failure with volume overload. N Engl J Med. 2022;387:1185–95.
41. Mullens W, Damman K, Harjola VP, et al. The use of diuretics in heart failure with congestion—a position statement from the Heart Failure Association of the European Society of Cardiology. Eur J Heart Fail. 2019;21:137–55.
42. Luckraz H, Giri R, Wrigley B, et al. Reduction in acute kidney injury post cardiac surgery using balanced forced diuresis: a randomized, controlled trial. Eur J Cardiothorac Surg. 2021;59:562–9.
43. Verbrugge FH, Grieten L, Mullens W. New insights into combinational drug therapy to manage congestion in heart failure. Curr Heart Fail Rep. 2014;11:1–9.
44. Schulze PC, Bogoviku J, Westphal J, et al. Effects of early empagliflozin initiation on diuresis and kidney function in patients with acute decompensated heart failure (EMPAG-HF). Circulation. 2022;146:289–98.
45. Gaudry S, Hajage D, Martin-Lefevre L, et al. Comparison of two delayed strategies for renal replacement therapy initiation for severe acute kidney injury (AKIKI 2): a multicentre, open-label, randomised, controlled trial. Lancet. 2021;397:1293–300.
46. Bagshaw SM, Wald R, Adhikari NKJ, et al. Timing of initiation of renal-replacement therapy in acute kidney injury. N Engl J Med. 2020;383:240–51.
47. Wald R, Beaubien-Souligny W, Chanchlani R, et al. Delivering optimal renal replacement therapy to critically ill patients with acute kidney injury. Intensive Care Med. 2022;48:1368–81.
48. Costanzo MR, Ronco C, Abraham WT, et al. Extracorporeal ultrafiltration for fluid overload in heart failure: current status and prospects for further research. J Am Coll Cardiol. 2017;69:2428–45.
49. Zarbock A, Kellum JA, Schmidt C, et al. Effect of early vs delayed initiation of renal replacement therapy on mortality in critically ill patients with acute kidney injury: the ELAIN Randomized Clinical Trial. JAMA. 2016;315:2190–9.
50. Schaubroeck HA, Gevaert S, Bagshaw SM, Kellum JA, Hoste EA. Acute cardiorenal syndrome in acute heart failure: focus on renal replacement therapy. Eur Heart J Acute Cardiovasc Care. 2020;9:802–11.

# Part VIII

# The Microcirculation and Metabolism

# 28 Update on the Microcirculatory Assessment of the Critically Ill Patient

S. H. Kuo, B. Ergin, and C. Ince

## 28.1 Introduction

One of the primary goals of intensive care medicine is to ensure that sufficient oxygen is delivered to the mitochondria to ensure adequate energy production needed for cell survival and function. To this end, it is key to ensure that sufficient oxygen-carrying blood reaches the microcirculation of the organs. The microcirculation is one of the main components of the circulation responsible for delivering oxygen, nutrients, hormones, and electrolytes to the organs and their parenchymal cells. It has been well established that deterioration of the microcirculation can lead to tissue hypoxia, cell death, and ultimately organ failure. However, in clinical practice, the focus is on the normalization of systemic hemodynamic parameters, such as arterial pressure, cardiac output, or left ventricular (LV) filling pressure, and the microcirculation has not been taken into account as a diagnostic parameter or target for treatment strategies, as yet. Early experimental studies suggested that the origin of the disease resided in the pathological heterogeneity of blood flow in the microcirculation, resulting in a defect in the oxygen extraction capacity of the parenchymal cells [1, 2]. Clinical introduction of orthogonal polarization spectral (OPS) imaging [3] enabled for the first time

S. H. Kuo
Department of Critical Care Medicine, Kaohsiung Veterans General Hospital, Kaohsiung, Taiwan

Department of Intensive Care, Erasmus MC, University Medical Center, Rotterdam, The Netherlands

B. Ergin · C. Ince (✉)
Department of Intensive Care, Erasmus MC, University Medical Center, Rotterdam, The Netherlands
e-mail: c.ince@erasmusmc.nl



J.-L. Vincent (ed.), *Annual Update in Intensive Care and Emergency Medicine 2023*, Annual Update in Intensive Care and Emergency Medicine,
https://doi.org/10.1007/978-3-031-23005-9_28

direct observation of the microcirculation of internal organs during neurosurgery. OPS imaging was further applied to the observation of the sublingual microcirculation in septic patients where severe alterations in capillary flow were observed [4, 5]. These studies unleashed a large number of studies that revealed the importance of the microcirculation in states of critical illness [6]. In parallel to the improvement in hand-held vital microscopes, image-capturing techniques and image analysis software provided deeper insight into the cause of a wide range of conditions in intensive care medicine.

Hand-held vital microscopy was thus introduced by the development of OPS imaging devices in 1999, whereby the microcirculatory system could be directly observed at the bedside. The technique was accomplished by illuminating tissue with light of a wavelength of 548 nm and linearly polarized light through a light guide with a magnifying lens at its tip, and then collecting backscattered light from the illuminated tissue through an orthogonal polarizer onto a charge-coupled device video camera system [3]. The green light used is absorbed by the red blood cells (RBCs) thus enabling the observation of RBCs flowing in the arterioles, capillaries, and venules of the organ's surface on which the light guide is placed. A next-generation, improved device was introduced called a sidestream dark field (SDF) imaging device (with a central light guide accompanied by concentrically placed light emitting diodes (LEDs)). By illuminating light of wavelength 530 nm from the outer core of the SDF light guide, tissue was illuminated from the side and reflected light collected by a centrally located light guide lens system, which was optically isolated from the illuminating outer ring to prevent the contamination by tissue surface reflections of illuminating light. The SDF image device enabled better observation of the microcirculatory system than its predecessor [7, 8] and has been used in many studies in the microcirculatory research field over the last decade. Subsequent, third-generation devices are referred to as incident dark field illumination (IDF) devices based on an early optical design by Sherman and Cook [9]. To date, IDF devices have provided the best images, revealing an additional 30% more visible capillaries than the previous generation devices [10]. In addition to IDF illumination associated with a high-grade magnification lens, the use of high-brightness LEDs with extremely short pulse time synchronized with the image acquisition enabled such sharp microcirculation images to be detected [11]. The use of IDF imaging can be regarded as the current state-of-the-art in clinical microcirculation research.

Despite limitations imposed by the technology for obtaining high quality video, and the long duration required for off-line software-based analysis, microcirculatory assessment of critically ill patients has provided detailed new insight into the origin of disease and the response to therapies. In this chapter, we would like to highlight the importance of the need to monitor the microcirculation at the bedside and update recent findings related to clinical microcirculation measurements in intensive care patients.

## 28.2 What Microcirculatory Measurement Has Taught Us About Pathophysiology

The second consensus on the assessment of sublingual microcirculation formulated by a European Society of Intensive Care Medicine (ESICM) task force provided a cornerstone for the clinical introduction of bedside monitoring of the microcirculation [12]. This consensus reviewed the need for better image acquisition and quality, and standardized image analysis and interpretation, and addressed the future requirements that needed to be met for the routine clinical introduction of microcirculatory measurement [12]. Specific patterns of microcirculatory vasculature alterations enable a differential diagnosis to be made to identify the cause of a loss of hemodynamic coherence between the systemic circulation and the microcirculation, in which normalized systemic variables are insufficient to identify the presence of microcirculatory dysfunction leading to parenchymal cell injury [13]. Four types of microcirculatory alterations can be identified, all associated with the development of reduced oxygen transport to the tissues by the microcirculation: heterogeneity, hemodilution, constriction/tamponade, and edema. The presence of heterogeneity in the perfusion of the microcirculation with the presence of plugged vessels next to patent vessels has been found to be specific to sepsis and associated with a high degree of sensitivity and specificity for mortality greater than those provided by systemic circulatory parameters [14, 15]. The consensus also identified the manner in which the different types of shock could be distinguished, how to perform a differential diagnosis on the types of microvascular alterations, and what to expect after interventions. Based on the foundation set by the consensus document, the assessment of the sublingual microcirculation has evolved beyond critical care. Currently, the state-of-the-art is focused on optimizing individualized care by microcirculation-targeted resuscitation and on early identification of medical treatment or interventions to optimize treatment response and prognosis. The inclusion of the ability to monitor the presence and activation of leukocytes [16] has in addition provided a unique monitoring platform to assess endothelial and inflammatory abnormalities in conjunction with the microhemodynamics associated with critical illness. From this point of view, bedside assessment of the (patho)physiological status of the microcirculation allows a personalized approach to be implemented in clinical practice by targeting resuscitation based on the normalization of the microcirculation in which differential diagnosis, identification and titration of treatment therapy, and (most importantly) evaluation of the efficacy of the therapy to normalize the microcirculation can be implemented.

## 28.3 Fluid Status

Administration of fluids is a cornerstone of the treatment of critically ill patients with hypovolemia or hypotension. Microcirculatory measurement during fluid therapy has been performed in various perioperative and intensive care studies. The need for the administration of fluids in response to the presence of hypovolemia can be assessed at the bedside by observation of reduced functional capillary density (FCD). FCD is defined by the total vessel density (TVD) and perfused vessel density (PVD) as a measure of diffusive capacity, and microvascular flow index (MFI) or RBC velocity (RBCv) as an indicator of the convective capacity of the microcirculation [12, 17]. Microcirculatory assessment found that the changes in afterload status were not directly related to the proportion of perfused vessels in microvascular perfusion [18] as expected, but were more related to preload [19]. In experimental and clinical studies, it was shown that colloids were more effective in recruiting the microcirculation than were crystalloids [20]. An optimal hemoglobin concentration for recruiting the microcirculation was investigated [21]. Recently a study suggested the presence of a possible coherent point (defined as mean circulatory filling pressure analog (Pmca)) between systemic hemodynamics and the microcirculatory system [22].

## 28.4 Sepsis

The mechanisms underlying the progress of sepsis to organ failure have been a source of speculation. A key role in this respect has been attributed to the pathogenesis of microcirculatory dysfunction leading to parenchymal injury. Several functional parameters of the microcirculation have been identified in sepsis patients, including alterations in FCD, TVD, PVD, MFI, and RBCv. Specifically, the heterogeneity index and space-time frames per vessel measuring perfusion abnormalities have been found to be altered, with their properties being different in different phases of the disease course and during resuscitation [12, 17, 23]. Such studies have shown that microcirculatory assessment in sepsis patients can predict the progress of the disease and the associated prognosis and mortality [10, 23, 24]. Assessment of parameters related to the function of the microcirculation may also provide insight into the efficacy of treatment, and even into the specific target for individualized treatment, which can lead to more effective treatment options, and more precise interventions and timing for effective control of sepsis [25–28]. By applying microcirculation assessment, it may also be possible to distinguish early on the development of sepsis from other forms of infection and shock [29, 30], thus providing a more sensitive window of opportunity to treat sepsis.

## 28.5 COVID-19

The coronavirus disease 2019 (COVID-19) pandemic has resulted in catastrophic casualties since late 2019, approaching 615 million confirmed diagnoses and resulting in 6.54 million deaths to date. COVID-19 has had not only a huge health issue-related impact but also a large socioeconomic burden. It is generally accepted that the endothelium is central in defining the pathophysiology of COVID-19 [31], which directly suggests the potential importance of microcirculatory monitoring for assessment of the presence and nature of the disease.

In a multicenter international study in COVID-19 patients, we investigated whether there were signs of microcirculatory alterations as are seen in sepsis [32]. Analysis of the microcirculation revealed the presence of increased microcirculatory leukocytes and microthrombi in agreement with the general finding of the inflammatory response known to occur in COVID-19 patients (Fig. 28.1). However, in this study we found, contrary to the microcirculatory alterations found in bacterial sepsis, increased TVD accompanied by a shift in RBC availability from the systemic circulation to the microcirculation as evidenced by a decrease in systemic hematocrit with a concomitant increase in microcirculatory hematocrit. These findings indicated the activation of an adaptive mechanism to enhance the oxygen extraction capacity of the microcirculation by decreasing diffusion distances between capillaries (increased TVD) and increasing convection of RBCs (increased RBC flow) in response to the COVID-19-induced hypoxia. A similar microcirculatory response to hypoxia has been shown to occur in healthy mountain climbers at high altitude conditions [33, 34]. This finding in COVID-19 patients explained the clinical condition described as "happy hypoxia" found in these patients [35]. Interestingly, this adaptive mechanism we found in COVID 19 patients was not present in patients who had sequential organ failure assessment (SOFA) scores >10 [32]. A well-described case study illustrating the various microcirculatory aspects of the COVID-19 patient, including recovery, was reported by Grewal and his colleagues [36] in a patient with subcutaneous emphysema, venous thrombosis, and pneumomediastinum. Microcirculatory images showed increases in PVD and RBCv as the disease became more severe indicating a need to recruit the microcirculation in response to hypoxia. Values returned to normality upon amelioration of the disease state.

Similar results as described above with variable properties have been found by other authors [32, 37]. Taken together, the loss of coherence between the systemic circulation and the microcirculation might serve as a predictor of the severity of disease and possibly be a prognosis factor for COVID-19 patients, a hypothesis which would need further study. In addition, the findings of multifocal microthrombosis and leukocyte recruitment might be a signal of activation of the inflammatory response [32, 38, 39]. The above findings support the idea that assessment of the microcirculation may provide a promising point-of-care modality for COVID-19 patients.

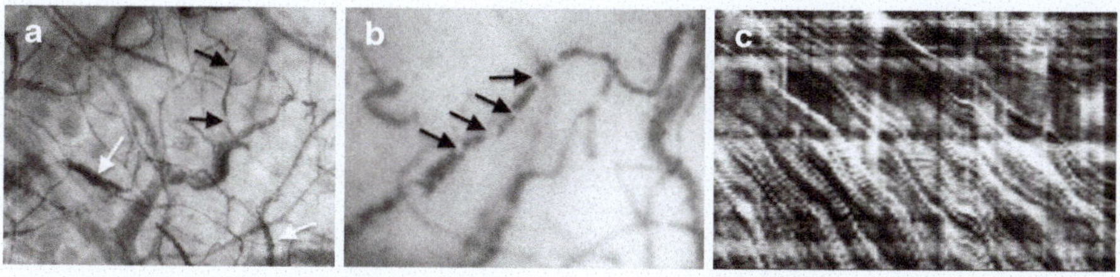


**Fig. 28.1** Sublingual microcirculatory images obtained from incident dark field illumination (IDF) camera in patients with coronavirus disease 2019 (COVID-19). Panel (**a**): Sublingual microcirculation with microthrombi (white arrow) and leukocytes (black arrow). Panel (**b**): Rolling leukocytes (black arrow). Panel (**c**): Space-time diagram showing the rolling leukocytes

## 28.6 Analysis of Microcirculatory Images and MicroTools as a Point-of-Care Tool for Microcirculatory Assessment at the Bedside

The analysis of microcirculatory images obtained from a hand-held vital microcirculation device has been challenging. Obtaining clinically significant functional microcirculatory parameters from vasculature mapping and flow calculation analysis has conventionally been done manually (AVA software), which was extremely time-consuming. A key requirement for reliable analysis to be made is that images are of sufficient quality for analysis. Quality can be assessed by the application of Massey's score, which requires five quality dimensions, including illumination, duration, focus, content, stability, and the presence of a pressure artifact [40]. For real-time clinical applications, there was a need for automatic analysis software. The first attempt for such a tool was provided by development of the so-called Automatic Vascular Analysis (Microvision Medical BV, Amsterdam, the Netherlands) [41]. This software was semi-automatic and had to be applied offline. It was a great step forward for clinical application because it allowed the calculation of quantitative variables related to the function of the microcirculation.

A major limitation impeding the introduction of microcirculatory assessment as a routine clinical technique has been the unavailability of quantitative automatic analysis software for real-time quantitative evaluation of the microcirculation. Such a development is essential to identify the quality of measurements and identify states of disease in need of therapy and ultimately to introduce microcirculatory-guided resuscitation where titration of therapy is indicated based on changes in the microcirculation [42].

Recently, we developed and clinically validated an automatic image analysis software platform for the analysis of microcirculation images for providing a quantitative assessment of microcirculatory variables, called MicroTools (Active Medical BV, Leiden, The Netherlands). We clinically validated MicroTools in an international database of 267 adult and pediatric patients in various states of disease [43], comparing analysis using MicroTools to analysis using the gold standard manual analysis and found a perfect correlation. Whereas manual analysis required in excess of 400 h to analyze the whole cohort, MicroTools was able to analyze the whole data set in under 45 min, supporting the idea that MicroTools can be used as a point-of-care tool at the bedside to implement microcirculation guided therapy (Fig. 28.2).

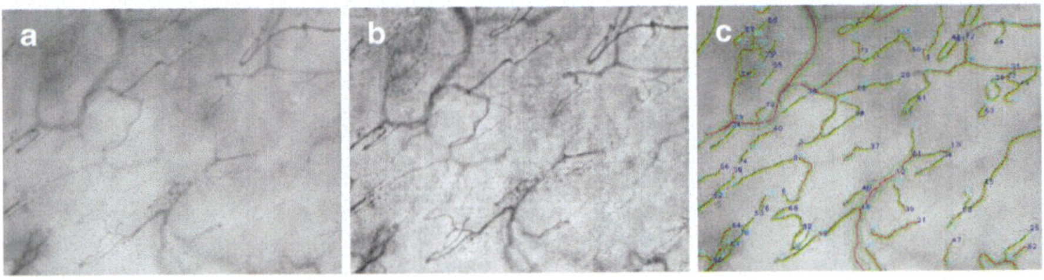


**Fig. 28.2** (**a–c**) Steps of sublingual microcirculatory analysis obtained from the fully automatic image analysis software, MicroTools (Active Medical BV, Leiden, The Netherlands)

Using MicroTools, the two main determinants of oxygen transport to tissue by the microcirculation can be quantified and distinguished, mainly the ability to quantify microcirculatory diffusion and its convection capacity. This ability enabled us to develop a new resuscitation parameter, which we termed tissue RBC perfusion (tRBCp) [44], which combined the diffusive and convective capacity of the microcirculation into a single parameter. We propose that this parameter might be a promising target to optimize microcirculatory tissue oxygen delivery in a resuscitation setting in critically ill patients [44].

## 28.7 Database Deep Learning and Artificial Intelligence

Gradually accumulating microcirculatory data in different states of disease and resuscitation have led to the suggestion that deep learning and artificial intelligence could be used to analyze images and extract clinically useful information from microcirculatory images [45].

Such an approach requires the availability of a large dataset to enable learning algorithms to be applied. To this end, we extended the previous data set we described in our clinical validation of MicroTools [43] to over 600 patients including information about their clinical status and their microcirculatory images. Using a subset of this database, we included four international, multicenter cohorts of critically ill COVID-19 patients and healthy volunteers and applied neuronal network training and internal validation on this data set. In addition, we quantified functional microcirculatory hemodynamic variables using MicroTools. Our results showed a slight advantage of artificial intelligence over MicroTools to distinguish COVID from healthy patients but when artificial intelligence analysis was combined with MicroTools, there was a high sensitivity and specificity to identify COVID-19 patients from microcirculatory images with an AUC of 0.84 [45]. This first such artificial intelligence study shows great promise for machine learning approaches for analysis of microcirculation images.

## 28.8 Future Developments

Current developments are ongoing to make microcirculation measurements more reliable and easier to perform. Such developments include optimizing image acquisition [46], introduction of educational programs [47], and the use of image stabilizers [48]. Further developments in the hardware investigated the potential use of other wavelengths showing improved image quality [49]. In addition, Kurata and co-workers proposed the use of dual-wavelength imaging to also obtain images of oxygen availability [50].

## 28.9 Conclusion

There is a severe lack of diagnostic tools at the bedside providing detailed information regarding the nature of disease and response to therapy. Such techniques are currently limited to the assessment of systemic hemodynamic variables and blood analysis whereas, outside of biomarkers, there is little to no information about the pathophysiological conditions of the parenchymal cells of the various organ systems. The nature of critical illness however is much more complex than systemic variables, which is why the introduction of microcirculatory analysis has had a significant impact on our understanding of the nature of critical illness over the last decade. Most importantly, these microcirculation studies have revealed the dissassociation between the macro- and microcirculations, especially in states of inflammation. These observations have provided valuable, personalized insight into critically ill patients. Microcirculatory assessment is a promising tool for the future that should be integrated with other bedside diagnostic tools. It is anticipated that receiving such detailed information about the origin of disease at the level of the microcirculation and its response to therapy will truly enable personalized medicine to be practiced at the bedside.

## References

1. Ince C, Ashruf JF, Avontuur JA, Wieringa PA, Spaan JA, Bruining HA. Heterogeneity of the hypoxic state in rat heart is determined at capillary level. Am J Physiol Heart Circ Physiol. 1993;264:H294–301.
2. Ince C, Sinaasappel M. Microcirculatory oxygenation and shunting in sepsis and shock. Crit Care Med. 1999;27:1369–77.
3. Groner W, Winkelman JW, Harris AG, et al. Orthogonal polarization spectral imaging: a new method for study of the microcirculation. Nat Med. 1999;5:1209–12.
4. De Backer D, Creteur J, Preiser JC, Dubois MJ, Vincent JL. Microvascular blood flow is altered in patients with sepsis. Am J Respir Crit Care Med. 2002;166:98–104.
5. Spronk PE, Ince C, Gardien MJ, Mathura KR, Oudemans-van Straaten HM, Zandstra DF. Nitroglycerin in septic shock after intravascular volume resuscitation. Lancet. 2002;360:1395–6.
6. Ince C. The microcirculation unveiled. Am J Respir Crit Care Med. 2002;166:1–2.
7. Ince C. The microcirculation is the motor of sepsis. Crit Care. 2005;9(Suppl 4):S13–9.
8. Goedhart PT, Khalilzada M, Bezemer R, Merza J, Ince C. Sidestream Dark Field (SDF) imaging: a novel stroboscopic LED ring-based imaging modality for clinical assessment of the microcirculation. Opt Express. 2007;15:15101–14.
9. Sherman H, Klausner S, Cook WA. Incident dark-field illumination: a new method for microcirculatory study. Angiology. 1971;22:295–303.
10. Yajnik V, Maarouf R. Sepsis and the microcirculation: the impact on outcomes. Curr Opin Anaesthesiol. 2022;35:230–5.
11. Aykut G, Veenstra G, Scorcella C, Ince C, Boerma C. Cytocam-IDF (incident dark field illumination) imaging for bedside monitoring of the microcirculation. Intensive Care Med Exp. 2015;3:40.
12. Ince C, Boerma EC, Cecconi M, et al. Second consensus on the assessment of sublingual microcirculation in critically ill patients: results from a task force of the European Society of Intensive Care Medicine. Intensive Care Med. 2018;44:281–99.

13. Ince C. Hemodynamic coherence and the rationale for monitoring the microcirculation. Crit Care. 2015;19(Suppl 3):S8.
14. De Backer D, Hollenberg S, Boerma C, et al. How to evaluate the microcirculation: report of a round table conference. Crit Care. 2007;11:R101.
15. Dobbe JG, Streekstra GJ, Atasever B, van Zijderveld R, Ince C. Measurement of functional microcirculatory geometry and velocity distributions using automated image analysis. Med Biol Eng Comput. 2008;46:659–70.
16. Uz Z, van Gulik TM, Aydemirli MD, et al. Identification and quantification of human microcirculatory leukocytes using handheld video microscopes at the bedside. J Appl Physiol. 2018;124:1550–7.
17. Moore JP, Dyson A, Singer M, Fraser J. Microcirculatory dysfunction and resuscitation: why, when, and how. Br J Anaesth. 2015;115:366–75.
18. Bond O, De Santis P, Iesu E, et al. Relationship between microcirculatory perfusion and arterial elastance: a pilot study. Crit Care Res Pract. 2019;2019:3256313.
19. Bouattour K, Teboul JL, Varin L, Vicaut E, Duranteau J. Preload dependence is associated with reduced sublingual microcirculation during major abdominal surgery. Anesthesiology. 2019;130:541–9.
20. Komori M, Samejima Y, Okamura K, et al. Effects of crystalloids and colloids on microcirculation, central venous oxygen saturation, and central venous-to-arterial carbon dioxide gap in a rabbit model of hemorrhagic shock. J Anesth. 2019;33:108–17.
21. Dyer WB, Simonova G, Chiaretti S, et al. Recovery of organ-specific tissue oxygen delivery at restrictive transfusion thresholds after fluid treatment in ovine haemorrhagic shock. Intensive Care Med Exp. 2022;10:12.
22. Chalkias A, Xenos M. Relationship of effective circulating volume with sublingual red blood cell velocity and microvessel pressure difference: a clinical investigation and computational fluid dynamics modeling. J Clin Med. 2022;11:4885.
23. Zhang XL, Li L, Peng QY, et al. [A preliminary study on the classification and prognosis of microcirculation alterations in patients with septic shock]. Zhonghua Nei Ke Za Zhi. 2021;60:898–903.
24. Holley AD, Dulhunty J, Udy A, et al. Early sequential microcirculation assessment in shocked patients as a predictor of outcome: a prospective observational cohort study. Shock. 2021;55:581–6.
25. Domizi R, Adrario E, Damiani E, et al. IgM-enriched immunoglobulins (Pentaglobin) may improve the microcirculation in sepsis: a pilot randomized trial. Ann Intensive Care. 2019;9:135.
26. Potter EK, Hodgson L, Creagh-Brown B, Forni LG. Manipulating the microcirculation in sepsis - the impact of vasoactive medications on microcirculatory blood flow: a systematic review. Shock. 2019;52:5–12.
27. Chen SH, Chan WS, Liu CM, et al. Effects of endotoxin adsorber hemoperfusion on sublingual microcirculation in patients with septic shock: a randomized controlled trial. Ann Intensive Care. 2020;10:80.
28. Duran S, Miedema D, Ergin B, Ince C. Sublingual microcirculatory evaluation of extracorporeal hemoadsorption with CytoSorb® in abdominal sepsis: a case report. Blood Purif. 2022;51:634–8.
29. Rovas A, Sackarnd J, Rossaint J, et al. Identification of novel sublingual parameters to analyze and diagnose microvascular dysfunction in sepsis: the NOSTRADAMUS study. Crit Care. 2021;25:112.
30. Fabian-Jessing BK, Massey MJ, Filbin MR, et al. In vivo quantification of rolling and adhered leukocytes in human sepsis. Crit Care. 2018;22:240.
31. Varga Z, Flammer AJ, Steiger P, et al. Endothelial cell infection and endotheliitis in COVID-19. Lancet. 2020;395:1417–8.
32. Favaron E, Ince C, Hilty MP, et al. Capillary leukocytes, microaggregates, and the response to hypoxemia in the microcirculation of coronavirus disease 2019 patients. Crit Care Med. 2021;49:661–70.

33. Gilbert-Kawai E, Coppel J, Phillip H, Grocott M, Ince C, Martin D. Changes in labial capillary density on ascent to and descent from high altitude. F1000Res. 2016;5:2107.
34. Hilty MP, Merz TM, Hefti U, Ince C, Maggiorini M, Pichler Hefti J. Recruitment of non-perfused sublingual capillaries increases microcirculatory oxygen extraction capacity throughout ascent to 7126 m. J Physiol. 2019;597:2623–38.
35. Couzin-Frankel J. The mystery of the pandemic's 'happy hypoxia'. Science. 2020;368:455–6.
36. Grewal S, Harjo B, Aykut G, et al. Case report: sublingual microcirculatory alterations in a Covid-19 patient with subcutaneous emphysema, venous thrombosis, and pneumomediastinum. Front Med (Lausanne). 2020;7:624695.
37. Hutchings SD, Watchorn J, Trovato F, et al. Microcirculatory, endothelial, and inflammatory responses in critically ill patients with COVID-19 are distinct from those seen in septic shock: a case control study. Shock. 2021;55:752–8.
38. do Espírito Santo DA, Lemos ACB, Miranda CH. In vivo demonstration of microvascular thrombosis in severe COVID-19. J Thromb Thrombolysis. 2020;50:790–4.
39. Bottari G, Ince C, Confalone V, et al. Case report: mMicrocirculatory leukocytes in a pediatric patient with severe SARS-CoV-2 pneumonia. Findings of leukocytes trafficking beyond the lungs. Front Pediatr. 2022;10:978381.
40. Massey MJ, Larochelle E, Najarro G, et al. The microcirculation image quality score: development and preliminary evaluation of a proposed approach to grading quality of image acquisition for bedside videomicroscopy. J Crit Care. 2013;28:913–7.
41. Bezemer R, Dobbe JG, Bartels SA, et al. Rapid automatic assessment of microvascular density in sidestream dark field images. Med Biol Eng Comput. 2011;49:1269–78.
42. Dilken O, Ergin B, Ince C. Assessment of sublingual microcirculation in critically ill patients: consensus and debate. Ann Transl Med. 2020;8:793.
43. Hilty MP, Akin S, Boerma C, et al. Automated algorithm analysis of sublingual microcirculation in an international multicentral database identifies alterations associated with disease and mechanism of resuscitation. Crit Care Med. 2020;48:e864–75.
44. Hilty MP, Ince C. Automated quantification of tissue red blood cell perfusion as a new resuscitation target. Curr Opin Crit Care. 2020;26:273–80.
45. Hilty MP, Favaron E, Wendel Garcia PD, et al. Microcirculatory alterations in critically ill COVID-19 patients analyzed using artificial intelligence. Crit Care. 2022;26:311.
46. Bruno RR, Schemmelmann M, Wollborn J, Kelm M, Jung C. Evaluation of a shorter algorithm in an automated analysis of sublingual microcirculation. Clin Hemorheol Microcirc. 2020;76:287–97.
47. Stankiewicz J, Jeyaraju M, Deitchman AR, Verceles AC, Grazioli A, McCurdy MT. Feasibility of tele-training to acquire sublingual microcirculatory images. ATS Sch. 2022;3:99–111.
48. Balestra GM, Bezemer R, Boerma EC, et al. Improvement of sidestream dark field imaging with an image acquisition stabilizer. BMC Med Imaging. 2010;10:15.
49. Liu B, He H, Feng X, et al. Sublingual microcirculation: comparison between the 415 nm blue light and 520 nm green light of sidestream dark field videomicroscopes. J Clin Monit Comput. 2023;37:297–302.
50. Kurata T, Li Z, Oda S, Kawahira H, Haneishi H. Impact of vessel diameter and bandwidth of illumination in sidestream dark-field oximetry. Biomed Opt Expr. 2015;6:1616–31.

# Intracellular Measurements of Micronutrients in the Critically Ill

# 29

A. M. E. de Man, F. A. L. van der Horst, and X. Forceville

## 29.1 Introduction

Micronutrients have been an area of intense research for decades in critical care; however the assessment of their status in intensive care unit (ICU) patients remains difficult [1]. This is problematic, because an adequate micronutrient status is essential for critically ill patients, due to the crucial role of micronutrients in metabolic, antioxidant, endocrine, and immune functions and thus in patient recovery [2, 3]. Measurement of plasma concentrations is the most common way to estimate micronutrient status. Decreased plasma concentrations are associated with poor wound healing, muscle weakness, inadequate immune response, and organ failure [4]. In critically ill patients, plasma micronutrient concentrations can be decreased up to 90% (!) [5] due to real losses through body fluids or increased metabolic use and/or apparent deficiencies caused by altered protein

A. M. E. de Man (✉)
Department of Intensive Care Medicine, Amsterdam UMC, Vrije Universiteit Amsterdam, Amsterdam, The Netherlands
e-mail: ame.deman@amsterdamumc.nl

F. A. L. van der Horst
Department of Clinical Chemistry, Reinier Medical Diagnostic Center, Delft, The Netherlands

X. Forceville
Centre Hospitalier Universitaire (CHU) de Rennes, CIC 1414 (Centre d'Investigation Clinique de Rennes), Inserm, Rennes, France

 
J.-L. Vincent (ed.), *Annual Update in Intensive Care and Emergency Medicine 2023*, Annual Update in Intensive Care and Emergency Medicine,
https://doi.org/10.1007/978-3-031-23005-9_29

binding, dilution, or redistribution due to inflammation. Therefore, plasma concentrations frequently may not adequately represent body status. In addition, these measurements of plasma concentrations are complex and expensive and mostly only available once every 2 weeks in routine settings. Therefore, in most critical care settings micronutrients are pragmatically supplemented, without estimation of their concentrations. Guidelines for micronutrient provision during critical illness are largely empiric [3]. However, administration of micronutrients to patients without a real micronutrient deficiency is unlikely to yield benefit and may potentially be disadvantageous. For example, vitamins C and E may sometimes disturb immune homeostasis by increased production of pro-inflammatory cytokines [6]. Furthermore, pro-oxidants are necessary to overcome antioxidant production by pathogens in some settings [7–9]. Plasma concentrations may therefore not be helpful in the management of critically ill patients. Intracellular concentrations may reflect the functional micronutrient status more adequately in case of inflammation. Erythrocytes and leukocytes are readily accessible body cells to assess the micronutrient status with. However, interpretation of the functional status based on intracellular concentrations can be complex. For example, the selenium atom is always inserted by covalent liaison(s) in selenocompounds (such as selenocysteine at the active site of all selenoenzymes, selenite, and the storage form selenomethionine). It does not act as a cofactor and/or ion, which is a crucial difference with nearly all other trace elements, such as zinc [10].

In this chapter, we will discuss the effects of inflammation on micronutrient plasma levels and summarize the results of relevant clinical studies investigating simultaneously plasma and intracellular measurements of micronutrients in patients with inflammation and in critically ill patients.

## 29.2 Inflammation

Most critically ill patients develop systemic inflammation in the early phase of their ICU stay due to their underlying illness, such as sepsis, trauma, or post-cardiac arrest. Release of pro-inflammatory cytokines increases capillary permeability, leading to leakage of plasma constituents to the interstitium, including the carrier proteins albumin and retinol binding protein. In addition, the production of these carrier proteins in the liver is decreased during inflammation [5]. Furthermore, sequestration of several micronutrients in the liver and other organs is stimulated by pro-inflammatory cytokines [11]. All these factors result in decreased circulating levels of multiple micronutrients [5].

Estimating micronutrient body status by plasma concentrations assumes a static equilibrium between circulating, tissue, and storage pools. However, the concentrations in these compartments is dynamic, and strongly affected by systemic inflammation [12]. This redistribution of the micronutrients between the different pools may be of benefit to the host. For example, the hepatic sequestration of zinc may guarantee its availability for crucial processes such as synthesis of acute-phase proteins and prevention of microbial invasion. Deprivation of plasma iron and selenium [13] may hamper bacterial growth. Low plasma concentrations may therefore not indicate deficiency in these cases, but reflect a beneficial adaption [12].

The magnitude of the effect of inflammation on plasma concentrations of micronutrients is often substantial, especially when C-reactive protein (CRP) concentrations are high. The effect is also highly variable, making adjustment of plasma concentrations based on CRP concentrations unreliable. Despite extensive reporting in the literature, there remains a general lack of awareness of the impact of inflammation on plasma micronutrient concentrations in clinical medicine, including among the critical care society [5].

## 29.3 Real vs. Apparent Deficiency

In critically ill patients, 'deficiency' is mostly defined as plasma concentrations below a reference interval (as defined for healthy persons). However, decreased plasma micronutrient concentrations can be caused by apparent and/or real deficiency (Fig. 29.1). Apparent deficiency can be caused by systemic inflammation with redistribution, decrease in carrier proteins, and hemodilution due to fluid loading [14]. Real deficiency can result from pre-existent malnutrition, losses from body fluids (increased urinary excretion, transdermal fluid losses through burn or traumatic wounds, gastrointestinal fistulae) or continuous renal replacement therapy (water-soluble micronutrients), decreased intestinal absorption, insufficient intake, medication use, and increased metabolic consumption. It is impossible to quantify the contribution of each factor to the low plasma concentrations. The question is whether threshold levels can be defined below which *real* deficiency is certainly present irrespective of the systemic inflammation [5]. In addition, it is not always possible to measure all relevant levels of a biomarker in a routine setting to assess the physiological status. For example, in the case of selenium, plasma selenium concentration does not provide information about: (1) the concentration on selenoenzymes, which are the effectors of antioxidant action or intracellular redox potential control; (2) the selenium storage form, selenomethionine [13, 15–18]; (3) derivates of selenite in case of infusion or bolus administration [13, 15–18].

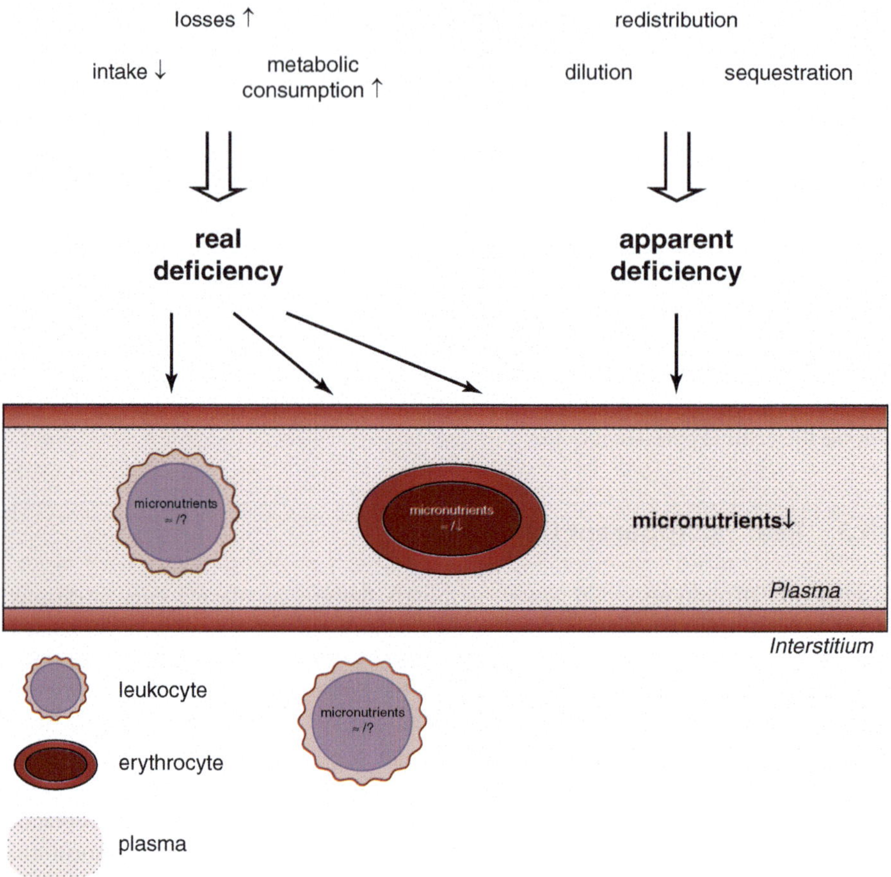


**Fig. 29.1** Real versus apparent deficiency of micronutrients

## 29.4 Elective Surgery as a Model for Inflammatory Response

Elective knee or hip arthroplasty induces a significant and reproducible systemic inflammatory response and therefore has been considered as an ideal model to examine the effect of inflammation on plasma micronutrient concentrations and their evolution when the systemic inflammatory response declines. In all studies investigating patients undergoing elective knee or hip surgery, postoperative CRP values peaked at 48 h [19–23]. In 10 patients who underwent knee arthroplasty plasma, flavin adenine dinucleotide (FAD, an indicator of B2) and pyridoxal-5′-phosphate (PLP, an indicator of B6) concentrations fell transiently ($p < 0.001$) by 37% and 48%, respectively, and had a time course inverse to that of CRP concentrations with their nadir after 48 h. Plasma FAD and PLP concentrations returned to pre-operative values by the seventh day post-operation without any dietary intervention, whereas CRP had substantially decreased by this time point but not fully returned to pre-operative levels [19]. In another study after knee arthroplasty (n = 11) mean plasma zinc concentrations fell by 40% ($p < 0.001$) at 24 h and selenium by 30% ($p < 0.001$) at 72 h. Both returned toward pre-operative values by 168 h without dietary intervention [20]. In a third study investigating 33 patients after knee arthroplasty, 25-hydroxyvitamin D (25(OH) D) concentrations decreased by 40% ($p < 0.001$) 6–12 h post-operation, and had not returned to pre-operative concentrations by day 5 ($p < 0.001$) [21].

In 11 adult patients after elective hip arthroplasty, plasma vitamin C fell substantially by 74% ($p < 0.01$) with the nadir on day 2–3, and vitamin E by 36% ($p < 0.01$) with the nadir on day 1–3, whereas CRP increased significantly by 160-fold with the peak on day 2 ($p < 0.01$) [22]. In 26 patients who underwent uncomplicated orthopedic operations (osteotomies, joint reconstructions, bone transplant/biopsies, arthrodesis), plasma vitamin A (↓40%), plasma vitamin E (↓27%), leukocyte vitamin C (↓41%), and plasma vitamin B6 (↓54%) mirrored the changes in CRP 48 h postoperatively, whereas serum folate (↓35%) and plasma vitamin C concentrations (↓40%) also decreased but followed a more random pattern [23].

## 29.5 Intracellular Measurements

Intracellular measurements could be a better reflection of micronutrient tissue status compared to plasma levels in ICU patients [24] and in other patients with inflammation, because they are less affected during times of acute illness and inflammation. Plasma concentrations of micronutrients are a short-term index, fluctuating over a shorter time-scale than intracellular concentrations [25]. Blood cells are readily accessible. Erythrocytes (life span 110 days) have limited metabolic activity including glycolysis, the Rapoport-Luebering shunt, the pentose phosphate pathway, antioxidant reactions, nucleotide metabolism reactions, and membrane transport processes. It is likely that erythrocyte concentrations will indicate long-term micronutrient status [26], whereas leukocytes may more accurately reflect acute changes in micronutrients status. Leukocytes have a higher metabolic activity, shorter life span (13–20 days), and are nucleated and therefore more likely to be representative of tissue cells [27]. However, leukocyte metabolism is strongly modified during sepsis and acute inflammation with an: (1) up to 100-fold oxygen consumption increase; (2) synthesis and excretion of reactive halogen and oxygen species; (3) and nevertheless an increased half-life [13].

### 29.5.1 Practical Issues: Erythrocytes

Erythrocytes are abundantly present and therefore simpler to separate and analyze than leukocytes [28]. Erythrocyte analytes are mostly expressed as a ratio of the hemoglobin concentration to correct for inaccuracy in pipetting packed red blood cells (RBCs). An attractive alternative option is expression as a ratio of the iron concentration (as a substitute for hemoglobin), which can be simultaneously measured with other trace elements by inductively coupled plasma mass spectrometry (ICP-MS). To make erythrocytes easier to use as a matrix for routine analysis, the decision can be made not to wash erythrocytes prior to analysis, although this will make the results less precise [20].

### 29.5.2 Practical Issues: Leukocytes

Considerable practical difficulties make leukocytes less attractive in a routine setting. A substantial volume of blood is needed and the blood samples have to be processed within 2 h after collection, because the concentrations of the leukocytes change quickly [26]. Furthermore, separation and isolation of leukocytes is laborious and requires skilled laboratory personnel. The standard methods of isolating leukocytes are prone to contamination with platelets, leading to variation in the relative contribution of platelets [29]. In addition, leukocyte populations may vary considerably in the relative proportions of granulocytes and mononuclear cells. Trying to avoid this by separation of granulocytes and mononuclear cells will be even more laborious and time consuming and there will always be some degree of contamination with other cell types [29]. Because of these issues, the leukocyte (buffy layer) estimation is rather crude and subject to considerable difficulty in interpretation.

## 29.6 Clinical Studies with Intracellular Measurements

In the last two decades, several studies have compared intracellular measurements of micronutrients with plasma concentrations, mostly in erythrocytes (Table 29.1).

### 29.6.1 Elective Knee Arthroplasty

Two studies investigated erythrocyte concentrations of micronutrients in patients having elective knee arthroplasty, as model for a significant and reproducible systemic inflammatory response. In 10 patients, erythrocyte thiamine diphosphate (TDP, an indicator of B1) concentration remained stable and within the reference range over the period of the study. TDP is largely located in the erythrocyte and as such is a recognized marker of tissue status. Erythrocyte FAD (an indicator of B2) and PLP (an indicator of B6) also remained stable and within reference intervals over the study period of 7 days. By contrast, plasma concentrations of FAD and PLP decreased below the reference range, inversely to the CRP-peak, and normalized at the end of the study period [19].

In a second study of 11 patients, mean plasma zinc and selenium concentrations decreased by 40% and 30%, respectively, with nadirs at 24 h for zinc and 72 h for selenium, and normalization of both by 168 h. The erythrocyte concentrations of zinc and selenium remained stable throughout the study period. These studies suggest that erythrocyte FAD, PLP, zinc, and selenium concentrations are not affected by the systemic inflammatory response [20].

**Table 29.1** Studies comparing intracellular measurements of micronutrients with plasma concentrations

| Micronutrient | Author [ref] | Population *Timepoint* | Plasma | Erythrocytes | Leukocytes |
|---|---|---|---|---|---|
| **Vitamin B1** | **Gray** [19] | **Knee arthroplasty** | | **TDP (ng/g Hb)** | |
| | n = 10 | *Baseline* | | 411 (351–549) | |
| | | *48 h* | | 462 (305–600) | |
| | | *168 h* | | 413 (353–552) | |
| | | Difference | | $p = 0.015$ | |
| **Vitamin B2** | **Gray** [19] | **Knee arthroplasty** | **FAD (nmol/l)** | **FAD (nmol/g Hb)** | |
| | n = 10 | *Baseline* | 62 (52–105) | 2.45 (1.70–3.90) | |
| | | *48 h* | 39 (24–76) | | |
| | | *168 h* | 66 (36–97) | 2.7 (1.9–3.8) | |
| | | Difference | $p < 0.001$ | $p = 0.115$ | |
| **Vitamin B6** | **Gray** [19] | **Knee arthroplasty** | **PLP (nmol/l)** | **PLP (pmol/g Hb)** | |
| | n = 10 | *Baseline* | 25 (17–36) | 295 (210–550) | |
| | | *48 h* | 13 (10–18) | | |
| | | *168 h* | 23 (13–29) | 320 (240–580) | |
| | | Difference | $p < 0.001$ | $p = 0.409$ | |
| | **Vasilaki** [28] | | **PLP (nmol/l)** | **PLP (pmol/g Hb)** | **PLP (pmol/$10^6$ cells)** |
| | n = 126 | **Healthy** | 52 (19–194) | 391 (234–815) | |
| | n = 96 | **Critically ill** | 20 (<2–333) | 261 (104–25,583) | 2.2 (0.4–8.2) |
| | | Difference | $p < 0.001$ | $p < 0.001$ | |
| **Vitamin C** | **Carr** [25] | | **Ascorbate (µmol/l)** | **Erythrocyte ascorbate (µmol/l)** | **Neutrophil ascorbate (nmol/$10^6$ cells)** |
| | n = 20 | **Healthy** | 88 (71–91) | 69 (65–110) | 0.35 (0.31–0.39) |
| | n = 18 | **Sepsis** | 14 (7.2–21) | 30 (17–42) | 0.33 (0.27–0.46) |
| | | Difference | $p < 0.001$ | $p = 0.002$ | $p > 0.05$ |
| **Vitamin E** | **Vasilaki** [30] | | **α-tocopherol (µmol/l)** | **α-tocopherol (nmol/g Hb)** | |
| | n = 67 | **Healthy** | 29 (14–47) | 18.5 (12–28) | |
| | n = 82 | **Critically ill** | 15 (4–41) | 18.6 (3.4–39.3) | |
| | | Difference | $p < 0.001$ | $p = 0.852$ | |

(continued)

**Table 29.1** (continued)

| Micronutrient | Author [ref] | Population<br>*Timepoint* | Plasma | Erythrocytes | Leukocytes |
|---|---|---|---|---|---|
| **Zinc** | **Ruocco** [11] | | **Zinc (µmol/l)** | **Zinc (µmol/l)** | |
| | n = 66 | **Critically ill** | 8.3 (SE 2.6) | 1.69 (SE 0.35) | |
| | n = 29 | **Sepsis** | 8.7 (SE 6.1) | 1.60 (0.48) | |
| | | Difference | p = 0.32 | p = 0.46 | |
| | **Oakes** [20] | **Knee arthroplasty** | **Zinc (µmol/l)** | **Zinc (µmol/mmol Fe)** | |
| | n = 11 | *Baseline* | 14.9 (13.1–17.9) | 10.2 (8.6–11.2) | |
| | | *24 h* | 9.3 (8.8–11.5) | | |
| | | *168 h* | 14.4 (12.4–20.3) | 10.6 (9.2–11.8) | |
| | | Difference | −40%, p < 0.001 (−32 to −44%) | | |
| | **Stefanowicz** [31] | | **Zinc (µmol/l)** | **Zinc (nmol/g Hb)** | |
| | n = 125 | Critically ill | 4.5 (0.6–27.0) | 581 (399–812) | |
| **Selenium** | **Ruocco** [11] | | **Selenium (µmol/l)** | **Selenium (µmol/l)** | |
| | n = 66 | **Critically ill** | 0.19 (SE 0.05) | 0.92 (SE 0.33) | |
| | n = 29 | **Sepsis** | 0.17 (SE 0.07) | 0.84 (SE 0.39) | |
| | | Difference | p = 0.02 | p = 0.05 | |
| | **Oakes** [20] | | **Selenium (µmol/l)** | **Selenium (µmol/mmol Fe)** | |
| | n = 11 | **Knee arthroplasty** | | | |
| | | Baseline | 0.89 (0.79–1.14) | 84 (69–136) | |
| | | 72 h | 0.66 (0.51–0.80) | | |
| | | 168 h | 0.87 (0.66–1.01) | 85.7 (66–135) | |
| | | Difference | −30% p < 0.001 (−22 to −36%) | | |
| | **Stefanowicz** [31] | | **Selenium (µmol/l)** | **Selenium (nmol/g Hb)** | |
| | n = 125 | Critically ill | 0.31 (0.01–5.68) | 5.3 (2.48–10.62) | |

*FAD* flavin adenine dinucleotide, *TDP* thiamine diphosphate, *PLP* pyridoxal-5′-phosphate

### 29.6.2 Critically Ill Patients

Two studies compared intracellular measurements in critically ill patients with values in healthy volunteers. In the first study (126 healthy volunteers and 96 critically ill patients), median plasma PLP was 62% lower in the critically ill group than in the healthy volunteers ($p < 0.001$), whereas the median red cell PLP was 33% lower ($p < 0.001$). White blood cell PLP concentrations could not be compared because they were not part of the original protocol and therefore not measured in the control group. These results support the hypothesis that erythrocyte PLP concentrations may be a more accurate reflection of tissue status than plasma measurements in critically ill patients [28]. In a second study (67 healthy volunteers and 82 critically ill patients), plasma α-tocopherol (an indicator of vitamin E) was significantly lower in critically ill patients compared with the controls ($p < 0.001$) with 41% of patients having concentrations below the reference interval. Erythrocyte α-tocopherol corrected for hemoglobin was similar ($p = 0.852$) in the critically ill patients and control subjects. The results of this study illustrated the discrepancy between vitamin E measurements in plasma and in erythrocytes [30].

In a study investigating 95 critically ill patients (29 with sepsis) in Brazil, mean selenium plasma and erythrocyte concentrations were significantly lower in patients with sepsis compared with the other critically ill patients. These results probably reflect two different mechanisms. Plasma selenium and selenoprotein-P decrease is associated with sepsis and its severity. In addition, there is a large selenium deficiency in Brazil that is likely to be implicated in low erythrocyte selenium concentration [11, 32]. These previously selenium-deficient patients are likely more susceptible to sepsis and oxidative stress than selenium-replete patients [13]. This pattern was not seen for zinc. Plasma zinc (84.2%), plasma selenium (100%) concentrations, and erythrocyte selenium concentration (82.6%) were below the reference interval for the healthy population [11]. In a second study focusing on critically ill patients ($n = 125$) in Scotland, plasma zinc and selenium concentrations at baseline were significantly below reference ranges, whereas erythrocyte zinc and selenium concentrations were normal [31].

In a recent study, plasma vitamin C concentrations were significantly lower in 18 patients with sepsis compared to 20 healthy volunteers ($p < 0.05$), whereas neutrophil ascorbate concentrations were comparable. In contrast, erythrocyte ascorbate concentrations from these septic patients were significantly lower than in healthy controls ($p = 0.002$), although 2.2-fold higher than the matched plasma concentrations in these patients ($p = 0.008$) [25]. This difference may be explained by increased generation of dehydroascorbic acid (DHA) in critically ill patients, accumulated in the erythrocytes by the glucose transporters and reduced back to ascorbate due to the presence of other antioxidants in the erythrocytes [33].

## 29.7 Discussion

Two small studies of patients having elective knee arthroplasty as a model for a significant and reproducible systemic inflammatory response showed that plasma concentrations of FAD, PLP, zinc, and selenium decreased transiently by 26–48% with their nadir at 48 h by contrast to the timing of the CRP peak. In contrast, erythrocyte concentrations remained stable.

In critically ill patients, plasma concentrations of vitamins B6, C, and E were decreased by 40–85% compared to healthy volunteers, and plasma zinc, selenium, and the major plasma selenoenzyme, selenoprotein-P, concentrations were below the reference range in 84–100% of the patients. In contrast to the plasma concentrations, the results of erythrocyte concentrations of the different micronutrients in critically ill patients were mixed. Erythrocyte vitamin E concentration remained stable, but there was a decrease in erythrocyte concentrations of vitamin B6 and vitamin C (33–57%), less pronounced compared to the decrease in plasma. Erythrocyte zinc concentrations were within the reference range for the healthy population, whereas the results for selenium were mixed, probably reflecting the impact of sepsis on plasma selenium and selenoprotein-P concentration and the importance of previous selenium status on erythrocyte selenium concentration (82% below reference range of normal).

Currently, micronutrient strategies vary hugely worldwide, with only 24% of the VITA-TRACE survey respondents actually performing some form of micronutrient monitoring [34]. Although high-dose micronutrient monotherapy is currently not advised due to lack of clinical benefit, repletion/administration of micronutrients at nutritional doses and in long-term infusions is recommended practice in major burns, high-output gastrointestinal fistulae and during continuous renal replacement therapy. For other critically ill patients, intravenously administered micronutrient bundles of moderately increased doses may improve clinical outcome, but (micro) nutrition requirements, although well-defined for healthy individuals, are largely unknown during critical illness [4]. These requirements will vary substantially between patients and with every phase of disease. One size will certainly not fit all. Furthermore, micronutrients never work alone, so should be viewed as a whole, as part of a complex and interconnected metabolic network [35]. The literature shows that plasma concentrations are unreliable to estimate micronutrient requirements in the critically ill; especially because not all relevant forms of a biomarker are available in a routine setting. For example, selenium is a required atom for selenoenzymes, so we have to move from selenium concentrations to selenocompounds concentrations and activity (e.g., selenoenzymes: selenoprotein-P and glutathione peroxidase 3 for plasma, and glutathione peroxidase 1 for erythrocytes; or selenite oxidant and pro-antioxidant compound depending on its concentration), and their actions as nutritional or therapeutic targets.

The results of clinical studies have shown that micronutrient concentrations in erythrocytes are unaffected by the acute inflammatory response after elective surgery. Micronutrient concentrations in erythrocytes are likely to better reflect tissue status in patients with critical illness, since almost all these patients will have systemic inflammation, but may also simultaneously have a true deficiency (due to real losses through body fluids, increased metabolic consumption or previous nutritional deficiency). These measurements may thus more reliably identify patients who may benefit from supplementation. The mixed results of the measurements of erythrocyte concentrations, but also of micronutrient supplementation in the critically ill [3] support this hypothesis. If erythrocyte concentrations are normal, supplementation may not be necessary and may even be disadvantageous for patients [8, 9]. Only two of the studies in Table 29.1 reported measurements of micronutrients in leukocytes. This is probably due to the more complex use of leukocytes, not only for research but also in a routine setting. However, these cell types might reflect the actual intracellular micronutrient status of a patient even better than erythrocytes, because they are metabolically more active. The feasibility of this approach, however, strongly depends on the development of easy to use isolation protocols for leukocytes.

Current results are not conclusive with regard to the potential of erythrocyte or leukocyte measurements as an index of tissue micronutrient status in critically ill patients. To be a useful indicator of tissue status, micronutrient concentrations in erythrocytes or leukocytes would be expected to decrease in patients developing deficiency and subsequently increase when supplementation is given [20]. Even more important, measurement of erythrocyte or leukocyte micronutrient concentrations is only useful if supplementation based on the results would yield better clinical outcomes. In that case, erythrocyte or leukocyte measurements could be used to guide personalized supplementation. These clinical studies have not been performed yet. In addition, the analytical capacities to measure not only plasma, but also intracellular concentrations of erythrocytes and possibly leukocytes, require facilities that are sporadically available worldwide. However, with current developments of modern laboratory equipment these tests might become available in a more routine setting in the coming years.

At this moment, the most common practice is to use CRP to estimate inflammatory status. In patients with CRP levels of more than 50 mg/l, plasma threshold values less than 20% of the lower reference range for the micronutrients may identify most deficient patients [4]. But, as demonstrated earlier, due to the substantial variability in the association between CRP and plasma micronutrients, this is only a rough estimation.

## 29.8 Conclusion

Plasma concentrations are the most frequently used estimators of the tissue status of micronutrients, but are unreliable due to systemic inflammation with redistribution, dilution, and decreased carrier protein concentrations. Well-defined reference intervals exist for healthy persons, but not for the critically ill. Erythrocytes and leukocytes may be an alternative matrix to assess tissue status in the critically ill. Until now, despite decreased plasma concentrations, administration of micronutrients during severe illness has given mixed results, and may even sometimes be disadvantageous [8, 9]. Measurement of plasma micronutrient concentrations in critically ill patients (or other patients with systemic inflammation) and comparing these with reference intervals for healthy persons will often be misleading and should generally be avoided [6]. Intracellular micronutrient concentrations in erythrocytes and/or leukocytes are promising as a more reliable estimate of tissue status than plasma measurements in critically ill patients.

Further studies are required to investigate whether deficiencies in erythrocyte or leukocyte concentrations of micronutrients are related to clinical outcome in critically ill patients and whether supplementation improves erythrocyte or leukocyte concentrations and clinical outcome in patients with probable micronutrient deficiencies. This approach is only feasible if advanced technologies are developed, such as multiparameter assays, to perform these measurements in daily clinical care for personalized medicine.

## References

1. Gudivada KK, Kumar A, Sriram K, et al. Antioxidant micronutrient supplements for adult critically ill patients: a bayesian multiple treatment comparisons meta-analysis. Clin Nutr ESPEN. 2022;47:78–88.
2. Casaer MP, Bellomo R. Micronutrient deficiency in critical illness: an invisible foe? Intensive Care Med. 2019;45:1136–9.
3. Berger MM, Shenkin A, Schweinlin A, et al. ESPEN micronutrient guideline. Clin Nutr. 2022;41:1357–424.
4. Berger MM, Manzanares W. Micronutrients early in critical illness, selective or generous, enteral or intravenous? Curr Opin Clin Nutr Metab Care. 2021;24:165–75.
5. Duncan A, Talwar D, McMillan DC, Stefanowicz F, O'Reilly DS. Quantitative data on the magnitude of the systemic inflammatory response and its effect on micronutrient status based on plasma measurements. Am J Clin Nutr. 2012;95:64–71.
6. Galloway P, McMillan DC, Sattar N. Effect of the inflammatory response on trace element and vitamin status. Ann Clin Biochem. 2000;37:289–97.
7. Gudivada KK, Kumar A, Shariff M, et al. Antioxidant micronutrient supplementation in critically ill adults: a systematic review with meta-analysis and trial sequential analysis. Clin Nutr. 2021;40:740–50.
8. Lamontagne F, Masse MH, Menard J, et al. Intravenous vitamin C in adults with sepsis in the intensive care unit. N Engl J Med. 2022;386:2387–98.
9. Heyland D, Muscedere J, Wischmeyer PE, et al. A randomized trial of glutamine and antioxidants in critically ill patients. N Engl J Med. 2013;368:1489–97.
10. Forceville X, Van Antwerpen P, Preiser JC. Selenocompounds and sepsis: redox bypass hypothesis for early diagnosis and treatment: part A-early acute phase of sepsis: an extraordinary redox situation (leukocyte/endothelium interaction leading to endothelial damage). Antioxid Redox Signal. 2021;35:113–38.
11. Cirino Ruocco MA, Pacheco Cechinatti ED, Barbosa F Jr, Navarro AM. Zinc and selenium status in critically ill patients according to severity stratification. Nutrition. 2018;45:85–9.
12. Prelack K, Sheridan RL. Micronutrient supplementation in the critically ill patient: strategies for clinical practice. J Trauma. 2001;51:601–20.
13. Forceville X, Van Antwerpen P, Annane D, Vincent JL. Selenocompounds and sepsis-redox bypass hypothesis: part B-selenocompounds in the management of early sepsis. Antioxid Redox Signal. 2022;37:998–1029.
14. Dao DT, Anez-Bustillos L, Cho BS, Li Z, Puder M, Gura KM. Assessment of micronutrient status in critically ill children: challenges and opportunities. Nutrients. 2017;9:1185.

15. Gladyshev VN, Arnér ES, Berry MJ, et al. Selenoprotein gene nomenclature. J Biol Chem. 2016;291:24036–40.
16. Lopes Junior E, Leite HP, Konstantyner T. Selenium and selenoproteins: from endothelial cytoprotection to clinical outcomes. Transl Res. 2019;208:85–104.
17. Brigelius-Flohé R, Arnér ESJ. Selenium and selenoproteins in (redox) signaling, diseases, and animal models - 200 year anniversary issue. Free Radic Biol Med. 2018;127:1–2.
18. Vacchina V, Bierla K, Szpunar J, Lobinski R. Quantification of SeMet and SeCys in biological fluids and tissues by liquid chromatography coupled to inductively coupled plasma mass spectrometry (HPLC-ICP MS). Methods Mol Biol. 2018;1661:153–62.
19. Gray A, McMillan DC, Wilson C, Williamson C, O'Reilly DS, Talwar D. The relationship between plasma and red cell concentrations of vitamins thiamine diphosphate, flavin adenine dinucleotide and pyridoxal 5-phosphate following elective knee arthroplasty. Clin Nutr. 2004;23:1080–3.
20. Oakes EJ, Lyon TD, Duncan A, Gray A, Talwar D, O'Reilly DS. Acute inflammatory response does not affect erythrocyte concentrations of copper, zinc and selenium. Clin Nutr. 2008;27:115–20.
21. Reid D, Toole BJ, Knox S, et al. The relation between acute changes in the systemic inflammatory response and plasma 25-hydroxyvitamin D concentrations after elective knee arthroplasty. Am J Clin Nutr. 2011;93:1006–11.
22. Conway FJ, Talwar D, McMillan DC. The relationship between acute changes in the systemic inflammatory response and plasma ascorbic acid, alpha-tocopherol and lipid peroxidation after elective hip arthroplasty. Clin Nutr. 2015;34:642–6.
23. Louw JA, Werbeck A, Louw ME, Kotze TJ, Cooper R, Labadarios D. Blood vitamin concentrations during the acute-phase response. Crit Care Med. 1992;20:934–41.
24. McMillan DC, Maguire D, Talwar D. Relationship between nutritional status and the systemic inflammatory response: micronutrients. Proc Nutr Soc. 2019;78(1):56–67.
25. Carr AC, Bozonet S, Pullar J, Spencer E, Rosengrave P, Shaw G. Neutrophils isolated from septic patients exhibit elevated uptake of vitamin C and normal intracellular concentrations despite a low vitamin C milieu. Antioxidants (Basel). 2021;10:1607.
26. Bates CJ. Vitamin analysis. Ann Clin Biochem. 1997;34:599–626.
27. Hinks LJ, Clayton BE, Lloyd RS. Zinc and copper concentrations in leucocytes and erythrocytes in healthy adults and the effect of oral contraceptives. J Clin Pathol. 1983;36:1016–21.
28. Vasilaki AT, McMillan DC, Kinsella J, Duncan A, O'Reilly DS, Talwar D. Relation between pyridoxal and pyridoxal phosphate concentrations in plasma, red cells, and white cells in patients with critical illness. Am J Clin Nutr. 2008;88:140–6.
29. Evans RM, Currie L, Campbell A. The distribution of ascorbic acid between various cellular components of blood, in normal individuals, and its relation to the plasma concentration. Br J Nutr. 1982;47:473–82.
30. Vasilaki AT, Leivaditi D, Talwar D, et al. Assessment of vitamin E status in patients with systemic inflammatory response syndrome: plasma, plasma corrected for lipids or red blood cell measurements? Clin Chim Acta. 2009;409:41–5.
31. Stefanowicz F, Gashut RA, Talwar D, et al. Assessment of plasma and red cell trace element concentrations, disease severity, and outcome in patients with critical illness. J Crit Care. 2014;29:214–8.
32. Watanabe LM, Navarro AM, Seale LA. Intersection between obesity, dietary selenium, and statin therapy in Brazil. Nutrients. 2021;13:2027.
33. Kuhn V, Diederich L, Keller TCS 4th, et al. Red blood cell function and dysfunction: redox regulation, nitric oxide metabolism, anemia. Antioxid Redox Signal. 2017;26:718–42.
34. Vankrunkelsven W, Gunst J, Amrein K, et al. Monitoring and parenteral administration of micronutrients, phosphate and magnesium in critically ill patients: the VITA-TRACE survey. Clin Nutr. 2021;40:590–9.
35. Berger MM. Nutrition and micronutrient therapy in critical illness should be individualized. JPEN J Parenter Enteral Nutr. 2020;44:1380–7.

# Optimal Glycemic Targets in Critically Ill Patients with Diabetes

# 30

A. P. Poole, M. Horowitz, and A. Deane

## 30.1 Introduction

Admission to an intensive care unit (ICU) can be precipitated by a variety of illnesses and injuries. Pre-existing diabetes markedly increases the risk of many of these illnesses [1]. Even in the absence of pre-existing diabetes, critically ill patients frequently develop hyperglycemia and insulin resistance, which has been termed 'stress hyperglycemia' [2]. Stress hyperglycemia is in part a reflection of the endogenous response to the illness or injury, including the secretion of counter-regulatory hormones, and treatments administered, including catecholamines, nutrition, and steroids, which exacerbate any disordered glucose metabolism induced by the illness or injury [3].

The rationale for treating hyperglycemia in the critically ill is underpinned by observational data consistently reporting strong associations between hyperglycemia and adverse outcomes, including increased mortality [4]. Whether such associations represent an epiphenomenon of critical illness or a causative relationship remains contentious [3].

A. P. Poole (✉)
Discipline of Acute Care Medicine, University of Adelaide, Adelaide, SA, Australia

School of Public Health and Preventive Medicine, Monash University, Melbourne, VIC, Australia
e-mail: Alexis.Poole@adelaide.edu.au

M. Horowitz
Discipline of Medicine, University of Adelaide, Adelaide, SA, Australia

Department of Endocrinology, Royal Adelaide Hospital, Adelaide, SA, Australia

A. Deane
Department of Intensive Care, The Royal Melbourne Hospital, Melbourne, VIC, Australia

Department of Critical Care, Melbourne Medical School, The University of Melbourne, Melbourne, VIC, Australia



J.-L. Vincent (ed.), *Annual Update in Intensive Care and Emergency Medicine 2023*, Annual Update in Intensive Care and Emergency Medicine,
https://doi.org/10.1007/978-3-031-23005-9_30

There are observational data that glycemic variability, a metric describing the magnitude of glucose fluctuations over time, is an independent predictor of morbidity and mortality [5–7]. While a reduction in variability may be a surrogate marker for better provision of intensive care, these adverse outcomes could also reflect the harmful impact of rapidly fluctuating blood glucose concentrations, which is to induce apoptosis and increase cytokine production and oxidative stress [8, 9].

There are also well described relationships between hypoglycemia and adverse outcomes, and the impact of these physiological responses may be synergistic during episodes of critical illness. Hypoglycemia (<4.0 mmol/l) or even a single episode of severe hypoglycemia (<2.2 mmol/l) are independently associated with a greater risk of dying [10, 11].

The management of hyperglycemia in the ICU frequently involves administration of intravenous insulin [12], with the inherent risk of causing hypoglycemia as well as increased glycemic variability [13]. This is compounded by other risk factors such as, but not limited to, renal failure, sepsis, and calorie intake [14].

In this chapter, we review the management of hyperglycemia in critically ill adult patients with type 2 diabetes, which will be referred to as diabetes throughout. The following areas are the focus: early trials of glucose control during critical illness, current management guidelines, glucose metrics modified by diabetes, prevalence of diabetes in critically patients, personalized approach to glycemic control, and recommendation for future research directions.

## 30.2 Early Trials of Glucose Control During Admission to the ICU

The apparent strong association between hyperglycemia and adverse outcomes in critically ill patients provided the rationale for a single center, open-label, parallel-group, randomized clinical trial of so-called 'intensive insulin therapy' in patients after major surgery admitted to an ICU [15]. Subsequently, large trials reported between 2001 and 2009 included patients irrespective of the presence of pre-existing diabetes. In the first trial [15], the intervention was 'intensive insulin therapy', which involved the strict treatment of hyperglycemia to maintain a blood glucose between 4.4 and 6.1 mmol/l with intravenous insulin. The investigators planned to include 2500 adult patients who required mechanical ventilation and primary outcome was all-cause mortality in the ICU, with secondary outcomes including in-hospital mortality and duration of ICU admission. The trial was stopped after 1548 participants due to a reduction in mortality in patients assigned intensive insulin therapy (intensive: 35 of 765 (4.6%) vs. comparator: 63 of 783 (80%); adjusted $p < 0.04$). Interim analyses were repeated at 3-month intervals and the trial stopped after the fourth analysis. While adjusting for repeated analysis, the p value did meet the set point for statistical significance; however, it should be appreciated that even with statistical adjustments for repeated analyses the risk of bias in an open-label trial remains [16]. The same investigators then conducted a single center, open-label, parallel-group, randomized clinical trial of 1200 patients from a medical ICU. Again, patients were eligible irrespective of previous diabetes. Between groups there was no statistically significant difference in the primary outcome of all-cause hospital mortality. A pre-planned analysis in those with greater exposure to the intervention (defined as 3 days or more) was undertaken [17]; in this subgroup a reduction in in-hospital mortality was evident in those assigned intensive insulin therapy (intensive: 121 of 386 (31.3%) vs. comparator: 145 of 38.1%); $p = 0.05$). When interpreting this observation it should be appreciated that post-randomization identification of a subgroup can be problematic, as conventional statistical methods are invalid when the post-randomization factor, in this case duration of exposure, is affected by the intervention being studied [16]. The studies included 407 patients with pre-existing diabetes; there was no significant difference in the primary outcome of hospital mortality (intensive: 48 of 207 (23.2%) vs. comparator: 44 of 200 (22.0%)) in these patients [18].

Glucontrol was a multicenter, open-label, parallel-group, randomized clinical trial comparing an intervention of intensive insulin therapy aiming for a blood glucose range of 4.4–6.1 mmol/l and a comparator group with a target blood glucose range of 7.8–10 mmol/l [19]. The trial was planned to enroll 3500 patients, but recruitment was terminated by the data safety monitoring board at the first interim analysis because of unintended protocol violations and time spent with blood glucose readings out of range. The trial was stopped after 1101 patients, with a three-fold increase in the proportion of patients having a hypoglycemia event (<2.2 mmol/l, intensive: 8.7% vs. comparator: 2.7%) and no statistical difference in 28-day mortality (intensive: 100 of 536 (18.7%) vs. comparator: 83 of 542 (15.3%); $p = 0.14$) [19].

The Efficacy of Volume Substitution and Insulin Therapy in Severe Sepsis (VISEP) study was a multicenter randomized clinical trial that incorporated a two-by-two factorial design. One of the interventions tested was an intensive insulin regimen (commenced >6.1 mmol/l maintained between 4.4 and 6.1 mmol/l); in the comparator group, insulin was commenced at >11.1 mmol/l, aiming to maintain a blood glucose between 10 and 11.1 mmol/l. This branch of the study stopped following the first safety analysis at 488 participants [20]. The intensive insulin therapy component was terminated because the data safety monitoring committee observed a substantial increase in the risk of hypoglycemia, defined as ≤2.2 mmol/l, with the intervention (intensive: 30 of 247 (12.1%) and comparator: 5 of 241 (2.1%)) [20]. All-cause day 90 mortality was not significantly different (intensive: 98 of 247 (39.7%) vs. comparator: 102 of 288 (35.4%) $p = 0.31$), including in the sub-group of patients with diabetes (intensive 29/72 (40.3%) vs. comparator 38/91 (41.8%) $p = 0.85$) [20].

While the results of subsequent trials appeared incongruent with the initial Leuven trial [15], they also demonstrated that maintaining blood glucose within strict ranges across multiple sites was particularly challenging. The Normoglycemia in Intensive

Care Evaluation-Survival Using Glucose Algorithm Regulation (NICE-SUGAR) trial was a multicenter, open-label, parallel-group, randomized trial evaluating intensive insulin therapy to achieve a blood glucose of (4.5–6.0 mmol/l) with a comparator group with a blood glucose <10.0 mmol/l [21]. The trial included 6100 participants and the primary outcome was all-cause mortality at day 90. In this trial, intensive insulin therapy increased 90-day mortality (intensive: 829 of 3010 (27.5%) and comparator: 751 of 3012 (24.9%); $p = 0.02$) and episodes of hypoglycemia (≤2.2 mmol/l) (206 of 3016 (6.8%) and 15 of 3014 (0.5%)) [21]. Subsequent analysis of the NICE-SUGAR study data indicated that even with adjustment for baseline and post-randomization confounders, the association of moderate and severe hypoglycemia with mortality remained significant in the sub-group of patients with diabetes (intensive 195/615 (31.7%) vs. comparator 165/596 (27.7%); $p = 0.60$) [22].

Taken together, these earlier randomized clinical trials suggest that, at least outside of specialized centers, trying to achieve blood glucose concentrations consistent with the fasting state (<6 mmol/l) using intensive insulin therapy increases the risk of morbidity and mortality in critically ill patients irrespective of whether they have pre-existing diabetes [15, 21, 22].

## 30.3 Clinical Practice Guidelines

The 2021 American Diabetes Association (ADA) clinical practice guidelines for hospitalized patients include a recommendation that insulin is commenced when a blood glucose of 10 mmol/l or more persists, and the blood glucose range that is targeted with treatment is 7.8–10.0 mmol/l [23]. The recommendations suggest possible alternative goals for critically ill patients with diabetic ketoacidosis, other hyperosmolar states, and cardiac surgical patients—all of which should be achieved without significant hypoglycemia.

The 2012 Society of Critical Care Medicine (SCCM) guideline [24] for management of hyperglycemia in critically ill patients suggests an insulin infusion should be initiated when the blood glucose is ≥8.3 mmol/l and titrated to maintain blood glucose <10.0 mmol/l in a way that limits the risk of hypoglycemia (<4.0 mmol/l). The quality of evidence that supports these guidelines was rated as very low, due to the limitations of the included trials [24]. Collectively, the authors of the ADA and SCCM guidelines also recognize the limitations in the current literature in relation to specific populations, recommending that future research should focus on sub-populations of critically ill patients [23, 24].

## 30.4 Prevalence of Diabetes in Patients Admitted to the ICU

Diabetes, particularly type 2 diabetes, is a prevalent chronic health condition [25]. As a result of high prevalence and complications associated with the disease, diabetes represents a major financial burden to the healthcare system and consumes a considerable proportion of healthcare expenditure [25]. The prevalence of patients with diabetes admitted to hospital is greater than in the general population, with estimates ranging between 11% and 35% of all patients [1]. The prevalence of critically ill patients with pre-existing diabetes is comparable to that of hospitalized patients at between 12% and 40%, and this has been established though observational and interventional studies that report diabetes as co-existing disease present on admission [26, 27]. These estimates of prevalence should be viewed circumspectly as, in the context of randomized trials, selection bias may occur to increase or decrease representation.

Diabetes that existed before ICU admission but had not been diagnosed is termed unrecognized diabetes and occurs in 6–16% of ICU admissions [27–30]. It is likely that an even greater proportion of critically patients have diabetes than are identified in studies or trials that depend on self-identification of diabetes, and more routine measurement may be warranted.

## 30.5 Evaluation of Previous Randomized Clinical Trials When Focusing on Patients with Pre-existing Diabetes

As described, the cohorts participating in earlier trials evaluating intensive insulin therapy included patients both with and without pre-existing diabetes. Analysis according to pre-existing diabetes has the potential to easily identify different phenotypes, with response to acute dysglycemia being dependent on pre-existing diabetes.

In a *post hoc* analysis of the two Leuven studies, the signal for benefit with intensive insulin therapy was confined to those without pre-existing diabetes [18]. In patients with pre-existing diabetes, a greater reduction in blood glucose was associated with greater in-hospital mortality, albeit not reaching pre-defined statistical significance (26.2% for <6.1 mmol/l, 21.6% for 6.1–8.3 mmol/l, and 21.2% for >8.3 mmol/l) [18]. In the NICE-SUGAR study there was increased mortality with intensive insulin therapy in patients with pre-existing diabetes (intensive 31.7% vs. control 27.6%) [21]. Results from these subgroups, and more recent retrospective and prospective analyses of cohorts with pre-existing diabetes have provided insights into the impact of hypoglycemia, hyperglycemia and glycemic variability in patients without diabetes [31–33]. With the heterogeneity of treatment effect observed across critically ill patients, these results raise the possibility that those with pre-existing diabetes should be considered a separate phenotype than patients with stress hyperglycemia.

## 30.6 Pre-existing Diabetes Relationship to Blood Glucose Metrics

Hyperglycemia in its most acute uncontrolled form has been clearly demonstrated to cause harm [34]. However, the threshold blood glucose concentration that is associated with harm remains to be determined. This certainly appears to be the case in patients with pre-existing chronic glycemia (i.e., those with a HbA1c ≥7%) who appear to demonstrate a blunted or absent response to acute hyperglycemia [35, 36].

Greater glycemic variability is associated with morbidity and mortality in patients with diabetes but associations between glycemic variability and outcomes are inconsistent. In part this may reflect low patient numbers, variability or pre-morbid glycemic control, and/or lack of power to detect a relationship [37]. It would not be surprising that diabetic patients have adapted somewhat to glycemic variability and developed protection. To determine whether glycemic variability is indeed harmful to patients with diabetes a suitably powered and conducted study is required [38].

Hypoglycemia is strongly associated with increased morbidity and mortality in critically ill patients with or without diabetes, but the effect is more marked in those without pre-existing diabetes [4, 18, 31, 39, 40].

## 30.7 Rationale for a Personalized Approach to Glycemic Control

A 'personalized' approach to acute glycemic control, which takes into consideration an individual's pre-existing glucose metabolism when determining an appropriate target glycemic range during a period of acute illness, has been suggested as a concept [1, 38, 41]. Results from observational and exploratory studies indicate that outcomes for patients with diabetes are different in relation to the impacts of hypoglycemia, hyperglycemia, and glycemic variability (Table 30.1) [4, 27, 31, 42–44]. Egi and colleagues reported that patients with a higher HbA1c on ICU admission were more likely to survive if they had blood glucose concentrations >10 mmol/l during their ICU admission [31]. Subsequently, several studies have made similar observations (Table 30.2) [4, 27, 42–44]. Although patients with diabetes appear to have some underlying protection against acute hyperglycemia, hypoglycemia has consistently been shown to be harmful and the threshold blood glucose for harm may even be slightly higher than for non-diabetic patients [11, 48].

Whilst these observational studies suggest that the threshold for harm is dependent on pre-morbid glycemic control, the outcomes are insufficient to affect practice. They have, however, informed further research into the use of such a 'personalized' approach to glycemic control for critically ill patients with diabetes.

**Table 30.1** Rationale for personalized blood glucose levels

| Author [ref] | Year | Study design | Number of sites | n | Diabetes n (%) | Results/main points |
|---|---|---|---|---|---|---|
| Egi [31] | 2008 | Retrospective observational | Multicenter | 4946 | 728 (14.7) | No association between hyperglycemia and ICU mortality in diabetic patients. |
| Plummer [27] | 2014 | Prospective observational | Single center | 1000 | 275 (27.5) | Hyperglycemia was not associated with mortality in patients with premorbid hyperglycemia. |
| Egi [42] | 2016 | Retrospective observational | Multicenter | 3084 | 1057 (34.3) | The higher the pre-morbid hyperglycemia, the greater the risk of death in patients experiencing any hypoglycemic episode. |
| Krinsley [43] | 2017 | Retrospective observational | Two centers | 6387 | 1872 (29.3) | No relationship between mean BG level and mortality in patients with diabetes. Hypoglycemia <4.0 mmol/l was associated with mortality in all patients. |
| Lin [44] | 2020 | Retrospective observational | Multicenter | 33,680 | 8701 (25.8) | In patients with diabetes, an elevated admission glucose did not appear to be associated with 28-day mortality. |
| Krinsley [4] | 2020 | Retrospective observational | Single center | 5567 | 1161 (20.1) | Increased BG increased mortality for patients with HbA1c <6.5%, but decreased mortality for patients with HbA1c ≥8.0% |
| Ma [37] | 2022 | Retrospective observational | Single center | 958 | 238 (24.8) | Greater glycemic variability and a higher rate of hypoglycemia was associated with mortality in patients with diabetes. Impact of hyperglycemia on mortality was nonsignificant in diabetics. |

*BG* blood glucose, *HbA1c* glycated hemoglobin

**Table 30.2** Studies of personalized blood glucose control

| Author [ref] | Year | Design | Sites | n | Diabetes n (%) | Intervention target range (mmol/l) | Control target range (mmol/l) |
|---|---|---|---|---|---|---|---|
| Di Muzio [45] | 2016 | Sequential period | Single center | 80 | 80 (100) | 10.0–14.0 | 6.0–10.0 |
| Kar [32] | 2016 | Sequential period | Single center | 83 | 83 (100) | 10.0–14.0 | 6.0–10.0 |
| Krinsley [46] | 2017 | Retrospective observational | Single center | 1979 | 406 (20.5) | 6.1–8.9 | 5.0–6.7 |
| Luethi [33] | 2018 | Sequential period | Single center | 700 | 700 (100) | 10.0–14.0 | 6.0–10.0 |
| Bohé [30] | 2021 | RCT | Multicenter | 1917 | 468 (24.4) | See Fig. 30.1 | |
| Poole [47] | 2022 | RCT | Multicenter | 434 | 434 (100) | 10.0–14.0 | 6.0–10.0 |

*RCT* randomized controlled trial

## 30.8 Studies of More Personalized Approach to Glucose Control

There are only a few studies of a 'personalized' approach to blood glucose based on the presence of diabetes and allowing mild to moderate hyperglycemia (≥10 mmol/l). Kar and colleagues [32] conducted a prospective, single center, sequential period study in adult patients with diabetes and chronic hyperglycemia (HbA1c ≥7%). During the initial 'standard care' period, insulin was commenced when blood glucose concentrations reached >10 mmol/l and titrated to maintain them between 6 and 10 mmol/l. During the liberal period, insulin administration was started once blood glucose was >14 mmol/l, and was then titrated to target blood glucose concentrations between 10 and 14 mmol/l. The 'standard care' period included 52 participants, the liberal period included 31 participants: peak blood glucose concentrations where comparable between the groups (standard group 15.8 (3.5) vs. 16.2 (3.9) mmol/l). During the liberal phase, the time-weighted blood glucose concentrations were predictably higher. During the standard care period, 18 patients (35%) had an episode of moderate-severe hypoglycemia (13 patients had moderate hypoglycemia and five had severe hypoglycemia) and during the liberal period five patients (16%) had an episode of hypoglycemia (four moderate and one patient severe). After adjustment for varying periods of observation, there was a tendency for fewer episodes of moderate-severe hypoglycemia during the liberal period [relative risk 0.47 (95% CI 0.19–1.13), p = 0.09]. Recurrent hypoglycemia was more common in the standard care phase, with 10 patients having recurrent moderate-severe hypoglycemia compared to only one patient in the liberal phase. No signal for harm was observed and patient-centered outcomes were similar in the two groups.

Luethi and colleagues [33] conducted a larger single center, sequential period study. They included 350 consecutively admitted patients with diabetes in whom the blood glucose target was 6–10 mmol/l during the standard care period. During the liberal period, a further 350 patients with diabetes received insulin once blood glucose levels were >14 mmol/l, with the insulin titrated to maintain a blood glucose between 10 and 14 mmol/l. The diagnosis of diabetes was determined pragmatically from medical records, or patient or relative report. In the liberal phase, median time-weighted average blood glucose concentrations were again greater than during the control period (11.0 [IQR 8.7–12.0] vs. 9.6 [IQR 8.5–11.0] mmol/l, p = <0.001). Fewer patients received insulin in the liberal compared with the control period (132 (37.7%) vs. 188 (53.7%) p = <0.001). In the sub-group of patients with chronic hyperglycemia (HbA1c >7%), the liberal approach was associated with a reduction in the number of episodes of hypoglycemia (≤3.9 mmol/l) (liberal: 9 (3%) vs. control: 22 (7%) p = 0.03).

Recently, Bohé and colleagues reported results from the CONTROLING trial; which was a blinded randomized clinical trial of a 'personalized approach' to blood glucose management based on the admission HbA1c [30]. The trial included 1917 patients and made use of a blinded, computer-generated algorithm to guide nursing staff on management of glycemia. In the comparator group, blood glucose concentrations were managed once they exceeded 10 mmol/l. The intervention group, who received the 'personalized approach', included patients with HbA1c ≤4.96% where the blood glucose target range was more stringent, i.e., 6.2 mmol/l compared to 12.1 mmol/l for those with HbA1c of ≥8.67% (Fig. 30.1). Implementation of such a complex intervention across multiple sites to patients with dynamic disease processes and interventions is challenging, and, not surprisingly, the target range was only achieved half of the time. However, the treatment separation was modest with only a small difference in time-weighted mean blood glucose levels in the reported cohort of 1828 (it was just 0.7 mmol/l). As could be expected, insulin administration

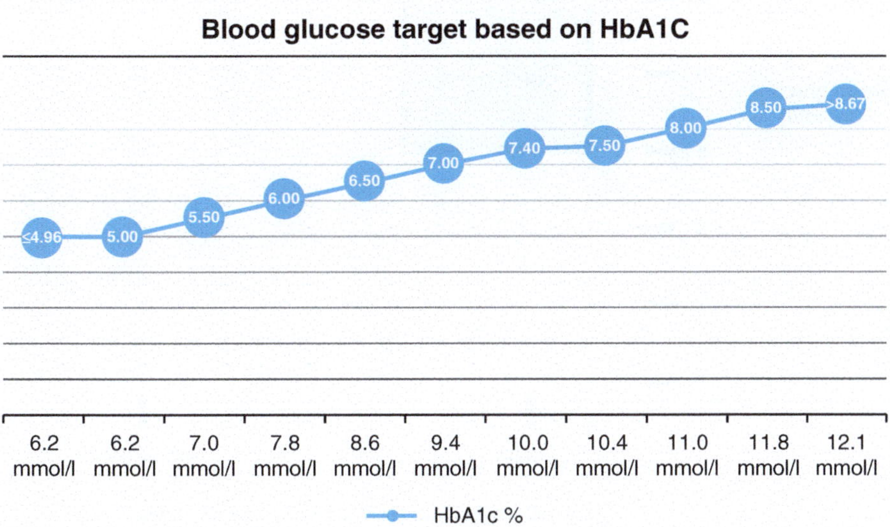


**Fig. 30.1** Personalized blood glucose targets used for intervention group in the CONTROLING study [30]. HbA1c: glycated hemoglobin

was greater in the personalized group, with 25% more patients receiving insulin. Episodes of severe hypoglycemia, defined as <2.2 mmol/l, were not statistically different between groups (personalized: 37 of 942 (3.9%) vs. comparator: 24 of 975 (2.5%); p = 0.09). However, hypoglycemia, defined as <4 mmol/l, was more frequent with the intervention (personalized: 294 of 942 (31.2%) vs. comparator: 154 of 975 (15.8%) p = <0.0001). As with previous studies, moderate and severe hypoglycemia were associated with increased mortality; with the low likelihood of benefit from the intervention in terms of 90-day mortality, the data safety monitoring committee recommended early trial cessation. The study predominantly included participants that did not have diabetes, and, of those with diabetes, only 14% had an HbA1c >7%. Accordingly, while this study reaffirms that hypoglycemia is harmful, patients with pre-existing diabetes only represented a small proportion of the participants.

More recently, we published the LUCID trial, a multicenter, open label, randomized clinical trial conducted in critically ill patients with pre-existing diabetes. With the liberal approach, insulin was commenced at >14.0 mmol/l and in the comparator group insulin was commenced at >10.0 mmol/l (Fig. 30.2) [47]. This is the first

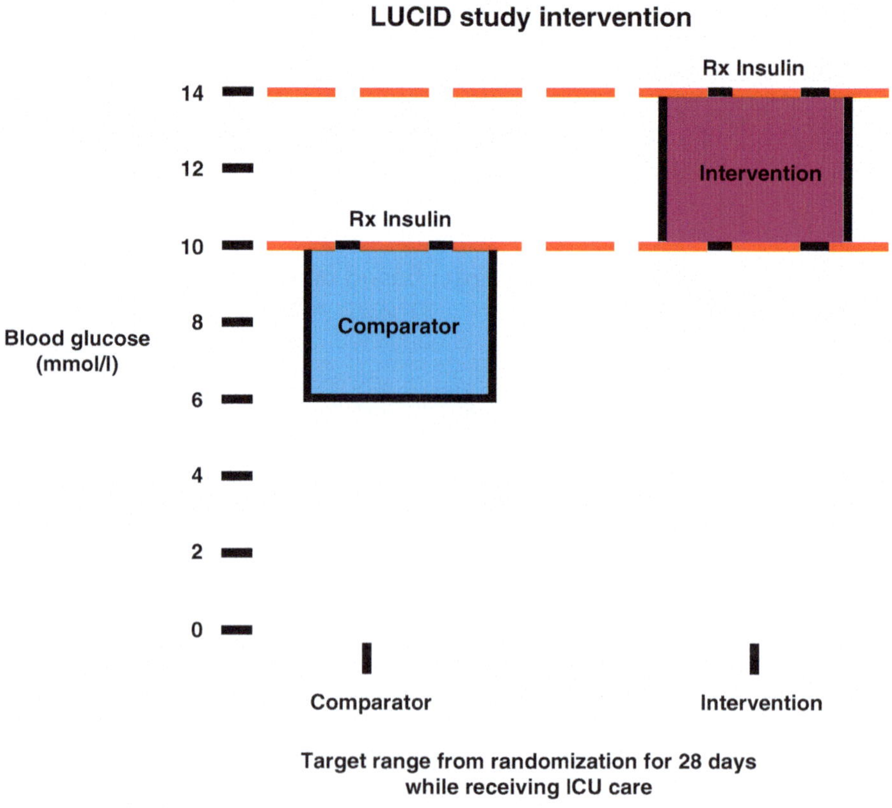


**Fig. 30.2** Blood glucose target ranges used in the LUCID study [47]

randomized trial to explore a liberal approach in critically ill patients with pre-existing diabetes. The study randomized 434 patients with diabetes, irrespective of their HbA1c (at randomization the median HbA1c was 7.3% in both groups). The median blood glucose was 11.8 mmol/l in the intervention group compared to 9.3 mmol/l in the comparator group. As with several other pragmatic trials, blood glucose concentrations were outside the target range about 50% of the time. The primary endpoint of the study was 28-day incidence of hypoglycemia, defined as <4.0 mmol/l, which was significantly lower in the intervention group (10 (5%) versus 38 (18%), IRR 0.36, 95% CI 0.11–1.14). Although the trial was not powered for patient-centered outcomes, 90-day mortality was numerically greater in the intervention arm. Accordingly, these findings suggest that a liberal approach should not be implemented outside of a well-designed clinical trial, and further consideration of admission HbA1c and use of technology to improve time-in-range may also be beneficial.

## 30.9 Future Research

Information from retrospective and prospective observational studies and from interventional studies, has provided considerable insight into critically ill patients with pre-existing diabetes and supports future exploration of a more personalized approach to glycemic control. The most recent studies—CONTROLING and LUCID—have provided insight into optimal study designs for future investigation of blood glucose management in critically ill patients with diabetes. With the recent advent of various technologies, such as continuous glucose monitoring, point-of-care HbA1c machines, and close-loop continuous glucose monitoring, we suggest further adequately powered trials in patients with the phenotype of diabetes are warranted. Outside of specific target ranges and methods for achieving these, investigations into alternative nutrition formulas have commenced, and may represent a method to reduce the amount of insulin required [49]. Given the consistent evidence that hypoglycemia and mortality are related in this population, glucose lowering therapies that are less likely to induce hypoglycemia would appear to be worthy of further investigation. A number of small studies have explored the use of these incretin-based therapies to reduce blood glucose with a lower risk of hypoglycemia [50]. They could potentially be used alone or in combination with insulin, as is the case in ambulatory type 2 diabetes.

## 30.10 Conclusion

The optimal blood glucose target for critically ill patients with pre-existing diabetes remains uncertain, as outcomes of recent trials are neither definitive nor practice changing. Future studies are required to provide clinical insight, as a more personalized approached is intuitively likely to be more effective. Future approaches to management of hyperglycemia should minimize the potential for hypoglycemia.

## References


1. Kar P, Jones KL, Horowitz M, Deane AM. Management of critically ill patients with type 2 diabetes: the need for personalised therapy. World J Diabetes. 2015;6:693–706.
2. Deane AM, Plummer MP, Ali Abdelhamid Y. Update on glucose control during and after critical illness. Curr Opin Crit Care. 2022;28:389–94.
3. Krinsley JS, Brownlee M, Schwartz MW, et al. Blood glucose targets in the critically ill: is one size fits all still appropriate? Lancet Diabetes Endocrinol. 2022;10:555–7.
4. Krinsley JS, Rule P, Pappy L, et al. The interaction of acute and chronic glycemia on the relationship of hyperglycemia, hypoglycemia, and glucose variability to mortality in the critically ill. Crit Care Med. 2020;48:1744–51.
5. Egi M, Bellomo R, Stachowski E, French CJ, Hart G. Variability of blood glucose concentration and short-term mortality in critically ill patients. Anesthesiology. 2006;105:244–52.
6. Krinsley JS. Glycemic variability: a strong independent predictor of mortality in critically ill patients. Crit Care Med. 2008;36:3008–13.
7. Hanna M, Balintescu A, Glassford N, et al. Glycemic lability index and mortality in critically ill patients—a multicenter cohort study. Acta Anaesthesiol Scand. 2021;65:1267–75.
8. Monnier L, Mas E, Ginet C, et al. Activation of oxidative stress by acute glucose fluctuations compared with sustained chronic hyperglycemia in patients with type 2 diabetes. JAMA. 2006;295:1681–7.
9. Quagliaro L, Piconi L, Assaloni R, Martinelli L, Motz E, Ceriello A. Intermittent high glucose enhances apoptosis related to oxidative stress in human umbilical vein endothelial cells. The role of protein kinase C and NAD(P)H-oxidase activation. Diabetes. 2003;52:2795–804.
10. Krinsley JS, Rule PR, Roberts GW, et al. Relative hypoglycemia and lower hemoglobin A1c-adjusted time in band are strongly associated with increased mortality in critically ill patients. Crit Care Med. 2022;50:e664–e73.
11. Guo JY, Chou RH, Kuo CS, et al. The paradox of the glycemic gap: does relative hypoglycemia exist in critically ill patients? Clin Nutr. 2021;40:4654–61.
12. Poole AP, Anstey J, Bellomo R, et al. Opinions and practices of blood glucose control in critically ill patients with pre-existing type 2 diabetes in Australian and New Zealand intensive care units. Aust Crit Care. 2019;32:361–5.
13. Ali Abdelhamid Y, Bernjak A, Phillips LK, et al. Nocturnal hypoglycemia in patients with diabetes discharged from ICUs: a prospective two-center cohort study. Crit Care Med. 2021;49:636–49.
14. Doola R, Preiser JC. Nutritional therapy in critically ill patients with diabetes. Curr Opin Clin Nutr Metab Care. 2022;25:93–8.
15. Van den Berghe G, Wouters P, Weekers F, et al. Intensive insulin therapy in critically ill patients. N Engl J Med. 2001;345:1359–67.
16. Schulz KF, Grimes DA. Multiplicity in randomized trials II: subgroup and interim analyses. Lancet. 2005;365:1657–61.
17. Van den Berghe G, Wilmer A, Hermans G, et al. Intensive insulin therapy in the medical ICU. N Engl J Med. 2006;354:449–61.
18. Van den Berghe G, Wilmer A, Milants I, et al. Intensive insulin therapy in mixed medical/surgical intensive care units: benefit versus harm. Diabetes. 2006;55:3151–9.
19. Preiser JC, Devos P, Ruiz-Santana S, et al. A prospective randomised multi-centre controlled trial on tight glucose control by intensive insulin therapy in adult intensive care units: the Glucontrol study. Intensive Care Med. 2009;35:1738–48.
20. Brunkhorst FM, Engel C, Bloos F, et al. Intensive insulin therapy and pentastarch resuscitation in severe sepsis. N Engl J Med. 2008;358:125–39.
21. Finfer S, Chittock DR, Su SY, et al. Intensive versus conventional glucose control in critically ill patients. N Engl J Med. 2009;360:1283–97.
22. Finfer S, Liu B, Chittock DR, et al. Hypoglycemia and risk of death in critically ill patients. N Engl J Med. 2012;367:1108–18.

23. American Diabetes Association. 15. Diabetes care in the hospital: standards of medical care in diabetes–2021. Diabetes Care. 2021;44(Suppl 1):S211–20.
24. Jacobi J, Bircher N, Krinsley J, et al. Guidelines for the use of an insulin infusion for the management of hyperglycemia in critically ill patients. Crit Care Med. 2012;40:3251–76.
25. Shaw JE, Sicree RA, Zimmet PZ. Global estimates of the prevalence of diabetes for 2010 and 2030. Diabetes Res Clin Pract. 2010;87:4–14.
26. Krinsley JS. Glycemic control, diabetic status, and mortality in a heterogeneous population of critically ill patients before and during the era of intensive glycemic management: six and one-half years experience at a university-affiliated community hospital. Semin Thorac Cardiovasc Surg. 2006;18:317–25.
27. Plummer MP, Bellomo R, Cousins CE, et al. Dysglycaemia in the critically ill and the interaction of chronic and acute glycaemia with mortality. Intensive Care Med. 2014;40:973–80.
28. Carpenter DL, Gregg SR, Xu K, Buchman TG, Coopersmith CM. Prevalence and impact of unknown diabetes in the ICU. Crit Care Med. 2015;43:e541–e50.
29. van Vught LA, Wiewel MA, Klein Klouwenberg PMC, et al. Admission hyperglycemia in critically ill sepsis patients: association with outcome and host response. Crit Care Med. 2016;44:1338–46.
30. Bohé J, Abidi H, Brunot V, et al. Individualised versus conventional glucose control in critically-ill patients: the CONTROLING study-a randomized clinical trial. Intensive Care Med. 2021;47:1271–83.
31. Egi M, Bellomo R, Stachowski E, et al. Blood glucose concentration and outcome of critical illness: the impact of diabetes. Crit Care Med. 2008;36:2249–55.
32. Kar P, Plummer MP, Bellomo R, et al. Liberal glycemic control in critically ill patients with type 2 diabetes: an exploratory study. Crit Care Med. 2016;44:1695–703.
33. Luethi N, Cioccari L, Biesenbach P, et al. Liberal glucose control in ICU Patients with diabetes: a before-and-after study. Crit Care Med. 2018;46:935–42.
34. Krinsley JS, Meyfroidt G, van den Berghe G, Egi M, Bellomo R. The impact of premorbid diabetic status on the relationship between the three domains of glycemic control and mortality in critically ill patients. Curr Opin Clin Nutr Metab Care. 2012;15:151–60.
35. Krinsley JS, Deane AM, Gunst J. The goal of personalized glucose control in the critically ill remains elusive. Intensive Care Med. 2021;47:1319–21.
36. Balintescu A, Mårtensson J. Hemoglobin A1c and permissive hyperglycemia in patients in the intensive care unit with diabetes. Crit Care Clin. 2019;35:289–300.
37. Ma H, Yu G, Wang Z, Zhou P, Lv W. Association between dysglycemia and mortality by diabetes status and risk factors of dysglycemia in critically ill patients: a retrospective study. Acta Diabetol. 2022;59:461–70.
38. Krinsley JS, Preiser JC. Is it time to abandon glucose control in critically ill adult patients? Curr Opin Crit Care. 2019;25:299–306.
39. Egi M, Bellomo R, Stachowski E, et al. Hypoglycemia and outcome in critically ill patients. Mayo Clin Proc. 2010;85:217–24.
40. Krinsley JS, Grover A. Severe hypoglycemia in critically ill patients: risk factors and outcomes. Crit Care Med. 2007;35:2262–7.
41. Plummer MP, Hermanides J, Deane AM. Is it time to personalise glucose targets during critical illness? Curr Opin Clin Nutr Metab Care. 2022;25:364–9.
42. Egi M, Krinsley JS, Maurer P, et al. Pre-morbid glycemic control modifies the interaction between acute hypoglycemia and mortality. Intensive Care Med. 2016;42:562–71.
43. Krinsley JS, Maurer P, Holewinski S, et al. Glucose control, diabetes status, and mortality in critically ill patients: the continuum from intensive care unit admission to hospital discharge. Mayo Clin Proc. 2017;92:1019–29.
44. Lin S, He W, Zeng M. Association of diabetes and admission blood glucose levels with short-term outcomes in patients with critical illnesses. J Inflamm Res. 2020;13:1151–66.
45. Di Muzio F, Presello B, Glassford NJ, et al. Liberal versus conventional glucose targets in critically ill diabetic patients: an exploratory safety cohort assessment. Crit Care Med. 2016;44:1683–91.

46. Krinsley JS, Preiser JC, Hirsch IB. Safety and efficacy of personalized glycemic control in critically ill patients: a 2-year before and after interventional trial. Endocr Pract. 2017;23:318–30.
47. Poole AP, Finnis ME, Anstey J, et al. The effect of a liberal approach to glucose control in critically ill patients with type 2 diabetes: a multicenter, parallel-group, open-label, randomized clinical trial. Am J Respir Crit Care Med. 2022;206:874–82.
48. Lou R, Jiang L, Wang M, Zhu B, Jiang Q, Wang P. Association between glycemic gap and mortality in critically ill patients with diabetes. J Intensive Care Med. 2022;38:42.
49. Doola R, Deane AM, Barrett HL, et al. The impact of a modified carbohydrate formula, and its constituents, on glycaemic control and inflammatory markers: a nested mechanistic sub-study. J Hum Nutr Diet. 2022;35:455–65.
50. Hulst AH, Plummer MP, Hollmann MW, et al. Systematic review of incretin therapy during peri-operative and intensive care. Crit Care. 2018;22:299.

# Part IX

# A Look Back at COVID-19

# Hydroxychloroquine: Time for Reappraisal of Its Effect in COVID-19 Patients

31

V. Cés de Souza Dantas, J. P. Cidade, and P. Póvoa

## 31.1 Introduction

Coronaviruses are subdivided into four genera: alphacoronavirus, betacoronavirus (βCoV), gammacoronavirus, and deltacoronavirus; they infect birds and mammals, such as the Malayan pangolin, Himalayan and Asian palm civets, and bats. Human coronaviruses generally cause respiratory and intestinal infections of low severity, with exceptions that occurred in 2002, 2012, and 2019 [1].

An unusual atypical pneumonia emerged in Foshan, Guangdong Province, mainland China, in November 2002. In February and March 2003, the disease spread to Hong Kong and then to Vietnam, Singapore, Canada, and more than 26 countries within a year, infecting more than 8000 people with a reported mortality rate of 10%. The new disease was named the severe acute respiratory syndrome (SARS) [2].

In 2012, the Middle East respiratory syndrome (MERS) coronavirus emerged [3], causing 2494 cases of infection and 858 deaths as of December 2019 in the

V. C. de Souza Dantas (✉)
Instituto D'or de Pesquisa e Ensino, Rio de Janeiro, Brazil

Grupo de Pesquisa Clínica, Hospital Naval Marcílio Dias, Rio de Janeiro, Brazil
e-mail: vicente.dantas@idor.org

J. P. Cidade
Intensive Care Unit-4, Department of Intensive Care, Hospital de São Francisco Xavier, CHLO, Lisbon, Portugal

P. Póvoa
Intensive Care Unit-4, Department of Intensive Care, Hospital de São Francisco Xavier, CHLO, Lisbon, Portugal

NOVA Medical School, New University of Lisbon, Lisbon, Portugal

Center for Clinical Epidemiology and Research Unit of Clinical Epidemiology, OUH Odense University Hospital, Odense, Denmark



J.-L. Vincent (ed.), *Annual Update in Intensive Care and Emergency Medicine 2023*, Annual Update in Intensive Care and Emergency Medicine,
https://doi.org/10.1007/978-3-031-23005-9_31

regions of or near the Arabian Peninsula [3]. The severe acute respiratory syndrome coronavirus-2 (SARS-CoV-2), which appeared in December 2019 is the seventh human coronavirus found to cause respiratory infection and belongs to the βCoV genus originating from bats.

## 31.2 SARS-CoV-2

In late 2019, the first case of a novel pneumonia caused by a previously unknown pathogen appeared in China [4]. On 12 January 2020, the World Health Organization (WHO) named this virus, SARS-CoV-2, as the cause of the novel coronavirus infectious disease 2019 (COVID-19) [4]. The COVID-19 pandemic has affected more than 593 million persons so far and led to over six million deaths around the world [5]. Although almost all literature considers bats as the source of SARS-CoV-2, direct evidence is still lacking [4]. However, enough arguments for bat involvement are available, based mainly on four approaches: (1) experience gathered from previous βCoV epidemics where all known human coronavirus pandemics originated from bats; (2) phylogenic relationship of SARS-CoV-2 and related clades; (3) data obtained through artificial infection of bats with SARS-CoV-2; and (4) computerized models of SARS-CoV-2 evolution.

The structure of coronaviruses, including SARS-CoV-2, is comprised of a spike glycoprotein, a hemagglutinin-esterase dimer, a membrane glycoprotein, the nucleocapsid protein, and the RNA genome (Fig. 31.1) [6]. SARS-CoV-2 upregulates angiotensin-converting enzyme 2 (ACE2) expression in tissues, thus virus

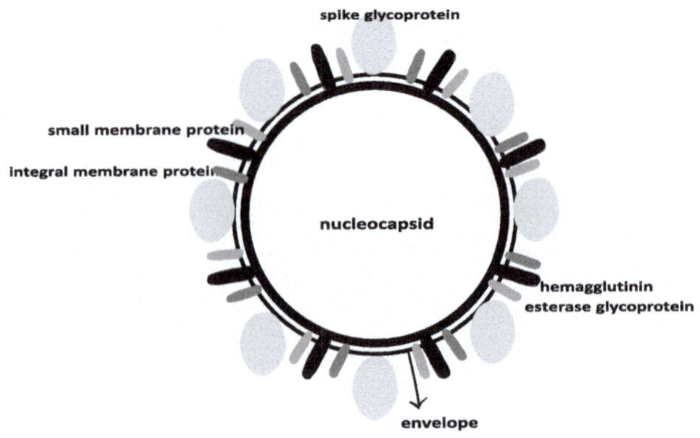


**Fig. 31.1** Schematic of the coronavirus structure

replication may increase. Binding to the ACE2 receptor triggers conformational changes in the glycoprotein, which inhibits virus neutralization by antibodies (Fig. 31.2) [6]. The spike glycoprotein enters the endoplasmic reticulum and binds to receptors of the human host cell. The glycoprotein determines the tissue tropism of the virus [6].

In 2003, at the time of the SARS-associated coronavirus epidemic [7], several drugs had been evaluated for their effectiveness on this virus; one of them was chloroquine [7]. No study demonstrated high *in vivo* chloroquine activity, and studies that demonstrated *in vitro* activity were forgotten with the disappearance of SARS-CoV [7].

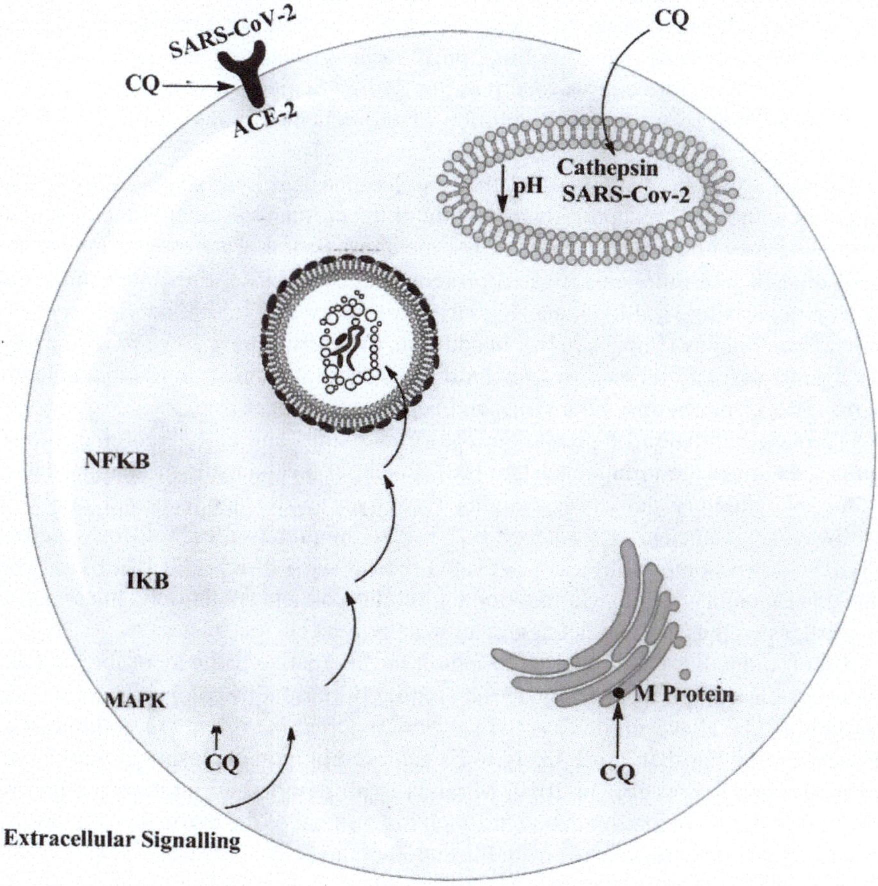


**Fig. 31.2** Possible effects of chloroquine on the severe acute respiratory syndrome coronavirus-2 (SARS-CoV-2) replication cycle. *ACE* angiotensin converting enzyme, *CQ* chloroquine, *MAPK* mitogen-activated protein kinase, *NFKB* nuclear factor kappa-B

## 31.3 Aminoquinolones

Chloroquine is an aminoquinolone derivative first developed for the treatment of malaria [7]. Chloroquine may also be used to treat extra-intestinal amebiasis [7]. Hydroxychloroquine is the other 4-aminoquinoline derivative antimalarial drug [8]. These agents are also used to treat rheumatic diseases, mainly systemic lupus erythematosus and rheumatoid arthritis [8].

Chloroquine has been a widely used, effective antimalarial therapy for decades. Chloroquine exerts its antimalarial effect during the blood stages or liver stages of the life cycle of the parasite [9]. As a protonated, weakly basic drug, chloroquine increases pH and accumulates in the food vacuole of parasites, where the host erythrocyte hemoglobin degrades, leading to the release of toxic products. It also inhibits the polymerization and detoxification of hematin and interferes with the degradation of host hemoglobin, preventing growth of *Plasmodium* [9]. Chloroquine therefore causes accumulation of free hematin, which is highly toxic to *Plasmodium*, resulting in dissolution of the cell membrane and death of the parasites [9].

*In vitro* studies have suggested that chloroquine and hydroxychloroquine can interfere with ACE2 receptor glycosylation of the coronavirus, increase endosomal pH, interfere with post-translational modification of viral proteins, and inhibit the activation of p38 mitogen-activated protein kinase (MAPK), thus inhibiting viral fusion, decreasing viral load, altering virion assembly, and inhibiting virus replication and autophagy (Fig. 31.2) [8]. In addition, these drugs have some *in vitro* activity against several other viruses, including influenza A, human immunodeficiency virus (HIV), enterovirus, Zika virus, and hepatitis C virus [8].

Through regulation of pro-inflammatory cytokines and cell signaling, chloroquine can affect the immune system [10]. Potential mechanisms of action include immunomodulatory activity via sigma-1 receptor (S1R) agonism and non-S1R pathways (e.g., nuclear factor-kappa B [NF-κB], inflammasomes, Toll-like receptor [TLR]4, peroxisome proliferator-activated receptor-γ [PPARγ]) [10], antiviral and anti-inflammatory actions via functional inhibition of acid sphingomyelinase activity [10], as well as antiplatelet aggregation activity [11].

Chloroquine has been reported to inhibit the alternative pathway of the complement system as well as to abrogate the clotting of plasma by calcium chloride and thrombin [11]. However, these activities were reported *in vitro* at chloroquine concentrations higher than those likely to be achieved in human plasma at therapeutically acceptable dosages. In 2019, Miranda et al. reported an inhibitory effect of chloroquine on coagulation *in vivo* through impairment of the extrinsic pathway, by impairing tissue factor release from the endothelium [12].

Because of its low therapeutic index and pharmacological activities of its metabolites, assessment of chloroquine pharmacokinetics is necessary for optimal clinical use. Drug disposition across different compartments proceeds in three phases—distribution from blood to tissues, equilibration between blood and tissues, and release from tissues back into blood [13]. These phases have half-lives of 3–8 h, 40–216 h, and 30–60 days, respectively [13]. The peak plasma concentration after an oral dose of chloroquine is reached in 3–12 h [13]. Thirty-three to 70% of the drug in plasma is protein-bound [13]. The most commonly quoted median value for the terminal elimination half-life is 40 days [13]. Chloroquine and hydroxychloroquine accumulate in different tissues in varying concentrations [13]. High concentrations of these drugs are found in the cardiac tissue, lungs, kidneys, liver, skeletal muscle, skin, and eye [13].

### 31.3.1 *In Vitro* Studies

Early in the pandemic, hydroxychloroquine was acclaimed as both a preventive and a therapeutic treatment for COVID-19, but subsequent clinical trials have not found any benefit, and some pointed to potential harm [14]. It is important to note that a possible explanation for this failure is based on the pharmacokinetic characteristics of these drugs. Because of significant interindividual pharmacokinetic variability, variable tissue concentrations might be found after administration of standardized doses [14]. In addition, the full effects of chloroquine and hydroxychloroquine may take 3–6 months to develop since it takes a long time to reach tissue steady state concentrations [14]. Some have attributed this to a pharmacodynamic mechanism involving an immune process that requires a long time to develop. However, the effect is predictable based on pharmacokinetics and the time required to saturate lysosomes [15]. The delayed onset of therapeutic effect of chloroquine and hydroxychloroquine can be shortened by using a higher loading dose in the first weeks to months at the price of an increased frequency of gastrointestinal side effects and other potentially dangerous cardiac toxicity.

Yao et al. [16] compared the *in vitro* antiviral activity of chloroquine and hydroxychloroquine against SARS-CoV-2 using a physiological pharmacokinetics model methodology that enabled five different dosing regimens to be simulated with the aim of predicting the safest dose of these drugs for lung tissue concentrations. This *in vitro* model showed that hydroxychloroquine was more potent than chloroquine. Based on the study results, they would recommend administering a loading dose of 400 mg of hydroxychloroquine sulfate orally twice daily, followed by a maintenance dose of 200 mg twice daily for 4 days for SARS-CoV-2 [16].

Wang et al. [17] studied the antiviral activity of chloroquine in Vero E6 cells. They showed that the 90% effective concentration of chloroquine against SARS-CoV-2 was similar to that in patients with rheumatoid arthritis who were receiving chloroquine 500 mg daily long-term [17].

Liu et al. [18] studied the *in vitro* anti-SARS-CoV-2 activity of hydroxychloroquine finding that it efficiently inhibited SARS-CoV-2 infection. In addition, the study confirmed that hydroxychloroquine inhibited the entry of SARS-CoV-2 into cells as well as inhibiting stages following SARS-CoV-2 entry; chloroquine had similar effects [18].

Due to this *in vitro* anti-viral activity, renewed interest in chloroquine and hydroxychloroquineas therapeutic options emerged in COVID-19 patients, along with the need for robust evidence to support this indication and its therapeutic safety.

### 31.3.2 Clinical Studies

Initial clinical studies, including two randomized clinical trials, reported conflicting results on clinical outcomes (in-hospital mortality rate, the rate of viral conversion and even the reduction of disease length) with use of hydroxychloroquine in COVID-19 [19–25]. However, these studies had methodological flaws and inconsistent data that compromised the robustness of the results.

The majority of the previously identified benefits and positive results from hydroxychloroquine were not reproduced in subsequent and more robust randomized clinical trials. In the RECOVERY open-label trial, an interim analysis of the patients in the hydroxychloroquine arm showed no impact on the 28-day all-cause mortality compared to usual care [26, 27]. The results further suggested that hydroxychloroquine treatment was associated with a lower likelihood of being discharged from the hospital alive at day 28 than was usual care (59.6% vs. 62.9%, relative risk [RR] 1.14, 95% confidence interval [CI] 1.03–1.27). These findings led to the immediate revocation of the Emergency Use authorization emitted by the FDA [28].

These data were reproduced by the Solidarity trial, which documented that hydroxychloroquine therapy had no effect on overall hospital mortality, initiation of ventilation, or length of hospital stay in hospitalized COVID-19 patients [29]. Moreover, the TOGETHER trial failed to support any significant benefit of hydroxychloroquine in the reduction of COVID-19-associated hospitalization rate or for the secondary outcome of viral clearance through day 14 [30].

Several reports also emerged focusing on the combination of hydroxychloroquine with macrolides, considering a potential therapeutic benefit on COVID-19 patients through combining the anti-viral properties of both drugs. However, in addition to the aforementioned RECOVERY trial, the ProPAC-COVID double-blinded placebo-controlled trial (n = 226) further confirmed that the combination of azithromycin and hydroxychloroquine did not improve survivability or reduce the length of hospitalization [31]. The results even favored stopping enrollment due to futility, considering that there were no differences in the primary outcome (days alive and discharged from hospital within 14 days; median [IQR]; 9.0 (3–11) days in the hydroxychloroquine plus azithromycin group versus 9.0 (7–10) days in the placebo group (p = 0.91)).

Randomized clinical trials focusing on hydroxychloroquine in non-hospitalized patients have also drawn substantial attention considering the burden of hospitalization and the relevant impact on financial resources and hospital bed shortages. The Brazilian COPE-Coalition V double-blind, multicenter, randomized, controlled trial showed that, in non-hospitalized patients with mild or moderate COVID-19, the use of hydroxychloroquine did not reduce the risk of hospitalization compared to placebo control (44 hospitalizations [6.4%] and 57 hospitalizations [8.3%], respectively, RR 0.77, 95% CI 0.52–1.12), and, consequentially, its routine use could not be recommended [32]. This evidence was further complemented by a meta-analysis which suggested that hydroxychloroquine had no significant benefit in reducing hospitalization among patients with positive tests (RR 0.77, 95% CI 0.57–1.04) [32]. These results followed the previously collected data by the Coalition Covid-19

Brazil I trial which had already documented that hydroxychloroquine did not improve clinical status at day 15 compared to standard care [33].

Considering its widespread use, several issues regarding hydroxychloroquine and chloroquine safety were raised, especially the known cardiac toxicity, during acute treatment of COVID-19 [34, 35]. The most common adverse effects of hydroxychloroquine and chloroquine relate to gastrointestinal symptoms and anorexia. However, a significant prolongation of the QT interval is a known side effect of taking hydroxychloroquine or chloroquine [36] and, although considered rare, long-term and high-dose intakes of these medications have been described as possible causes of irreversible damage to the cardiovascular and neurological systems [34, 37].

As azithromycin and hydroxychloroquine can work as senolytics *in vitro*, we should be more cautious about cardiovascular disorders as cardiac cells become more senescent with aging [37]. More recently, studies found that hydroxychloroquine plus azithromycin increased the risk of corrected QTc prolongation and cardiac arrhythmias in COVID-19 patients [36]. Patients receiving combined hydroxychloroquine and azithromycin should be monitored for cardiovascular and ophthalmological toxicity, especially older patients.

In this regard, important insights on the safety profile of hydroxychloroquine stemmed from a cohort study of patients with COVID-19 pneumonia [36]. The results showed that patients who had been treated with hydroxychloroquine had a high risk of QTc prolongation, with or without concurrent treatment with a macrolide (median baseline QTc was 455 [IQR 430–474] milliseconds versus 473 [454–487] milliseconds in the hydroxychloroquine treatment group and 442 [427–461] milliseconds in the hydroxychloroquine and azithromycin treatment group [$p < 0.001$]) [36].

A recent meta-analysis grouped and summarized the data collected in randomized trials investigating hydroxychloroquine or chloroquine as treatment for COVID-19 [28]. The results shed more light on these therapies, offering useful insight for a challenging health situation. The combined odds ratio (OR) on all-cause mortality for hydroxychloroquine was 1.11 (95% CI 1.02, 1.2; $I^2 = 0\%$; 26 trials; 10,012 patients) and for chloroquine 1.77 (95% CI 0.15, 21.13, $I^2 = 0\%$; 4 trials; 307 patients) and no subgroup effects were identified. Treatment with hydroxychloroquine is therefore associated with increased mortality in COVID-19 patients, and there is no benefit from treatment with chloroquine based on currently available randomized trial data [38–40].

## 31.4 Conclusion

Emerging evidence-based medicine proves, once again, the need to perform good clinical research and good randomized clinical trials to assess the true value of a drug before recommending its widespread clinical use. This is the only way to protect patients against useless and dangerous treatments, ensuring that only effective therapies are delivered, despite the pressure of high expectations in pandemic settings, namely from social media. The discrepant results between the early studies, showing a positive effect on patient outcomes, and the more recent randomized clinical trials, proving a higher mortality rate of COVID-19 patients treated with hydroxychloroquine, further endorse the need to rethink and review clinical indications as new evidence emerges, to provide the best care and survival chance to patients in an already serious situation.

## References

1. Lu H, Stratton CW, Tang YW. Outbreak of pneumonia of unknown etiology in Wuhan, China: the mystery and the miracle. J Med Virol. 2020;92:401–2.
2. Chan-Yeung M, Xu RH. SARS: epidemiology. Respirology. 2003;8(Suppl 1):S9–14.
3. Zaki AM, van Boheemen S, Bestebroer TM, et al. Isolation of a novel coronavirus from a man with pneumonia in Saudi Arabia. N Engl J Med. 2012;367:1814–20.
4. Wu F, Zhao S, Yu B, et al. A new coronavirus associated with human respiratory disease in China. Nature. 2020;579:265–9.
5. COVID-19 coronavirus pandemic coronavirus cases. Available at: https://www.worldometers.info/coronavirus. Accessed 22 Aug 2022.
6. Lu R, Zhao X, Li J, et al. Genomic characterisation and epidemiology of 2019 novel coronavirus: implications for virus origins and receptor binding. Lancet. 2020;395:565–74.
7. Keyaerts E, Vijgen L, Maes P, et al. In vitro inhibition of severe acute respiratory syndrome coronavirus by chloroquine. Biochem Biophys Res Commun. 2004;323:264–8.
8. McChesney EW. Animal toxicity and pharmacokinetics of hydroxychloroquine sulfate. Am J Med. 1983;75:11–8.
9. Tse EG, Korsik M, Todd MH. The past, present and future of anti-malarial medicines. Malar J. 2019;18:93.
10. Seitz M, Valbracht J, Quach J, et al. Gold sodium thiomalate and chloroquine inhibit cytokine production in monocytic THP-1 cells through distinct transcriptional and posttranslational mechanisms. J Clin Immunol. 2003;23:477–84.
11. Ramanathan VD, Sengupta U. In vitro inhibition of the activation of the human complement and coagulation systems by chloroquine. Int J Immunopharmacol. 1985;7:769–73.
12. Miranda S, Billoir P, Damian L, et al. Hydroxychloroquine reverses the prothrombotic state in a mouse model of antiphospholipid syndrome: role of reduced inflammation and endothelial dysfunction. PLoS One. 2019;14:e0212614.
13. Iredale J, Fieger H, Wainer IW. Determination of the stereoisomers of hydroxychloroquine and its major metabolites in plasma and urine following a single oral administration of racemic hydroxychloroquine. Semin Arthritis Rheum. 1993;23:74–81.
14. Ducharme J, Farinotti R. Clinical pharmacokinetics and metabolism of chloroquine. Clin Pharmacokinet. 1996;31:257–74.
15. Rowland M, Tozer TN. Clinical Pharmacokinetics and Pharmacodynamics. Concepts and Applications. Philadelphia: Wolters Kluwer; 2011. p. 579.
16. Yao X, Ye F, Zhang M, et al. In vitro antiviral activity and projection of optimized dosing design of hydroxychloroquine for the treatment of severe acute respiratory syndrome coronavirus 2 (SARS-CoV-2). Clin Infect Dis. 2020;71:732–9.
17. Wang M, Cao R, Zhang L, et al. Remdesivir and chloroquine effectively inhibit the recently emerged novel coronavirus (2019-nCoV) in vitro. Cell Res. 2020;30:269–71.
18. Liu J, Cao R, Xu M, Wang X, Zhang H, Hu H, et al. Hydroxychloroquine, a less toxic derivative of chloroquine, is effective in inhibiting SARS-CoV-2 infection in vitro. Cell Discov. 2020;6:16.
19. Chen J, Liu D, Liu L, et al. A pilot study of hydroxychloroquine in treatment of patients with moderate COVID-19 [in Chinese]. Zhejiang Da Xue Xue Bao Yi Xue Ban. 2020;49:215–9.
20. Chen Z, Hu J, Zhang Z, et al. Efficacy of hydroxychloroquine in patients with COVID-19: results of a randomized clinical trial. medRxiv. 2020. https://doi.org/10.1101/2020.03.22.20040758.

21. Yu B, Wang DW, Li C. Hydroxychloroquine application is associated with a decreased mortality in critically ill patients with COVID-19. medRxiv. 2020. https://doi.org/10.1101/2020.04.27.20073379.
22. Rosenberg ES, Dufort EM, Udo T, et al. Association of treatment with hydroxychloroquine or azithromycin with in-hospital mortality in patients with COVID-19 in New York State. JAMA. 2020;323:2493–502.
23. Lee JE, Lee SO, Heo J, et al. Comparative outcomes of lopinavir/ritonavir and hydroxychloroquine for the treatment of coronavirus disease 2019 with mild to moderate severity. Antivir Ther. 2021;26:34–42.
24. Geleris J, Sun Y, Platt J, et al. Observational study of hydroxychloroquine in hospitalized patients with COVID-19. N Engl J Med. 2020;382:2411–8.
25. Mallat J, Hamed F, Balkis M, et al. Hydroxychloroquine is associated with slower viral clearance in clinical COVID-19 patients with mild to moderate disease. Medicine (Baltimore). 2020;99:e23720.
26. Abaleke E, Abbas M, Abbasi S, et al. Azithromycin in patients admitted to hospital with COVID-19 (RECOVERY): a randomised, controlled, open-label, platform trial. Lancet. 2021;397:605–12.
27. Horby P, Mafham M, Linsell L, et al. Effect of hydroxychloroquine in hospitalized patients with Covid-19. N Engl J Med. 2020;383:2030–40.
28. Axfors C, Schmitt AM, Janiaud P, et al. Mortality outcomes with hydroxychloroquine and chloroquine in COVID-19 from an international collaborative meta-analysis of randomized. Nat Commun. 2021;12:2349.
29. Pan H, Peto R, Henao-Restrepo AM, et al. Repurposed antiviral drugs for Covid-19 - interim WHO solidarity trial results. N Engl J Med. 2021;384:497–511.
30. Reis G, Silva EASM, Silva DCM, et al. Effect of early treatment with hydroxychloroquine or lopinavir and ritonavir on risk of hospitalization among patients with COVID-19: the TOGETHER randomized clinical trial. JAMA Netw Open. 2021;4:e216468.
31. Sivapalan P, Ulrik CS, Lapperre TS, et al. Azithromycin and hydroxychloroquine in hospitalised patients with confirmed COVID-19: a randomised double-blinded placebo-controlled trial. Eur Respir J. 2022;59:2100752.
32. Avezum A, Oliveira GBF, Oliveira H, et al. Hydroxychloroquine versus placebo in the treatment of non-hospitalised patients with COVID-19 (COPE – Coalition V): A double-blind, multicentre, randomised, controlled trial. Lancet Reg Health Am. 2022;11:100243.
33. Cavalcanti AB, Zampieri FG, Rosa RG, et al. Hydroxychloroquine with or without azithromycin in mild-to-moderate Covid-19. N Engl J Med. 2020;383:2041–52.
34. Giudicessi JR, Noseworthy PA, Friedman PA, et al. Urgent guidance for navigating and circumventing the QTc-prolonging and torsadogenic potential of possible pharmacotherapies for coronavirus disease 19 (COVID-19). Mayo Clin Proc. 2020;95:1213–21.
35. Lane JC, Weaver J, Kostka K, et al. Risk of hydroxychloroquine alone and in combination with azithromycin in the treatment of rheumatoid arthritis: a multinational, retrospective study. Lancet Rheumatol. 2020;2:e698–711.
36. Mercuro NJ, Yen CF, Shim DJ, et al. Risk of QT interval prolongation associated with use of hydroxychloroquine with or without concomitant azithromycin among hospitalized patients testing positive for coronavirus disease 2019 (COVID-19). JAMA Cardiol. 2020;5:1036–41.
37. Wu CI, Postema PG, Arbelo E, et al. SARS-CoV-2, COVID-19, and inherited arrhythmia syndromes. Heart Rhythm. 2020;17:1456–62.
38. Oscanoa TJ, Romero-Qrtuno R, Carvajal A, et al. A pharmacological perspective of chloroquine in SARS-CoV-2 infection: An old drug for the fight against a new coronavirus? Int J Antimicrob Agents. 2020;56:106078.
39. Xu J, Cao B. Lessons learnt from hydroxychloroquine/azithromycin in treatment of COVID-19. Eur Respir J. 2022;59:2102002.
40. Saghir SAM, Algabri NA, Alagawany MM, et al. Chloroquine and hydroxychloroquine for the prevention and treatment of COVID-19: a fiction, hope or hype? An updated review. Ther Clin Risk Manag. 2021;17:371–87.

# Blood Purification in COVID-19 in the Absence of Acute Kidney Injury

# 32

P. M. Honoré, S. Blackman, and E. Perriens

## 32.1 Introduction

During the rush of the coronavirus disease 2019 (COVID-19) pandemic, hemofiltration was proposed as a potential treatment for severe COVID-19. It was initially thought that removing the inflammatory 'storm' generated during COVID-19, which worsened acute respiratory distress syndrome (ARDS), would be beneficial [1]. Hemofiltration can also efficiently eliminate viruses [2], nucleocapsids [3], and endotoxins [4]. In this chapter, we will describe the functions of blood purification use in detail, as well as the studies that evaluated their effectiveness during the pandemic [5].

## 32.2 Tackling the Inflammatory Storm Initiated by COVID-19

### 32.2.1 Sorbents

Several studies have evaluated the impact of reducing the cytokine storm during severe COVID-19 [6]. When interleukin-6 (IL-6) levels in septic shock and COVID-19 inflammatory storms are compared, they are about 100,000 pg/ml during septic shock versus 40–80 ng/ml during a COVID-19 inflammatory storm [7], demonstrating that the term "cytokine storm" is a misnomer [8, 9].

P. M. Honoré (✉)
ICU Department, Centre Hospitalier Universitaire Brugmann, Brussels, Belgium

ICU Department, CHU UCL Godinne, UCLouvain Medical School, Yvoir, Belgium
e-mail: patrick.honore@chuuclnamur.uclouvain.be

S. Blackman · E. Perriens
ICU Department, Centre Hospitalier Universitaire Brugmann, Brussels, Belgium



J.-L. Vincent (ed.), *Annual Update in Intensive Care and Emergency Medicine 2023*,
Annual Update in Intensive Care and Emergency Medicine,
https://doi.org/10.1007/978-3-031-23005-9_32

The correct timing of the hemofiltration is important in this setting. IL-6 has both pro- and anti-inflammatory properties, depending on the pathway of transduction: the classic signaling pathway, mediated by the membrane-bound form of the IL-6 receptor, is believed to be anti-inflammatory, whereas the trans-signaling pathway, mediated by the soluble form of the IL-6 receptor, is believed to be pro-inflammatory [10]. In patients with COVID-19, it is important to preserve the regenerative and anti-inflammatory properties of the classic IL-6 pathway and block only the pro-inflammatory actions [11]. This is a major limitation with blood purification, as it is non-selective, and may explain why the results from studies exploring blood purification for COVID-19 cytokine storm have been disappointing [12].

The removal of excess cytokines using sorbent was studied in patients with severe COVID-19 requiring extracorporeal membrane oxygenation (ECMO) [13]. This single-center, randomized controlled trial (RCT) investigated serum IL-6 concentrations after 72 h of ECMO and 30-day survival in a control group and a group treated with CytoSorb (CytoSorbents Corporation, Monmouth Junction, NJ, USA). Adjusted mean log IL-6 concentrations after 72 h were higher in the cytokine adsorption group than in the controls (95% CI –0.70 to 1.30, $p = 0.54$) [13]. Survival after 30 days was 18% with cytokine adsorption and 76% without cytokine adsorption ($p = 0.0016$) [13]. The authors concluded that early initiation of cytokine adsorption in patients with severe COVID-19 and veno-venous ECMO (VV-ECMO) did not reduce serum IL-6 concentrations and actually had a negative effect on survival [13].

In a single-center pilot trial, the effect of extracorporeal cytokine reduction using CytoSorb was studied in patients with COVID-19-associated vasoplegic shock [14]. The 50 patients were randomized into a control group and a group receiving treatment with CytoSorb. All patients required norepinephrine >0.2 μg/kg/min to maintain mean arterial pressure (MAP) ≥65 mmHg, had C-reactive protein (CRP) levels >100 mg/l, and acute kidney injury (AKI) stage 3 with need for continuous renal replacement therapy (CRRT) [14]. Time until resolution of vasoplegic shock, mortality, IL-6 concentrations, and catecholamine requirements were measured [14]. There were no significant differences between the groups in hemodynamic improvement or mortality rate at 30 and 90 days [14]. The authors concluded that CytoSorb treatment did not improve resolution of vasoplegic shock compared with standard therapy [14]. This lack of effect on IL-6 levels and hemodynamic status using CytoSorb raises questions regarding the mechanisms underlying the use of sorbents in treating inflammation in COVID-19 [14].

A recent systematic review of 11 articles also showed a lack of clinical evidence of efficacy of CytoSorb in patients with COVID-19 and concluded that the use of hemoperfusion in these patients does not seem to be supported outside of clinical trials [7], as also discussed in recent narrative reviews on extracorporeal blood purification in patients with COVID-19 [15, 16].

### 32.2.2 Therapeutic Plasma Exchange

The benefits of therapeutic plasma exchange as an adjunctive therapy for cytokine-mediated inflammation in COVID-19 remain theoretical [17]. The causal relationship between cytokine release syndrome and the development and progression of ARDS, multiple organ failure (MOF), and septic shock remains to be proven. Therapeutic plasma exchange not only removes pro-inflammatory cytokines, but also anti-inflammatory mediators and host defense factors, such as immunoglobulins [17]. Some authors assert that therapeutic plasma exchange is unique because it offers benefits on multiple levels by removing inflammatory cytokines, stabilizing endothelial membranes, and resetting hypercoagulable states [18]. The major difference between therapeutic plasma exchange and modern extracorporeal adsorption strategies is the exchange of septic shock plasma with fresh frozen plasma (FFP), which may prevent non-selective depletion of pro- and anti-inflammatory cytokines and instead replenish protective factors (within FFP) that have been consumed by sepsis [19]. The magnitude of the inflammatory response does not justify non-selective removal of components of the inflammatory response, especially considering that some of them may be beneficial. Therapeutic plasma exchange also has the potential to cause harm by diluting or attenuating the host's adaptive response to infection by depleting immunoglobulins and complement components 3 and 4 in individuals treated with plasmapheresis [20]. In the context of the severe acute respiratory syndrome coronavirus 2 (SARS-CoV-2) outbreak, therapeutic plasma exchange removed protective antibodies formed by the patient, which is not desirable [20] (Fig. 32.1). However, other extracorporeal blood filtration techniques, such as the oXiris filter (Baxter International, Deerfield, IL, USA), are now under investigation [21].

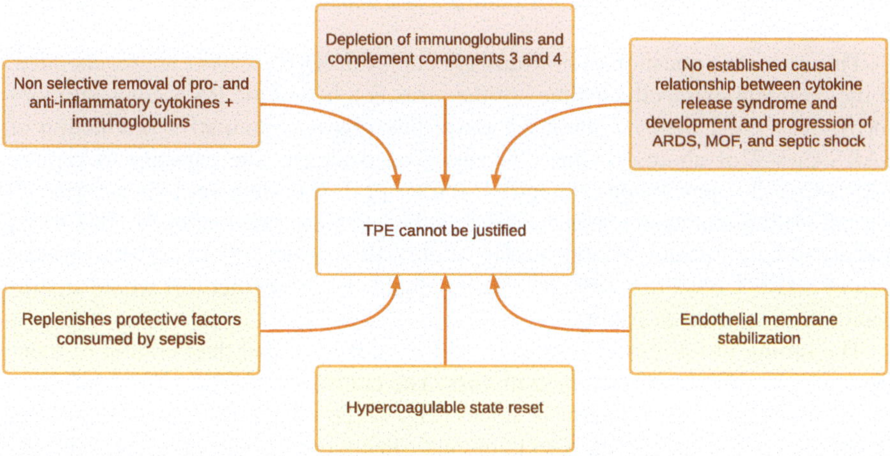


**Fig. 32.1** Is therapeutic plasma exchange (TPE) justified for the treatment of coronavirus disease 2019 (COVID-19)? *ARDS* acute respiratory distress syndrome, *MOF* multiple organ failure

## 32.3 Removing SARS-CoV-2 and Nucleocapsids

### 32.3.1 SARS-CoV-2 Removal by Seraph® 100

The new sorbent, Seraph® 100 (ExThera Medical, Martinez, CA, USA), contains ultrahigh molecular weight polyethylene beads with end-point-attached heparin [2, 22]. This filter is approved by the USA Food and Drug Administration (FDA) for the removal of pathogens such as bacteria, viruses, and toxins from the bloodstream, by binding irreversibly to the immobilized heparin column [2, 22]. In pre-clinical studies, the system was not only able to reduce the amount of Zika virus from the blood by 87%, but also cytomegalovirus CMV (79%) and adenoviruses (62%) [2]. In this study, Seffer et al. claimed that the Seraph® 100 could remove COVID-19 virus, but did not specify to what extent [2].

Olson et al. evaluated the capacity of the Seraph® 100 to remove SARS-CoV-2 in an infected patient [23]. They extrapolated that one Seraph-100 device should clear up to 100 billion SARS-CoV-2 virions [23]. In a patient with a blood volume of 5 l, this would translate to 18,000,000 viral copies/ml [23]. This seems to be an impressive amount; however several questions arise. Is this amount significantly greater than the production of SARS-CoV-2 copies in the human body? What is the best moment for the removal of SARS-CoV-2 virions in an infected patient? Finally, is this removal correlated with significant clinical improvement? Is virus reduction correlated with improved survival?

Using the best available knowledge, researchers estimated the total number and mass of SARS-CoV-2 virions in body fluids and host tissues in an infected person [24]. They estimated that each infected person carries $10^9$ to $10^{11}$ virions during the peak of infection, with a total mass in the range of 1–100 μg. This amounts to roughly 100 billion virions, corresponding to the capacity of removal of one Seraph® 100 filter [22, 24].

This raises the question of how quickly copies of SARS-CoV-2 are regenerated. If the "resident extracellular time" of the virus is 8 h, and the RNA concentrations for SARS-CoV-2 peak at about 2.7 days, this gives a cumulative production of SARS-CoV-2 of about 30 times the observed peak and the capacity to capture SARS-CoV-2 copies by one Seraph® 100 filter [25]. If these assertions are true, 30 Seraph® 100 filters would be needed over 3 days to clear a patient of SARS-CoV-2, and use of a single Seraph® 100 per day would only remove 10% of the total production of SARS-CoV-2 that day [26], raising doubts as to whether this would significantly help an infected patient.

The timing of the therapy, the peak of the viral load, and the duration of treatment are also important factors to discuss. The course of a SARS-CoV-2 infection can be divided into three phases or stages (Fig. 32.2): stage I refers to the beginning of the infection, stage II refers to pulmonary involvement with or without hypoxemia, and stage III refers to the systemic inflammation [27, 28]. Virus production peaks during stage I while the infection settles in the lungs and the patient remains asymptomatic [27]. In this first phase, if the patient is paucisymptomatic but has a positive polymerase chain reaction (PCR) test, the only biological modifications

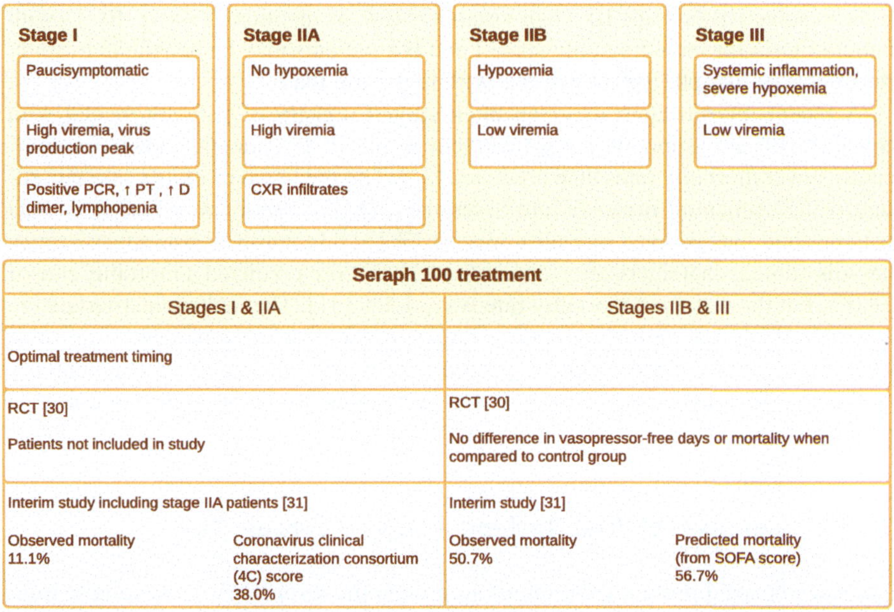


**Fig. 32.2** Evolution of the four stages of severe acute respiratory syndrome coronavirus 2 (SARS-CoV-2) infection and proposed ideal timing for Seraph 100 treatment. *PCR* polymerase chain reaction, *PT* prothrombin time, *CXR* chest X-ray, *RCT* randomized controlled trial, *SOFA* sequential organ failure assessment

include lymphopenia, raised D-dimer concentrations, and increased prothrombin time; CRP and IL-6 concentrations are not yet altered [27] and chest X-rays are normal [27]. In stage IIA, there is no hypoxemia, however there are pulmonary infiltrates on the chest X-ray. In stage IIB, the patient becomes hypoxemic and is hospitalized; however, viremia is low [27]. During stage III, systemic inflammation and severe hypoxemia remain, and most of these patients are hospitalized in the intensive care unit (ICU).

If treated according to a patient's degree of viremia, the optimal timing for Seraph® 100 treatment would therefore be during stage I or IIA, which would be difficult to achieve [27]. The only way to do this would be to measure the viral load immediately after a positive PCR test in an asymptomatic patient [29]. If the viral count was high, the patient would be sent to the hospital for Seraph® 100 treatment. The duration of the treatment would depend on the moment of the 3-day peak. If the patient is in stage IIB or stage III, a Seraph® 100 procedure would be of no benefit as there is a small to no viral load during these phases [27].

One large multicenter study evaluated clinical improvement after the use of Seraph® 100, comparing 53 treated patients with 53 controls [30]. There was no difference in vasopressor-free days in patients treated with Seraph® 100 compared to those who were not. The average difference in mortality between treated and control subjects was also not significant [30]. However, all patients included in the study were in stage IIB or stage III when viremia is low, as mentioned above. RCTs with better criteria for including only stage I and IIA patients may be beneficial to study the effects of Seraph® 100 in patients with high viral load.

A recent interim analysis of an international registry of patients treated with Seraph® 100 also supports early treatment in non-ICU patients, showing significantly lower mortality rates than predicted [31]. The predicted mortality rate according to the sequential organ failure assessment (SOFA) score was 56.7% in ICU patients, and the observed mortality was 50.7% [31]. In non-ICU patients, the coronavirus clinical characterization consortium (4C) score predicted a mortality rate of 38.0%, but the observed mortality rate was 11.1% [31]. The inclusion criteria were a positive PCR test and pneumonia, which suggests that these patients were most likely in stage IIA during which the viral load is still significant, thus potentially explaining the efficacy of Seraph® 100 on decreasing 30-day mortality in non-ICU patients [31].

### 32.3.2 Removal of Viral Nucleocapsids by Seraph® 100

The nucleocapsid protein (N-protein) surrounds the viral RNA, protecting it from the host cell environment and facilitating RNA transcription, an essential step for viral replication [3, 32]. It is abundantly expressed inside cells infected with SARS-CoV-2. Seraph® 100 decreased SARS-CoV-2 nucleocapsid protein in the blood of patients with COVID-19 [3, 32], although this finding has not yet been correlated to clinical improvement. It would be interesting to evaluate the clinical effect of the concomitant removal of the virions and the N-proteins to determine whether the effect is additional or synergetic.

## 32.4 Removing Endotoxin During Severe COVID-19 Infection

Sirivongrangson et al. studied 19 patients with severe COVID-19; 13 of the patients were admitted to the ICU and 10 were receiving mechanical ventilation [33]. Eight patients had high endotoxin activity assay (EAA) values and more of these patients required mechanical ventilation than did the patients with low EAA values (62.5% vs. 45.5%) [33]. The proportion of patients requiring vasopressors, prone positioning, and ECMO did not differ between EAA groups, which is perhaps surprising as endotoxin has strong vasoplegic effects. The study concluded that endotoxemia, presumably from the gut, may complicate COVID-19 [33]. In another study of 32 patients, EEA was measured in patients with MOF [34]. Twenty-six patients had intermediate (0.40–0.59) or high (≥0.6) levels of EAA despite a low incidence of superimposed Gram-negative bacteria (6% of patients), supporting the hypothesis of Sirivongrangson et al. suggesting gut translocation as the origin for the majority of endotoxins in severe COVID-19 [34].

Finally, the role of endotoxin in severe COVID-19 and whether it should be treated should be discussed [35] (Fig. 32.3). A recent article showed a high-affinity

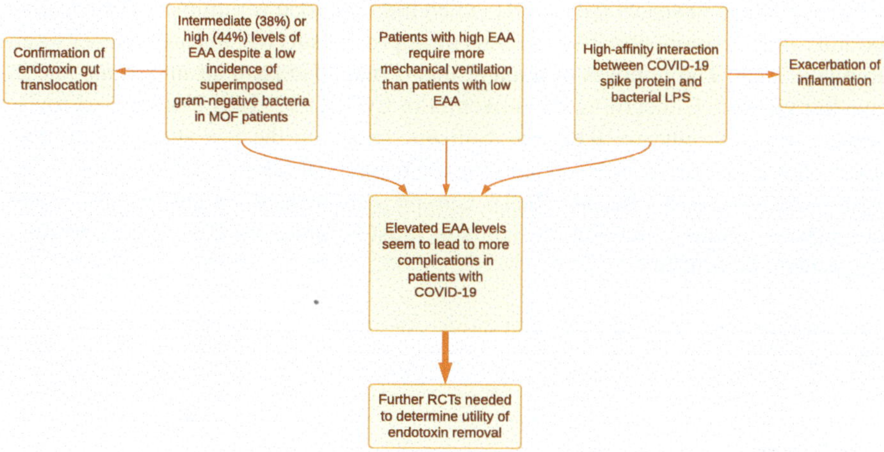


**Fig. 32.3** Role of endotoxin in severity of coronavirus disease 2019 (COVID-19) and its origin, based on data from [34]. *EAA* endotoxin activity assay, *MOF* multiple organ failure, *LPS* lipopolysaccharide, *RCT* randomized controlled trial

interaction between the COVID-19 spike (S) protein and bacterial lipopolysaccharide (LPS), leading to an exacerbation of inflammation and linking the metabolic syndrome to COVID-19 [36]. In an observational study from Japan, 12 COVID-19 patients who required oxygen support underwent endotoxin removal by polymyxin B direct hemoperfusion (PMX-DHP) [37]. The authors concluded that PMX-DHP was more effective in patients with intermediate severity COVID-19 who were receiving high levels of oxygen than in patients receiving mechanical ventilation or ECMO [37]. In another study, PMX-DHP was used in 12 patients with COVID-19 receiving invasive mechanical ventilation [38]. The SOFA score improved in the 120 h following the intervention, and the EAA decreased from 0.78 to 0.60 although this result was not statistically significant [38]. The contradictory results from these two studies confirm the need for larger RCTs.

## 32.5 Conclusion

Blood purification in patients with severe COVID-19 can currently be viewed from three approaches: first, removal of the cytokine storm—a misnomer—by new sorbents; second, the use of a special sorbent, Seraph® 100, a cartridge that may remove billions of SARS-CoV-2 virions and nucleocapsids; third, the removal of endotoxin. Regarding the removal of excess inflammation during severe COVID-19, results are disappointing with no difference or an increase in mortality in treated patients. Therapeutic plasma exchange has several adverse effects and cannot be recommended either. Concerning the removal of viruses and the nucleocapsid, doubts remain regarding efficacy. It is unsure whether use of one cartridge per day is able to extract significant copies of SARS-CoV-2. Timing is also an issue, as the studies included patients in stages IIB and III, when the viral load is minimal. The Seraph® 100 filter may be more effective in terms of improved survival in early phases when viremia is high. The removal of nucleocapsids may also have an important role in reducing viremia. Concerning endotoxemia in COVID-19, LPS binding and translocation from the gut are likely mechanisms, based on the few studies available. However, we have no answers concerning the benefits of removing these endotoxins on clinical outcomes. Before RCTs can be commenced to study these three approaches, it is clear that the mechanisms must be understood to be able to fully comprehend their utility.

**Acknowledgements** We would like to thank Ibrahim Bousbiat for his incredible help in the manuscript.

## References

1. Kang K, Luo Y, Gao Y, et al. Continuous renal replacement therapy with oXiris filter may not be an effective resolution to alleviate cytokine release syndrome in non-AKI patients with severe and critical COVID-19. Front Pharmacol. 2022;13:817793.
2. Seffer MT, Cottam D, Forni LG, et al. Heparin 2.0: a new approach to the infection crisis. Blood Purif. 2021;50:28–34.
3. Kielstein JT, Borchina DN, Fühner T, et al. Hemofiltration with the Seraph® 100 Microbind® Affinity filter decreases SARS-CoV-2 nucleocapsid protein in critically ill COVID-19 patients. Crit Care. 2021;25:190.
4. Peerapornratana S, Sirivongrangson P, Tungsanga S, et al. Endotoxin adsorbent therapy in severe COVID-19 pneumonia. Blood Purif. 2022;51:47–54.
5. Ronco C, Navalesi P, Vincent JL. Coronavirus epidemic: preparing for extracorporeal organ support in intensive care. Lancet Respir Med. 2020;8:240–1.
6. Rampino T, Gregorini M, Perotti L, et al. Hemoperfusion with CytoSorb as adjuvant therapy in critically ill patients with SARS-CoV2 pneumonia. Blood Purif. 2021;50:566–71.
7. Sanfilippo F, Martucci G, La Via L, et al. Hemoperfusion and blood purification strategies in patients with COVID-19: a systematic review. Artif Organs. 2021;45:1466–76.
8. Bonnet B, Cosme J, Dupuis C, et al. Severe COVID-19 is characterized by the co-occurrence of moderate cytokine inflammation and severe monocyte dysregulation. EBioMedicine. 2021;73:103622.
9. Sinha P, Matthay MA, Calfee CS. Is a "cytokine storm" relevant to COVID-19? JAMA Intern Med. 2020;180:1152–15.
10. Honore PM, Barreto Gutierrez L, et al. Inhibiting IL-6 in COVID-19: we are not sure. Crit Care. 2020;24:463.
11. Scheller J, Chalaris A, Schmidt-Arras D, et al. The pro- and anti-inflammatory properties of the cytokine interleukin-6. Biochim Biophys Acta. 2011;1813:878–88.
12. Kielstein JT, Zarbock A. Is this the beginning of the end of cytokine adsorption? Crit Care Med. 2022;50:1026–9.
13. Supady A, Weber E, Rieder M, et al. Cytokine adsorption in patients with severe COVID-19 pneumonia requiring extracorporeal membrane oxygenation (CYCOV): a single centre, open-label, randomised, controlled trial. Lancet Respir Med. 2021;9:755–62.
14. Stockmann H, Thelen P, Stroben F, et al. CytoSorb rescue for COVID-19 patients with vasoplegic shock and multiple organ failure: a prospective, open-label, randomized controlled pilot study. Crit Care Med. 2022;50:964–76.
15. Koc S, Uysal H. Literature review of hemadsorption therapy in severe COVID-19 cases: a narrative review. Clin Lab. 2022;68. https://doi.org/10.7754/Clin.Lab.2021.210839.

16. Kashani K, Forni LG. Extracorporeal blood purification is appropriate in critically ill patients with COVID-19 and multiorgan failure: CON. Kidney360. 2021;3:419–22.
17. Lu W, Kelley W, Fang DC, et al. The use of therapeutic plasma exchange as adjunctive therapy in the treatment of coronavirus disease 2019: a critical appraisal of the current evidence. J Clin Apher. 2021;36:483–91.
18. Keith P, Day M, Perkins L, et al. A novel treatment approach to the novel coronavirus: an argument for the use of therapeutic plasma exchange for fulminant COVID-19. Crit Care. 2020;24:128.
19. Knaup H, Stahl K, Schmidt BMW, et al. Early therapeutic plasma exchange in septic shock: a prospective open-label nonrandomized pilot study focusing on safety, hemodynamics, vascular barrier function, and biologic markers. Crit Care. 2018;22:285.
20. Honore PM, Mugisha A, Kugener L, et al. Therapeutic plasma exchange as a routine therapy in septic shock and as an experimental treatment for COVID-19: we are not sure. Crit Care. 2020;24:226.
21. Niazi NS, Nassar TI, Stewart IJ, et al. A review of extracorporeal blood purification techniques for the treatment of critically ill coronavirus disease 2019 patients. ASAIO J. 2022;68:1219–27.
22. Eden G, Schmidt JJ, Büttner S, et al. Safety and efficacy of the Seraph® 100 Microbind® Affinity Blood Filter to remove bacteria from the blood stream: results of the first in human study. Crit Care. 2022;26:181.
23. Olson SW, Oliver JD, Collen J, et al. Treatment for severe coronavirus disease 2019 With the Seraph-100 Microbind Affinity blood filter. Crit Care Explor. 2020;2:e0180.
24. Sender R, Bar-On YM, Gleizer S, et al. The total number and mass of SARS-CoV-2 virions. Proc Natl Acad Sci U S A. 2021;118:e2024815118.
25. Wang S, Pan Y, Wang Q, et al. Modeling the viral dynamics of SARS-CoV-2 infection. Math Biosci. 2020;328:108438.
26. Hattaf K, Yousfi N. Dynamics of SARS-CoV-2 infection model with two modes of transmission and immune response. Math Biosci Eng. 2020;17:5326–40.
27. Aguilar RB, Hardigan P, Mayi B, et al. Current understanding of COVID-19 clinical course and investigational treatments. Front Med (Lausanne). 2020;7:555301.
28. Siddiqi HS, Mehra MR. COVID-19 illness in native and immunosuppressed states: a clinical therapeutic staging proposal. J Heart Lung Transplant. 2020;39:405–7.
29. Kissler SM, Fauver JR, Mack C, et al. Viral dynamics of acute SARS-CoV-2 infection and applications to diagnostic and public health strategies. PLoS Biol. 2021;19:e3001333.
30. Chitty SA, Mobbs S, Rifkin BS, et al. A multicenter evaluation of the Seraph 100 microbind affinity blood filter for the treatment of severe COVID-19. Crit Care Explor. 2022;4:e0662.
31. Schmidt JJ, Borchina DN, Van't Klooster M, et al. Interim analysis of the COSA (COVID-19 patients treated with the Seraph® 100 Microbind® Affinity filter) registry. Nephrol Dial Transplant. 2022;37:673–80.
32. Rifkin BS, Stewart IJ, et al. Seraph-100 hemoperfusion in SARS-CoV-2-infected patients early in critical illness: a case series. Blood Purif. 2022;51:317–20.
33. Sirivongrangson P, Kulvichit W, Payungporn S, et al. Endotoxemia and circulating bacteriome in severe COVID-19 patients. Intensive Care Med Exp. 2020;8:72.
34. Khan S, Bolotova O, Sahib H, et al. Endotoxemia in critically ill patients with COVID-19. Blood Purif. 2022;51:513–9.
35. Honore PM, Redant S, De Bels D. Is an EAA > 0.6 in severe COVID-19 patients synonymous with a toxic and pro-inflammatory endotoxin profile, and should we treat it? Intensive Care Med Exp. 2021;9:16.
36. Petruk G, Puthia M, Petrlova J, et al. SARS-CoV-2 spike protein binds to bacterial lipopolysaccharide and boosts proinflammatory activity. J Mol Cell Biol. 2020;12:916–32.
37. Katagiri D, Izumi S, Takano H. When should polymyxin B-immobilized polystyrene column be introduced to improve COVID-19 prognosis? Ther Apher Dial. 2022;26:550–1.
38. De Rosa S, Cuteli SL, Ferrer R, et al. Polymyxin B hemoperfusion in coronavirus disease 2019 patients with endotoxic shock: case series from EUPHAS2 registry. Artif Organs. 2021;45:E187–94.

# Part X

# Neurologic Considerations

# 33 Epidemiology, Outcomes, and Costs of Pediatric Traumatic Brain Injury Treated in the ICU

E. Mikkonen, R. Raj, and M. B. Skrifvars

## 33.1 Introduction

Up to 1% of children and young adults attend medical services annually following traumatic brain injury (TBI) [1, 2], and over a quarter of all TBI cases are in patients younger than 15 years [2]. The incidence rates follow a U-shaped curve, peaking in early childhood and adolescence. In childhood, falls are the leading injury mechanism, whereas motor vehicle accidents are the leading cause in adolescence [1, 3]. Few head injuries sustained by children and adolescents require hospitalization, and fewer yet require admission to the intensive care unit (ICU). However, the sequelae of TBI sustained in childhood and adolescence can be devastating. Globally, TBI is a significant cause of mortality and morbidity in the pediatric population [4]. Pediatric TBI also has major societal impacts, and it has been estimated to be the fifth most expensive pediatric hospital diagnosis in the United States [3]. Despite its huge personal and societal impact, little is known about this population. The physiological changes from infancy to adolescence and the effect these have on injury characteristics and recovery remain, to a large extent, open questions. In contrast to the adult population, where recovery to the previous level of function is considered desirable, the ambition in the pediatric TBI population is for the young developing central nervous system (CNS) to keep meeting

E. Mikkonen
Department of Perioperative Medicine and Intensive Care, Karolinska University Hospital, Stockholm, Sweden

R. Raj
Department of Neurosurgery, Helsinki University Hospital, University of Helsinki, Helsinki, Finland

M. B. Skrifvars (✉)
Department of Emergency Care and Services, Helsinki University Hospital, University of Helsinki, Helsinki, Finland
e-mail: markus.skrifvars@hus.fi



J.-L. Vincent (ed.), *Annual Update in Intensive Care and Emergency Medicine 2023*,
Annual Update in Intensive Care and Emergency Medicine,
https://doi.org/10.1007/978-3-031-23005-9_33

developmental milestones after injury. It has therefore been suggested that children might actually "grow into their disabilities," as the full magnitude of a disability might not manifest until the patient fails to acquire future skills [5].

The first treatment guidelines for severe pediatric TBI were published in 2003, and the latest revision in 2019 [6]. These treatment guidelines remain largely consensus-based due to a lack of evidence. Although the treatment principles follow those of adult TBI (i.e., optimizing cerebral oxygenation and perfusion to limit secondary injury), target values and best practices to reach these goals have been difficult to establish. The field has gained significant attention in recent years, yet much remains to be elucidated to help this vulnerable and understudied population.

## 33.2 Epidemiology

In the USA, over 140,000 children and adolescents are estimated to be living with long-lasting social, emotional, cognitive, and physical sequelae of TBI [7] Pediatric TBI is a significant global public health issue affecting populations in high- and low-income countries [4]. Falls and traffic accidents are the leading cause of TBI in both adult and pediatric populations [4]. Falls tend to cause milder TBI, whereas traffic accidents are the most common cause of severe TBI. In Asia and Africa, traffic-related pediatric TBI patients are more often pedestrians, whereas in high-income countries, they tend to be passengers [4], highlighting the importance of infrastructural road safety measures to prevent TBI, such as sidewalks and traffic lights. Public awareness concerning, for example, bicycle helmets, might also reduce the incidence of pediatric TBI [8]. Sex differences in incidence rates in early childhood are small; however, with increasing age, males surpass females by almost double the incidence [4]. Globally, TBI due to recreational sports seems to be more frequent in high-income English-speaking countries, possibly due to the preference for contact sports, such as rugby and American football [4]. Furthermore, injuries peak during the summer months and on weekends, possibly due to more time spent outdoors and on recreational activities [4]. Abusive head injuries in infants represent a distinct entity, often affecting children under 6 months of age. Injuries are characterized by rotational acceleration/deceleration forces, multiple lesions, a delay in seeking medical attention, and usually a very poor prognosis [9]. Unfortunately, social inequality is mirrored in pediatric TBI incidence and outcomes. Children from families of lower socioeconomic classes and families with psychiatric morbidities seem to have an increased risk of sustaining TBI [10]. A recent study from the USA found that children in less affluent areas are more likely to suffer ballistic TBI and to die from TBI than their peers living in wealthier areas [11].

The most severely injured TBI patients are admitted to the ICU. However, even patients with milder TBI may be admitted to the ICU due to extracranial injuries or a lack of intermediary units, for example. A recent study from the multinational Collaborative European NeuroTrauma Effectiveness Research in TBI (CENTER-TBI) project reported a median Glasgow Coma Scale (GCS) score of 11 (interquartile range [IQR] 6–14) among pediatric TBI patients admitted to ICUs and, perhaps more notably, that 38% of patients admitted to the ICU had mild TBI (GCS 1–15). ICU-admitted pediatric patients had a 6-month mortality rate of 5% compared to 21% for adults [12, 13].

According to open access data from the Swedish Intensive Care Registry, 39% of TBI-related ICU admissions of patients under the age of 16 between 2008 and mid-2022 had simple concussion as their primary diagnosis. During this period, there were 1981 TBI-related ICU admissions (some patients could have had multiple admissions due to, e.g., readmissions or hospital transfers), with an ICU mortality of only 2% (33 patients). We observed similar numbers in a multicenter study of ICU-treated pediatric TBI in Finland: 40% of the patients had mild TBI (GCS 13–15), but a slightly higher 6-month mortality rate at 9% [14]. Thus, at least in the European context, the ICU-treated pediatric TBI population is very heterogeneous in severity, and mortality rates seem low, which is at least partly explained by the low injury severity. Some patients with mild TBI may be admitted to the ICU due to the lack of intermediary units; that is, patients who only need observation after, for example, concussion to avoid unnecessary computed tomography (CT) scans. In these cases, the introduction of laboratory biomarkers of severe intracranial pathology, such as the S100b or glial fibrillary acid protein, could circumvent this problem and save resources. However, the ICU admission of patients with mild injuries is not unique to the pediatric population. A CENTER-TBI study of the adult population found that 36% of adult TBI patients treated in ICUs were admitted with a GCS >13 [13].

## 33.3 Pediatric Anatomy and Physiology

Infants are born with large heads relative to their body size. Furthermore, facial structures are small, offering little protection to the brain against external forces, and the skull bones are thinner and more flexible, exposing the underlying cortex to more energy at impact (Fig. 33.1). The thin infant skull is also more prone to fractures than that of adults. Conversely, in very young infants, flexible bones together

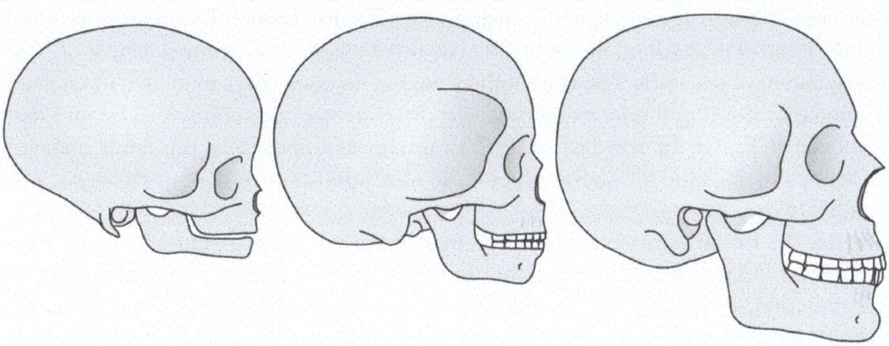

**Fig. 33.1** Small facial structures and a protruding forehead predispose the infant skull to more external force compared to older children and adults

with open fontanels can offer some protection against the buildup of intracranial pressure (ICP) [15]. The infant brain contains up to 90% water, which decreases to 75% with increasing myelinization throughout childhood and adolescence [16]. Experimental data also suggest that young children have stiffer brain parenchyma compared to adults, possibly altering the conduction of external forces in the brain parenchyma [15]. Moreover, the weak neck muscles supporting the relatively large head could further increase the likelihood of rotational forces and diffuse injury [15].

Normal physiological values change during development. Some of these, such as blood pressure, heart rate, and respiratory rate, are well established. However, some values relevant to the treatment of TBI have yet to be elucidated. Cerebral blood flow seems to be low in early infancy, to increase during childhood, and to drop to adult levels during adolescence. The implications of these changes for TBI treatment remain unknown [17]. Recently, a retrospective study of pediatric TBI patients identified threshold cerebral perfusion pressure (CPP) values as associated with increased mortality, yet there is scant evidence to base treatment recommendations on [18].

Children have also been observed to suffer more seizures associated with head injuries, many of which may remain subclinical [16]. The exact mechanism behind this susceptibility is unclear. Underrecognition and failure to treat these subclinical seizures can cause increased metabolic failure in the injured brain and further aggravate secondary injury.

## 33.4 Treatment

The Guidelines for the Management of Pediatric Severe Traumatic Brain Injury were first published by the Brain Trauma Foundation in 2003 with subsequent revisions in 2012 and 2019 [6]. Due to a lack of evidence, they remain largely consensus-based, with very few high-quality randomized controlled trials (RCTs) to guide decision-making [6]. Treatment of pediatric TBI follows the same principles as the treatment of adult TBI; that is, mitigating secondary injury mainly through control of cerebral substrate delivery and consumption [19]. Thus, treatment has revolved around ICP control, adequate mean arterial pressure (MAP), blood oxygenation, and the control of cerebral metabolism. The most extensively studied aspect of ICU management of pediatric TBI is hypothermia, but no conclusive evidence in favor of prophylactic cooling therapies has been reported. However, cooling can be initiated to reduce ICP. ICP targets are set to 20 mmHg, as opposed to the adult updated guidelines of 22 mmHg, and a target CPP of a minimum of 40 mmHg is recommended [6].

After the initial injury, several molecular pathways, such as mitochondrial dysfunction, oxidative stress, blood–brain barrier dysfunction, excitotoxicity, and inflammation, contribute to secondary injury causing irreversible tissue damage. Despite some promising preclinical data, no neuroprotective pharmaceutical treatments to mitigate these processes have made it to the clinical setting. Some of the agents that have failed in adult TBI studies include, but are not limited to, progesterone, statins, and erythropoietin [20]. One reason for the failure of promising experimental data to translate to the clinical setting could be the extreme heterogeneity of TBI and a historical tendency to focus on neurons, with less attention being paid to, for example, astrocytes, microglia, endothelial cells, etc.

## 33.5 Outcomes and Sequelae

Pediatric TBI patients have long been thought to benefit from the increased plasticity of the CNS. This plasticity refers to structural and functional changes at the synaptic and network levels that allow the CNS to adapt to new environmental challenges, be that harder complexity of schoolwork or a focal brain insult [21]. However, the plastic advantage in brain injury suggested by early studies was observed in the context of focal lesions [5]. TBI, in contrast, is often diffuse in nature, raising concerns regarding the generalizability of these findings. Some evidence supports the opposing view that younger children are more vulnerable and have poorer outcomes than their older peers. This has been explained, for example, by the disrupted development of necessary networks that enable the acquisition of future skills [5]. It could be the case that children go through developmental phases of particular vulnerability to injury [5]. However, due to the extreme heterogeneity of the condition (injury type, severity, localization, and patient age), large longitudinal studies need to be conducted to elucidate the complex relationships between developmental phases, injury characteristics, and outcomes. More crude outcome measures, such as mortality, have yielded conflicting results [22–24]. Some large observational studies have noted higher mortality rates in the very young. Anatomical differences that predispose young infants to more external forces could be one explanation. High mortality in pediatric TBI populations could also be explained by abusive head trauma ("shaken baby syndrome"), a condition of often extreme diffuse injuries and poor prognosis [9].

Functional outcomes after TBI are often measured using different scales. The Glasgow Outcome Scale (GOS) [25] is a five-point scale (1 = dead to 5 = no or minor disability) developed in the 1970s and is familiar to many adult ICU physicians. Definitions such as "independent in daily living" have some inherent problems in the youngest populations, and the GOS might thus not always apply in the pediatric context. Some outcome scales have been developed specifically for the pediatric population, such as the Pediatric Cerebral Performance Category (PCPC) scale [26] for short-term outcome measurement (Table 33.1). The PCPC is a six-point scale with similarities to the GOS scale, with an emphasis on deviation from age-appropriate development. The GOS has also been developed to give the GOS-extended (GOS-E), providing a more nuanced and granular picture of disability, and further to the GOS-E pediatric, which considers the specific developmental characteristics of children [27]. However, in the literature, the outcome is often dichotomized as either favorable or unfavorable at a chosen cutoff, usually between moderate and severe disability. In these cases, the normal GOS scale has often been used.

**Table 33.1** Comparison of the Pediatric Cerebral Performance Category (PCPC) Scale and the original Glasgow Outcome Scale (GOS)

| PCPC (at ICU discharge) [26] | GOS [25] |
|---|---|
| **1 Normal**: at age-appropriate level; school-age child attending regular school classroom | **5 Good recovery**: resumption of normal life with only minor neurological or psychological deficits |
| **2 Mild disability**: Conscious, alert, and able to interact at age-appropriate level; school-age child attending regular school classroom but grade perhaps not appropriate for age; possibility of mild neurologic deficit | |
| **3 Moderate disability**: Conscious; sufficient cerebral function for age-appropriate independent activities of daily life; school-age child attending special education classroom and/or learning deficit present | **4 Moderate disability**: disabled but independent in daily living |
| **4 Severe disability**: Conscious; dependent on others for daily support because of impaired brain function | **3 Severe disability**: conscious but dependent for daily support |
| **5 Coma or vegetative state**: Any degree of coma without the presence of all brain death criteria; unawareness, even if awake in appearance, without interaction with environment; cerebral unresponsiveness and no evidence of cortex function (not aroused by verbal stimuli); possibility of some reflexive response, spontaneous eye-opening, and sleep-wake cycles | **2 Persistent vegetative state**: can open eyes and show sleep patterns; no communication, no movement |
| **6 Brain death**: Apnea, areflexia, and/or electroencephalographic silence | **1 Dead**: attributable to brain injury, either direct or indirect |

### 33.5.1 Neurological Sequelae

Seizures are well-known complications of head trauma. Seizures can be categorized as immediate (<24 h after injury), early (24 h to 1 week after injury), and late (>1 week after injury). Immediate and early seizures are thought to be pathophysiologically different; immediate and early seizures are caused by acute metabolic failure, disrupted ion balance, and excitotoxicity, whereas late seizures are thought to be caused by, for example, synaptic loss and pathological rewiring, leading to chronically elevated seizure susceptibility [28]. The mechanisms and biomarkers of post-traumatic epileptogenesis have not been fully elucidated. Prophylactic treatment with antiepileptic drugs has not been shown to prevent the development of late seizures. A large population-based study by Christensen et al. of children and young adults showed an increased risk of post-traumatic epilepsy over 10 years after injury, even after mild TBI [29]. Studies have suggested that 1–9% of childhood epilepsies are preceded by head injury [30, 31]. Similar results have been found in the adult population [32]. Childhood epilepsy can have devastating social and emotional effects on patients and their families. These patients seem to have adverse outcomes regarding social and educational achievement in adulthood and a reduced lifespan if refractory to treatment [33, 34].

Motor and cerebellar disorders, such as tremor, ataxia, spasticity, and muscle weakness, are not uncommon after TBI. The prevalence rates of motor and cerebellar disorders at long-term follow-up were both 14% in a French cohort of severely injured TBI patients. However, children and adolescents seem to recover better from motor deficits than adults [9].

### 33.5.2 Cognitive and Psychiatric Sequelae

Many cognitive sequelae after TBI may take years to detect, as the complexity of environmental demands increases and the failed development of attention, language, executive functioning, and problem-solving skills becomes more evident [35]. A longitudinal study of survivors of preschool moderate-to-severe TBI found that only a third of patients maintained full employment as adults [36].

Commonly reported behavioral sequelae of pediatric TBI include mood disorders, anxiety, lack of emotional control, disinhibition, and difficulties with interpersonal skills. The risk factors for psychiatric morbidity after pediatric TBI are probably multifactorial, with hereditary, environmental, and injury-related factors contributing to post-traumatic psychiatric morbidity. Critical illness and ICU stays have been linked to mood disorders; however, compared to orthopedically injured peers, pediatric TBI patients seem to have more mood disorders [37]. White matter disruption in the frontal lobe has been found to independently increase the likelihood of novel psychiatric disorders after pediatric TBI [38]. The frontal lobes are particularly vulnerable in TBI, as the brain moves inside the skull following external force, pressing the orbitofrontal and inferior temporal cortex against the bony protrusion in the anterior and temporal skull base [39]. The frontal cortex is home to many of the evolutionarily late features of brain functioning, such as reasoning, emotional control, social cognition, and planning. Thus, it is hardly surprising that TBI often causes problems in these domains. Further, many of these functions are underdeveloped in the young brain, as the frontal cortex continues to develop well into early adulthood [39]. How early injury to these areas affects normal frontal maturation is still incompletely understood.

Post-traumatic psychopharmacology has gained some attention in the adult population, yet few studies have been conducted in the pediatric population [40]. Post-traumatic pediatric cognitive dysfunction is problematic in the sense that there is no or very little experience of some drugs for the treatment of similar symptoms of other etiologies compared to the adult population in which dopaminergic agonists like amantadine are used, for example, in dementia. Stimulants, however, have been widely studied and prescribed to children and adolescents for a long time. Stimulants have also proved to be of some benefit in adults for the treatment of cognitive decline after TBI by improving attention [41]. By improving attention, other cognitive sequelae, such as impaired memory and executive function, could also be mitigated. Antidepressants have been studied in the adult population, but the evidence after pediatric TBI is scant. Sertraline seems to be the safest and most effective option [40]. Some psychopharmacologic strategies, such as off-label use of antipsychotics to control behavioral problems, can be especially problematic due to their tendency to sedate, reduce seizure thresholds, and have adverse cognitive effects in the already vulnerable post-traumatic brain [41]. Antiepileptic drugs, such as valproic acid, carbamazepine, and lamotrigine, could also be used to treat agitation, although there is currently only a pediatric indication for the treatment of seizures or bipolar disorder [40]. In a study by our group, 45% of adolescents (age >12 years) with a moderate disability (GOS score of 4) were prescribed some psychotropic drugs during follow-up [42]. The same study found no injury-related risk factors associated with the utilization of psychopharmaceuticals after discharge.

### 33.5.3 Endocrinological Dysfunction

Due to its localization at the base of the skull, the hypothalamus and pituitary glands are vulnerable to damage in TBI. TBI usually causes only brief disruptions in pituitary function; however, some children and adolescents can experience chronic symptoms. The immediate effects of posterior lobe insults are familiar to many intensivists through the disturbances of antidiuretic hormone secretion and subsequent fluid balance disruption. The anterior pituitary controls multiple hormonal axes (somatotropic, thyrotropic, adrenotropic, lactotropic, and gonadotropic) that are important for normal growth and development in youth and puberty. However, little is known about the epidemiology and long-term consequences of disruptions in these systems after pediatric TBI. Temporal trends can be unpredictable, and symptoms can be subtle and hard to detect. The literature suggests that somatotropic, gonadotropic, and adrenotropic disturbances are the most common chronic insufficiencies, increasing the risk of reduced growth, delayed or absent puberty, and adrenal insufficiency. No conclusive evidence on the risk factors for endocrinopathies after TBI exists, with high-quality studies of radiological biomarkers lacking. Abusive head trauma has been suggested as a high-risk mechanism for post-TBI hypopituitarism, although even mild TBIs can be the trigger [9, 39].

## 33.6 Prognostication After Pediatric TBI

Prognosis has always played an important part in the communication between healthcare providers and patients or their relatives. Historically, prognostication was based on experience or clinical intuition. However, the increased availability of patient data and the sophistication of statistical models have led to the identification of prognostic variables and the development of prognostic models. Prognostic variables in TBI have been thoroughly investigated in the adult population. Injury severity measured by, for example, the GCS score and pupillary light reactivity has proven very useful in the prognostication of outcome in adult TBI patients [43]. Low GCS scores, particularly low motor scores, indicate severe disruptions of consciousness and damage to the vital basal parts of the brain. Pupillary light reactivity, conversely, is an indirect measure of compression on the oculomotor nerve caused by impending uncial herniation following a mass-occupying lesion or diffuse edema in the confined space of the cranium. In the adult population, increasing age has consistently shown a strong correlation with poorer outcomes. As outlined in the previous section, the relationship between age and outcome in pediatric TBI is less clear. By analyzing different radiological findings on admission CT scans, several radiological prognostic models have been developed for the adult population, such as the Marshall, Rotterdam, and Helsinki CT scoring models [44]. Patients can have very low GCS scores due to different etiologies, some of which may respond very well to treatment. This is recognized by some CT scoring models, such as the Rotterdam and Helsinki CT scores, which give patients a more favorable prognosis if an epidural hematoma is present. Patients with epidural hematomas can present with very low GCS scores and possibly die, but given urgent adequate surgical treatment, may recover fully with very little parenchymal damage. In these cases, GCS can give an overly pessimistic prognosis compared to CT findings.

The predictive performance of a prognostic model is commonly expressed using two values: discrimination (i.e., the model's tendency to assign a higher risk to patients with a certain outcome) and calibration (i.e., how well the model's assigned likelihood matches the actual observed likelihood of an outcome). Discrimination is often described graphically with an area under the receiver operating characteristic curve (AUROC or often just AUC) or C-statistic. An AUC or C-statistic score of 0.5 indicates that the model performs no better than a flip of a coin, whereas 1.0 indicates perfect discrimination. The AUC or C-statistic score does not separate between specificity and sensitivity and is thus not useful as such for diagnostic tests, for example, where the cutoffs for sensitivity and specificity may vary depending on the clinical context in which the test is used. Another useful measure of model performance is $R^2$ (or various pseudo-$R^2$ tests for dichotomous outcomes). $R^2$ indicates how much of the observed variation in outcomes is explained by the model; for example, if GCS explains 50% of the variability in observed mortality after TBI, the $R^2$ score of GCS would be 0.5 [43].

Many of the available models have been validated in the pediatric population. Perhaps surprisingly, these models developed for the adult population seem to perform better in the pediatric TBI population [14] (Table 33.2). This could be because pediatric TBI patients are less likely to suffer from confounding diseases, such as

**Table 33.2** Discriminatory power of existing prediction models in the adult and pediatric populations

| | Marshall CT classification | Rotterdam CT score | Helsinki CT score |
|---|---|---|---|
| *Adult population* | | | |
| AUC mortality | 0.61–0.67 | 0.68–0.75 | 0.74–0.75 |
| AUC functional outcome | 0.58–0.63 | 0.62–0.68 | 0.72–0.75 |
| *Pediatric population* | | | |
| AUC mortality | 0.78 | 0.84–0.85 | 0.81 |
| AUC functional outcome | 0.66 | 0.75 | 0.72 |

An area under the curve (AUC) of 0.5 indicates that the model performs no better than chance, while >0.7 is considered satisfactory, >0.8 is considered good, and >0.9 is considered excellent. An AUC of 1.0 would indicate 100% specificity and sensitivity cardiovascular or lung diseases, than adult and elderly TBI patients. Thus, they are more discrete TBI patients, making it easier for prognostic models to predict outcomes based on TBI-relevant data, such as the GCS score or head CT scans. These findings indicate that existing prognostic models could also be utilized for baseline stratification and propensity score matching in the pediatric TBI population.

## 33.7 Costs

Pediatric TBI has a huge societal impact. As mentioned earlier, pediatric TBI is considered one of the most expensive pediatric hospital diagnoses. This only accounts for direct health care costs. Given the possibly lifelong sequelae, with productivity losses both for the parents and the patient in the future, pediatric TBI can constitute an enormous preventable burden on society [45]. A study of adult mild-to-moderate TBI found that 84% of the total cost at 1 year was due to productivity losses [46]. In a study by our group, the average total 1-year cost of pediatric TBI treated in Finnish university ICUs was €48,719, of which two-thirds were hospital admission costs, 27% were rehabilitation unit costs, and 7% were social security reimbursement costs [47]. Higher injury severity measured by admission GCS, pupillary light reactivity, and CT scan findings, as well as major extracranial injury, correlated with increased total costs. Compared to a study of adult TBI patients in a similar setting, the mean cost per patient was higher in our pediatric cohort (€37,528 per adult patient). Higher resource utilization in the pediatric population could be explained by relative unwillingness to, for example, withdraw care when treating pediatric patients. However, in the pediatric cohort, 69% of the resources were spent on patients with favorable functional outcomes, compared to 45% in the adult cohort, suggesting better resource allocation and that children benefited more from treatment. In the adult population, a larger proportion of costs was spent on rehabilitation and social security reimbursement at 1 year (index hospital 44%, rehabilitation unit 42%, and social security costs 14%, respectively), suggesting better rehabilitation potential in pediatric patients. Neurocritical care in general can be resource-intensive, with multiple novel multimodal monitoring modalities and long ICU stays. However, a study from the United States found that adherence to current treatment guidelines for severe pediatric TBI did not increase total hospital or ICU costs [48]. Unfortunately, data on the costs and cost-effectiveness of TBI rehabilitation are scarce, and the Centers for Disease Control and Prevention (CDC) have specifically highlighted the importance of cost-effectiveness analyses of rehabilitation strategies [35]. Multiple studies have found the importance of family-related factors for pediatric TBI outcomes: socioeconomic factors predispose children to both injury itself and poorer recovery [9, 10]. Rehabilitation and recovery from pediatric TBI can be financially stressful for families due to workdays lost and out-of-pocket health care expenditure. Legislative measures to mitigate the financial burden on families could be a societal cost worth considering, to improve the recovery environment for children and adolescents.

## 33.8 Future Perspectives

Severe pediatric TBI is a very heterogeneous disease, and there is little good evidence to guide clinical decision-making in critically ill pediatric TBI patients. As mentioned, during almost 15 years of nationwide registration in Sweden, only 33 pediatric TBI patients died during their ICU stay. These data suggest two recommendations: treatment should be highly centralized to maintain clinical competence, and multinational collaboration will be essential in future studies to reach statistical power. Today, most RCTs have been small or single center [49]. The hypothermia study by Hutchison et al. included 225 patients and, to our knowledge, is the largest multicenter RCT in severe pediatric TBI [50]. Further, only a few new RCTs are registered at ClinicalTrials.gov. It has been argued that for future RCTs in pediatric TBI to be more effective, injury characterization needs more attention, as, for example, a low GCS score in the setting of an acute epidural hematoma vs. diffuse edema means two completely different things concerning prognosis and treatment strategies. Furthermore, the effectiveness of RCTs in improving outcomes in critical care in general has also been questioned [51]. Thus, other paths to improved knowledge and efficient treatment guidelines have been sought. Comparative effectiveness research uses observational data to compare the effectiveness of different treatment strategies using real-world data and sophisticated statistical analyses. Two important examples are the Collaborative European NeuroTrauma Effectiveness Research in TBI (CENTER-TBI) project and the Approaches and Decisions in Acute Pediatric TBI (ADAPT) Trial [52, 53]. The CENTER-TBI project enrolled both adult and pediatric TBI patients of all severities, whereas the ADAPT trial recruited 1000 pediatric patients with severe TBI. The hope is that these large prospective, observational, multinational collaborations will help fill some of the knowledge gaps that, perhaps, RCTs will never elucidate in pediatric TBI. Technological advancements and improved multimodal monitoring could provide new insights into the nature of the disease and guide the search for novel therapies and treatment strategies for both adult and pediatric TBI.

## 33.9 Conclusion

Pediatric TBI remains a concerning global public health issue, disproportionately affecting vulnerable groups. Most injuries are mild in nature, yet injuries of all severities can have lifelong debilitating neurologic, cognitive, behavioral, and social sequelae. In addition to personal suffering, pediatric TBI has a substantial societal impact due to treatment costs and productivity losses. Contrary to popular belief, younger children do not seem to have better outcomes than adolescents and adults, with some evidence suggesting the opposite. The physiology of pediatric TBI is incompletely understood, and more research is needed to understand the complex interaction between normal development and various types of TBI. As with adult TBI, no neuroprotective pharmacological treatments have made it to the clinical setting. TBIs of all severities are admitted to ICUs, with over a third of pediatric TBI patients admitted to ICUs in Europe suffering from mild injuries. By optimizing treatment to mitigate acute secondary injury, an ICU stay can offer a great opportunity to change the patient's trajectory away from lifelong sequelae. Today, medical management in the ICU is similar to that of adult patients, optimizing the supply and demand of oxygen and nutrients with some variation in target values. However, the guidelines for the treatment of the most severely injured patients lack good evidence and are mostly consensus-based. Well-powered RCTs have been notoriously hard to conduct in this population, but alternative study designs, together with multimodal monitoring, might help breach some of the knowledge gaps needed to improve the outcomes of this understudied population.

## References


1. McKinlay A, Grace RC, Horwood LJ, Fergusson DM, Ridder EM, MacFarlane MR. Prevalence of traumatic brain injury among children, adolescents and young adults: prospective evidence from a birth cohort. Brain Inj. 2009;22:175–81.
2. Feigin VL, Theadom A, Barker-Collo S, et al. Incidence of traumatic brain injury in New Zealand: a population-based study. Lancet Neurol. 2013;12:53–64.
3. Schneier AJ, Shields BJ, Hostetler SG, Xiang H, Smith GA. Incidence of pediatric traumatic brain injury and associated hospital resource utilization in the United States. Pediatrics. 2006;118:483–92.
4. Dewan MC, Mummareddy N, Wellons JC, Bonfield CM. Epidemiology of global pediatric traumatic brain injury: qualitative review. World Neurosurg. 2016;91:497–509.e1.
5. Anderson V, Spencer-Smith M, Wood A. Do children really recover better? Neurobehavioural plasticity after early brain insult. Brain. 2011;134:2197–221.
6. Kochanek P, Tasker RC, Carney N, et al. Guidelines for the management of pediatric severe traumatic brain injury, third edition: update of the Brain Trauma Foundation Guidelines. Pediatr Crit Care Med. 2019;20:1–82.
7. Zaloshnja E, Miller T, Langlois AJ, Selassie AW. Prevalence of long-term disability from traumatic brain injury in the civilian population of the United States, 2005. J Head Trauma Rehabil. 2005;23:394–400.
8. Sarmiento K, Haileyesus T, Waltzman D, Daugherty J. Emergency department visits for bicycle-related traumatic brain injuries among children and adults — United States, 2009–2018. Morb Mortal Wkly Rep. 2021;70:693–7.
9. Chevignard M, Câmara-Costa H, Dellatolas G. Pediatric traumatic brain injury and abusive head trauma. In: Gallagher A, Bulteau C, Cohen D, Michaud JL, editors. Handbook of clinical neurology, vol. 3. Amsterdam: Elsevier; 2020. p. 451–84.
10. Schachar RJ, Park LS, Dennis M. Mental health implications of traumatic brain injury (TBI) in children and youth. J Can Acad Child Adolesc Psychiatry. 2015;24:100–8.
11. Pelletier JH, Rakkar J, Simon D, et al. Association between pediatric TBI mortality and median family income in the United States: a retrospective cohort study. Lancet Reg Heal Am. 2022;5:100–64.
12. Riemann L, Zweckberger K, Unterberg A, El Damaty A, Younsi A. Injury causes and severity in pediatric traumatic brain injury patients admitted to the ward or intensive care unit: a Collaborative European Neurotrauma Effectiveness Research in Traumatic Brain Injury (CENTER-TBI) study. Front Neurol. 2020;11:345.
13. Steyerberg EW, Wiegers E, Sewalt C, et al. Case-mix, care pathways, and outcomes in patients with traumatic brain injury in CENTER-TBI: a European prospective, multicentre, longitudinal, cohort study. Lancet Neurol. 2019;18:923–34.

14. Mikkonen ED, Skrifvars MB, Reinikainen M, et al. Validation of prognostic models in intensive care unit–treated pediatric traumatic brain injury patients. J Neurosurg Pediatr. 2019;24:330–7.
15. Figaji AA. Anatomical and physiological differences between children and adults relevant to traumatic brain injury and the implications for clinical assessment and care. Front Neurol. 2017;8:685.
16. Duhaime AC, Rindler RS. Special considerations in infants and children. In: Grafman J, Salazar AM, editors. Handbook of clinical neurology, vol. 3. Amsterdam: Elsevier; 2015. p. 219–42.
17. Udomphorn Y, Armstead WM, Vavilala MS. Cerebral blood flow and autoregulation after pediatric traumatic brain injury. Pediatr Neurol. 2009;38:225–34.
18. Woods KS, Horvat CM, Kantawala S, et al. Intracranial and cerebral perfusion pressure thresholds associated with inhospital mortality across pediatric neurocritical care. Pediatr Crit Care Med. 2021;22:135–46.
19. Meyfroidt G, Bouzat P, Casaer MP, et al. Management of moderate to severe traumatic brain injury: an update for the intensivist. Intensive Care Med. 2022;48:647–66.
20. Zoerle T, Carbonara M, Zanier ER, et al. Rethinking neuroprotection in severe traumatic brain injury: toward bedside neuroprotection. Front Neurol. 2017;8:354.
21. Griesbach GS, Hovda DA. Cellular and molecular neuronal plasticity. In: Grafman J, Salazar AM, editors. Handbook of clinical neurology, vol. 3. Amsterdam: Elsevier; 2015. p. 681–90.
22. Morrison WE, Arbelaez JJ, Fackler JC, De Maio A, Paidas CN. Gender and age effects on outcome after pediatric traumatic brain injury. Pediatr Crit Care Med. 2004;5:145–51.
23. Ducrocq SC, Meyer PG, Orliaguet GA, et al. Epidemiology and early predictive factors of mortality and outcome in children with traumatic severe brain injury: experience of a French pediatric trauma center. Pediatr Crit Care Med. 2006;7:461–7.
24. Sarnaik A, Ferguson NM, O'Meara AI, et al. Age and mortality in pediatric severe traumatic brain injury: results from an international study. Neurocrit Care. 2018;28:302–13.
25. Jennett B, Bond M. Assessment of outcome after severe brain damage. A practical scale. Lancet. 1975;1:480–4.
26. Fiser DH. Assessing the outcome of pediatric intensive care. J Pediatr. 1992;121:68–74.
27. Beers SR, Wisniewski SR, Garcia-Filion P, et al. Validity of a pediatric version of the Glasgow Outcome Scale–Extended. J Neurotrauma. 2012;29:1126–39.
28. Hunt RFI, Boychuk JA, Smith BN. Neural circuit mechanisms of post–traumatic epilepsy. Front Cell Neurosci. 2013;7:89.
29. Christensen J, Pedersen MG, Pedersen CB, Sidenius P, Olsen J, Vestergaard M. Long-term risk of epilepsy after traumatic brain injury in children and young adults: a population-based cohort study. Lancet. 2009;73:1105–10.
30. Kurtz Z, Tookey P, Ross E. Epilepsy in young people: 23 year follow up of the British national child development study. BMJ. 1998;316:339–42.
31. Aaberg KM, Surén P, Søraas CL, et al. Seizures, syndromes, and etiologies in childhood epilepsy: the International League Against Epilepsy 1981, 1989, and 2017 classifications used in a population-based cohort. Epilepsia. 2017;58:1880–91.
32. Hauser WA, Annegers JF, Kurland LT. Incidence of epilepsy and unprovoked seizures in Rochester, Minnesota: 1935–1984. Epilepsia. 1993;34:453–8.
33. Sillanpää M, Jalava M, Kaleva O, Shinnar S. Long-term prognosis of seizures with onset in childhood. N Engl J Med. 2009;338:1715–22.
34. Cianchetti C, Messina P, Pupillo E, et al. The perceived burden of epilepsy: impact on the quality of life of children and adolescents and their families. Seizure. 2015;24:93–101.
35. Frieden TR, Houry D, Baldwin G. Report to Congress on traumatic brain injury in the United States: epidemiology and rehabilitation. Available at: https://www.cdc.gov/traumaticbraininjury/pdf/TBI_Report_to_Congress_Epi_and_Rehab-a.pdf. Accessed 8 Nov 2022.
36. Nybo T, Sainio M, Müller K. Stability of vocational outcome in adulthood after moderate to severe preschool brain injury. J Int Neuropsychol Soc. 2004;10:719–23.
37. Laliberté Durish C, Pereverseff RS, Yeates KO. Depression and depressive symptoms in pediatric traumatic brain injury: a scoping review. J Head Trauma Rehabil. 2018;33:E18–30.

38. Max JE, Wilde EA, Bigler ED, et al. Neuroimaging correlates of novel psychiatric disorders after pediatric traumatic brain injury. J Am Acad Child Adolesc Psychiatry. 2012;51:1208–17.
39. Rostami E, Figaji A, Adelson PD. Pediatric TBI - current state of the art and future perspective. Front Neurol. 2021;12:649676.
40. Pangilinan PH, Giacoletti-Argento A, Shellhaas R, Hurvitz EA, Hornyak JE. Neuropharmacology in pediatric brain injury: a review. Pediatr Rehabil Dev Disabil. 2010;2:1127–40.
41. Polich G, Iaccarino MA, Zafonte R. Psychopharmacology of traumatic brain injury. In: Reus VI, Lindqvist D, editors. Handbook of Clinical Neurology, vol. 3. Amsterdam: Elsevier; 2019. p. 253–67.
42. Mikkonen ED, Skrifvars MB, Reinikainen M, et al. Psychotropic medication after intensive care unit–treated pediatric traumatic brain injury. Pediatr Neurol. 2020;112:64–70.
43. Maas AIR, Lingsma HF, Roozenbeek B. Predicting outcome after traumatic brain injury. In: Grafman J, Salazar AM, editors. Handbook of Clinical Neurology, vol. 3. Amsterdam: Elsevier; 2015. p. 455–74.
44. Raj R, Siironen J, Skrifvars MB, Hernesniemi J, Kivisaari R. Predicting outcome in traumatic brain injury: development of a novel computerized tomography classification system (Helsinki Computerized Tomography Score). J Neurotrauma. 2014;75:632–47.
45. Schulman J, Sacks J, Provenzano G. State level estimates of the incidence and economic burden of head injuries stemming from non-universal use of bicycle helmets. Inj Prev. 2002;8:47–52.
46. Howe EI, Andelic N, Fure SCR, et al. Cost-effectiveness analysis of combined cognitive and vocational rehabilitation in patients with mild-to-moderate TBI: results from a randomized controlled trial. BMC Health Serv Res. 2022;22:1–13.
47. Mikkonen ED, Skrifvars MB, Reinikainen M, et al. One-year costs of intensive care in pediatric patients with traumatic brain injury. J Neurosurg Pediatr. 2020;27:79–86.
48. Graves JM, Kannan N, Mink RB, et al. Guideline adherence and hospital costs in pediatric severe traumatic brain injury. Pediatr Crit Care Med. 2016;17:438–44.
49. Appavu B, Foldes ST, Adelson PD. Clinical trials for pediatric traumatic brain injury: definition of insanity? J Neurosurg Pediatr. 2019;23:661–9.
50. Hutchison JS, Ward RE, Lacroix J, et al. Hypothermia therapy after traumatic brain injury in children. N Engl J Med. 2008;358:2447–56.
51. Santacruz CA, Pereira AJ, Celis E, Vincent JL. Which multicenter randomized controlled trials in critical care medicine have shown reduced mortality? A systematic review. Crit Care Med. 2019;47:1680–91.
52. CENTER-TBI. Available at: https://www.center-tbi.eu/. Accessed 8 Nov 2022.
53. Approaches and Decisions in Acute Pediatric TBI (ADAPT) Trial. Available at: https://www.adapttrial.org/. Accessed 8 Nov 2022.

# Quality Improvement in the Determination of Death by Neurologic Criteria Around the World

# 34

A. Lewis, M. P. Kirschen, and R. Badenes

## 34.1 Introduction

Public trust in the determination of brain death/death by neurologic criteria is contingent upon prevention of false positive determinations [1]. Unfortunately, although brain death/death by neurologic criteria is accepted throughout much of the world as equivalent to death by circulatory–respiratory criteria, numerous studies have reported variability across national and hospital policies, practice, and documentation for brain death/death by neurologic criteria determination [2–9]. Most recently, a 2020 study by Lewis et al. demonstrated inconsistency across 78 national policies [2]. This variability has the potential to lead to inaccurate brain death/death by neurologic criteria determinations.

A. Lewis
Department of Neurology and Neurosurgery, NYU Langone Medical Center, New York, NY, USA

M. P. Kirschen
Department of Anesthesiology and Critical Care Medicine, The Children's Hospital of Philadelphia, Perelman School of Medicine at the University of Pennsylvania, Philadelphia, PA, USA

R. Badenes (✉)
Department of Anesthesiology and Surgical-Trauma Intensive Care, Hospital Clinic Universitari, Valencia, Spain

Department of Surgery. Anesthesiology and Critical Care, School of Medicine, University of Valencia, Valencia, Spain
e-mail: rbadenes@uv.es



J.-L. Vincent (ed.), *Annual Update in Intensive Care and Emergency Medicine 2023*, Annual Update in Intensive Care and Emergency Medicine,
https://doi.org/10.1007/978-3-031-23005-9_34

The World Brain Death Project (WBDP), an international consensus statement, establishes minimum requirements for brain death/death by neurologic criteria determination in an effort to facilitate consistency, both within and between countries [10]. The WBDP was endorsed by five world federations—(1) the World Federation of Critical Care Nurses, (2) the World Federation of Intensive and Critical Care, (3) the World Federation of Neurology, (4) the World Federation of Neurosurgical Societies and (5) the World Federation of Pediatric Intensive and Critical Care Societies. The intent of the WBDP is for its minimum requirements for brain death/death by neurologic criteria determination to guide revision or creation of national policies for brain death/death by neurologic criteria determination around the world, after which hospital policies can be written or revised to reflect national policies. However, the WBDP questions what quality improvement measures can be put into place to ensure consistent and thorough brain death/death by neurologic criteria determination and eliminate the risk of false positive determinations [11].

Quality improvement efforts to promote accuracy and consistency in brain death/death by neurologic criteria determination must focus on updating national and hospital policies (which describe what clinicians should do) and addressing the discrepancy between policies and clinical practice (what clinicians actually do). This requires (1) medical society or governmental healthcare organizations to (a) align national brain death/death by neurologic criteria policies with the minimum requirements outlined by the WBDP and (b) facilitate regulation of hospital policies on brain death/death by neurologic criteria determination and credentialing of clinicians involved in brain death/death by neurologic criteria determination; (2) hospitals to ensure their policies are consistent with national policies; and (3) clinicians to be educated about the nuances of brain death/death by neurologic criteria determination [1].

The WBDP recommends that clinicians involved in brain death/death by neurologic criteria determination should (1) be licensed, (2) have completed training, and (3) be trained in brain death/death by neurologic criteria determination and in counseling families at the end-of-life [10]. The best way to evaluate and validate training programs and clinician competence in brain death/death by neurologic criteria determination is unknown. However, it is imperative that clinicians involved in brain death/death by neurologic criteria determination are familiar with conditions that could confound the evaluation (i.e., evaluate prerequisites for brain death/death by neurologic criteria determination), and with performance of the clinical examination and apnea test and the appropriate use of ancillary testing to prevent false positive brain death/death by neurologic criteria determinations. The WBDP statement includes a thorough review of this information including a checklist and flow diagram [10].

The goal of this chapter is to provide quality improvement guidance to prevent false positive brain death/death by neurologic criteria determinations and ensure patient safety during brain death/death by neurologic criteria determination. The chapter addresses: (1) brain death/death by neurologic criteria mimics, (2) confounders that interfere with the clinical brain death/death by neurologic criteria evaluation, (3) prevention of complications during the apnea test, (4) ancillary testing confounders and limitations, and (5) special considerations for brain death/death by neurologic criteria determination in pediatric patients.

**Table 34.1** Mimics of brain death/death by neurologic criteria [10]

| Condition |
|---|
| Botulism |
| Cervical cord injury |
| Fulminant Guillain-Barré syndrome |
| Hypokalemia |
| Leptomeningeal carcinomatosis |
| Organophosphate poisoning |
| Rabies encephalitis |
| Snake bite |

## 34.2 Brain Death/Death by Neurologic Criteria Mimics

The WBDP specifies that brain death/death by neurologic criteria determination requires identification of "an established neurological diagnosis, the nature and severity of which is capable of resulting in the irreversible loss of the capacity for consciousness, the irreversible loss of all brainstem reflexes and the irreversible loss of the ability to spontaneously breathe in the face of a carbon dioxide and acidosis challenge" [10]. Diagnoses that most often lead to brain death/death by neurologic criteria include hypoxic ischemic brain injury, stroke (ischemic stroke, subarachnoid hemorrhage, or intracerebral hemorrhage) and traumatic brain injury [12]. Other diagnoses that can lead to brain death/death by neurologic criteria include infections of the central nervous system (meningitis, encephalitis, abscesses), neoplasms, obstructive hydrocephalus, and edema secondary to severe metabolic derangements, such as acute hyponatremia, hyperammonemia or liver failure.

It is important to recognize there are a number of potentially reversible conditions that mimic brain death/death by neurologic criteria. Because of this, if the etiology of a patient's neurologic state is unknown, or any of the conditions that can mimic brain death/death by neurologic criteria may be present, clinicians should not perform an evaluation for brain death/death by neurologic criteria (Table 34.1).

## 34.3 Confounders That Interfere with the Clinical Brain Death/Death by Neurologic Criteria Evaluation

Even if a patient has a catastrophic brain injury from an etiology that can lead to brain death/death by neurologic criteria, there are a number of confounding conditions that have the potential to interfere with the brain death/death by neurologic criteria evaluation and could make a person appear as though they fulfil criteria, when they in fact do not (Table 34.2) [10, 13]. The WBDP defines "confounders" as "circumstances during which a diagnostic test or clinical evaluation may become unreliable and require repetition over time or application of an alternative test" [10]. The WBDP provides guidance about how to minimize the likelihood that confounders will lead to a false positive brain death/death by neurologic criteria determination.

**Table 34.2** Confounding factors for the clinical brain death/death by neurologic criteria evaluation (from [13] with permission)

| Disease process | Possible exam components confounded |
|---|---|
| Hypothermia | Complete exam |
| Muscular paralysis | Complete exam |
| Sedation/analgesia | Complete exam |
| Hypoxia | Complete exam |
| Hypotension | Complete exam |
| Hypoglycemia | Complete exam |
| Endocrine or metabolic abnormality | Complete exam |
| Basal skull fracture with hemotympanum | Oculovestibular reflex |
| Facial trauma | Pupillary response, oculovestibular, and oculocephalic reflexes, cranial pain response |
| Pulmonary injury/disease | Apnea test |
| Cervical spine injury | Corporal pain response, apnea test |
| Anophthalmia | Pupillary, corneal, oculovestibular, and oculocephalic reflexes |

### 34.3.1 Hypothermia

Hypothermia can temporarily blunt brain activity leading to reversible coma, brainstem areflexia, and inability to breathe spontaneously [14]. Hypothermia may be induced environmentally or intentionally for therapeutic benefit through use of targeted temperature management (TTM) or may result from severe brain injury due to loss of sympathetic regulation and catecholamine release (41–100% of patients develop hypothermia in the setting of brain death/death by neurologic criteria) [15]. Despite this, Lewis et al. found that only 78% of national brain death/death by neurologic criteria policies addressed the minimum temperature for brain death/death by neurologic criteria determination, and it ranged from 32 to 36 °C [2]. Additionally, only 10% of national policies included information about brain death/death by neurologic criteria determination after hypothermia and only two national policies clearly specified the minimum duration to observe patients for neurologic recovery after rewarming before conducting the evaluation for brain death/death by neurologic criteria (both advised waiting at least 24 h after rewarming).

To ensure temperature does not confound brain death/death by neurologic criteria determination, the WBDP suggests a minimum core temperature of 36 °C (defined by esophageal, bladder, rectal, or central venous or arterial catheter temperature measurement) [10]. The WBDP advises use of a warming blanket, an automated temperature regulation device, a thermal mattress, warmed fluids, and/or warmed oxygen to achieve this temperature, if needed. The WBDP also provides detailed guidance about timing of the brain death/death by neurologic criteria evaluation after rewarming. This includes waiting a period of at least 24 h after rewarming to observe for neurologic recovery and a low threshold to perform ancillary testing to evaluate brain blood flow in addition to completion of the clinical brain death/death by neurologic criteria examination and apnea test.

### 34.3.2 Muscle Paralysis

Muscle paralysis due to pharmacological paralytics or a neuromuscular disorder can interfere with the assessment for irreversible loss of brain-mediated motor responses, brainstem reflexes and the ability to breathe spontaneously. However, Lewis et al. found that only 63% of national brain death/death by neurologic criteria policies noted that the effects of pharmacological paralytics must be excluded prior to brain death/death by neurologic criteria determination [2]. The WBDP recommends use of a train-of-four stimulator or demonstration of the presence of deep tendon reflexes prior to performance of an evaluation for brain death/death by neurologic criteria [10]. The WBDP also notes that ancillary testing should be performed in addition to completion of the clinical examination and apnea test for patients with a severe neuromuscular disorder, like amyotrophic lateral sclerosis, given that lack of motor responses in these patients cannot definitively be attributed solely to their catastrophic brain injury.

### 34.3.3 Sedation/Analgesia

Sedation and analgesia can depress the central nervous system (CNS), as can a number of other medications, including antibiotics, baclofen, bupropion, tricyclic antidepressants, and valproic acid [13]. Clearance of these medications can be delayed in the setting of renal or hepatic dysfunction, obesity or hypothermia. Although Lewis et al. found that the majority of national brain death/death by neurologic criteria policies (82%) noted the need to exclude the effects of drugs or medications that depress the CNS before conducting the evaluation for brain death/death by neurologic criteria, this was not uniformly specified (51% mentioned sedation and 31% mentioned analgesia) [2]. Pharmacological derangements were included as an indication for ancillary testing in 36% of national brain death/death by neurologic criteria policies.

The WBDP recommends excluding the effects of drugs or medications prior to evaluation for brain death/death by neurologic criteria (1) using a toxicology screen if there is concern for toxic exposure; (2) via measurement of drug levels, if able, to ensure they are within or below the therapeutic range and are not felt to have the potential to confound the evaluation; or (3) by ensuring five elimination half-lives have passed, assuming normal hepatic and renal function [10]. If there is concern that drug elimination cannot be confirmed prior to evaluation for brain death/death by neurologic criteria, ancillary testing should be performed in addition to the clinical examination and apnea test.

### 34.3.4 Hypoxia

Hypoxic-ischemic brain injury can temporarily blunt brain activity, but Lewis et al. found that very few national brain death/death by neurologic criteria policies (17%) specified the need for an observation period after hypoxic-ischemic brain injury before evaluation for brain death/death by neurologic criteria [2, 16]. These policies all noted it was necessary to observe for at least 24 h after resuscitation to confirm there had been no neurologic recovery before initiating the evaluation for brain death/death by neurologic criteria [2]. Additionally, 7% of national brain death/death by neurologic criteria policies recommended performance of ancillary testing for patients with hypoxic-ischemic brain injury.

The WBDP recommends that patients should be observed for at least 24 h after hypoxic-ischemic brain injury, with consideration for ancillary testing in the setting of hypothermia after resuscitation following hypoxic-ischemic brain injury (as discussed above) [10].

### 34.3.5 Hypotension

Hypotension occurs in 65–97% of patients with catastrophic brain injury due to loss of hypothalamic function, loss of central vasomotor regulation of sympathetic tone, decreased cardiac contractility, hypovolemia, or other causes of shock [15]. Although systemic hypotension results in brain hypoperfusion, which can cause transient reversible loss of brain function, Lewis et al. found that only 44% of national brain death/death by neurologic criteria policies addressed the minimum blood pressure for brain death/death by neurologic criteria determination [2]. Some policies required normotension or absence of shock or hemodynamic instability, whereas other policies specified the minimum acceptable blood pressure (mean arterial pressure [MAP] >60 mmHg, MAP >70 mmHg, systolic blood pressure [SBP] >90 mmHg, SBP >100 mmHg, or other threshold). Cardiovascular instability was noted to be an indication for ancillary testing in 7% of national brain death/death by neurologic criteria policies.

The WBDP suggests a minimum MAP of 60 mmHg or SBP of 100 mmHg (and age appropriate targets in pediatric patients) prior to evaluation for brain death/death by neurologic criteria [10].

### 34.3.6 Hypoglycemia or Other Endocrine or Metabolic Abnormality

Hypoglycemia can lead to reversible loss of brain function, but there is no established lower limit of glucose for brain death/death by neurologic criteria determination [10, 17]. However, in a survey of 84 physicians in the Neurocritical Care Society, Lerner et al. found that 33% of respondents reported that their institution stipulated the minimum glucose for evaluation for brain death/death by neurologic criteria [17]. Respondents also commented on the laboratory thresholds they personally found acceptable for brain death/death by neurologic criteria determination. The median lower glucose threshold accepted among respondents was 60 mg/dl (interquartile range (IQR) 50–69 mg/dl).

Other endocrine or metabolic abnormalities could also impact the evaluation for brain death/death by neurologic criteria. Lewis et al. found that the need to rule out electrolyte, acid/base or endocrine derangements before brain death/death by neurologic criteria determination was addressed in 72% of national policies, though very few provided specific values (8% indicated specific electrolyte values, 5% included a specific acid/base threshold, and 1% noted specific endocrine values) [2]. Metabolic derangements were noted to be an indication for ancillary testing in 19% of national brain death/death by neurologic criteria policies.

The aforementioned survey by Lerner et al. demonstrated that there were varying perspectives on the specific metabolic values that preclude brain death/death by neurologic criteria determination. In addition to glucose, arterial pH and sodium were considered the most important variables to check [17]. The median personal lower and upper pH thresholds were 7.25 (IQR 7.1–7.3) and 7.55 (IQR 7.5–7.6), respectively, while the median personal lower and upper sodium thresholds were 125 mEq/l (IQR 120–130 mEq/l) and 160 mEq/l (IQR 155–170 mEq/l), respectively.

The WBDP recommends correction of severe metabolic, acid-base, and endocrine derangements, when feasible, and performance of ancillary testing to augment the clinical evaluation if these derangements cannot be corrected, but does not provide specific lower or upper limits for laboratory values [10].

### 34.3.7 Basal Skull Fracture with Hemotympanum

Lewis et al. noted variable guidance across national brain death/death by neurologic criteria policies about whether the oculovestibular reflex can be tested in the setting of basal skull fracture; 19% indicated a ruptured eardrum precluded the assessment, 9% indicated a ruptured eardrum does not preclude the assessment, and 5% specified that a skull fracture could blunt the response [2]. The need for ancillary testing in patients with a ruptured eardrum was required in 7% of national brain death/death by neurologic criteria policies.

The WBDP recommends ancillary testing in addition to completion of the clinical examination and apnea test for patients with a fracture of the base of the skull or petrous temporal bone given the potential for this type of injury to make the oculovestibular reflex unreliable on the side of the fracture [10]. It also notes that presence of a ruptured tympanic membrane does not negate evaluation of the reflex, but that this could lead to an increased risk of meningitis.

### 34.3.8 Facial Trauma

Lewis et al. found that national brain death/death by neurologic criteria policies provided inconsistent guidance about the ability to perform a complete brain death/death by neurologic criteria evaluation in patients with facial trauma; 25% noted this was an indication for ancillary testing [2].

The WBDP advises that facial trauma could interfere with assessment of the pupillary, oculovestibular, and oculocephalic reflexes or the motor response of the face, necessitating ancillary testing in addition to completion of the clinical examination and apnea test [10].

### 34.3.9 Pulmonary Injury/Disease

Acute lung injury or chronic pulmonary disease has the potential to interfere with the apnea test [10]. Lewis et al. found that 50% of national brain death/death by neurologic criteria policies noted that inability to complete the apnea test warranted ancillary testing [2]. Safety considerations for performance of the apnea test are discussed in detail below.

### 34.3.10 Cervical Spine Injury

Cervical spine injury has the potential to interfere with evaluation of motor responses, the oculocephalic reflex, the cough reflex, and the apnea test [10]. Lewis et al. found that 32% of national brain death/death by neurologic criteria policies indicated that cervical spine injury should be ruled out before assessment of the oculocephalic reflex, 3% indicated this should be ruled out before assessment of the cough reflex, and 5% indicated this should be ruled out before the apnea test; 9% specified that ancillary testing should be performed in patients with cervical spine injury [2].

The WBDP advises that the oculocephalic reflex should not be tested in patients with a cervical spine injury, but that if the oculovestibular reflex is performed and there are no extraocular movements, ancillary testing is not required as long as the rest of the clinical examination and the apnea test are completed and consistent with brain death/death by neurologic criteria [10]. However, it also notes that high spinal cord injuries can impact the efferent limb of the cough reflex and the apnea test and therefore recommends performance of ancillary testing.

### 34.3.11 Anophthalmia

In the setting of anophthalmia, the pupillary, corneal, oculovestibular, and oculocephalic reflexes on the side without an eye cannot be evaluated. Lewis et al. found that 14% of national brain death/death by neurologic criteria policies specified that ancillary testing should be performed in patients with only one eye [2].

The WBDP recommends ancillary testing in addition to completion of the clinical examination and the apnea test for patients with anophthalmia [10].

## 34.4 Considerations for Performance of the Clinical Examination

After ruling out the aforementioned mimics and confounders for the evaluation of brain death/death by neurologic criteria, the clinical examination can be performed. The steps for performance of the clinical examination for brain death/death by neurologic criteria determination, responses consistent with brain death/death by neurologic criteria, and special considerations enumerated by the WBDP are summarized in Table 34.3 [10].

**Table 34.3** Technique and considerations for the performance of the clinical brain death/death by neurologic criteria (BD/DNC) examination (from [10] with permission)

| Component | Test | Response consistent with BD/DNC | Considerations |
|---|---|---|---|
| Coma | Apply maximal external stimulation (including noxious visual, auditory, and tactile stimulation) to assess for arousal or awareness | There is no evidence of arousal or awareness to maximal external stimulation (including noxious visual, auditory, and tactile stimulation) | |
| Motor responses of the face and limbs | • Apply deep pressure to all of the following:<br>1. the condyles at the level of the temporomandibular joints<br>2. the supraorbital notch bilaterally<br>3. the sternal notch<br>4. all four extremities, both proximally and distally<br>• Insert a cotton swab on a stick in each nostril to perform "nasal tickle" testing | • Noxious stimuli should not produce grimacing, facial muscle movement, or a motor response of the limbs other than spinally mediated reflexes<br>• Noxious stimuli above the foramen magnum should not produce any movement in the face or body. Noxious stimuli below the foramen magnum should not produce any movement in the face but may elicit spinally mediated peripheral motor reflexes | • The clinical differentiation of spinal from brain-mediated motor responses requires expertise. Consultation with an experienced practitioner is recommended if the origin of a response is unclear. Alternatively, if interpretation is unclear, ancillary testing is recommended<br>• Ancillary testing is recommended if a person has a preexisting severe neuromuscular disorder, such as amyotrophic lateral sclerosis or a preexisting severe sensory neuropathy<br>• Ancillary testing is not required if a person does not have all four limbs; absence of a limb does not preclude motor testing to pain on that side of the body<br>• Severe facial trauma or swelling may preclude evaluation of facial motor response, so ancillary testing is recommended in this setting |
| Pupillary reflex | Shine a bright light into each of the person's eyes, looking for pupillary constriction and measuring the diameter of the pupils (use of a magnifying glass and/or pupillometer is suggested) | There should be absence of ipsilateral and contralateral pupillary response, with pupils fixed in a midsize or dilated position ($\approx$4–6 mm), in both eyes | • Constricted pupils are not consistent with BD/DNC and suggest the possibility of drug intoxication or locked-in syndrome<br>• Pupils can be any shape (round/oval/irregular)<br>• Corneal trauma or prior ophthalmic surgery may influence pupillary reactivity and preclude adequate evaluation, necessitating ancillary testing<br>• Ocular instillation of drugs may artificially produce transiently nonreactive pupils<br>• In the setting of anophthalmia or inability to see the pupils, ancillary testing is recommended |

| | | | |
|---|---|---|---|
| Oculocephalic (OCR) and oculovestibular (OVR) reflexes | • OCR: Rotate the head briskly horizontally to both sides. There should be no movement of the eyes relative to head movement. Testing vertically is optional<br>• OVR: Examine the auditory canal for patency and an intact tympanic membrane. Elevate the head to 30° to place the horizontal semicircular canals in the correct vertical position. Irrigate with at least 30 ml of ice water for at least 60 s using a syringe or a syringe attached to a catheter placed inside the canal. Test both sides separately, with a 5-min interval between to allow the endolymph temperature to equilibrate | There should be absence of extraocular movements. Detection of any extraocular movements is not compatible with BD/DNC | • Confirm the integrity of the cervical spine before proceeding with the OCR test. If the OCR cannot be performed, but the OVR is performed and there are no extraocular movements, ancillary testing is not required<br>• Ensure the integrity of the tympanic membrane. Presence of a ruptured tympanic membrane does not negate the clinical testing but may risk introducing infections in the ear<br>• A fracture of the base of the skull or petrous temporal bone may obliterate the response on the side of the fracture, and ancillary testing is recommended in this instance<br>• Severe orbital or scleral edema or chemosis may affect the free motion of the globes, and ancillary testing is recommended in this instance<br>• In the setting of anophthalmia, ancillary testing is recommended |
| Corneal reflex | Touch the cornea of both eyes with a cotton swab on a stick at the external border of the iris, applying light pressure and observing for any eyelid movement | No eyelid movement should be seen | • Care should be taken to avoid damaging the cornea<br>• In the setting of anophthalmia, severe orbital edema, prior corneal transplantation, or scleral edema or chemosis, ancillary testing is recommended |
| Gag and cough reflexes | • Gag reflex: stimulate the posterior pharyngeal wall bilaterally with a tongue depressor or suction catheter<br>• Cough reflex: stimulate the tracheobronchial wall to the level of the carina with deep endotracheal placement of a suction catheter | Absence of gag and cough | The efferent limb for the cough reflex includes the phrenic nerve, which may be injured in persons with high cervical cord injuries, so ancillary testing is recommended in this setting |

## 34.5 Apnea Test Safety Considerations

Safety considerations for performance of the apnea test are discussed here, but a detailed discussion of the procedure for performance of the apnea test can be found in the WBDP summary and supplemental documents [10]. The WBDP advises that the brain death/death by neurologic criteria evaluation should not begin until it has been determined that the patient is not taking any spontaneous breaths when the ventilator is in spontaneous breathing mode and that the apnea test should only be conducted after the clinical examination has been completed and found to be consistent with brain death/death by neurologic criteria. Further, the WBDP recommends that ventilator requirements and pulmonary status be assessed prior to the apnea test to determine whether the patient is likely to tolerate the test.

Although the apnea test is generally considered safe, induction of a hypercarbic acidemic state can lead to complications (Table 34.4). Reviews of the literature have demonstrated that the apnea test needs to be aborted due to hemodynamic instability in 1–20% of patients, particularly those of younger age, with lower pre-test pH, hypotension, a high arterial-alveolar gradient, or polytrauma [10, 18, 19]. However, the risks of the apnea test can be minimized through strict adherence to guidance on ensuring prerequisites are met prior to the apnea test.

**Table 34.4** Apnea test safety considerations [10, 15, 18]

| Complication | Prevention techniques |
|---|---|
| Hypotension | • Ensure MAP >60 mmHg or SBP >100 mmHg before testing is initiated<br>• Use fluids/vasopressors/inotropes as needed<br>• Ensure euvolemia/hypervolemia prior to testing<br>• Ensure temperature is >36 °C<br>Abort testing for MAP <60 mmHg or SBP <100 mmHg |
| Hypoxemia | • Preoxygenate with 100% oxygen for 10-min prior to testing<br>• Consider checking arterial blood gas to ensure $PaO_2$ >200 mmHg<br>• Consider use of CPAP or a PEEP valve<br>Abort testing for sustained desaturation <85% |
| Pneumothorax, pneumomediastinum, and pneumoperitoneum | • Ensure insufflation catheter tip is in the distal third of the endotracheal tube<br>• Ensure insufflation catheter is not too wide compared to the diameter of the endotracheal tube<br>• Minimize oxygen flow rate through insufflation catheter |
| Arrhythmia/cardiac arrest | • Prevent hypotension and hypoxemia<br>• Correct electrolyte derangements<br>• Ensure temperature is >36 °C |

*MAP* mean arterial pressure, *SBP* systolic blood pressure, *CPAP* continuous positive airway pressure, *PEEP* positive end-expiratory pressure

Nonetheless, because of the potential for complications during the apnea test, the WBDP notes that it should be performed by clinicians with experience in cardiopulmonary resuscitation (CPR) [10]. The WBDP advises that if the apnea test is aborted, ancillary testing should be performed or the apnea test should be repeated after waiting additional time for resolution of hemodynamic instability. If the apnea test is aborted due to hypoxemia, consideration can be given to repeating it after improvement in pulmonary dysfunction (perhaps via performance of recruitment maneuvers) or using continuous positive airway pressure (CPAP) or a positive end-expiratory pressure (PEEP) valve to minimize the risk of hypoxemia or induction of hypercarbia with carbogen to reach the target $PaCO_2$ and pH faster.

### 34.5.1 Hypotension

Patients may develop hypotension during the apnea test as a result of either the acidosis itself or preexisting conditions; these include arteriolar vasodilation, decreased preload, or depressed myocardial contractility [10, 18]. A review of complications during the apnea test by Busl et al. found that the incidence of hypotension during the apnea test was 7–39% [18]. Despite this, only 14% of national brain death/death by neurologic criteria policies recommended aborting the apnea test if hypotension occurred [2].

To minimize the risk of hypotension during an apnea test and ensure the evaluation is not impacted by hypoperfusion of the medullary chemoreceptors, the WBDP suggests a minimum MAP of 60 mmHg or SBP of 100 mmHg (and age appropriate targets in pediatric patients) be maintained for the apnea test through use of fluids, vasopressors, or inotropes as needed [10]. Further, it recommends aborting the test for MAP <60 mmHg or SBP <100 mmHg.

### 34.5.2 Hypoxemia

The apnea test can lead to hypoxemia due to atelectasis [10, 18]. Busl et al. found that the incidence of hypoxemia during the apnea test was 4–6% [18]. Despite this, only 23% of national brain death/death by neurologic criteria policies recommended that the apnea test be aborted in case of hypoxemia [2].

To decrease the risk of hypoxemia during an apnea test, the WBDP suggests that patients be preoxygenated with 100% oxygen for at least 10-min prior to the apnea test and that use of CPAP or a PEEP valve be considered to prevent atelectasis [10]. Some national brain death/death by neurologic criteria policies specified that the apnea test should only be performed after an arterial blood gas demonstrates the $PaO_2$ is $\geq$200 mmHg [2]. The WBDP also recommends aborting the apnea test for sustained desaturation <85% [10].

### 34.5.3 Pneumothorax, Pneumomediastinum and Pneumoperitoneum

Barotrauma can lead to pneumothorax, pneumomediastinum or pneumoperitoneum during the apnea test [10, 18]. This can develop due to a number of mechanisms. If an insufflation catheter is used and the catheter is placed too deep, there can be tracheal perforation or if the catheter is too wide, gas flow can be obstructed. Secretions can also obstruct oxygenation or gas outflow. Finally, barotrauma can develop if oxygen flow is too high. Busl et al. reported that barotrauma during the apnea test was very rare [18]. To prevent these complications, it has been suggested that the oxygen insufflation catheter tip be in the distal third of the endotracheal tube, the catheter diameter be <50–70% of the endotracheal tube diameter, and hyperoxygenation be avoided (<6 l/min is generally advised) [2, 10].

### 34.5.4 Arrhythmia/Cardiac Arrest

An arrhythmia or cardiac arrest can occur during the apnea test as a consequence of hypotension, hypoxemia or acidosis. Busl et al. found that the incidence of arrhythmia during the apnea test was 1% and the incidence of cardiac arrest was <1% [18]. The recommendation to abort the apnea test due to a dysrhythmia was only mentioned in 21% of national brain death/death by neurologic criteria policies [2]. The WBDP recommends aborting the apnea test if an unstable arrhythmia occurs [10].

## 34.6 Ancillary Testing Confounders/Limitations

Lewis et al. found variability in ancillary testing across national brain death/death by neurologic criteria policies; this included variability in (1) the accepted ancillary tests, (2) guidance on performance and interpretation of the tests, and (3) an explanation of the confounders/limitations associated with ancillary testing [2, 20]. Of the national brain death/death by neurologic criteria policies that included an assessment of brain blood flow, <10% described confounders/limitations that could impact interpretation of the results [20]. Of the national policies that included electroencephalography (EEG) as an acceptable ancillary test, 20% noted the potential for artifact, 18% noted it could be affected by sedatives, 16% noted it could be affected by hypothermia, 11% noted it could be affected by metabolic derangements, and 11% noted it predominantly assessed the cortex.

The WBDP recommends ancillary testing is required if the clinical examination and apnea test cannot be completed, confounding conditions cannot be resolved, or there is uncertainty about interpretation of spinal-mediated reflexes [10]. The WBDP includes three acceptable ways to evaluate for the absence of brain blood flow for the purposes of brain death/death by neurologic criteria determination: (1) digital subtraction angiography, (2) radionuclide angiography/scintigraphy, and (3) transcranial Doppler ultrasonography [10]. The WBDP suggests against routine use of EEG as an ancillary test since it does not provide information about brainstem function, and advises that other tests to evaluate brain blood flow (e.g., computed tomography angiography or magnetic resonance angiography) or electrical activity (e.g., evoked potentials) should not be utilized. Confounders and limitations for each ancillary test are summarized in Table 34.5 [10, 23, 24].

**Table 34.5** Ancillary testing confounders/limitations [10, 20–22]

| Test | Confounder/limitation[a] | Sensitivity/ specificity |
|---|---|---|
| Brain blood flow | | |
| *Computed tomography angiography* | • Requires transport to the scanner<br>• Image variability based on injection technique<br>• Potential to miss a slow flow state<br>• Risk of nephrotoxicity | 52–97%/100% |
| *Digital subtraction angiography*[b] | • Requires transport to angiography suite<br>• Risk of nephrotoxicity<br>• Image variability based on injection technique | 100%/100% |
| *Magnetic resonance angiography* | • Requires transport to the scanner<br>• Image variability based on injection technique | 93–100%/100% |
| *Radionuclide angiography*[b] | • Limited evaluation of brainstem | 99%/56% |
| *Radionuclide scintigraphy*[b] | • Requires transport to the scanner<br>• Planar imaging may have limited evaluation of brainstem | Planar: 78%/100%<br>SPECT: 88%/100% |
| *Transcranial Doppler ultrasonography*[b] | • Potential for technical difficulties in performance<br>• Potential for lack of windows | 90%/98% |
| Electrophysiological function | | |
| *Electroencephalography* | • Risk of environmental artifact<br>• Confounded by sedation, hypothermia and toxic-metabolic derangements<br>• Predominantly provides information about cortical function | 53–80%/97% |
| *Evoked potentials-auditory* | • Can be absent in comatose patients with other intact brainstem reflexes<br>• Confounded by sedation, hypothermia, isolated eighth nerve and brainstem lesions<br>• Only evaluates auditory pathways<br>• Performance/interpretation may be limited by experience | NA/NA |
| *Evoked potentials-somatosensory* | • Can be absent in comatose patients with ongoing brain function<br>• Confounded by cervical spine injury, isolated brainstem lesions, sedation and hypothermia<br>• Only evaluates somatosensory pathways<br>• Performance/interpretation may be limited by experience | 100%/78% |

(continued)

**Table 34.5** (continued)

| Test | Confounder/limitation[a] | Sensitivity/ specificity |
|---|---|---|
| *Evoked potentials-visual* | • Can be absent in comatose patients with ongoing brain function<br>• Confounded by sedation, retinal or optic nerve lesions<br>• Only evaluates visual pathways<br>• Performance/interpretation may be limited by experience | NA/NA |

*NA* not available
[a] Performance/interpretation of all ancillary tests may be limited by experience
[b] Accepted by the World Brain Death Project (WBDP)

## 34.7 Special Considerations for Brain Death/Death by Neurologic Criteria Determination in Pediatric Patients

In some nations, brain death/death by neurologic criteria policies vary based on age to account for physiologic and anatomic differences in younger patients that necessitate a higher degree of conservatism [2, 20, 25]. For example, the USA has different brain death/death by neurologic criteria policies for adults and infants/children [26, 27]. Where pediatric specific guidance is provided, it addresses prerequisites for the brain death/death by neurologic criteria evaluation, the clinical examination, the apnea test, and ancillary testing [2].

First, drug metabolism can be different in pediatric patients compared to adults, so this should be accounted for when assessing fulfilment of prerequisites for brain death/death by neurologic criteria determination.

Second, serial examinations with a specified observation period between them to ensure there is no recovery of neurologic function, and/or a longer observation period prior to brain death/death by neurologic criteria determination, is sometimes required for pediatric patients [2]. This is particularly important for infants after cardiac arrest, since their brainstem may be more resistant to hypoxic-ischemic brain injury than older children and adults [25]. Infants with open fontanelles also may not have the same consequences of intracranial pressure and herniation as adults. While the WBDP suggests that a single evaluation is the minimum standard for brain death/death by neurologic criteria determination in adults, two clinical examinations and apnea tests are considered the minimum standard for brain death/death by neurologic criteria determination in pediatric patients [10]. Additionally, the WBDP recommends a "cautious approach with serial examinations and an adequate observation period" to minimize the risk of diagnostic error. However, the WBDP questions whether a single examination may be practical and safe for brain death/death by neurologic criteria determination in children [11].

Third, the WBDP recommends that tracheal insufflation should not be used for the apnea test in newborns, infants, and young children [10]. CPAP can be used in children to prevent atelectasis; this has a low adverse event rate [19]. The WBDP also suggests that ancillary testing be performed *in lieu* of the apnea test in patients with chronic hypoxemia due to cyanotic heart disease [10].

Finally, the WBDP recommends a radionuclide cerebral blood flow study as the preferred ancillary test and suggests that EEG is a valid ancillary study in infants and children and can be used in certain jurisdictions [10]. The WBDP also recommends that transcranial Doppler ultrasonography not be used in pediatric patients due to lack of data.

## 34.8 Conclusion

Quality improvement in brain death/death by neurologic criteria determination is needed to prevent false positive determinations and subsequent loss of public trust in brain death/death by neurologic criteria. This improvement requires education of clinicians involved in brain death/death by neurologic criteria determination and revision of national and hospital brain death/death by neurologic criteria policies to meet the minimum requirements described by the WBDP [10]. Clinicians involved in brain death/death by neurologic criteria determination must be knowledgeable about (1) brain death/death by neurologic criteria mimics, (2) confounders that interfere with the clinical brain death/death by neurologic criteria evaluation, (3) prevention of complications during the apnea test, (4) ancillary testing confounders/limitations, and (5) special considerations for brain death/death by neurologic criteria determination in pediatric patients. Education about brain death/death by neurologic criteria determination can be found in the Neurocritical Care Society's Brain Death Determination Course, an online continuing medical education module endorsed by the American Academy of Neurology, which reviews components of the evaluation, prerequisites, the clinical examination, the apnea test, ancillary testing, documentation, and communication [28, 29]. Finally, other institutional or national systems to prevent false positive brain death/death by neurologic criteria determinations include requiring credentialing of clinicians involved in brain death/death by neurologic criteria determination and oversight of hospital brain death/death by neurologic criteria policies by regulatory authorities [1, 30]. However, it is unknown what is the best (1) way to evaluate and validate the quality and efficacy of brain death/death by neurologic criteria training programs, (2) way to assess for clinician competence in brain death/death by neurologic criteria determination, and (3) means to certify and recertify clinicians for brain death/death by neurologic criteria determination [10]. Quality improvement research related to optimization of the accuracy and consistency of brain death/death by neurologic criteria determinations is needed.

## References


1. Lewis A, Bernat JL, Blosser S, et al. An interdisciplinary response to contemporary concerns about brain death determination. Neurology. 2018;90:423–6.
2. Lewis A, Bakkar A, Kreiger-Benson E, et al. Determination of death by neurologic criteria around the world. Neurology. 2020;95:e299–309.
3. Wijdicks EFM. Brain death worldwide: accepted fact but no global consensus in diagnostic criteria. Neurology. 2002;58:20–5.
4. Wahlster S, Wijdicks E, Patel P, Greer D, Hemphill J, Carone M, Mateen F. Brain death declaration: practices and perceptions worldwide. Neurology. 2015;84:1870–9.
5. Greer DM, Wang HH, Robinson JD, Varelas PN, Henderson GV, Wijdicks EFM. Variability of brain death policies in the United States. JAMA Neurol. 2016;73:213–8.
6. Braksick SA, Robinson CP, Gronseth GS, Hocker S, Wijdicks EFM, Rabinstein AA. Variability in reported physician practices for brain death determination. Neurology. 2019;92:e888–94.
7. Mathur M, Petersen L, Stadtler M, et al. Variability in pediatric brain death determination and documentation in southern California. Pediatrics. 2008;121:988–93.
8. Varelas PN, Goldenberg F, Greer D, et al. Documentation of brain death/death by neurologic criteria. Supplement 9 of Determination of brain death/death by neurologic criteria: the World Brain Death Project. JAMA. 2020;324:1078–97.
9. Francoeur C, Weiss MJ, Macdonald JM, et al. Variability in pediatric brain death determination protocols in the United States. Neurology. 2021;97:e310–9.
10. Greer D, Shemie S, Lewis A, et al. Determination of brain death/death by neurologic criteria: the World Brain Death Project. JAMA. 2020;324:1078–97.
11. Greer D, Shemie S, Lewis A, et al. Questions that address knowledge gaps to facilitate development of a research agenda about brain death/death by neurologic criteria. Supplement 17 of Determination of brain death/death by neurologic criteria: the world brain death project. JAMA. 2020;324:1078–97.
12. Hoppe A, Bleck T, Lewis A, et al. The science of brain death/death by neurologic criteria. Supplement 2 of Determination of brain death/death by neurologic criteria: the world brain death project. JAMA. 2020;324:1078–97.
13. Varelas P, Goldenberg F, Lewis A, et al. Minimum clinical criteria for determination of brain death/death by neurologic criteria. Supplement 4 of Determination of brain death/death by neurologic criteria: the World Brain Death Project. JAMA. 2020;324:1078–97.
14. Lewis A, Souter M, Greer D, Sung G, Torrance S, Shemie SD. Determination of brain death/death by neurologic criteria after treatment with targeted temperature management. Supplement 8 of Determination of brain death/death by neurologic criteria after treatment with targeted temperature management. JAMA. 2020;324:1078–97.
15. Lewis A, Souter M, Baldessari M, et al. Somatic support after brain death/death by neurologic criteria for organ donation and other special circumstances. Supplement 11 of Determination of brain death/death by neurologic criteria: the world brain death project. JAMA. 2020;324:1078–97.
16. Carroll E, Lewis A. Neuroprognostication after Cardiac arrest: who recovers? who progresses to brain death? Semin Neurol. 2021;41:606–18.
17. Lerner DP, Bassil R, Tadevosyan A, et al. Metabolic values precluding clinical death by neurologic criteria/brain death: survey of neurocritical care society physicians. J Clin Neurosci. 2021;88:16–21.
18. Busl KM, Lewis A, Varelas PN. Apnea testing for the determination of brain death: a systematic scoping review. Neurocrit Care. 2021;34:608–20.
19. Puccetti DF, Morrison W, Francoeur C, Mai M, Kirschen MP. Apnea testing using continuous positive airway pressure when determining death by neurologic criteria in children. Pediatr Crit Care Med. 2020;21:e1152–6.
20. Lewis A, Liebman J, Kreiger-Benson E, et al. Ancillary testing for determination of death by neurologic criteria around the world. Neurocrit Care. 2021;34:473–84.

21. Wijdicks EFM. The case against confirmatory tests for determining brain death in adults. Neurology. 2010;75:77–83.
22. Academy of Medical Royal Colleges. A code of practice for the diagnosis and confirmation of death. 2008. Available at: https://www.aomrc.org.uk/reports-guidance/ukdec-reports-and-guidance/code-practice-diagnosis-confirmation-death/. Accessed 11 Nov 2022.
23. Souter M, Alexandrov A, Topcuoglu MA, et al. Beyond minimum clinical determination of brain death/death by neurologic criteria. Supplement 5 of Determination of brain death/death by neurologic criteria: the World Brain Death Project. JAMA. 2020;324:1078–97.
24. Greer D, Shemie S, Lewis A, et al. A checklist for determination of brain death/death by neurologic criteria. Supplement 15 of Determination of brain death/death by neurologic criteria: the World Brain Death Project. JAMA. 2020;324:1078–97.
25. Nakagawa TA, Jacobe S, Greer D, et al. Pediatric and neonatal brain death/death by neurologic criteria. Supplement 6 of Determination of brain death/death by neurologic criteria: the World Brain Death Project. JAMA. 2020;324:1078–97.
26. Wijdicks EFM, Varelas PN, Gronseth GS, Greer DM. Evidence-based guideline update: determining brain death in adults. Neurology. 2010;74:1911–8.
27. Nakagawa TA, Ashwal S, Mathur M, Mysore M, Committee for Determination of Brain Death in Infants and Children. Guidelines for the determination of brain death in infants and children: an update of the 1987 task force recommendations-executive summary. Ann Neurol. 2012;71:573–85.
28. The Neurocritical Care Society Brain Death Determination Course. Available at: https://www.neurocriticalcare.org/higherlogic/s/p/cm/ld/fid=1101. Accessed 9 Dec 2022.
29. Rubin MA, Kirschen MP, Lewis A. The Neurocritical Care Brain Death Determination Course: purpose, design, and early findings. Neurocrit Care. 2021;35:913–5.
30. Thomson D, Varelas PN, Goldenberg FD, et al. Qualifications for and education on determination of brain death/death by neurologic criteria. Supplement 10 of Determination of brain death/death by neurologic criteria: the World Brain Death Project. JAMA. 2020;324:1078–97.

# Part XI

# Obstetric Issues

# COVID-19 ARDS in Pregnancy: Implications for the Non-COVID Era

# 35

M. Di Nardo, M. C. Casadio, and V. M. Ranieri

## 35.1 Introduction

Acute respiratory distress syndrome (ARDS) is a form of respiratory failure characterized by pulmonary edema due to pulmonary inflammation, decreased lung compliance, and severe hypoxemia. The Berlin definition is currently used to diagnose ARDS, and its severity is evaluated using three oxygenation thresholds [1]. Although data on ARDS during pregnancy are limited to case reports and case series [2], there is a consistent agreement that: (a) ARDS is a major mortality and morbidity factor for both the mother and the fetus; (b) ARDS is the most frequent cause of intensive care unit (ICU) admission during pregnancy [3]. The frequency of ARDS in the non-pregnant population ranges between 5 and 80 cases per 100,000 people per year [4], whereas the incidence of ARDS during pregnancy is higher (70–120 cases per 100,000 deliveries) [5] indicating that pregnancy may increase the risk of ARDS. The mortality rate of ARDS in the general population is around 40%, while in pregnancy it is variable and ranges between 25% and 50% [4, 6] with significant morbidity continuing even after the initial ARDS recovery [7].

The coronavirus disease 2019 (COVID-19) pandemic has dramatically increased the number of patients with ARDS requiring ICU admission for ventilatory support. While in 2016, 20% of patients admitted to the ICU had ARDS [8], in 2020, 60% of patients admitted to the ICU had COVID-19-induced ARDS [9]. Consistent with these data, a dramatic increase in COVID-19-induced ARDS was observed in

M. Di Nardo
Pediatric Intensive Care Unit, Ospedale Pediatrico Bambino Gesù, IRCCS, Rome, Italy

M. C. Casadio · V. M. Ranieri (✉)
Dipartimento di Scienze Mediche e Chirurgiche (DIMEC), Anesthesia and Intensive Care Medicine, Policlinico di Sant'Orsola, IRCCS, Alma Mater Studiorum University of Bologna, Bologna, Italy
e-mail: m.ranieri@unibo.it



J.-L. Vincent (ed.), *Annual Update in Intensive Care and Emergency Medicine 2023*, Annual Update in Intensive Care and Emergency Medicine,
https://doi.org/10.1007/978-3-031-23005-9_35

pregnant women. Early data from China and the USA showed that the risk of severe COVID-19 and ARDS in pregnant women was similar to that of the general population [10–12]. However, this first enthusiasm was dampened by other data showing that pregnant women with COVID-19 had a higher risk of hospitalization than non-pregnant women [13]. Symptomatic pregnant women with COVID-19 have an increased risk of ICU admission and adverse maternal and neonatal outcomes [14–16] compared with symptomatic non-pregnant females. A multicenter international study conducted in 32 ICUs in France, Belgium, and Switzerland showed that among the 2480 pregnant women with COVID-19, 187 (8%) were admitted to the ICU for severe pneumonia due to the severe acute respiratory syndrome coronavirus 2 (SARS-CoV-2), and 73 (39%) patients had required intubation [17].

Considering the large amount of data gathered during the COVID-19 pandemic, we will review the evidence to provide tools for a better understanding and clinical management of ARDS during pregnancy in the non-COVID era.

## 35.2 Pregnancy, ARDS, and SARS-CoV-2 Infection

Several physiologic changes related to pregnancy may increase the risk of ARDS (Table 35.1) [18, 19]. For example, as the uterus enlarges, the functional residual capacity (FRC) may reduce significantly favoring the development of atelectasis. The increase in plasma volume coupled with a decrease in oncotic pressure may contribute to pulmonary edema [6]. Pregnancy-specific conditions, such as pulmonary edema due to preeclampsia, amniotic fluid embolism, tocolytic-associated pulmonary edema, and obstetric sepsis (e.g., chorioamnionitis and endometritis), may increase the risk of ARDS [6]. Alterations in cell-mediated immunity may predispose the patient to pulmonary infections with higher fatality rates than in the general population [19]. Delayed stomach emptying caused by progesterone, may increase intra-abdominal pressure and favor gastric acid aspiration, increasing the risk of ARDS. Increase in the human placental growth hormone during late pregnancy results in airway hyperemia and edema and increased respiratory drive and minute ventilation (20–40% over baseline by term). The major mechanism behind the increase in minute ventilation is the increase in the tidal volume of approximately 30–35% above baseline. Due to all these changes, arterial blood gases during pregnancy show respiratory alkalosis with a compensatory renal excretion of bicarbonate; as a result, the partial pressure of carbon dioxide ($PaCO_2$) is lower than normal (28–32 mmHg) as is the plasma bicarbonate (18–21 mEq/l) [20].

Of note, the mother's oxygen intake and carbon dioxide output increase during pregnancy, reaching 20–33% over baseline by the third trimester. Therefore, pregnant patients are more vulnerable to hypoxia than non-pregnant patients in case of hypoventilation or apnea. Additionally, severe alkalosis and acidosis (metabolic or respiratory) may decrease uterine blood flow and negatively impact fetal oxygenation [2, 6]. Consequently, maintenance of high levels of perfusion (cardiac index >4–5 l/min/m$^2$) to the uterus and adequate values of gas exchange (oxygen partial pressure ($PaO_2$) $\geq$70 mmHg, $PaCO_2$ <45 mmHg with a pH >7.30) are essential for

**Table 35.1** Physiologic changes during pregnancy

| System | Physiologic change |
|---|---|
| Respiratory changes | Increase in oxygen demand |
| | Increase in minute ventilation |
| | Hyperventilation (↑ $PO_2$ and ↓ $PCO_2$) |
| | Reduction in functional residual capacity |
| Cardiovascular changes | Increase in cardiac output (up to 40%) |
| | Reduction in systemic vascular resistance due to peripheral vasodilatation (up to 25–30%) |
| | Reduction in venous return, mainly because of inferior vena cava compression |
| | Reduction in colloid osmotic pressure/pulmonary capillary wedge pressure gradient, with high risk of pulmonary edema |
| Hematological changes | Increase in plasma volume (up to 10% above baseline by 7 weeks of gestation, plateau by 32 weeks at 45–50%), parallel but weaker increase in red blood cell mass (18–25%), determining dilutional anemia |
| | Increase in white cell count |
| | Reduction in platelet count (dilutional effect and/or increased consumption secondary to endothelial-mediated activation) |
| | Increase in coagulation factors (fibrinogen, factor VII, VIII, IX, X, XII) and von Willebrand factor circulating levels, maintenance or slight decrease in natural anticoagulant levels (antithrombin III, protein C, protein S), reduction in fibrinolytic activity (increase in plasminogen activator inhibitors 1 and 2); thus, defining a pro-coagulable state |
| Immunological changes | Increase in complement system molecules (C3, C4, C5, C9) and regulatory proteins (factor H) |
| | Increase in neutrophil count, though less active (e.g., lower phagocytosis) |
| | Reduced natural killer cells, T-helper-cells and T-cytotoxic cells (increased susceptibility to viral and fungal pneumonias) |
| | Diversion of Th1/Th2 immunological responses towards a Th2 specific response |
| | Reduction in B-cell count ("physiological" B cell lymphopenia), especially innate B-1 cell levels (major source of "innate" IgM antibodies), and function (e.g. loss of responsiveness to mitogens) |
| | Increase in IgG1 and IgG3 levels (third trimester), stable IgG2 and IgG4 levels |
| | Increased proportion of T-regulatory-cells (peak in second trimester) |
| | Increase in CD19+CD24hiCD27+ B-regulatory-cell (first trimester, important role in maternal Th1 responses suppression) |

fetal well-being [6, 18]. Clinically, the signs and symptoms of ARDS reflect the underlying disease process [21]. However, critical patients may exhibit classical generic signs and symptoms of acute hypoxemic respiratory failure, such as worsening dyspnea, tachypnea, tachycardia, cyanosis, restlessness, and confusion. Chest auscultation can detect diffuse bilateral crackles or wheezing at the bases of the lungs.

Over the last 20 years, various definitions of "obstetric-related ARDS" have been proposed, including ARDS during pregnancy or occurring within 7 days after delivery, or within a month after delivery [6]. However, as the majority of pregnancy-related physiological changes persist for 6 weeks after birth, it could be more appropriate to include the postpartum period in the definition [6, 7]. According to the Berlin definition, ARDS requires the presence of bilateral pulmonary infiltrates on chest X-ray or computed tomography (CT) scan; thus, both imaging techniques should be used to finalize diagnosis. However, these techniques require ionizing radiation and may have adverse effects on the fetus depending on the maternal gestational age [22]. These adverse effects include teratogenicity, abnormal neurological development, and an increased risk of childhood leukemia [23]. Fetal teratogenicity risks are higher during the first trimester and are related to the total dose of radiation administered (usually requiring >50 mGy). However, the risk of fetal teratogenicity with low radiation exposure (<50 mGy) is minimal. For this reason, maternal examinations should not be withheld when necessary for the diagnosis and clinical management of ARDS in pregnancy.

Several physiologic adaptations to pregnancy may increase maternal susceptibility to infections and to SARS-CoV-2 infection, including changes in the maternal immune system function, impairment of the respiratory function, and the hypercoagulability state (Table 35.1) [24, 25]. Maternal changes in immune function consist of a hormone-mediated shift from a T helper 1 to T helper 2 cell response with a decrease in CD4+ and CD8+ T cells. This asset produces an important immunomodulation associated with an anti-inflammatory cytokine profile to prevent rejection of the fetus [25]. These changes, associated with the reduction in the FRC, make pregnant women more susceptible to respiratory infections [24, 25]. Moreover, the hypercoagulable state typical of physiological pregnancy, is amplified by SARS-CoV-2 infection. SARS-CoV-2 causes a significant activation of coagulation pathways and fibrinolysis and endothelial damage (thrombotic microangiopathy) [26]. Consequently, pregnant women with COVID-19 may have synergistic factors that may increase the risk of thrombosis and thromboembolic events (pulmonary embolism) and pre-eclampsia [24, 27].

SARS-CoV-2 infection in pregnant women can be asymptomatic (most of the cases) or symptomatic [24]. The most common clinical manifestations [24] are cough, dyspnea, and fever, and symptoms do not appear to differ based on gestational age [28]. Symptomatic pregnant women can be classified as mild, moderate, severe, and critical (Table 35.2) according to the severity of the respiratory disease and the presence of multiorgan failure and are generally admitted to the hospital in the late second or third trimester [29]. Risk factors for severe COVID-19 disease in

**Table 35.2** Classification of coronavirus disease 2019 (COVID-19) by severity

| Classification | Definition |
|---|---|
| Asymptomatic | Positive SARS-CoV-2 testing, but no symptoms |
| Mild | Fever, cough, but no shortness of breath, dyspnea or abnormal imaging on chest X-ray |
| Moderate | Clinical or radiographic evidence of mild pneumonia ($O_2$ saturation >93% on room air at sea level) |
| Severe | Dyspnea, respiratory rate >30/min, $O_2$ saturation <93%, $PaO_2/FiO_2$ <300 or >50% lung infiltrates |
| Critical | Respiratory failure requiring invasive mechanical ventilation, septic shock and/or multiorgan dysfunction |

pregnancy include older age, black or Hispanic race, obesity, systemic hypertension, and diabetes [14, 24]. Adverse maternal and neonatal outcomes are reported in pregnant patients with severe or critical COVID-19 [14]. Differential diagnoses for symptomatic respiratory failure due to COVID-19 in pregnancy can be wide-ranging and include pulmonary embolism, cardiomyopathy, pre-eclampsia, and other etiologies of viral/bacterial pneumonia.

Respiratory failure associated with COVID-19, despite meeting the Berlin criteria for ARDS in most cases, may present distinctive features, including severe hypoxemia often associated with "near normal" respiratory system compliance (phenotype L) [30]. This combination is uncommon in 'typical' ARDS and may require different bedside management. Recent data suggest that SARS-CoV-2 infection leads to an interstitial pneumonia (ground-glass lesions) associated with relatively little gasless tissue at the beginning of the infection. Consequently, loss of hypoxic vasoconstriction may be responsible for the hypoxemia [30]. Compared to non-pregnant women, these features generally cause an increase in the respiratory drive, which is clinically manifest by an increase in the respiratory rate, rather than an increased tidal volume, which is already increased during pregnancy. In many COVID-19 pregnant patients, this phenotype of ARDS can stabilize and improve, whereas in others, either because of disease severity or suboptimal treatment, it may assume the characteristics of typical ARDS (phenotype H). This H phenotype presents extensive lung consolidations and higher lung weight on CT scan. In these patients, potential lung recruitment with positive end-expiratory pressure (PEEP) is high. A meta-analysis of 42 studies including 247 pregnant women with COVID-19 showed that a focal (unilateral or bilateral) ground-glass pattern (interstitial edema) was more frequent in asymptomatic mild cases, while diffuse ground-glass densities, consolidations (alveolar edema), subpleural lesions, and pleural effusions were more frequent in severe cases [31].

Several key factors may be responsible for the worsening of this form of respiratory failure: (a) the natural evolution of COVID-19 disease in an immunocompromised host; (b) bacterial superinfections; and (c) the depth of the negative intrathoracic pressure during spontaneous breathing [30]. All these features may increase lung inflammation, interstitial edema, lung weight, and consequently the amount of atelectasis. The increase in atelectasis, as well as in D-dimer levels, which reflects the endothelial injury caused by COVID-19, may contribute to hypoxemia increasing the death space.

## 35.3 Maternal Management of COVID-19 ARDS

The first and immediate goal in all ARDS cases involving pregnant women with COVID-19, is to maintain an adequate maternal $PaO_2$ (>70 mmHg) and $PaCO_2$ (<45 mmHg) [32]. In the early phases of ARDS, these targets may be achieved simply with low flow oxygen administration (e.g., venti-mask). However, as the disease worsens, oxygen supplementation may be delivered by different devices, including high-flow nasal-cannula (HFNC) oxygenation, continuous positive airway pressure

(CPAP), and non-invasive ventilation (NIV) [33]. Optimal non-invasive respiratory support, time of intubation, and mechanical ventilation settings are still controversial in COVID-19 patients [34]. Whereas the indications for invasive mechanical ventilation are the same as for non-COVID-19 pregnant women, they also include altered mental status, progressive or refractory hypoxemia, signs of respiratory maternal fatigue, and acidosis [34].

HFNCs are the most common technique to provide oxygen supplementation in ARDS patients. HFNCs provide a heated and humidified oxygen flow up to 60 l/min and a $FiO_2$ up to 100% [2]. This technique may improve the $CO_2$ wash out from the upper airways and may generate a modest PEEP (2–5 $cmH_2O$). HFNC oxygen may minimize mucosal injury, improve secretion clearance, and reduce transpulmonary driving pressure. HFNCs are generally considered comfortable by patients and associated with a higher compliance than other non-invasive devices or techniques, such as facial masks, helmet CPAP, or NIV through a ventilator [35]. When HFNC oxygenation fails, CPAP or NIV through a ventilator can be used for short-term ventilatory support. CPAP may be administered with different devices (facial mask or helmet) [35, 36]. However, NIV should be attempted with caution in pregnant patients before endotracheal intubation due to the risk of gastric acid aspiration [36]. Decreased tone of the lower esophageal sphincter, increased abdominal pressure, and decreased gastric emptying may put pregnant women at risk of aspiration. This risk is further increased during NIV, which may lead to gastric distension. Additionally, potential development of high inspiratory efforts during NIV can generate large tidal volumes, that may induce self-induced lung injury (SILI) with NIV failure and barotrauma (i.e., pneumothorax and pneumomediastinum) [30].

In pregnant women failing NIV, invasive positive pressure mechanical ventilation is essential to improve gas exchange and reduce the work of breathing. Intubation in pregnant patients should be performed by experienced staff, since the risk of failed intubation is higher compared to non-pregnant women, due to the anatomical changes related to pregnancy (e.g., airway edema) [2, 6, 15, 32]. Once intubated, current guidelines suggest that pregnant patients should be treated as classic ARDS patients with low tidal volume (6 ml/kg of predicted body weight [PBW]) and a plateau pressure ($P_{Plat}$) limited to 28–30 $cmH_2O$ [30]. However, since the cause of ventilator-induced lung injury (VILI) is not the pressure applied to the whole respiratory system (Paw), but that applied to the lung (i.e., the transpulmonary pressure), a $P_{Plat}$ value of 28–30 $cmH_2O$ may not be sufficient to counterbalance a reduced chest wall compliance of the pregnant patient [37] and may favor atelectasis development. Actually, the relationship between the airway pressure and the transpulmonary pressure in an individual patient is strictly linear and follows the formula: $P_L = Paw \times (E_L/E_{tot})$ [38]. The transpulmonary pressure ($P_L$) equals the applied airway pressure (Paw) times the ratio of lung elastance to total respiratory system elastance ($E_L/E_{tot}$). In the general population, this ratio averages 0.7; however, in ARDS, it may vary between 0.2 and 0.8 [38]. Thus, the 'safe' 30 $cmH_2O$ may result in a transpulmonary pressure as low as 6 $cmH_2O$ causing hypoxemia or as high as 24 $cmH_2O$ causing lung overdistension. In pregnant women, the $E_L/E_{tot}$ is generally low as in obese patients (e.g. 0.2), therefore, even a Paw of 28–30 $cmH_2O$ may generate a low transpulmonary pressure causing hypoventilation and severe hypoxemia [37]. In these patients, hypoxemia may be easily reversed by safely increasing tidal volume till a transpulmonary pressure of between 22 and 24 $cmH_2O$. In general, COVID-19 patients with a L phenotype, generally have a low response to PEEP (low potential for lung recruitment) and should be treated with low PEEP levels (5–8 $cmH_2O$) [39], while patients with a H phenotype (high potential for lung recruitment), may require higher PEEP levels to counterbalance the increased weight of the lung due to edema. There are several methods to personalize PEEP in ARDS patients [40]. Generally, the main goal is to achieve a PEEP level that allows reduction of the driving pressure ($<15$ $cmH_2O$) with the best respiratory system compliance. However, caution should be taken in pregnant patients, since high PEEP levels may reduce maternal venous return and cardiac output, and consequently affect the oxygen delivery to the fetus. For this reason, close maternal and fetal assessment is essential in pregnant patients receiving high PEEP levels.

Recently, Péju and coworkers showed that obesity, pregnancy-related complications, more advanced term of pregnancy, and NIV use were more frequent in patients who required to be intubated. When the authors performed a multivariate analysis, obesity (hazard ratio [HR] 2.00, 95% confidence interval [CI] 1.05–3.80, $p = 0.03$), term of pregnancy (HR 1.07, 95% CI 1.02–1.10, per + 1 week gestation, $p = 0.01$), extent of CT scan abnormalities >50% (HR 2.69, 95% CI 1.30–5.60, $p < 0.01$), and NIV use (HR 2.06, 95% CI 1.09–3.90, $p = 0.03$) were associated with a higher risk of intubation [17].

### 35.3.1 Prone Position

Prone positioning is generally recommended to manage severe ARDS with a $PaO_2/FiO_2$ <150 mmHg [41]. Repeated cycles of prone positioning, lasting at least 12–16 h, may improve ventral-dorsal pleural pressure gradient and reduce alveolar shunt. In COVID-19 patients with significant consolidation in the dependent zones, prone positioning has been recommended to improve oxygenation [30, 42]. Several reports have described its feasibility and safety also in COVID-19 pregnant patients with ARDS [43]. However, prone positioning in pregnant women requires appropriate supports to sustain the large gravid abdomen and the fetal heart rate should be carefully monitored during the procedure to identify any deterioration in clinical status (Fig. 35.1) [44]. Pregnant women should be kept in the prone position as long as they can tolerate it. Prone positioning should be discontinued if there is no gas exchange improvement, in the presence of acute derangements of fetal heart rate tracing or maternal hemodynamic worsening, or in the presence of significant gas exchange improvement when the patient is returned to the supine position. Furthermore, particular attention should be paid to prevent complications associated with prone positioning, including vascular line and endotracheal tube displacement, facial edema, pressure sores, corneal abrasions, and brachial plexus injury [43, 44].

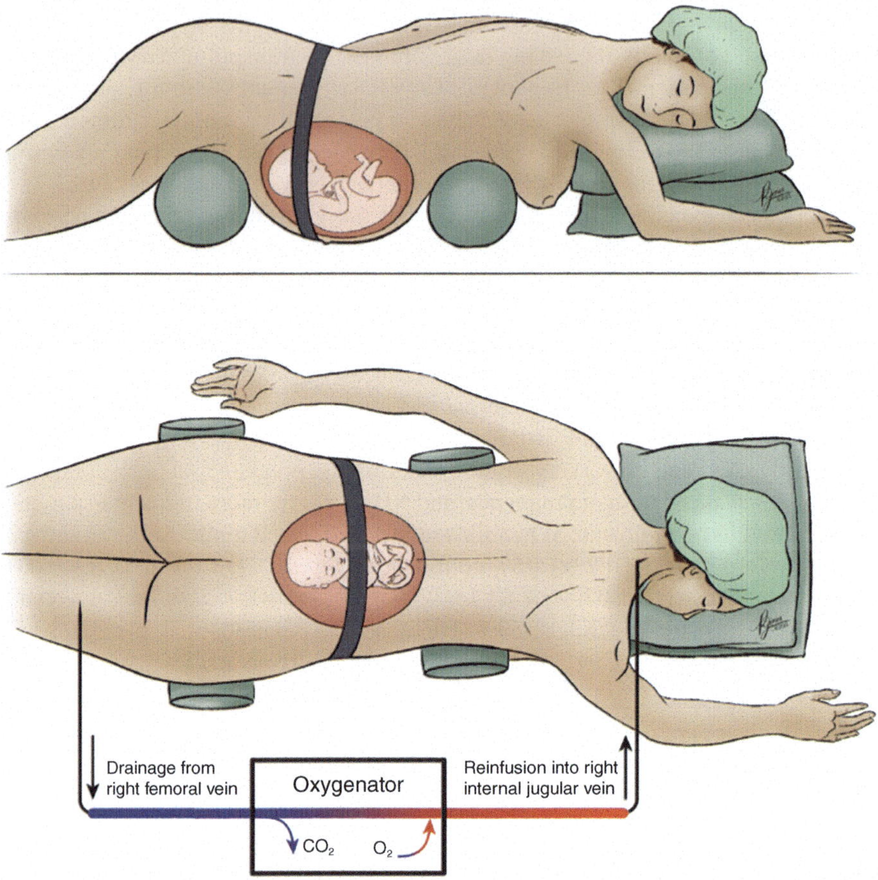


**Fig. 35.1** Prone positioning in pregnant patients with and without extracorporeal membrane oxygenation (ECMO) support

### 35.3.2 Extracorporeal Membrane Oxygenation (ECMO)

Veno-venous extracorporeal membrane oxygenation (VV-ECMO) is an invasive strategy to support patients with refractory respiratory failure [45]. Indications for VV-ECMO in the general population are: $PaO_2/FiO_2$ <50 mmHg for >3 h or $PaO_2/FiO_2$ <80 mmHg for >6 h; pH <7.25 with $PaCO_2$ >60 mmHg for >6 h with a respiratory rate up to 35 breaths/min, along with plateau pressure >30 $cmH_2O$ [45]; these indications are also used during pregnancy. Veno-arterial (VA-ECMO) is commonly used in the postpartum period rather than antenatally to manage peripartum cardiomyopathy, pulmonary embolism, amniotic fluid embolism, cardiac arrest, and septic shock. During the 2009 H1N1 pandemic, ECMO was successfully used to rescue pregnant women with refractory hypoxemia [46, 47]. Positive results were found also during the COVID-19 pandemic [48–50]. In a recent retrospective cohort study including 100 COVID-19 pregnant/peripartum patients supported with VV-ECMO, survival to hospital discharge was higher and ECMO-related complications were lower than those of non-pregnant women supported with VV-ECMO for ARDS [48].

ECMO management for COVID-19 ARDS is not significantly different from that of other forms of ARDS in pregnancy [47]. Since maternal cardiac output increases by the third trimester, ECMO flows should be kept higher (100–120 ml/kg/min) than for non-pregnant patients to grant an adequate fetal oxygenation as reflected by a maternal $SaO_2$ >90%. Hypercapnia and hypocapnia should be avoided and a range of $PaCO_2$ between 28 and 32 mmHg should be pursued to create a favorable partial pressure gradient for fetal $CO_2$ elimination and oxygen intake. Native lung management is generally provided with 'lung rest settings', which includes a plateau pressure between 20 and 25 $cmH_2O$, PEEP between 10 and 15 $cmH_2O$, $FiO_2$ between 30% and 40%, and a respiratory rate between 5 and 10 breaths/min.

Continuous fetal heart tracing is mandatory during ECMO to detect early signs of decompensation. As in the general population, optimal anticoagulation management in pregnant patients has not yet been established, however, in COVID-19 patients, higher levels of anticoagulation should be used; in selected patients at high risk of bleeding, ECMO without systemic anticoagulation has been successfully used.

Currently, the guidelines from the Society for Maternal-Fetal Medicine suggests the use of ECMO as rescue for COVID-19 ARDS in postpartum and pregnant women <32 weeks gestation to facilitate *in utero* fetal development [51].

### 35.3.3 Pharmacological Treatment

A variety of treatment options has been evaluated for COVID-19 patients and although some of them (e.g., dexamethasone, remdesivir, tocilizumab, etc.) have shown clinical benefits (e.g., decreasing duration of hospital stay, improving overall morbidity, etc.), their use is controversial in pregnant women, who have often been excluded from clinical trials. The Recovery trial [52] demonstrated that a daily dose 6 mg of dexamethasone for 10 days may decrease the risk of mortality in COVID-19 patients requiring oxygen therapy and mechanical ventilation. Of note, since this dose was previously shown not to be teratogenic in pregnant women, this trial also included pregnant and breastfeeding women. Importantly, when steroids are used to speed up fetal lung maturity, a dose of 6 mg of dexamethasone every 12 h for 48 h is recommended followed by 10 days of daily 6 mg doses.

Remdesivir has been shown to reduce the duration of disease in patients receiving oxygen therapy, and current guidelines recommend its use in hospitalized patients with an $SpO_2$ <94%. There are no data available from pregnant women. However, no known teratogenic effects of remdesivir have been reported in previous experiments, so remdesivir may be considered an optional treatment for severe COVID-19 ARDS in pregnancy [53].

As COVID-19 patients have a higher risk of thromboembolic events due to the direct endothelial damage caused by SARS-COV-2, thromboprophylaxis is strongly recommended in hospitalized pregnant patients [53].

## 35.4 Timing and Delivery of the Fetus

The care of a critically ill pregnant woman with COVID-19 requires a multidisciplinary team consisting of obstetricians, intensivists, cardiothoracic surgeons, perfusionists, anesthesiologists, neonatologists, physiotherapists, and nurses.

Because there are few data supporting the optimal timing and mode of delivery (vaginal vs. Cesarean) in pregnant women with severe COVID-19, to individualize treatment the whole team should carefully evaluate the fetus gestational age and its clinical condition as well as the maternal health status and its likelihood of recovery with delivery [6, 15]. In the case of acute changes in maternal respiratory/hemodynamic status, continuous fetal monitoring should be promptly initiated. Emergency Cesarean section may be considered in case of fetal distress, critical maternal deterioration including septic shock and multiorgan failure, or poor progression in labor [15]. However, before a viable gestational age is reached, delivery is not an option and every attempt should be made to postpone delivery [6]. In such cases, the use of VV-ECMO has been advocated to improve maternal gas exchange while awaiting for the fetus to reach an adequate gestational age (32–34 weeks) [50, 51]. In late pregnancy, elective delivery may improve maternal status (reduction of the oxygen consumption, improvement in diaphragmatic excursion, reduction in intrathoracic pressure, and resolution of the aortocaval compression) [15]. After delivery, immediate clamping of the umbilical cord and separation of the newborn from the mother is recommended to reduce the risk of vertical SARS-CoV-2 infection [15, 32].

## 35.5 Conclusion

The extensive clinical experience gained during the pandemic in the treatment of pregnant patients with ARDS [17] coupled with acquisition of the knowledge that COVID-19 ARDS does not differ substantially in terms of pathophysiology and treatment from conventional ARDS [54], leads us to conclude that clinical knowledge acquired during the pandemic can be transferred to the management of pregnant patients with ARDS not due to COVID.

Management requires a multidisciplinary team composed of intensivists, gynecologists, neonatologists, midwives, and obstetric nurses. Low flow oxygen therapy or HFNC oxygenation can be used in the early management of patients with hypoxemia while NIV is recommended only for short-term periods. Invasive mechanical ventilation should be considered in case of failing NIV and tailored according to the lung and chest wall elastance. Severe hypoxemia refractory to maximal medical management should be treated with careful use of prone-positioning first. ECMO may also be implemented until a viable gestational age is reached. Pharmacological treatment in more severe cases is controversial since pregnant women have been excluded from several trials; however, the use of steroids in patients requiring oxygen support or mechanical ventilation may be recommended as well as thromboprophylaxis. Timing and mode of delivery should be individualized according to the maternal/fetal condition.

## References


1. Ranieri VM, Rubenfeld GD, Thompson BT, et al. Acute respiratory distress syndrome: the Berlin Definition. JAMA. 2012;307:2526–33.
2. Lapinsky SE. Management of acute respiratory failure in pregnancy. Semin Respir Crit Care Med. 2017;38:201–7.
3. Pollock W, Rose L, Dennis CL. Pregnant and postpartum admissions to the intensive care unit: a systematic review. Intensive Care Med. 2010;36:1465–74.
4. Pham T, Rubenfeld GD. Fifty years of research in ARDS. The epidemiology of acute respiratory distress syndrome. A 50th birthday review. Am J Respir Crit Care Med. 2017;195:860–70.
5. Vasquez DN, Estenssoro E, Canales HS, et al. Clinical characteristics and outcomes of obstetric patients requiring ICU admission. Chest. 2007;131:718–24.
6. Cole DE, Taylor TL, McCullough DM, Shoff CT, Derdak S. Acute respiratory distress syndrome in pregnancy. Crit Care Med. 2005;33(10 Suppl):S269–78.
7. Catanzarite V, Willms D, Wong D, Landers C, Cousins L, Schrimmer D. Acute respiratory distress syndrome in pregnancy and the puerperium: causes, courses, and outcomes. Obstet Gynecol. 2001;97:760–4.
8. Bellani G, Laffey JG, Pham T, et al. Epidemiology, patterns of care, and mortality for patients with acute respiratory distress syndrome in intensive care units in 50 countries. JAMA. 2016;315(8):788–800.
9. Tzotzos SJ, Fischer B, Fischer H, Zeitlinger M. Incidence of ARDS and outcomes in hospitalized patients with COVID-19: a global literature survey. Crit Care. 2020;24:516.
10. Chen L, Li Q, Zheng D, et al. Clinical characteristics of pregnant women with Covid-19 in Wuhan, China. New Engl J Med. 2020;382:e100.
11. Breslin N, Baptiste C, Miller R, et al. Coronavirus disease 2019 in pregnancy: early lessons. Am J Obstet Gynecol MFM. 2020;2:100111.
12. Lokken EM, Huebner EM, Taylor GG, et al. Disease severity, pregnancy outcomes, and maternal deaths among pregnant patients with severe acute respiratory syndrome coronavirus 2 infection in Washington State. Am J Obstet Gynecol. 2021;225:77.e71–14.
13. Lokken EM, Taylor GG, Huebner EM, et al. Higher severe acute respiratory syndrome coronavirus 2 infection rate in pregnant patients. Am J Obstet Gynecol. 2021;225:75.e71–16.
14. Brandt JS, Hill J, Reddy A, et al. Epidemiology of coronavirus disease 2019 in pregnancy: risk factors and associations with adverse maternal and neonatal outcomes. Am J Obstet Gynecol. 2021;224:389.e381–9.
15. Kumar R, Yeni CM, Utami NA, et al. SARS-CoV-2 infection during pregnancy and pregnancy-related conditions: concerns, challenges, management and mitigation strategies-a narrative review. J Infect Public Health. 2021;14:863–75.
16. Levitus M, Shainker SA, Colvin M. COVID-19 in the critically ill pregnant patient. Crit Care Clin. 2022;38:521–34.
17. Péju E, Belicard F, Silva S, et al. Management and outcomes of pregnant women admitted to intensive care unit for severe pneumonia related to SARS-CoV-2 infection: the multicenter and international COVIDPREG study. Intensive Care Med. 2022;48:1185–96.
18. Hegewald MJ, Crapo RO. Respiratory physiology in pregnancy. Clin Chest Med. 2011;32:1–13.
19. Bandi VD, Munnur U, Matthay MA. Acute lung injury and acute respiratory distress syndrome in pregnancy. Crit Care Clin. 2004;20:577–607.

20. Lucius H, Gahlenbeck H, Kleine HO, Fabel H, Bartels H. Respiratory functions, buffer system, and electrolyte concentrations of blood during human pregnancy. Respir Physiol. 1970;9:311–7.
21. Rush B, Martinka P, Kilb B, McDermid RC, Boyd JH, Celi LA. Acute respiratory distress syndrome in pregnant women. Obstet Gynecol. 2017;129:530–5.
22. Guilbaud L, Beghin D, Dhombres F, et al. Pregnancy outcome after first trimester exposure to ionizing radiations. Eur J Obstet Gynecol Reprod Biol. 2019;232:18–21.
23. Lowe S. Diagnostic imaging in pregnancy: making informed decisions. Obstet Med. 2019;12:116–22.
24. Boushra MN, Koyfman A, Long B. COVID-19 in pregnancy and the puerperium: a review for emergency physicians. Am J Emerg Med. 2021;40:193–8.
25. Wastnedge EAN, Reynolds RM, van Boeckel SR, et al. Pregnancy and COVID-19. Physiol Rev. 2021;101:303–18.
26. Bahraini M, Dorgalaleh A. The impact of SARS-CoV-2 infection on blood coagulation and fibrinolytic pathways: a review of prothrombotic changes caused by COVID-19. Semin Thromb Hemost. 2022;48:19–30.
27. Mendoza M, Garcia-Ruiz I, Maiz N, et al. Pre-eclampsia-like syndrome induced by severe COVID-19: a prospective observational study. BJOG. 2020;127:1374–80.
28. Liu D, Li L, Wu X, Zheng D, Wang J, Yang L, Zheng C. Pregnancy and perinatal outcomes of women with coronavirus disease (COVID-19) pneumonia: a preliminary analysis. AJR Am J Roentgenol. 2020;215:127–32.
29. Knight M, Bunch K, Vousden N, et al. Characteristics and outcomes of pregnant women admitted to hospital with confirmed SARS-CoV-2 infection in UK: national population based cohort study. BMJ. 2020;369:m2107.
30. Gattinoni L, Chiumello D, Caironi P, et al. COVID-19 pneumonia: different respiratory treatments for different phenotypes? Intensive Care Med. 2020;46:1099–102.
31. Galang RR, Chang K, Strid P, Snead MC, et al. Severe coronavirus infections in pregnancy: a systematic review. Obstet Gynecol. 2020;136:262–72.
32. Lapinsky SE. Acute respiratory failure in pregnancy. Obstet Med. 2015;8:126–32.
33. Navas-Blanco JR, Dudaryk R. Management of respiratory distress syndrome due to COVID-19 infection. BMC Anesthesiol. 2020;20:177.
34. Bhatia PK, Biyani G, Mohammed S, Sethi P, Bihani P. Acute respiratory failure and mechanical ventilation in pregnant patient: a narrative review of literature. J Anaesthesiol Clin Pharmacol. 2016;32:431–9.
35. Raoof S, Nava S, Carpati C, Hill NS. High-flow, noninvasive ventilation and awake (nonintubation) proning in patients with coronavirus disease 2019 with respiratory failure. Chest. 2020;158:1992–2002.
36. Al-Ansari MA, Hameed AA, Al-jawder SE, Saeed HM. Use of noninvasive positive pressure ventilation during pregnancy: case series. Ann Thorac Med. 2007;2:23–5.
37. Tonetti T, Vasques F, Rapetti F, et al. Driving pressure and mechanical power: new targets for VILI prevention. Ann Transl Med. 2017;5:286.
38. Gattinoni L, Marini JJ, Collino F, et al. The future of mechanical ventilation: lessons from the present and the past. Crit Care. 2017;21:183.
39. Pan C, Chen L, Lu C, et al. Lung recruitability in COVID-19-associated acute respiratory distress syndrome: a single-center observational study. Am J Respir Crit Care Med. 2020;201:1294–7.
40. Mauri T, Spinelli E, Scotti E, et al. Potential for lung recruitment and ventilation-perfusion mismatch in patients with the acute respiratory distress syndrome from coronavirus disease 2019. Crit Care Med. 2020;48:1129–34.
41. Guérin C, Albert RK, Beitler J, et al. Prone position in ARDS patients: why, when, how and for whom. Intensive Care Med. 2020;46:2385–96.
42. Liu L, Xie J, Wang C, et al. Prone position improves lung ventilation-perfusion matching in non-intubated COVID-19 patients: a prospective physiologic study. Crit Care. 2022;26:193.

43. Tolcher MC, McKinney JR, Eppes CS, et al. Prone positioning for pregnant women with hypoxemia due to coronavirus disease 2019 (COVID-19). Obstet Gynecol. 2020;136:259–61.
44. Cavalcante FML, Fernandes CDS, Rocha LDS, Galindo-Neto NM, Caetano J, Barros LM. Use of the prone position in pregnant women with COVID-19 or other health conditions. Rev Lat Am Enfermagem. 2021;29:e3494.
45. Combes A, Peek GJ, Hajage D, et al. ECMO for severe ARDS: systematic review and individual patient data meta-analysis. Intensive Care Med. 2020;46:2048–57.
46. Jamieson DJ, Rasmussen SA. An update on COVID-19 and pregnancy. Am J Obstet Gynecol. 2021;226:177.
47. Wong MJ, Bharadwaj S, Galey JL, Lankford AS, Galvagno S, Kodali BS. Extracorporeal membrane oxygenation for pregnant and postpartum patients. Anesth Analg. 2022;135:277–89.
48. O'Neil ER, Lin H, Shamshirsaz AA, et al. Pregnant/peripartum women with COVID-19 high survival with ECMO: an extracorporeal life support organization registry analysis. Am J Respir Crit Care Med. 2022;205:248–50.
49. Malfertheiner SF, Brodie D, Burrell A, et al. Extracorporeal membrane oxygenation during pregnancy and peripartal. An international retrospective multicenter study. Perfusion 2022. https://doi.org/10.1177/02676591221090668. Epub ahead of print.
50. Mohammed Bamasood O, Shamsah M, et al. Extracorporeal membrane oxygenation in pregnant women with COVID-19. ASAIO J. 2022;68:471–7.
51. Society for Maternal-Fetal Medicine (SFMF). Management considerations for pregnant patients with COVID-19. 2021. Available at: https://s3.amazonaws.com/cdn.smfm.org/media/2734/SMFM_COVID_Management_of_COVID_pos_preg_patients_2-2-21_(final).pdf. Accessed 16 Nov 2022.
52. Horby P, Lim WS, Emberson JR, et al. Dexamethasone in hospitalized patients with Covid-19. N Engl J Med. 2021;384:693–704.
53. D'Souza R, Ashraf R, Rowe H, et al. Pregnancy and COVID-19: pharmacologic considerations. Ultrasound Obstet Gynecol. 2021;57:195–203.
54. Grasselli G, Tonetti T, Protti A, et al. Pathophysiology of COVID-19-associated acute respiratory distress syndrome: a multicentre prospective observational study. Lancet Respir Med. 2020;8:1201–8.

# Amniotic Fluid Embolism

# 36

E. LaFond and J. Bakker

## 36.1 Introduction

Amniotic fluid embolism is one of the most devastating complications in obstetrics. It is characterized by the sudden onset of hypotension, hypoxia, and coagulopathy during, or immediately after, delivery. The coagulopathy can lead to profound postpartum hemorrhage. While rare in an absolute sense, amniotic fluid embolism is identified as the leading cause of maternal mortality in many developed countries [1, 2]. Most clinicians and institutions have limited experience with the management of amniotic fluid embolism. Intensivists are often called upon to co-manage cases of suspected amniotic fluid embolism with our colleagues in obstetrics and anesthesia, so familiarity with this condition is imperative.

E. LaFond
Division of Pulmonary & Critical Care, New York University Grossman School of Medicine, New York, NY, USA

J. Bakker (✉)
Division of Pulmonary & Critical Care, New York University Grossman School of Medicine, New York, NY, USA

Division of Pulmonary, Allergy, and Critical Care Medicine, Columbia University College of Physicians & Surgeons, New York, NY, USA

Department of Intensive Care Adults, Erasmus MC University Medical Center, Rotterdam, Netherlands

Department of Intensive Care, Pontificia Universidad Católica de Chile, Santiago, Chile
e-mail: jan.bakker@nyulangone.org



J.-L. Vincent (ed.), *Annual Update in Intensive Care and Emergency Medicine 2023*, Annual Update in Intensive Care and Emergency Medicine,
https://doi.org/10.1007/978-3-031-23005-9_36

## 36.2 Pathophysiology

The pathogenesis of amniotic fluid embolism is unclear. Historically, it was believed to result from mechanical obstruction of the maternal pulmonary circulation by fetal squamous cells, leading to cardiopulmonary collapse. However, subsequent research has suggested that the pathophysiology involves the abnormal release of pro-inflammatory mediators in response to fetal antigens, similar to the systemic inflammatory response syndrome (SIRS), where the abnormal host response, rather than the inciting antigen itself, is responsible for the subsequent clinical manifestations [2–4]. The physical breach between the maternal and fetal compartments is thought to occur at the level of endocervical veins, placental attachment sites, and uterine trauma sites, creating a pressure gradient for amniotic fluid to move from the uterus to the maternal circulation [5]. This hypothesis is supported by the increased risk of amniotic fluid embolism among patients with placental pathology, instrumented vaginal deliveries, Cesarean section, and cervical or uterine lacerations [5, 6].

These inflammatory mediators and endogenous catecholamines induce pulmonary hypertension and acute cor pulmonale. Right ventricular (RV) dilation, RV systolic dysfunction, and a D-shaped septum have been observed on transesophageal echocardiography (TEE) performed during the hyperacute phase of amniotic fluid embolism (within 30 min) [7]. Right heart failure can subsequently lead to left ventricular (LV) failure. Studies performed using pulmonary artery catheters later in the early course of amniotic fluid embolism (1–2 h after onset of clinical signs) reported a high pulmonary artery occlusion pressure (PAOP) and LV dysfunction, supporting the hypothesis that there may be a bisphasic reaction in which early right-sided heart failure leads to the development of LV failure [2].

Disseminated intravascular coagulation (DIC) complicates up to 80% of cases of amniotic fluid embolism. The precise mechanism remains unclear. DIC is thought to develop when tissue factor in amniotic fluid binds factor VII, activating the extrinsic pathway. This activates factor X and the development of a consumptive coagulopathy [5]. Additional research has highlighted complement activation as another possible explanation [8].

There is considerable debate regarding whether a consumptive coagulopathy or massive fibrinolysis causes post-partum hemorrhage in DIC from amniotic fluid embolism. There is conflicting evidence, as case reports describing the use of thromboelastogram (TEG) or rotational thromboelastography (ROTEM) in amniotic fluid embolism have described findings consistent with both consumptive coagulopathy and massive fibrinolysis [9–11].

## 36.3 Incidence

The true incidence of amniotic fluid embolism is confounded by the absence of a gold-standard diagnostic test, the use of different diagnostic criteria, inconsistent reporting, and a clinical presentation that shares features with more common obstetric complications. However, the incidence of amniotic fluid embolism is estimated to be 1 per 40,000 deliveries [2] and the reported mortality rate is approximately 20% [12]. While rare in an absolute sense, amniotic fluid embolism is identified as the leading cause of maternal mortality in many developed countries [1, 2].

## 36.4 Clinical Features

Amniotic fluid embolism is characterized by the sudden onset of hypotension, hypoxia, and coagulopathy leading to hemorrhage. Additional clinical features can include cardiac arrest, cardiac dysrhythmia, altered mental status, and seizure. When cardiac arrest occurs, asystole, pulseless electrical activity (PEA), and ventricularly fibrillation (VF) or ventricular tachycardia (VT) have all been described [13]. Patients who survive amniotic fluid embolism can go on to develop multiorgan failure, acute respiratory distress syndrome (ARDS), and hypoxic brain injury [13].

The onset of amniotic fluid embolism usually occurs during labor and delivery or immediately following delivery (within 30 min). However, delayed amniotic fluid embolism has been reported as late as 48 h postpartum. There are also case reports of amniotic fluid embolism occurring after first or second trimester abortion, amniocentesis, and uterine or cervical trauma [5].

## 36.5 Diagnosis

The diagnosis of amniotic fluid embolism is a clinical diagnosis of exclusion. Diagnostic challenge arises in cases that do not present with the classic triad of hypotension, hypoxia, and coagulopathy. Amniotic fluid embolism can present with only hypotension and respiratory failure, and rarer still, DIC can be the presenting feature or can be absent altogether. Atypical presentations represent approximately 25% of all cases of amniotic fluid embolism [2]. Furthermore, hypotension, hypoxia, and coagulopathy are not unique to amniotic fluid embolism, and can be present in isolation or in varying combinations in other conditions that cause pregnant or postpartum patients to become critically ill, such as pulmonary embolism, peripartum cardiomyopathy, myocardial infarction, and septic shock (Table 36.1).

No single diagnostic test or biomarker for amniotic fluid embolism has been identified. Historically, the detection of fetal squamous cells in the maternal pulmonary circulation via pulmonary artery catheter was considered diagnostic, but further studies have demonstrated that these findings are also present in critically ill pregnant or postpartum patients without amniotic fluid embolism [2, 14]. Several studies have investigated potential biomarkers for amniotic fluid embolism, most notably insulin-like growth factor binding protein-1 (IGFBP-1), a protein found in high concentrations in the amniotic fluid. However, results of a recent retrospective multicenter cohort study were negative [15].

**Table 36.1** Amniotic fluid embolism: an overview

| Characteristic | Comment |
|---|---|
| Incidence | 1 in 40,000 births |
| Mortality | 20.4% |
| Risk factors | Advanced maternal age, placental pathology (placenta previa, accreta, or abruption), instrumented vaginal delivery, Cesarean section |
| Clinical features | Classic triad of hypotension, hypoxia, and coagulopathy during or immediately following delivery |
| Differential diagnosis | Pulmonary embolism, air embolism, high neuraxial anesthesia, myocardial infarction, peripartum cardiomyopathy, aortic dissection, aspiration, septic shock, anaphylactic shock, postpartum hemorrhage from another cause |
| Management | Advanced cardiac life support (ACLS), intubation and mechanical ventilation, correction of underlying coagulopathy, management of severe hemorrhage, consideration of VA-ECMO |

*VA-ECMO* veno-arterial extracorporeal membrane oxygenation

Results of additional laboratory and radiographic studies are nonspecific. The white blood cell count may be elevated. Patients with DIC will exhibit a low fibrinogen (<200 mg/dl), elevated D-dimer, thrombocytopenia, and a prolonged prothrombin time (PT) and international normalized ratio (INR). Additional non-specific findings include elevated cardiac enzymes, metabolic acidosis, and hypoxemia on arterial blood gas. Renal and hepatic dysfunction can arise in patients who survive amniotic fluid embolism and go on to develop multiorgan dysfunction.

Chest imaging is often normal in the earliest phases of the disease, but subsequently reveals diffuse bilateral alveolar infiltrates. While transthoracic or transesophageal echocardiogram can be helpful in ruling out other etiologies of cardiac arrest, it cannot distinguish between amniotic fluid embolism and pulmonary embolism, as both entities have similar findings of RV enlargement, hypokinesis, and bowing of the interventricular septum [7]. Depending on the stability of the patient, computed tomography (CT) of the chest with contrast can evaluate for the presence of pulmonary embolism, which is often in the differential diagnosis when amniotic fluid embolism is suspected. Perhaps the most helpful distinguishing factor between the two entities is the presence of DIC, which is seen in amniotic fluid embolism and not in pulmonary embolism. Other disorders that can mimic amniotic fluid embolism include hemorrhage from uterine atony, uterine and lower genital tract lacerations, retained placenta, complications of neuraxial anesthesia, anaphylactic shock, venous air embolism, and cardiogenic shock from peripartum cardiomyopathy or myocardinal infarction.

In an attempt to standardize diagnosis, reporting, and research efforts, the Society of Maternal-Fetal Medicine (SMFM) and the Amniotic Fluid Embolism Foundation proposed four diagnostic criteria, all of which must be met [16]:

- Sudden onset of cardiopulmonary arrest or hypotension (systolic blood pressure <90 mmHg) with respiratory compromise (defined as dyspnea, cyanosis, or peripheral oxygen saturation <90% breathing ambient air)

- DIC, using the following scoring system, modified for pregnancy, where a score of ≥3 is consistent with DIC:
  - Platelet count >100,000 = 0 points, <100,000 = 1 point, <50,000 = 2 points
  - Prolonged PT or INR <25% increase = 0 points, 25–50% increase = 1 point, >50% increase = 20 points
  - Fibrinogen level >200 mg/dl = 0 points, <200 mg/dl = 1 point
- Clinical onset during labor, or within 30 min of placental delivery
- Absence of fever during labor (>38 °C)

## 36.6 Management

Effective management of amniotic fluid embolism requires the coordinated delivery of supportive care by a multidisciplinary team consisting of maternal-fetal medicine, anesthesia, and critical care physicians in addition to respiratory therapists and nurses. Treatment is largely supportive and based on maintaining cardiac output and oxygenation while correcting the underlying coagulopathy.

When indicated, cardiopulmonary resuscitation (CPR) should be performed. Advanced cardiac life support (ACLS) guidelines should be followed. There are no modifications for a pregnant patient, and the administration of epinephrine, amiodarone, and defibrillation should be performed when indicated. However, there are a few unique features of cardiac arrest in a pregnant patient that are worth highlighting: manual lateral displacement of the uterus can help relieve aortocaval compression and improve hemodynamics in patients who have not yet delivered, and establishing intravenous access above the level of the diaphragm can improve drug delivery. If the patient is still pregnant with a viable fetus, a perimortem Cesarean section should be performed within 4 min.

Intubation and mechanical ventilation are often required. It should be noted that the pregnant and post-partum airway can be challenging secondary to edema and hyperemia of the upper airway mucosa, decreased functional residual capacity, and increased oxygen consumption leading to a lower tolerance of apnea, and an increased aspiration risk. Intubation should be performed by an experienced provider with multiple backup options available [17].

In patients with DIC, treatment of coagulopathy even without frank hemorrhage is warranted given the high risk of bleeding. Common transfusion thresholds include administering platelets if the platelet count is <50,000, administering fresh frozen plasma (FFP) if the PT or activated partial thromboplastin time (aPTT) are prolonged, and administering cryoprecipitate if the fibrinogen is <200 mg/dl. For patients with hemorrhage, activation of the massive transfusion protocol is often indicated.

For refractory cases of amniotic fluid embolism, the use of veno-arterial extraporeal membrane oxygenation (VA-ECMO) has been described in case reports, despite the extremely high bleeding risk in this population [18–22]. In nearly all cases, patients required use of a massive transfusion protocol. The majority of patients required hemostatic procedures such as arterial embolization or surgeries such as hysterectomy, often returning to the operating room multiple times for control of intra-abdominal bleeding. The average time on VA-ECMO was 4 days, and in all cases an upfront anticoagulation-free strategy was used [18]. Despite the high morbidity attributed to hemorrhage, 70% of patients survived, providing an argument that amniotic fluid embolism and severe DIC should not be considered an absolute contraindication to the use of VA-ECMO.

## 36.7 Conclusion

Amniotic fluid embolism is a catastrophic complication of labor and delivery whose pathogenesis is still poorly understood. As a rare entity without a specific diagnostic test or treatment, management is challenging. Familiarity with this condition and the prompt delivery of coordinated supportive care by obstetricians and intensivists is essential in obtaining optimal outcomes.

## References

1. McDonnell N, Knight M, Peek MJ, et al. Amniotic fluid embolism: an Australian-New Zealand population-based study. BMC Pregn Childb. 2015;15:352.
2. Clark SL. Amniotic fluid embolism. Obstet Gynecol. 2014;123:337–48.
3. Funk M, Damron A, Bandi V, Aagaard K, Szigeti R, Clark S. Pulmonary vascular obstruction by squamous cells is not involved in amniotic fluid embolism. Am J Obstet Gynecol. 2018;218:460–1.
4. Sultan P, Seligman K, Carvalho B. Amniotic fluid embolism: update and review. Curr Opin Anaesthesiol. 2016;29:288–96.
5. Conde-Agudelo A, Romero R. Amniotic fluid embolism: an evidence-based review. Am J Obstet Gynecol. 2009;201:445.e1–13.
6. Abenhaim HA, Azoulay L, Kramer MS, Leduc L. Incidence and risk factors of amniotic fluid embolisms: a population-based study on 3 million births in the United States. Am J Obstet Gynecol. 2008;199:49.e1–8.
7. Simard C, Yang S, Koolian M, Shear R, Rudski L, Lipes J. The role of echocardiography in amniotic fluid embolism: a case series and review of the literature. Can J Anaesth. 2021;68:1541–8.
8. Benson MD. A hypothesis regarding complement activation and amniotic fluid embolism. Med Hypotheses. 2007;68:1019–25.
9. Collins NF, Bloor M, McDonnell NJ. Hyperfibrinolysis diagnosed by rotational thromboelastometry in a case of suspected amniotic fluid embolism. Int J Obstet Anesth. 2013;22:71–6.
10. Fudaba M, Tachibana D, Misugi T, Nakano A, Koyama M. Excessive fibrinolysis detected with thromboelastography in a case of amniotic fluid embolism: fibrinolysis may precede coagulopathy. J Thromb Thrombolysis. 2021;51:818–20.
11. Loughran JA, Kitchen TL, Sindhakar S, Ashraf M, Awad M, Kealaher EJ. Rotational thromboelastometry (ROTEM®)-guided diagnosis and management of amniotic fluid embolism. Int J Obstet Anesth. 2019;38:127–30.
12. Benson MD. Amniotic fluid embolism mortality rate. J Obstet Gynaecol Res. 2017;43:1714–8.
13. Clark SL, Hankins GD, Dudley DA, Dildy GA, Porter TF. Amniotic fluid embolism: analysis of the national registry. Am J Obstet Gynecol. 1995;172:1158–67.

14. Lee W, Ginsburg KA, Cotton DB, Kaufman RH. Squamous and trophoblastic cells in the maternal pulmonary circulation identified by invasive hemodynamic monitoring during the peripartum period. Am J Obstet Gynecol. 1986;155:999–1001.
15. Bouvet L, Gariel C, Charvet A, Boisson-Gaudin C, Chassard D. Contribution of blood detection of insulin-like growth factor binding protein-1 for the diagnosis of amniotic-fluid embolism: a retrospective multicentre cohort study. BJOG. 2021;128:1966–73.
16. Clark SL, Romero R, Dildy GA, et al. Proposed diagnostic criteria for the case definition of amniotic fluid embolism in research studies. Am J Obstet Gynecol. 2016;215:408–12.
17. Toppozada H, Michaels L, Toppozada M, El-Ghazzawi I, Talaat M, Elwany S. The human respiratory nasal mucosa in pregnancy. An electron microscopic and histochemical study. J Laryngol Otol. 1982;96:613–26.
18. Aissi James S, Klein T, Lebreton G, et al. Amniotic fluid embolism rescued by venoarterial extracorporeal membrane oxygenation. Crit Care. 2022;26:96.
19. Wothe JK, Elfstrand E, Mooney MR, Wothe DD. Rotational thromboelastometry-guided venoarterial extracorporeal membrane oxygenation in the treatment of amniotic fluid embolism. Case Rep Obstet Gynecol. 2022;2022:9658708.
20. Gitman R, Bachar B, Mendenhall B. Amniotic fluid embolism treated with veno-arterial extracorporeal membrane oxygenation. Case Rep Crit Care. 2019;2019:4589636.
21. Viau-Lapointe J, Filewod N. Extracorporeal therapies for amniotic fluid embolism. Obstet Gynecol. 2019;134:989–94.
22. Adachi M, Adachi T, Fujita T, Hyuga S, Onishi Y, Okutomi T. Venoarterial extracorporeal membrane oxygenation as an early treatment for amniotic fluid embolism with cardiac arrest: a case report. J Obstet Gynaecol Res. 2021;47:3374–8.

# Part XII

# Pre- and Post-Intensive Care

# Remote Telehealth Aid During Humanitarian Crisis

# 37

J. A. Yelon, S. Subramanian, and L. J. Kaplan

## 37.1 Introduction

Disasters may be natural or manmade [1]. Natural disasters include weather-related events, such as earthquakes, volcanic eruptions, and hurricane-driven flooding. Manmade disasters include mass shootings, violent extremism, CBRNE (chemical, biologic, nuclear, radiologic and explosive) events, and humanitarian crises related to military conflict or war [2]. Whether natural or manmade, both have the potential to overwhelm local, regional, or national resources. Accordingly, external aid may be required to meet basic health needs, address infrastructure, or deliver supplies including food, water, and medical therapeutics. Military aid may be required to restore civil order or protect aid workers and their supplies.

External aid may flow from different sources including, but not limited to, bordering or remote countries, non-governmental organizations (NGOs), medical professional organizations (MPOs), healthcare centers with their own teams, as well as

J. A. Yelon
Division of Trauma, Surgical Critical Care and Emergency Surgery, Department of Surgery, Perelman School of Medicine, University of Pennsylvania, Philadelphia, PA, USA

F. Edward Hebert School of Medicine, Uniformed Services University of the Health Sciences, Bethesda, MD, USA

S. Subramanian
Omnicure, St. Louis, MO, USA

L. J. Kaplan (✉)
Division of Trauma, Surgical Critical Care and Emergency Surgery, Department of Surgery, Perelman School of Medicine, University of Pennsylvania, Philadelphia, PA, USA

Surgical Services, Section of Surgical Critical Care and Emergency General Surgery, Corporal Michael J Crescenz VA Medical Center, Philadelphia, PA, USA
e-mail: Lewis.Kaplan@pennmedicine.upenn.edu



J.-L. Vincent (ed.), *Annual Update in Intensive Care and Emergency Medicine 2023*, Annual Update in Intensive Care and Emergency Medicine,
https://doi.org/10.1007/978-3-031-23005-9_37

well-intentioned independent medical personnel or private individuals who may have had prior military medic or combatant training. In-country team member safety and team security is assumed to be uncertain during active events such as violent extremism, government unrest, or warfare. Therefore, deploying independent healthcare teams to active warzones, as well as sites potentially impacted by military weaponry or combatant teams may be quite ill-advised. Nonetheless, healthcare professionals and others evidence a strong desire to help those in crisis [3]. One potentially viable option is remote aid when cognitive assistance as well as materiel sourcing may be of benefit.

## 37.2 Methods of Remote Healthcare

In many ways, remote healthcare has become synonymous with telemedicine. Particularly during the severe acute respiratory syndrome coronavirus 2 (SARS-CoV-2) pandemic, telemedicine has arisen as a viable means to monitor patient care when hospitalization is not required, convalescence after acute inpatient care or emergency department (ED) management, and wound healing when care was rendered far from the site of residence [4]. Telemedicine has blossomed in military experience by providing military role-2 (limited resources military medical facility from which frontline care units transfer patients for damage-control interventions and stabilization for eventual evacuation) consultative services. A form of telemedicine, telecritical care, blossomed during the SARS-CoV-2 pandemic because of a host of interwoven factors [5]. Local facilities were unable to transfer SARS-CoV-2 patients due to patient surge at more complex facilities; transfer was often limited to those who needed extracorporeal membrane oxygenation (ECMO) rescue, or post-injury care. In the USA, only half of all acute care facilities are staffed with intensivists, leaving unstaffed facilities in need of cognitive aid. As hospitals ran out of licensed beds, novel care spaces were developed and were often staffed with non-intensivists and non-intensive care unit (ICU) nurses, and non-ICU respiratory therapists and PharmDs using a tiered staffing approach [6]. Finally, remote evaluation of the need for transfer to a more complex facility leveraged telecritical care in the ED and inpatient spaces for patients suffering stroke and injury. Often, consultation was accompanied by education as well.

## 37.3 Methods of Remote Education and Communication

When in-person meetings and travel for MPO educational offerings were halted during the SARS-CoV-2 pandemic, remote learning leveraged rapidly with platforms developing including CISCO WebEx, Go-To-Meeting, Microsoft TEAMS, ZOOM, Apple FaceTime, as well as the video features of Facebook Live, and WhatsApp. Notably, platforms such as Twitter and self-assembled, often specialty focused WhatsApp groups shared emerging medical news and science across countries, helping crystallize a truly global medical community. Digital platforms were also used for in-hospital consultation when non-essential clinicians were sheltered at home, especially in settings where a telecritical care system was already embedded. Similarly, those platforms were used for family meetings when visitation was suspended, an approach that allowed participants to see facial expressions that would have been concealed by a facemask and partly obscured by a faceshield [7]. Many platforms support multiple users, real-time video, screen sharing, and recording features. MPOs commonly used ZOOM and Teams for committee work and yearly educational congresses during SARS-CoV-2 pandemic years 1 and 2. Furthermore, telementoring during operative procedures also benefitted from the rapid growth of digital platforms [8].

## 37.4 Opportunities for Improvement with Remote Platforms

Using digital platforms to link remote parties requires all participants to use the same version. Depending on the specific needs being met, the display differences between desktop and handheld mobile device versions may be insurmountable (e.g., large volume of text, determining who wants to speak). Some platforms occasionally suffer from cross-device compatibility issues. All of the platforms remain subject to internet access and accessible bandwidth. For example, as schools moved to virtual education early in the pandemic, several platforms being used for telework, or telemedicine applications suffered repeated failures as a reflection of network overload. Moreover, session length may be subject to the license purchased, driving the need for creative scheduling to accommodate needs. Sessions may be readily recorded (with participant concordance) and repeatedly viewed, but are devoid of preplanned analytics (numbers of participants, poll data, time devoted to a specific activity, etc.). Furthermore, when used for telemedicine or telecritical care support, the data reviewed and recommendations generated do not easily integrate into the patient's existing electronic health record (EHR).

The desire to integrate the data from the recording, or the recording itself, in a seamless fashion remains elusive; incorporation as a non-searchable external document is currently achievable and not within all EHRs. Therefore, bidirectional data flow is not able to be met by any of the existing digital platforms, all of which would need to conform to Fast Healthcare Interoperability Resources (FHIR) interoperability standards as articulated by Health Level 7 (HL7), a standards development organization—standards which they were not designed to meet as their current use is an adaptation to an unforeseen healthcare need [9, 10]. FHIR standards are designed to facilitate the accurate and rapid exchange of clinical or administrative data to occur across different EHRs. Despite these limitations, digital platforms remain a viable option for providing remote aid during a humanitarian crisis.

## 37.5 Remote Aid During a Humanitarian Crisis

Regardless of the selected platform, digital linkage will need to find a mutually agreeable time to link parties across disparate time zones. This approach works well for planned conferences to discuss specific patients, review their care, and plan future care. Any of the conferencing solutions can meet this need. Groups will also benefit from establishing a roster of individuals who are willing to be available on-demand for impromptu consultation. This kind of linkage may occur across a conferencing platform, but may be more conveniently achieved across an app such as WhatsAPP that supports telephone conversation, face-to-face video calling, or text-based discourse for less critical exchanges.

A needs assessment is essential to match requested or desired aid with deployable resources including clinician specialties. For example, 'trauma surgery' in parts of the European Union may mean orthopedic surgery as opposed to what it means in the USA—a general surgeon trained in injury care and critical care. Additionally, translation between English and other languages may be required to facilitate aid. Desired aid may span five main domains: cognitive information (person-to-person), decision-making, care sequencing, technical advice, and published material (operative atlases, resource guides, textbooks, or other curated peer-reviewed literature). Providing informational material may be straightforward, especially with the prevalence of open access publications, as well as on-line texts. Rendering clinical care aid requires different approaches. Finally, cybersecurity concerns should be addressed, particularly when dealing with governmental entities.

### 37.5.1 Approaches to Providing Remote Aid During a Humanitarian Crisis

The easiest approach is voice communication by wired or wireless telephone. This option limits face-to-face discourse, enforces a limit on multi-person input, and precludes visual cues—an element that may be useful in addressing some differences between low-context and high-context cultures. Digital platforms may therefore offer specific advantages over voice only communication. Existing platforms have been previously mentioned and can clearly link participants, regardless of distance, for planned or impromptu discussion. However, all of them would benefit from a secure portal for data input for consultative team review ahead of that discussion. Such information may include deidentified patient information including images (radiologic and other) and may be shared across repositories such as Dropbox or a similar portal. Regardless of how that data is made available for the consultative team, current approaches do not support routine data analysis of uploaded information. Doing so requires a separate database and data entry person or persons. Data analysis is key to track major issues, follow a patient's clinical course, and to perform interim and summative assessments of the impact of guidance on outcome, resource utilization, and the scope of consultation.

All platforms rely on stable internet access—a foundation that is uniquely subject to infrastructure destruction during disasters of short (earthquake) or long duration (war) [11]. Relatedly, when the internet link is unstable, the platform will be unable to be effectively used during active interfacility transport, or during evacuation from a Role 1 facility, a battlefield, or the site of explosion-induced building collapse [12]. If the platform is linked to a desktop, it may be unable to be effectively used for intra-op consultation. Moreover, care suggestions must be separately recorded by those requesting consultation using a program (or paper) as the platform does not provide a mechanism for recording and then exporting such information. Additionally, the success of consultation with one team may lead to scope creep, further making it quite difficult to capture the breadth of consultative work and its impact on patient care. Unsurprisingly, multiple teams may desire consultation in the same time frame based on their facility workflow and their time zone. These competing sessions articulate the need for more than one consultative team leader, an individual who may ideally be the Chief Medical Officer—especially when they can help with consultation—and not only administrative needs or resource allocation. An alternative approach that offers more functionality may enhance rendering remote aid.

During the height of the SARS-CoV-2 pandemic, several technology companies worked with the US Army Telemedicine and Advanced Technology Research Center (TATRC) to develop a stand-alone acute telecritical care platform [13]. The driving need for such an approach was the lack of uniform intensivist coverage across US acute care facilities, as well as the dearth of intensivists in Indian Health Service facilities. This program is termed the National Emergency TeleCritical Care Network (NETCCN). Its key features include that it is a stand-alone cloud-hosted program and app that is compliant with the Health Insurance Portability and Accountability Act (HIPPA). It demonstrates a double encrypted security feature as a minimum software requirement. The NETCCN app is handheld device-friendly with deployable tablet and desktop applications. Most importantly, it is an EHR agnostic method of providing critical care consultation to an ICU team. Clinical data may be readily captured for concomitant or retrospective analysis. An operational dashboard for tracking system level operational metrics and clinician efficiency supports data analysis. From a human factors perspective, there are specific spaces for uploading physiologic, laboratory, radiology data, and photos as well as entering progress notes paralleling common EHR domains (Fig. 37.1). Therefore, built-in workflows used by clinicians for routine care establish minimum training requirements. Digital video capture supports 1:1 connectivity for intraoperative consultation, as well as built-in 'teams' functionality allowing multiple disciplines to collaborate in care delivery. Finally, there is a section for individual patient follow-up in a fashion asynchronous from the initial consultation.

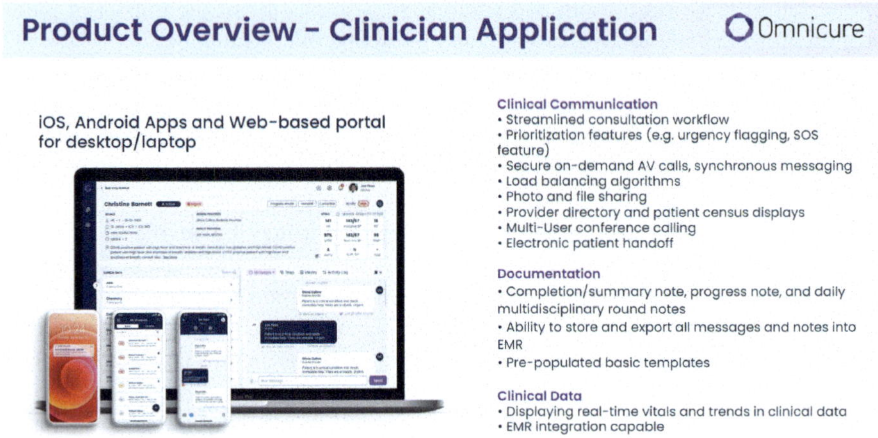


**Fig. 37.1** The National Emergency TeleCritical Care Network (NETCCN) telemedicine application. This screenshot depicts the unique features of the working NETCCN app by Omnicure. Reproduced with permission from Omnicure Inc.; replication of content in print or otherwise is unlawful and subject to legal penalties

### 37.5.2 Barriers to NETCCN Telemedicine Application Adaptation for Remote Humanitarian Aid

The NETCCN telemedicine App was not initially planned for multiple people (>6) online at once, but this capability is already under development. As it was initially designed for US use with English-language speaking users, it is not loaded for translation across multiple languages. While programs exist, there is a financial cost to them—a cost that is avoidable with live translation. Downloading the app requires enabling country specific downloading by the app owner—a quite minor barrier. However, a major consideration is the need to implement geofencing for operational security for patients and clinicians during a humanitarian crisis. Additionally, the use of such applications in the European Union requires compliance with the General Data Protection Regulation (GDPR), which can impact rapid technology deployment.

## 37.6 Providing Materiel Aid

Both MPO and healthcare institutions or healthcare systems may seek to send supplies or devices to a disaster site. It is essential to accurately understand precisely what those at the disaster location need and can use, compared to what might be available to send. Often basic supplies, including the kind that were in short supply during the pandemic, are essential as their transport for regular resupply may be disrupted. Alternative means of transportation such as humanitarian aid agency-supported delivery may be required. Accordingly, having an aid organization, and a

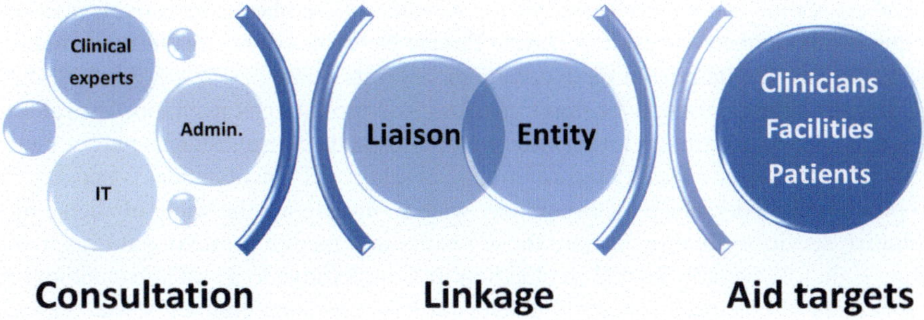


**Fig. 37.2** Key team members for providing remote aid. This graphic depicts essential, but not all, team members involved in rendering remote aid. *Admin* administration, *IT* information technology

point person who serves as a liaison to help coordinate outreach and delivery is key (Fig. 37.2). Specific devices may also be important including additional ambulances or radiology imaging equipment. These are more costly, and an individual facility in or near a disaster zone may not have access to government funds to purchase what they need. Generous donations, including those from healthcare technology or device corporations, help address this gap.

## 37.7 Patient Sharing

When the care needed by a specific patient, or group of patients—such as those with burn injury—cannot be provided in local facilities, there is an opportunity for international rescue [14]. The World Health Organization has some pathways to facilitate the evacuation of unique patients to accepting facilities in other countries [15]. Similar arrangements may be crafted by an institution engaged in rendering remote aid. This kind of patient sharing may clearly identify the destination facility, but will not identify that facility as one that is providing remote consultative aid. Issues in repatriation, financial remuneration for care, rehabilitation, and more are outside of the scope of this chapter but highlight that international patient sharing is a vast endeavor.

## 37.8 Operational Security Issues

Operational security issues may be quite different in the aftermath of a natural disaster as opposed to a manmade one such as military conflict or war. In a natural disaster there is no or little need to avoid geolocation but there is always a need for cybersecurity. During a manmade disaster such as a military conflict or war there is a strong imperative to foil geolocation and to ensure effective cybersecurity [16]. Furthermore, an additional layer of security is required to preserve the identity of: (1) those reaching out for non-national aid, (2) the care facility, (3) patients, and (4) clinician family members. Clinicians should be assigned code names or numbers, and patients may be sequentially numbered as well. A Virtual Private Network (VPN) should be routinely used to access the internet or other communication services.

Similar imperatives may be important for those providing consultation as well—a non-intuitive thought as clinicians commonly provide consultation as part of their workflow. Consultant facility information technology (IT) involvement is necessary to preserve network integrity. Some may wish to investigate the value of such consultative services—and then share those results in a medial professional organization venue followed by journal publication. It is imperative to avoid presentation or publication of potentially identifying data until after military conflict or war ceases. Some clinicians may also desire to travel to the disaster or crisis site to provide on-site aid. Such travel generally may require multi-level clearance including but not limited to the originating and host facilities, the traveler's government, and the disaster location's government. The individual's personal risk is high and should be evaluated in the context of a threat matrix [3]. Resources required for complex or even basic care may be depleted or absent; individual transportation of sufficient resources is not a viable approach based upon logistics, space, or cost. Since physical fitness is not an employment criteria for most hospital-based clinicians, individual or team physical fitness for austere environments may be lacking [17].

Individual travel places the clinician outside of the bounds of an official government or military asset. Therefore, official aid through embassy resources may be non-existent—especially if the embassy assets have already been evacuated. Therefore, safety and security issues abound and drive the need for contingency planning including evacuation, exfiltration, and potentially rescue. It is important to recall that highly trained clinicians from a remote country may be viewed as a high-value hostage and may be targeted for kidnapping as a means of exerting political pressure (especially if the travel is shared across accessible venues such as social media). Finally, one must beware of rendering advanced aid for which post-intervention resources may not exist (e.g., providing limb amputations in a setting where prostheses, rehabilitation, and ramp-based building access are not present) [18]. Despite the need for substantial operational security, there are a host of desirable outgrowths of remote aid collaborations that may come to fruition after the disaster has been resolved.

## 37.9 Potentially Desirable Outcomes

Certainly, scholarly investigations of tracked data provide an analysis and potential roadmap for future undertakings. More powerful is the opportunity for transnational and transcontinental collaboration enhancing education, clinician training (including exchange programs and fellowships), career advancement opportunities, and the development of a visiting scholar program. Regardless, perhaps the most impactful is participating in the reconstruction and reconfiguration of the infrastructure for local healthcare capability—an essential element of local regrowth after disaster-based destruction [19, 20].

## 37.10 Medical-Legal Considerations

Remote aid provides consultation, not direct medical or surgical care. As such, there are virtually no medical-legal considerations to address. Individuals who travel to disaster sites outside of an organizational structure engender many medical-legal concerns. Providing direct patient care outside of one's native country generally requires an appropriate license, or a waiver to needing that license, in order to engage in medical or surgical interventions. Failing to secure suitable permission to practice in another country generally leaves one individually liable for that care as unlicensed care in a non-native country typically falls outside of the boundaries of professional liability coverage. NGOs have pathways to navigate these considerations, and invited military members are covered by their armed forces policies. Since travel to a disaster zone may lead to personal injury, specific medical care coverage that also embraces medical evacuation is essential; many medical travel health insurance policies often cover *in situ* care including road traffic accidents but not transnational medical evacuation [3, 21]. Therefore, during protracted disasters such as war, remote aid is a particularly attractive approach to rendering humanitarian aid.

## 37.11 Conclusion

Remote aid during a humanitarian crisis is feasible and there are a variety of digital platforms that help individuals or teams to achieve that goal. Many of those platforms are currently integrated into social interactions as well as the business of medicine and medical professional organizations. The evolution and repurposing of existing telemedicine technology approaches that are clinical-friendly may offer significant advantages compared to current digital platforms but come at a small financial and large time cost. Time spent in reprogramming and reconfiguration may be substantial. Embedding translation programming that can work across multiple languages—as opposed to being purpose-built for two languages—is not yet standard. Every approach to rendering remote aid must embrace operational security for those providing as well as those receiving aid. In-person aid is a high-risk activity and benefits from specific planning and preparation that is quite challenging and may be insurmountable for an independent individual. There are a host of potential benefits to rendering remote aid that support and enhance local facilities that may blossom once the humanitarian crisis has been resolved.

## References


1. Kaplan LJ, Tisherman S. Disaster preparedness and management. In: Hidalgo J, Pérez-Fernández J, Rodríguez-Vega G (eds) Critical Care Administration. Cham: Springer; 2020. p. 159–75.
2. Coleman CN, Bader JL, Koerner JF, et al. Chemical, biological, radiological, nuclear, and explosive (CBRNE) science and the CBRNE science medical operations science support expert (CMOSSE). Disast Med Public Health Prepar. 2019;13:995–1010.
3. Bailey H, Kaplan LJ. Volunteerism during humanitarian crises: a practical guide. Crit Care. 2022;26:1–6.
4. Bruni T, Lalvani A, Richeldi L. Telemedicine-enabled accelerated discharge of patients hospitalized with COVID-19 to isolation in repurposed hotel rooms. Am J Respir Crit Care Med. 2020;202:508–10.
5. Krouss M, Allison MG, Rios S, et al. Rapid implementation of telecritical care support during a pandemic: lessons learned during the coronavirus disease 2020 surge in New York City. Crit Care Explor. 2020;2:e0271.
6. Harris GH, Baldisseri MR, Reynolds BR, et al. Design for implementation of a system-level ICU pandemic surge staffing plan. Crit Care Explor. 2020;2:e0136.
7. Rose L, Cook A, Onwumere J, et al. Psychological distress and morbidity of family members experiencing virtual visiting in intensive care during COVID-19: an observational cohort study. Intensive Care Med. 2022;48:1156–64.
8. Huang EY, Knight S, Guetter CR, et al. Telemedicine and telementoring in the surgical specialties: a narrative review. Am J Surg. 2019;218:760–6.
9. HealthIT.gov FHIR Fact Sheets. Available at: https://www.healthit.gov/topic/standards-technology/standards/fhir-fact-sheets. Accessed 15 Aug 2022.
10. HL7 International. FHIR Certification. Available at: www.hl7.org/certification/fhir.cfm. Accessed 15 Aug 2022.
11. Kadri F, Birregah B, Châtelet E. The impact of natural disasters on critical infrastructures: a domino effect-based study. J Homeland Secur Emerg Manag. 2014;11:217–41.
12. Olson LC Jr, Bailey CJ, Mabry LR, et al. Forward aeromedical evacuation: a brief history, lessons learned from the Global War on Terror, and the way forward for US policy. J Trauma Acute Care Surg. 2013;75:S130–6.
13. Scott BK, Miller GT, Fonda SJ, et al. Advanced digital health technologies for COVID-19 and future emergencies. Telemed e-Health. 2020;26:1226–33.
14. Almeland SK, Depoortere E, Jennes S, et al. Burn mass casualty incidents in Europe: a European response plan within the European union civil protection mechanism. Burns. 2022;48:1794.
15. World Health Organization. Emergencies. Available at: www.who.int/emergencies/operations. Accessed 20 Aug 2022.
16. Argaw ST, Troncoso-Pastoriza JR, Lacey D, et al. Cybersecurity of Hospitals: discussing the challenges and working towards mitigating the risks. BMC Med Infor Decis Mak. 2020;20:146.
17. Nicholson B, Neskey J, Stanfield R, et al. Integrating prolonged field care into rough terrain and mountain warfare training: the mountain critical care course. J Spec Oper Med. 2019;19:66–9.
18. Iezzoni LI, Ronan LJ. Disability legacy of the Haitian earthquake. Ann Intern Med. 2010;152:812–4.
19. Sword-Daniels VL, Twigg J, Rossetto T, Johnston DM. Unpacking long-term disaster recovery processes: a case study of the healthcare system in Montserrat, West Indies. Int J Mass Emerg Disast. 2016;34:113.
20. Shabsigh R, Nettleship JE. Recovery from crisis. In: Shabsigh R (ed) Health Crisis Management in Acute Care Hospitals. Cham: Springer; 2022. p. 315–31.
21. Caponecchia C, Tan DT. Exploring the traveler underinsurance problem. Ann Tour Res. 2019;76:343–5.

# Boarding in the Emergency Department: Challenges and Success Strategies to Mitigate the Current Crisis

38

H. Bailey

## 38.1 Introduction

Despite having life-threatening conditions that require critical care management, many patients remain in the emergency department (ED) for extended lengths of time. This process is termed 'boarding' and leaves the 'admitted' patient in an outpatient setting despite being critically ill. Moreover, this system issue either makes ED clinicians responsible for the critically ill or injured patient while managing other ED patients, or forces inpatient teams to manage patients in a remote fashion. Since neither situation is ideal—and may be unsafe—ED patient boarding unsurprisingly correlates with longer total length of stay, increasing staff stress, worsened burnout symptoms, and untoward patient outcomes including mortality [1, 2]. Unfortunately, boarding is not a new issue and it appears to be worsening [3]. Indeed, the coronavirus disease 2019 (COVID-19) pandemic has highlighted these longstanding issues and challenges and has underscored maladaptive processes, within and external to the hospital, that drive boarding [4]. It is essential to understand modifiable aspects of hospital practice to help address patient volume that is related to healthcare issues external to the acute care facility including regionalization induced reduced access to care [3, 5]. This chapter will explore the drivers and impact of boarding patients in the ED as well as potential repair strategies for the ED and hospital to improve patient flow and outcome.

H. Bailey (✉)
Department of Emergency Medicine, VA Medical Center, Durham, NC, USA
e-mail: Heatherlee.Bailey-Cooner@VA.gov



J.-L. Vincent (ed.), *Annual Update in Intensive Care and Emergency Medicine 2023*, Annual Update in Intensive Care and Emergency Medicine,
https://doi.org/10.1007/978-3-031-23005-9_38

## 38.2 ED Boarding Versus ED Crowding

Since ED boarding refers to patients who are awaiting admission to the hospital but for whom there are no in-patient beds available, the term is a misnomer—such patients have an identified alternate destination. Instead, ED crowding (or overcrowding) is a broader term that encompasses the total volume of ED patients including those awaiting: (1) initial evaluation, (2) completion of ongoing care prior to discharge, and (3) transport to their inpatient destination [6]. EDs are commonly evaluated using metrics that assess the timeliness of care. Therefore, in an attempt to rapidly assess and treat all presenting patients, patients are commonly evaluated and treated in diverse locations including traditional rooms, triage areas, and increasingly, hallways. The use of non-traditional care areas is anticipated to lead to increased staff stress that is exacerbated by staffing shortages [7]. Such stress may be expressed as fatigue, increased burnout symptoms, moral distress, and ultimately departure from the ED or healthcare entirely. Therefore, regardless of the term that is used, both boarding and crowding are symptoms of larger system issues.

## 38.3 Drivers of Boarding

ED patient boarding is driven by processes external to the hospital as well as local dynamics within the hospital (Fig. 38.1). EDs are increasingly used for primary care as well as the sequelae of lack of routine health maintenance. As small facilities close—an event hastened by the pandemic in some locales—access to care is more difficult. Regionalization has intensified the relocation of high intensity services to

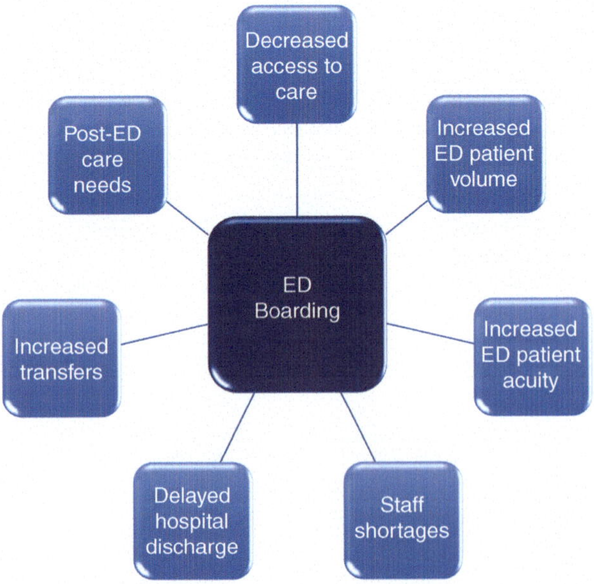


**Fig. 38.1** Key aspects that drive emergency department (ED) boarding

specific sites, many of which are urban. Routine health maintenance is also challenging to obtain for those who cross borders illegally, migrants, refugees, the unemployed, and those who have not engaged in national healthplans (where available). Therefore, EDs often serve as a site of last resort for routine as well as acute conditions [8, 9]. Accordingly, there has been an increase in the number of patients presenting to an ED by 25% in the last decade [10]. EDs are also the victims of complex care success in that patients may live longer despite complex comorbid disease (e.g., multivisceral solid organ transplantation, advanced malignancy care using chimeric antigen receptor T cells [CAR-T] therapy and the like). This has led to an increased severity of illness in patients presenting to the ED, most of whom will require inpatient admission to manage disease progression or care complications. To wit, patients requiring admission to an intensive care unit (ICU) from the ED have increased by 80% in the last decade [10, 11]. This need has led to an increased ED length of stay (LOS) that may range from 6 h to several days. Patients may await the discharge of a patient from the bed to which they have been assigned, or there may be an available bed that cannot be staffed.

The mismatch between the demand for hospital services and the facility's ability to deliver them has been termed hospital disequilibrium. In many ways, disequilibrium represents 'normal' ED operation as patients continuously present for care in numbers that exceed available ED beds or evaluation spaces, some of which are occupied by patients awaiting an inpatient bed. Exacerbating this disequilibrium is the common practice of inpatient discharge principally during daytime hours. Acute care unit discharges that await daytime hours to occur also impede ICU transfers to the acute care unit when occupancy is high; both delays contribute to ED crowding [12]. The processes related to inpatient discharge and intrafacility transfer create inherent delays as well.

Inpatients being discharged to home must have discharge orders and outpatient medications entered into the electronic health record (EHR); delays related to trainee order entry in teaching facilities are common, especially at the start of the academic year. Required equipment must be secured when required, and transportation must be arranged whether by commercial service or private vehicle. The process is quite similar for those being transferred to another facility for ongoing care, but is also subject to bed availability at the receiving facility, and generally does not engage private vehicle transportation. Finally, room disinfection and restocking are required prior to accepting a patient into that specific location—a process that may be prolonged when patients have high consequence infections such as with severe acute respiratory syndrome coronavirus 2 (SARS-CoV-2) [13]. Each of these interlinked elements impacts a facility's occupancy throughout each 24 h cycle.

The higher the hospital occupancy, the longer the anticipated time for patients to reach their inpatient bed. A hospital occupancy of 80% generally begins to impact ED LOS, making boarding more likely especially for the critically ill [14]. Pre-pandemic, high occupancy was often a problem for tertiary and quaternary referral centers. During the pandemic, community, rural as well as critical access facilities also demonstrated high occupancy as transfers to complex centers were problematic. As the pandemic recedes, smaller facilities continue to be impacted by the need to transfer patients to referral centers. Physician staffing in smaller facilities commonly occurs as a single physician. Dividing that physician's attention between all of the patients who need acute care, discharge from the ED, admission to the facility, and transfer to another location is challenging and impedes focused care [15].

Delay in transferring patients out of the ICU leads to admission delay from the ED or transfer in from outside facilities. This kind of delay is often related to the lack of an available acute care unit bed to which the patient may be moved, or the lack of a bed at a less complex facility such as a rehabilitation center. ICU discharge delay augments strain in that facility's ED as well as EDs in referring facilities. A recent study found that 12.8% of total ICU days, at a cost of 34 million US dollars (6.4% total ICU dollars spent), were attributed to patients waiting for transfer out of the ICU [16]. Importantly, delayed ICU transfer is increasingly common and may have adverse impact on patients [14, 16]. Patients awaiting transfer continue to be exposed to ICU stressors including, but not limited to, noise (alarms, routine care, emergencies) and disrupted sleep, which may contribute to acute sequelae such as delirium, or long term sequalae such as the post-intensive care syndrome (PICS). In response to ICU discharge delay, and to avoid overwhelming the ICU team if they are not limited to geographic coverage, some systems transfer care responsibility to a non-ICU team. Unless the ICU nursing team is well acquainted with this process, it may be unclear who they should contact for ongoing care issues for patients awaiting transfer when responsibility has been shifted to a non-ICU team. This approach seems intuitively attractive, but if not well executed, may contribute to care delays, especially since the responsible physician care team is remote from the patient and nurse [14].

High acuity ICUs are most commonly located in high acuity centers that serve as regional centers of excellence that provide complex care. Based upon the need for specific specialists, *de facto* regionalization often typifies care for injury, cardiac and vascular care, neurologic care (stroke, aneurysm, malignancy), and transplantation (solid and liquid organ). These centers serve as rescue sites for the rest of the hospitals in their region—unless they are also overwhelmed and on 'diversion'. These specialty patients frequently require advanced therapy, such as angioembolization, complex surgical intervention, and of course, critical care. Transplants centers also support pre-transplant patients with critical illness, some of whom require extracorporeal support techniques to manage organ failure while awaiting donor organ availability. Patients that require prolonged ICU LOS contribute to the lack of acute bed availability and notably include those with chronic critical illness [17]. The consequences of ED boarding impact all aspects of hospital operations, but most importantly, patients.

## 38.4 Impact of Boarding

When critically ill patients board in the ED, the usual processes that guide care towards recovery may be derailed. These processes include timely administration of therapeutic agents, adherence to institutional protocols or national care guidelines as ED clinicians must manage the entirety of the ED's patients, not just those with critical illness awaiting an inpatient bed. Relatedly, most ED clinicians do not engage in an inpatient practice, further distancing them from usual inpatient care practices. Moreover, consultation by specialty services, such as case management, physical therapy or occupational therapy, as well as therapeutic visitation by family is often absent or quite limited while patients are boarding. ED boarding of critically ill patients increases their overall hospital LOS and correlates with increased mortality [18]. After approximately 6 h of waiting for an ICU bed in the ED, critically ill patient mortality increases with ED boarding time serving as an independent risk factor for mortality [10, 19]. After 6 h, the number needed to harm is 1 in 82 patients for increased 30 day mortality. After 8 h, the number needed to harm reduces to 1 in 72 patients [20]. In large patient volume EDs these numbers are frequently reached in less than 24 h. Non-critically ill patients may be impacted as well, manifested as delays to diagnosis and treatment as ED clinicians remain engaged with boarding patients [21].

Importantly, the effects on staff, from physicians to nurses, is essential to explore. Boarding of critically ill or injured patients creates durable stress when it occurs on a regular basis. Moreover, that stress, and the perceived inequitable distribution of resources and access to specialized care ties to moral distress as well. In combination, high acuity, excess volume, and boarding is likely to exacerbate burnout syndrome as well as departure from healthcare [22]. The ED as a site of high burnout syndrome prevalence predates the pandemic and has been exacerbated by the sharp rise in firearm violence that seems to be persistent in many locations [23, 24]. Like burnout syndrome, in large part, boarding reflects system issues that are potentially modifiable.

## 38.5 System Barriers that Enable Boarding

It is imperative to identify the barriers to smooth patient flow that are unique to each aspect of the acute care health system since those barriers inadvertently enable boarding. Major barriers may be found in each of the following seven areas: ED, elective admission process, operating room (OR) schedule, ICUs, acute care units, out of hospital transfers, and the inpatient discharge process. In the ED, patient volume, especially around predictable events, should be met with appropriate staffing. A surge plan should be articulated to address excess patient volume that occurs in an unanticipated fashion. Since the ED is routinely assessed for care timeliness (arrival, evaluation, admission or discharge decision, therapy initiation, and time to departure), it is a key location from which to garner data to begin to explore barriers [25]. The hospital admission process should be reviewed as elective admissions for out-of-OR as well as OR procedure patients generally receive top priority in securing an inpatient bed. Critical care units may also have issues with boarding of patients whose acuity status has improved but remain in the ICU because of lack of inpatient bed availability. Less common is an unwillingness by the ICU team to transfer to the acute care floor. Instead, the admitting team (principally for surgical patients) may be opposed to transfer out of the ICU. This conflict needs to have a system-based resolution pathway so it does not rely on individual intervention. For a patient to move onto an acute care unit, nursing hand-off is required. Patients can be 'pushed' to those units (a less effective approach), or they may be 'pulled' by the receiving unit (much more effective and benefits from an incentive plan) [5, 14, 25]. With regard to discharge, the acute care unit staff may have trouble securing discharge orders, or the necessary supplies, medication, or transportation required for timely discharge. These delays are also mitigatable using systems-based approaches that are individual agnostic. For tertiary or quaternary referral centers, there is a constant stream of patients for whom transfer from another hospital is requested. A transfer center and direct attending-to-attending discourse is of immense aid in determining the urgency of transfer [15, 26]. During times of high occupancy, arbitration by a senior clinical administrator such as the Chief Medical Officer may be required—as occurred during SARS-CoV-2 patient surges in many facilities. Exploring these processes for opportunities for improvement will help craft a comprehensive approach to improving patient throughput and reducing ED boarding [5, 14].

## 38.6 Potential Repair Strategies

ED boarding has been a problem for decades. Accordingly, some healthcare systems have developed approaches besides improving patient flow processes to address boarding [5] (Fig. 38.2). One approach is to create a resuscitative care unit (RCU) in or adjacent to the ED to serve as an alternative critical care site while awaiting an inpatient bed. RCUs may function as typical ICUs (i.e., ED ICU), or they may have a more focused scope of capability. An ED ICU provides the full scope of critical care management within a dedicated space and with dedicated staff; trauma patients are not typically managed in this kind of unit as injury care benefits from a specifically focused ICU staff [18, 27]. Directed care may be implemented by an intensivist at the bedside or led by a clinician via telecritical care [27, 28]. Both ED ICUs and the utilization of telecritical care improves outcomes and reduces mortality in critically ill patients that are not yet assigned to a traditional

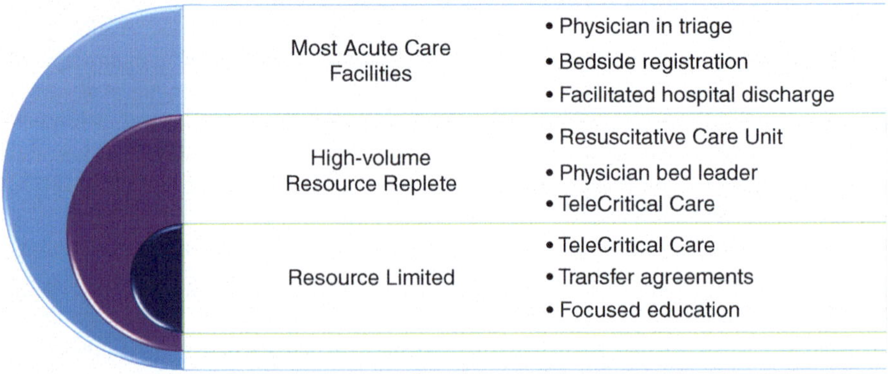


**Fig. 38.2** Potential ED boarding repair strategies

critical care bed [3, 10, 28]. Some RCU patients may resolve their ICU needs within 24 h (e.g., patients with diabetic ketoacidosis), while others continue receiving critical care until an inpatient ICU bed becomes available (e.g., severe community acquired pneumonia with acute respiratory failure) [18, 27]. A less intense type of RCU is an ICU observation unit. This RCU also has a dedicated space and team and may continue resuscitation, but is unable to deliver advanced care such as continuous renal replacement therapy (CRRT) or mechanical circulatory support. This kind of RCU offloads ED clinicians from managing critically ill patients while they await an inpatient bed. A third type of RCU is known as a rapid diagnosis unit. This unit is a temporary flex unit that is intended to expand ED capacity during periods of patient surge such as a disaster (or the recent pandemic) but is not an ICU [3, 10, 29, 30]. Linking all of the ICUs across a single healthcare system into a coordinated entity defines a critical care organization (CCO).

CCOs function as a collaborative in that they share similar protocols, guidelines, and in general, standardized equipment and medication profiles. However, the value of a CCO when there is patient surge, is that patients may be moved between institutions that are capable of rendering the required care. This function is known as "load balancing". CCOs also aid in apportioning incoming transfer patients across the entire system and not just a single institution. The emphasis of the CCO is on value-based care with the patient at the center of the structure, not the institution [31]. CCOs are led by an intensivist who interfaces with ICU leadership across all of the integrated ICUs, a position that fosters communication.

Relatedly, a facility bed leader who is typically a physician can interface with the admissions office, the transfer center, and the ED to help ensure appropriate patient admission, transfer, and bedding. Creating such a role favorably impacts ED LOS and reduces time to admission [32]. This individual may have key roles in utilization management and quality improvement committees for the acute care facility as well. A daily bed leader is more commonly found in large systems. In smaller hospitals, including those that serve as critical access facilities, other approaches are more fruitful.

Three approaches may be useful for smaller facilities: transfer agreements, affiliation with a larger hospital system, and telemedicine. It is imperative that transfer agreements are in place to assist clinicians who must transfer critically ill patients to a more complex facility regardless of time of day or patients' ability to pay. Joining an established hospital network as an affiliated site aids in transfer and repatriation of patients after their acute needs have been met. In-network transfers are readily accepted unless the receiving facility is operating in crisis mode. Even when the complex care facility is operating in crisis mode—such as during sequential waves of the pandemic—telemedicine consultation can help guide care at outlying facilities [15, 33]. Critical care guidance (telecritical care), stroke assessment and management (tele-stroke), and post-injury care have benefited from remote guidance by specialists [34]. The SARS-CoV-2 pandemic ably demonstrated that clinicians of all parent specialties may benefit from specific education regarding critical care.

## 38.7 Clinician and Team Education

Regardless of their discipline, clinicians needed to help care for those with critical illness during the pandemic. Often, non-ICU clinicians (physicians, nurses, respiratory therapists, pharmacists, and others) needed to help care for patients in novel ICUs under the supervision of skilled critical care professionals. This approach is known as the tiered staffing model and is useful during disasters as well [35]. In order to help non-ICU clinicians function well in that role, a variety of focused critical care educational resources were developed and deployed by major medical professional organizations as well as individual healthcare facilities [35, 36]. While useful during the pandemic, these educational training events underscore the opportunity to enhance critical care education as a routine. Such an approach would influence training curricula for every healthcare specialty and would take years to come to fruition. Importantly, enhanced residency exposure to critical care only serves to establish a foundation upon which time-sensitive training may be layered as needed [30]. Regular reinforcement of core critical care concepts, including those focused on recognition of critical illness and resuscitation, would aid in skill and knowledge retention. The goal of such training is to improve every clinician's ability to participate in critical care. Specifically, it would enhance ED clinicians' ability to provide more complex care in a seamless fashion for those who continue to board in the ED while awaiting an inpatient ICU bed. Regardless of the intensity of such training, it would not serve as a substitute for established fellowship training in critical care medicine. Those undertaking fellowship benefit from developing both system management and leadership skills—two key non-medical skills.

Devoting additional time during critical care medicine fellowship training to disaster management would enhance the intensivist's ability to lead during disasters, and help ICU team members to understand and fulfill their roles within a disaster command structure [37, 38]. This kind of education and training is essential to effectively deploy and manage novel ICUs or during a disaster response, but also has implications for ED boarding of critically ill patients—an undesirable event that may be viewed as a continual crisis in a global fashion.

## 38.8 Conclusion

ED boarding of patients reflects system issues with patient flow. Patients with critical illness who board in the ED are at high risk for untoward outcomes. Boarding creates stress for ED clinicians of all disciplines and contributes to burnout symptoms that may adversely impact the available workforce. System-based approaches to mitigating boarding are applicable to every facility, but deployable countermeasures will vary based upon facility complexity. Enhancing ED clinician critical care training will help improve the care of those who board in the ED while awaiting an inpatient ICU bed.

## References


1. Chalifn DB, Trzeciak S, Likourezos A, Baumann BM, Dellinger RF. Impact of delayed transfer of critically ill patients from the emergency department to the intensive care unit. Crit Care Med. 2007;35:1437–83.
2. Waters A. Government "missed opportunity" to tackle NHS and social care shortages. BMJ. 2022;376:0422.
3. Mohr NM, Wessman BT, Bassin B, et al. Boarding of critically ill patients in the emergency department. Crit Care Med. 2020;48:1180–7.
4. Lucero A, Sokol K, Hyun J, et al. Worsening of emergency department length of stay during the COVID-19 Pandemic. JACEP Open. 2021;2:e12489.
5. Morley C, Unwin M, Peterson GM, Stankovich J, Kinsman L. Emergency department crowding: a systematic review of causes, consequences, and solutions. PLoS One. 2018;13:e0203316.
6. McKenna P, Heslin SM, Vicellio P, Mallon WK, Hernandez C, Morley EJ. Emergency department and hospital crowding: causes, consequences and cures. Clin Exp Emerg Med. 2019;6:189–95.
7. Innes GD, Sivilotti MLA, Ovens H, et al. Emergency overcrowding and access block: a smaller problem than we think. CJEM. 2019;21:177–85.
8. Kellerman AL. Crisis in the emergency department. N Engl J Med. 2006;355:1300–3.
9. Christensen J. How the pandemic killed a record number of rural hospitals. Available at: https://www.cnn.com/2021/07/31/health/rural-hospital-closures-pandemic/index.html. Accessed 30 Aug 2022.
10. Wessman BT, Mohr NM. Emergency department ICUs add value. Crit Care Med. 2022;50:1265–7.
11. Herring AA, Ginde AA, Fahimi J, et al. Increasing critical care admissions from U.S. emergency departments, 2001-2009. Crit Care Med. 2013;41:1197–204.
12. Vermeulen MJ, Ray JG, Bell C, Cayen B, Stukel TA, Schull MJ. Disequilibrium between admitted and discharged hospitalized patients affects emergency department length of stay. Ann Emerg Med. 2009;54:794–804.
13. Welch S. Hospital wide strategies for reducing inpatient discharge delays and boarding. Available at: https://www.acepnow.com/article/hospital-wide-strategies-for-reducing-inpatient-discharge-delays-and-boarding/?singlepage=1&theme=print-friendly. Accessed 20 Jul 2022.
14. Ofoma UR, Montoya J, Saha D, et al. Associations between hospital occupancy, intensive care unit transfer delay and hospital mortality. J Crit Care. 2020;58:48–55.
15. Augustin JJ. Another COVID casualty: The Emergency Department transfer process. Available at: https://www.acepnow.com/article/another-covid-casualty-the-emergency-department-transfer-process/. Accessed 20 Jul 2022.
16. Bagshaw SM, Tran DT, Opgenorth D, et al. Assessment of costs of avoidable delays in Intensive Care Unit Discharge. JAMA Netw Open. 2020;3:e2013913.
17. Hirshberg EL, Wilson EL, Stanfield V, et al. Impact of critical illness on resource utilization: a comparison of use in the year before and after ICU admission. Crit Care Med. 2019;47:1497–504.
18. Weingart SD, Sherwin RL, Emlett LL, Tawil I, Mayglothling J, Rittenberger JC. ED intensivists and ED intensive care units. Am J Emerg Med. 2013;31:617–20.
19. Jayaprakash N, Pflaum-Carlson J, Gardner-Gray J, et al. Critical care delivery solutions in the emergency department: evolving models in caring for ICU boarders. Ann Emerg Med. 2020;76:709–16.
20. Jones S, Moulton C, Swift S, et al. Association between delays to patient admission from the emergency department and all cause 30-day mortality. Emerg Med. 2022;39:168–73.
21. van der Linden MC, Meester BEAM, van der Linden N. Emergency department crowding affects triage processes. Int Emerg Nurs. 2016;29:27–31.
22. Kelly LA, Gee PM, Butler RJ. Impact of nurse burnout on organizational and position turnover. Nurs Outlook. 2021;69:96–102.

23. Moskop JC, Geiderman JM, Marshall KD, et al. Another look at the persistent moral problem of emergency department crowding. Ann Emerg Med. 2019;74:357–64.
24. Abdallah HO, Zhao C, Kaufman E, et al. Increased firearm injury during the COVID-19 pandemic: a hidden urban burden. J Am Coll Surg. 2021;232:159–68.
25. Change AM, Cohen DJ, Lin A, et al. Hospital strategies for reducing emergency department crowding: a mixed-methods study. Ann Emerg Med. 2018;71:497–505.e4.
26. Franklin BJ, Vakili S, Huckman RS, et al. The inpatient discharge lounge as a potential mechanism to mitigate emergency department boarding and crowding. Ann Emerg Med. 2020;75:704–14.
27. Gunnerson KJ, Bassin BS, Harvey RA, et al. Association of emergency department based intensive care unit with survival and inpatient intensive care unit admissions. JAMA Netw Open. 2019;2:e197584.
28. Kadar RB, Amici DR, Hesse K, Bonder A, Ries M. Impact of telemonitoring of critically ill emergency department patients awaiting ICU transfer. Crit Care Med. 2019;47:1201–7.
29. Leibner E, Spiegel R, Hsu CH, et al. Anatomy of resuscitative care unit: expanding the borders of traditional intensive care units. Emerg Med J. 2019;36:364–8.
30. Bailey H, Kaplan LJ. Enhancing non-ICU clinician capability and ICU bed capacity to manage pandemic patient surge. In: Vincent JL (ed). Annual Update in Intensive Care and Emergency Medicine 2021. Cham: Springer Nature; 2021. p. 295–304.
31. Leung S, Gregg SR, Coopersmith CM, et al. Critical care organizations: business of critical care and value/performance building. Crit Care Med. 2018;46:1–11.
32. Matthews KS, Durst MS, Vargas-Tores C, Olsen AD, Mazumdar M, Richardson LD. Effect of emergency department and ICU occupancy on admission decisions and outcomes for critically ill patients. Crit Care Med. 2018;46:720–7.
33. Pamplin JC, Scott BJ, Quinn MT, et al. Technology and disasters: the evolution of the National Emergency Tele-Critical Care Network. Crit Care Med. 2021;49:1007–14.
34. Subramanian S, Pamplin JC, Hravnak M, et al. Tele-critical care: an update from the society of critical care medicine Tele-ICU Committee. Crit Care Med. 2020;48:553–61.
35. SCCM. Critical care for non-ICU clinicians. Available at: https://www.sccm.org/COVID19RapidResources/Resources/Critical-Care-for-Non-ICU-Clinicians-Expert-Panel. Accessed 21 Aug 2022.
36. ESICM. European Commission C19_SPACE (COVID 19 skills preparation course). Available at: https://www.esicm.org/covid-19-skills-preparation-course/. Accessed 21 Aug 2002.
37. Dichter JR, Devereaux AS, Sprung CL, et al. Mass critical care surge response during COVID-19. Implementation of contingency strategies – a preliminary report of findings from a Task Force for mass critical care. Chest. 2022;161:429–7.
38. Halpern NA, Tan KS. United States resource availability for COVID-19. Available at: https://sccm.org/Blog/March-2020/United-States-Resource-Availability-for-COVID-19?_zs=jxpjd1&_zl=w9pb6. Accessed 31 Aug 2022.

# Post-Intensive Care Syndrome Revisited in Light of the COVID-19 Pandemic

39

K. Kotfis, K. Lechowicz, and W. Dąbrowski

## 39.1 Introduction

The last 100 years have been characterized by numerous important discoveries in almost every field of life. These have involved advances within the medical field, including clinical (e.g., the discoveries of causes and treatments for diseases), pharmacological (new drugs and therapies), and technical (e.g., ventilators, advanced monitoring, dialysis equipment). The developments in medicine and improvement in the public's knowledge about health-promoting measures have contributed to a significant increase in life expectancy with new challenges that we, as physicians, must be ready for. The older age of our patients means an increased number of chronic diseases, multimorbidity, and prolonged convalescence due to reduced physiological capacity.

Each year, millions of critically ill patients are treated in intensive care units (ICUs) around the world, at least a third of whom require support for multiple organ functions [1]. The current state of knowledge has resulted in a growing population of so-called 'ICU survivors', i.e., patients who have survived critical illness through support in the ICU thus who have survived diseases that until recently were considered incurable. This is undoubtedly a significant success story, which should be closely monitored by follow-up care after hospitalization. After discharge from the ICU, many patients experience multilevel health problems that many clinicians not used to providing ICU care are unaware of.

K. Kotfis (✉) · K. Lechowicz
Department of Anesthesiology, Intensive Therapy and Acute Intoxications, Pomeranian Medical University in Szczecin, Szczecin, Poland
e-mail: katarzyna.kotfis@pum.edu.pl

W. Dąbrowski
Department of Anaesthesiology and Intensive Care, Medical University of Lublin, Lublin, Poland



J.-L. Vincent (ed.), *Annual Update in Intensive Care and Emergency Medicine 2023*, Annual Update in Intensive Care and Emergency Medicine,
https://doi.org/10.1007/978-3-031-23005-9_39

This problem has been brought to light by coronavirus disease 2019 (COVID-19), with many 'non-intensivist' physicians coming into contact with severely ill patients, whose chronic diseases have been destabilized by the severe acute respiratory syndrome coronavirus 2 (SARS-CoV-2) infection.

## 39.2 Definition and Epidemiology

In 2012, a panel of experts from the Society of Critical Care Medicine (SCCM) described the consequences of an ICU stay, including cognitive impairment, mental state disorders, and impaired physical capacity after leaving the unit, as the post-intensive care syndrome (PICS) [2]. This definition has contributed to considering the critically ill patient not only through their experience in the ICU, but in a longer term perspective that includes preparing the patient to reach a similar functioning level to that prior to the critical illness.

These long-term limitations in physical, mental, cognitive, and social zones affect up to 50% of patients who leave the ICU and are considered 'cured' [3]. Up to 40% of patients have generalized cognitive impairment, and in 26% of them the symptoms correspond to a mild form of Alzheimer's disease 3 months after leaving the ICU. After one year, these deficits decreased to 34% and 24%, respectively [3]. It has also been shown that a longer duration of severe state was independently associated with a worse prognosis [4]. The prevalence of depression, anxiety, or post-traumatic stress disorder (PTSD) ranges from 13 to 60%, and physical impairment (e.g., acquired muscle weakness, impaired lung spirometry volumes, and diffusion capacity) occurs in up to 40% of ICU survivors [3].

Mental disorders occurring due to a patient's treatment in the ICU can also affect family members and others close to the patient. This is due to the constant stress, anxiety, and concern about their condition, both during the illness itself and after death or discharge from the hospital, which is called post-intensive care syndrome-family (PICS-F). It has been shown that symptoms of stress, anxiety, or depression can be observed in up to 30% of family members of patients treated in the ICU [4].

The problems defined by PICS and its classical definition have recently been challenged due to numerous publications describing a wider range of complications of the ICU stay, expanding the concept of PICS as defined by the SCCM. Rousseau et al. proposed to broaden the current definition of PICS to include new components (i.e., osteopenia, chronic pain, sleep disorders, chronic fatigue, vulnerability, metabolic disorders, osteopenia, and endocrine dysfunction) along with contributing factors (i.e., baseline health and functional status, ICU-related factors, post-ICU condition, and care) and consequences (i.e., social problems, reduced health-related quality of life, increased costs, including readmissions to the ICU and the hospital) [5], as shown in Table 39.1.

**Table 39.1** Disorders included in post-intensive care syndrome (PICS) [3, 5]

| Post-intensive care syndrome | Type of disturbance |
|---|---|
| *PICS (Patient)* | |
| Adaptation disorders | Changes associated with new or worsened impairment<br>Deterioration in sense of one's own health (feelings of fragility)<br>Changes in lifestyle |
| Psychological disorders | Anxiety (acute stress syndrome)<br>PTSD<br>Depression<br>Fear/constant sense of danger<br>Sleep disorders (insomnia, nightmares)<br>Irritability<br>Sexual dysfunction |
| Cognitive impairments | Memory disorders<br>Attention and concentration disorders<br>Visual-spatial disorder<br>Slowing down of speed of thought processes<br>Executive function disorder<br>Dementia worsening<br>Disorders of the senses (sensing and interpretation) |
| Physical problems | Weakening of the respiratory system (pulmonary complications)<br>Neuromuscular disorders (ICU-AW, muscle atrophy, neuropathy)<br>A sense of exhaustion<br>Pain<br>Loss of weight<br>Loss of appetite<br>Dependence on other people |
| Failed social construction | Social isolation<br>Deterioration of interpersonal relationships<br>Deterioration of relationships within the family<br>Financial problems (increased employment problems, rehabilitation costs)<br>Altered personality and opinions |
| *PICS-F (Family)* | |
| Mental health | Anxiety (acute stress syndrome)<br>PTSD<br>Depression<br>Grief |
| Economic and social problems | Increased patient care costs<br>Reduction in working time, unemployment<br>Decreased social contact |

*PTSD* post-traumatic stress disorder, *ICU-AW* intensive care unit-acquired weakness

## 39.3 Association with Functional Outcome

It has been suggested that there is a relationship between the various components of PICS, with impairment of one function exacerbating impairment of another [6].

### 39.3.1 Cognitive Impairment

Cognitive impairment after critical illness in the ICU presents with variable severity. Mild changes may manifest as minor difficulties in performing complex tasks, while severe changes contribute to an inability to perform daily activities necessary for independent living. Several areas can be distinguished in which PICS plays an important role: attention and concentration, memory, speed of logical thinking, and executive functions [7]. Most often, impaired memory function contributes to impaired daily functioning and compliance with post-discharge instructions (e.g., keeping up with medication or medical appointments), further delaying full recovery. Cognitive impairment can reach the level of mild dementia up to 6 months after ICU discharge. Patients are characterized by impaired social and occupational function, difficulty performing mental tasks such as managing household finances, or multidimensional tasks like driving, among others [8].

Communication difficulties are also often observed in patients undergoing rehabilitation, making diagnosis more difficult and worsening treatment options for these disorders [9]. Cognitive impairment often remains undiagnosed due to communication difficulties in these patients, as well as low public awareness and low availability of formal diagnostic tests for dementia outside of specialized neurological rehabilitation facilities [10].

### 39.3.2 Psychiatric Symptoms

Mental disorders that remain after treatment in the ICU, which primarily include anxiety, depression, and PTSD, often cause disability, and impair the quality of life for both patients and family members [6]. The most frequent symptoms are irritability, restlessness, fatigue, appetite disorders, sleep problems (mainly insomnia), and alcohol abuse after returning home [11]. Depression combined with cognitive disorders also takes a toll on patients and their families financially. The SUPPORT study (The Study to Understand Prognoses and Preferences for Outcomes and Risks of Treatment) showed that about 30% of patients were unable to return to work after ICU treatment, and 20% of family members had to stop their own work to care for the patient or use professional medical care for an average of 17.4 h per week, which significantly affected the household budget [12]. Additionally, it may contribute to the avoidance of visits to healthcare professionals, which further delays the diagnosis and exacerbates the disorder.

### 39.3.3 Physical Impairment

Muscle weakness (ICU-acquired weakness) often occurs in ICU patients, and is the cause of decreased mobility, multiple falls, and even quadriplegia [13]. Muscle atrophy and disorders of the nature of myopathy or polyneuropathy have a multifactorial basis and affect all, not just patients who remained immobile for a longer time. In addition, muscle regeneration may also be reduced in these patients due to the reduced number of progenitor cells in patients after ICU treatment. These symptoms often interfere with daily living activities (ability to take medications independently and perform household chores), and necessitate months of rehabilitation, especially when accompanied by contractures, malnutrition, or impaired respiratory function [14]. Contractures are a relatively common complication, occurring at a rate of 34% in patients staying in the ICU for 14 days or longer [15].

The causes of PICS for each patient may be different. Table 39.2 lists the known risk factors for each component of PICS. Some authors note that this list of symptoms should be expanded to include numerous other complications that are observed after an ICU stay. These additionally include accelerated loss of bone mass and increased risk of fractures, swallowing disorders, endocrine and metabolic disorders (including newly diagnosed diabetes mellitus), and hormonal changes, as well as the presence of chronic pain syndromes not only of nociceptive but also neuropathic origin.

**Table 39.2** Risk factors for each component of post-intensive care syndrome (PICS)

| Symptom | Risk factor |
|---|---|
| Neuropathy, Myopathy | Hyperglycemia |
| | Systemic inflammatory response |
| | Sepsis |
| | Multi-organ failure |
| Muscle weakness | Steroid therapy |
| | Acquired diseases in the ICU |
| | Advanced age |
| | Lung damage |
| | Weakness before admission |
| Depression | Traumatic memories |
| | Psychiatric symptoms at discharge |
| | Weakening of physical functions |
| PTSD | Excessive sedation |
| | ICU delirium |
| Anxiety disorders | Unemployment |
| | Duration of mechanical ventilation |
| | Female |
| | Younger age |
| | Lower level of education |
| Cognitive impairments | Lower intelligence quotient (IQ) |
| | Delirium |
| | Excessive sedation |
| | Hypoxia |
| | Carbohydrate metabolism disorders |

## 39.4 Diagnostics

The diagnosis and recognition of PICS is one of the biggest challenges of modern critical care. In clinical practice, the tests used to identify the elements of PICS syndrome are not routinely performed, often leaving the syndrome unrecognized and underreported [7]. Testing patients for PICS is not common practice. According to SCCM recommendations aimed at detecting PICS in the year 2020, patients should be evaluated for cognitive, psychiatric, and physical impairment, not only at the end of treatment (2–4 weeks after ICU stay) but throughout hospitalization, which will allow for early detection of progressive changes and modifications to prevent worsening of impairment [16, 17].

Every patient should undergo a clinical evaluation and formal screening tests to detect cognitive deficits. Currently, there is no ideal tool for assessing long-term cognitive impairment [18]. Nevertheless, the MoCA scale (Montreal Cognitive Assessment), which is a validated test used to identify executive abilities often lacking in ICU patients, has been shown to have good efficacy in detecting mild cognitive impairment [19]. Screening should also be performed to identify depression, anxiety, or PTSD [20, 21]. The SCCM recommends the use of the Hospital Anxiety and Depression Scale (HADS) and the Impact of Event Scale-Revised (PTSD) to assess psychiatric disorders, and the 6-min walk and/or the EuroQol-5D-5L, health-related quality of life measure to assess physical capacity. Interactions during the ICU stay are important in the patient's physical assessment. To provide holistic care a specialized team of physiotherapists with extensive ICU experience should be involved in patient care to assess skeletal dysfunction and the presence of muscular atrophy. A similar assessment should be performed on every patient after leaving the hospital and during rehabilitation in the outpatient setting, which would identify those most in need of support [9]. The assessment of a patient's nutritional status is also of great importance as is the assessment of respiratory capacity, which should be performed routinely in all ICUs. Fundamental to the diagnosis of PICS is the exclusion of comorbidities that may produce similar symptoms.

## 39.5 Interventions

The most effective strategy for limiting PICS is prevention. A package of coordinated interventions has been developed to minimize the likelihood of developing PICS in mechanically ventilated patients, namely the ABCDEF bundle (Assessing Pain, Both Spontaneous Awakening and Breathing Trials, Choice of Drugs, Delirium Monitoring/Management, Early Exercise/Mobility, and Family Empowerment) [22, 23] that can be enhanced by good communication and reliable handout materials [24]. The effectiveness of the ABCDEF bundle was confirmed in a large prospective study involving more than 15,000 adult ICU patients, which found that the use of the ABCDEF method significantly reduced the risk of death within 7 days of admission, as well as the need for mechanical ventilation, physical restraint, and the risk of coma, delirium, or readmission to the ICU or another ward [25].

A correct approach to nutrition, balancing protein and caloric requirements adequate to the patient's current condition is also an important tool in the prevention of PICS. Inadequate dietary protein intake promotes catabolic processes and muscle mass reduction, which can exacerbate ICU-acquired weakness [26, 27]. Prevention of muscle mass loss also involves mobilizing these muscles and commencing physiotherapy as soon as possible. Active exercises are appropriate to the patient's condition, and in unconscious patients, electrostimulation of muscles (EMS) contributes to reducing muscle atrophy and thus improves the patient's overall condition [5].

The family plays an important role in the healing process, especially in the patient's return to full function, and separation from the family and loved ones can have long-term consequences on critically ill patients. A recent study by Moss et al. in a group of 14,344 patients showed that ICU family visitation was associated with a decreased risk of psychiatric disorders in critically ill patients up to 1 year after hospital discharge [28]. While still in the ICU, the patient's family or loved ones can take part in creating an ICU diary. This process involves writing a description of each day during the ICU stay, adding pictures and graphics, and thus reducing the guesswork for patients unable to recall these difficult events. The creation of ICU diaries that document patient experiences during critical illness has been shown to be effective in improving patient recovery. A recent meta-analysis showed that ICU diaries reduced the risk of depression and preserved the quality of life of patients after ICU admission, but did not seem to have any beneficial effect on the relatives of the patients [29]. It is not entirely certain whether their use significantly affects mental disorders in patients, however, studies report a significant (5 vs. 13%) reduction in the incidence of PTSD in patients [30, 31].

Multidisciplinary intensive-level patient care should not end after the patient is discharged from the ICU. In many countries, post-ICU in-patient and out-patient clinics are emerging. These facilities have been created for patients who have completed their treatment in the ICU and are geared toward helping the patients return to full function. Activities in such clinics include intensive rehabilitation and consultation by psychiatrists and psychologists with support for cognitive abilities and mental problems. Such facilities are ideal for diagnosing PICS in patients; however, there are no established uniform guidelines for these facilities. The PRaCTICaL randomized trial evaluated the usefulness of these clinics through rehabilitation and observational follow-up visits. It showed no significant differences between the control groups but recommended that more weight should be given to early physical rehabilitation, delirium, cognitive dysfunction, and relatives in recovery from critical illness [32].

## 39.6 Post-Intensive Care/Post-COVID-19 Syndrome

At the end of 2019, a worldwide crisis in global medical care emerged as the COVID-19 pandemic. Treating patients was a significant challenge due to the rapidity of symptom management, lack of causal treatment, and the significant infectivity of the virus, which contributed to significant mortality and many patients in the ICU. The pandemic also changed the profile of patients in the ICU. The incidence of PICS after COVID-19 varied widely, with 28–87% of cases showing physical impairment, 20–57% cognitive impairment, and 6–60% mental health problems 1–6 months after discharge [33]. Patients diagnosed with COVID-19 mainly struggled with respiratory failure and acute respiratory distress syndrome (ARDS), requiring intubation and mechanical ventilation. In these patients, pain management and sedation are the cornerstones of ensuring their comfort. This is important, especially when using a prone position, high-pressure ventilation, or extracorporeal membrane oxygenation (ECMO). In addition, the significant risk of spreading the disease with unplanned extubation exacerbated the widespread use of deeper sedation [33].

The COVID-19 pandemic has increased awareness of PICS and the long-term impairments that survivors of critical illness often experience. The World Health Organization (WHO) has estimated that 10%–20% of people who have COVID will develop post-COVID conditions, with more than 100 associated symptoms, the most common being fatigue, chronic general pain, sleep disturbances, shortness of breath, motor or sensory dysfunction, cognitive impairment, and mental health symptoms. Researchers also found that 9% of people were unable to return to work after three months. The features of long-COVID very much resemble and overlap with the symptoms of PICS [34]. In addition, deterioration in physical performance can be observed in patients after COVID-19 compared to PICS in other diseases. This may be due to numerous long-term pulmonary complications, such as pulmonary fibrosis, chronic respiratory failure, pulmonary thrombosis, bronchial dilatation, cavitary lung disease, and spontaneous pneumothorax [35, 36].

Numerous restrictions implemented during the COVID-19 pandemic also contributed to the difficult treatment and prevention of PICS in ICU patients. It was problematic to implement the ABCDEF bundle, which was only successful in part: A, 45%; B, 28%; C, 52%; D, 35%; E, 47%; and F, 16% [37]. A significant difference could be seen especially in aspects related to the family. Restrictions regarding family visits reduced the possibility of cooperation with the family to reduce the frequency of PICS and intensified the development of PICS-F [38]. These restrictions and the prohibition of visitation are hard to counteract. Many hospitals already have videoconferencing or online visits that make it possible to contact the patient with visiting restrictions [33].

A comparison of the incidence of PICS in patients after COVID-19 versus the 'usual ICU stay' showed that COVID-19 patients are more likely to have PICS-specific disorders. Among these symptoms, the incidence of anxiety disorders and PTSD was lower which may be related to the different characteristics of the group. Patients at high risk for severe complications of COVID-19 were usually older men, which stands in contrast to the risk factors for PTSD, i.e., young women [39]. Patients treated in the ICU for COVID-19 were significantly more likely to experience episodes of delirium, which may be related to the invasion of neural tissue by the virus [34].

Establishing a post-hospital care system related to COVID-19 can be a major challenge for health systems. Treatment of ICU-related complications may require the collaboration of numerous specialists, such as nurses, physiotherapists, occupational therapists, psychologists, nutritionists, and physicians. Their task will be to support patients in all areas of PICS, both through psychotherapy and treatment of psychiatric and cognitive disorders but also through rehabilitation and appropriate nutritional treatment. In the prevention of PICS, it is important to increase awareness of the syndrome not only for the patients and their families, but for the entire medical community. This can contribute to the introduction of interventions that will not necessarily incur significant direct costs but will prevent long-term social costs associated with numerous complications in patients [40].

Early mobilization of COVID-19 patients appears to be an effective, though not entirely easy method for reducing the risk of PICS and improving the ability to return to normal life. Many critically ill COVID-19 patients are very weak and refuse to move in and out of bed or perform any form of exercise. Moreover, many of them require mechanical ventilation, which is often associated with the need for sedation to improve gas exchange. Lack of active movement can cause a variety of disorders leading to muscle wasting, myopathy, and polyneuropathy that prolong treatment duration and increase the risk of death during and after the hospital stay [41, 42]. A rapid and massive increase in the levels of pro-inflammatory cytokines following infection-related inflammatory responses also impairs muscle activity and promotes skeletal muscle atrophy with reduced protein content and myotube diameter [43–45]. Another important mechanism leading to muscle weakness is direct viral infection of the muscle tissue with scattered necrosis of myofibers and mitochondrial abnormalities [46]. Early mobilization has been documented as a promising intervention to reduce muscle weakness and PICS [41, 47–49]. Maintenance of muscle strength correlates with an improvement in functional capacity, shorter duration of mechanical ventilation or support, and therefore shorter length of hospital treatment [47–49]. It has been documented that even short periods of active muscle activity are associated with profitable metabolic changes and better immune response [50–52]. Importantly, skeletal muscle is well-recognized as an important organ producing various molecules with vital functions. These molecules, commonly known as myokines, are produced and secreted only during muscle activity and have been described as peptides, cytokines, and growth factors [53, 54]. The level of myokines negatively correlates with the weakness of critically ill patients and has been proposed as a sensitive biomarker of frailty [54]. Even short but regular active mobilization with a cycle ergometer enhances recovery of functional exercise capacity, reduces the risk of delirium, and improves gastrointestinal function and functional status at the time of discharge from the ICU [50, 55]. Noteworthy, several studies have documented that each type of early mobilization, including with a cycle ergometer, is safe, feasible, and well tolerated in critically ill patients, and endotracheal intubation is not a contraindication to this kind of activity (Fig. 39.1) [41, 47, 48, 50–55]. Hence, early mobilization, defined as mobilization within 72 h after admission to the ICU, should be implemented as the standard treatment of critically ill patients to improve the quality of patient care.

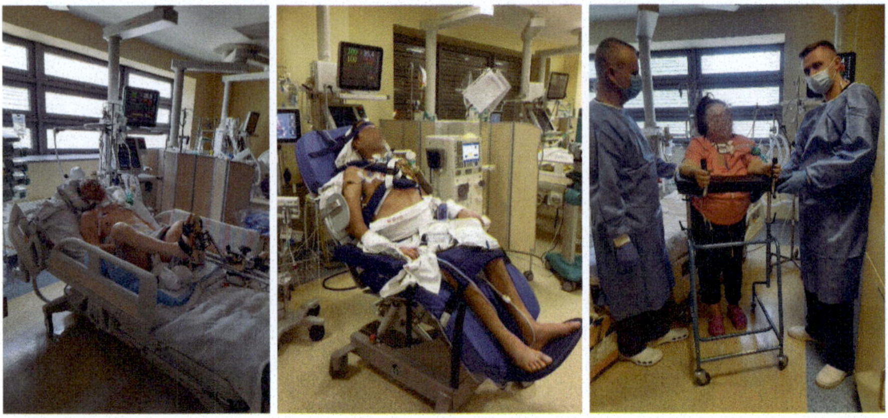

**Fig. 39.1** Example of three mechanically ventilated patients managed with early mobilization. All these patients were discharged from the intensive care unit (ICU) in good clinical condition and none was readmitted to the ICU. Post-intensive care syndrome was not identified in any of them, and they all returned to normal life after discharge from the hospital. (Photos from the authors' collections)

## 39.7 Conclusion

Recent advances within the field of critical care medicine have contributed to an increase in the percentage of patients who survive and are discharged from ICUs despite suffering from severe illness. These patients are, however, often living with the burden of PICS, which occurs in half of ICU survivors. PICS can have multidimensional adverse effects both in patients discharged from the ICU, but also in their families, affecting their integrative social function. Although the syndrome has been widely discussed in the literature it is still inadequately diagnosed, conceptualized, and treated. Recently more people are suffering from long-term mental, physical, and cognitive dysfunction due to the consequences of the global COVID-19 pandemic. The quality of ICU care has been challenged during the pandemic, mainly through an overwhelming use of deeper sedation, inadequate physiotherapy, and lack of family support. All aspects of PICS can be actively treated through cognitive and physical exercises and psychological support, but purpose-built facilities and programs are necessary to support patients and their families.

## References


1. Yende S, Austin S, Rhodes A, et al. Long-term quality of life among survivors of severe sepsis: analyses of two international trials. Crit Care Med. 2016;44:1461–7.
2. Needham DM, Davidson J, Cohen H, et al. Improving long-term outcomes after discharge from intensive care unit: report from a stakeholders' conference. Crit Care Med. 2012;40:502–9.
3. Yuan C, Timmins F, Thompson DR. Post-intensive care syndrome: a concept analysis. Int J Nurs Stud. 2021;114:103814.

4. Davidson JE, Jones C, Bienvenu OJ. Family response to critical illness: postintensive care syndrome-family. Crit Care Med. 2012;40:618–24.
5. Rousseau AF, Prescott HC, Brett SJ, et al. Long-term outcomes after critical illness: recent insights. Crit Care. 2021;25:108.
6. Bienvenu OJ, Colantuoni E, Mendez-Tellez PA, et al. Cooccurrence of and remission from general anxiety, depression, and posttraumatic stress disorder symptoms after acute lung injury: a 2-year longitudinal study. Crit Care Med. 2015;43:642–53.
7. Marra A, Pandharipande PP, Girard TD, et al. Co-occurrence of post-intensive care syndrome problems among 406 survivors of critical illness. Crit Care Med. 2018;46:1393–401.
8. Sukantarat KT, Burgess PW, Williamson RCN, Brett SJ. Prolonged cognitive dysfunction in survivors of critical illness. Anaesthesia. 2005;60:847–53.
9. Szylińska A, Listewnik M, Rotter I, et al. The efficacy of inpatient vs. home-based physiotherapy following coronary artery bypass grafting. Int J Environ Res Public Health. 2018;15:2572.
10. Pandharipande P. Long-term cognitive impairment after critical illness: commentary. J Pain Symptom Manage. 2014;369:1306–16.
11. Davydow DS, Gifford JM, Desai SV, Bienvenu OJ, Needham DM. Depression in general intensive care unit survivors: a systematic review. Intensive Care Med. 2009;35:796–809.
12. Myers EA, Smith DA, Allen SR, Kaplan LJ. Post-ICU syndrome: rescuing the undiagnosed. J Am Acad Physician Assist. 2016;29:34–7.
13. De Jonghe B, Sharshar T, Lefaucheur JP, et al. Paresis acquired in the intensive care unit: a prospective multicenter study. JAMA. 2002;288:2859–67.
14. Jackson JC, Pandharipande PP, Girard TD, et al. Depression, post-traumatic stress disorder, and functional disability in survivors of critical illness in the BRAIN-ICU study: a longitudinal cohort study. Lancet Respir Med. 2014;2:369–79.
15. Clavet H, Hébert PC, Fergusson D, Doucette S, Trudel G. Joint contracture following prolonged stay in the intensive care unit. CMAJ. 2008;178:691–7.
16. Mikkelsen ME, Still M, Anderson BJ, et al. Society of critical care medicine's international consensus conference on prediction and identification of long-term impairments after critical illness. Crit Care Med. 2020;48:1670–9.
17. Mikkelsen ME, Christie JD, Lanken PN, et al. The adult respiratory distress syndrome cognitive outcomes study: long-term neuropsychological function in survivors of acute lung injury. Am J Respir Crit Care Med. 2012;185:1307–15.
18. Narváez-Martínez MA, Gómez-Tovar LO, Henao-Castaño ÁM. Scales to measure post intensive care syndrome, a scoping review. Enferm Clin (Engl Ed). 2022;32:440–50.
19. Nasreddine ZS, Phillips NA, Bédirian V, et al. The Montreal Cognitive Assessment, MoCA: a brief screening tool for mild cognitive impairment. J Am Geriatr Soc. 2005;53:695–9.
20. Zigmond AS, Snaith RP. The hospital anxiety and depression scale. Acta Psychiatr Scand. 1983;67:361–70.
21. Stoll C, Kapfhammer HP, Rothenhäusler HB, et al. Sensitivity and specificity of a screening test to document traumatic experiences and to diagnose post-traumatic stress disorder in ARDS patients after intensive care treatment. Intensive Care Med. 1999;25:697–704.
22. Kotfis K, Zegan-Barańska M, Strzelbicka M, Safranow K, Żukowski M, Ely EW. Validation of the Polish version of the Critical Care Pain Observation Tool (CPOT) to assess pain intensity in adult, intubated intensive care unit patients: the POL-CPOT study. Arch Med Sci. 2018;14:880–9.
23. Kotfis K, Strzelbicka M, Zegan-Barańska M, et al. Validation of the behavioral pain scale to assess pain intensity in adult, intubated postcardiac surgery patients: a cohort observational study—POL-BPS. Medicine. 2018;97:e12443.
24. Inoue S, Hatakeyama J, Kondo Y, et al. Post-intensive care syndrome: its pathophysiology, prevention, and future directions. Acute Med Surg. 2019;6:233.
25. Pun BT, Balas MC, Barnes-Daly MA, et al. Caring for critically ill patients with the ABCDEF bundle: results of the ICU Liberation Collaborative in over 15,000 adults. Crit Care Med. 2019;47:3–14.

26. Preiser JC, Ichai C, Orban J-C, Groeneveld ABJ. Metabolic response to the stress of critical illness. Br J Anaesth. 2014;113:945–54.
27. Rousseau AF, Foidart-Desalle M, Ledoux D, et al. Effects of cholecalciferol supplementation and optimized calcium intakes on vitamin D status, muscle strength and bone health: a one-year pilot randomized controlled trial in adults with severe burns. Burns. 2015;41:317–25.
28. Moss SJ, Rosgen BK, Lucini F, et al. Psychiatric outcomes in ICU patients with family visitation: a population-based retrospective cohort study. Chest. 2022;162:578–87.
29. Barreto BB, Luz M, Rios MNDO, Lopes AA, Gusmao-Flores D. The impact of intensive care unit diaries on patients' and relatives' outcomes: a systematic review and meta-analysis. Crit Care. 2019;23:1–10.
30. Mehlhorn J, Freytag A, Schmidt KB, et al. Rehabilitation interventions for postintensive care syndrome: a systematic review. Crit Care Med. 2014;42:1263–71.
31. Ullman AJ, Aitken LM, Rattray J, et al. Intensive care diaries to promote recovery for patients and families after critical illness: a cochrane systematic review. Int J Nurs Stud. 2015;52:1243–53.
32. Cuthbertson BH, Rattray J, Campbell MK, et al. The PRaCTICaL study of nurse led, intensive care follow-up programmes for improving long term outcomes from critical illness: a pragmatic randomised controlled trial. BMJ. 2009;339:1016.
33. Nakanishi N, Liu K, Kawakami D, et al. Post-intensive care syndrome and its new challenges in coronavirus disease 2019 (COVID-19) pandemic: a review of recent advances and perspectives. J Clin Med. 2021;10:3870.
34. Vrettou CS, Mantziou V, Vassiliou AG, Dimopoulou I, Orfanos SE, Kotanidou A. Post-intensive care syndrome in survivors from critical illness including COVID-19 patients: a narrative review. Life (Basel). 2022;12:107.
35. Lechowicz K, Drożdżal S, Machaj F, et al. COVID-19: The potential treatment of pulmonary fibrosis associated with SARS-CoV-2 infection. J Clin Med. 2020;9:1–21.
36. Al-Jahdhami I, Al-Mawali A, Bennji SM. Respiratory complications after COVID-19. Oman Med J. 2022;37:e343.
37. Liu K, Nakamura K, Katsukawa H, et al. ABCDEF bundle and supportive ICU practices for patients with coronavirus disease 2019 infection: an international point prevalence study. Crit Care Explor. 2021;3:e0353.
38. Amass T, Van Scoy LJ, Hua M, et al. Stress-related disorders of family members of patients admitted to the intensive care unit with COVID-19. JAMA Intern Med. 2022;182:624–33.
39. Weidman K, LaFond E, Hoffman KL, et al. Post-intensive care unit syndrome in a cohort of COVID-19 survivors in New York City. Ann Am Thorac Soc. 2022;19:1158–68.
40. Jaffri A, Jaffri UA. Post-intensive care syndrome and COVID-19: crisis after a crisis? Heart Lung. 2020;49:883–4.
41. Zhang L, Hu W, Cai Z, et al. Early mobilization of critically ill patients in the intensive care unit: a systematic review and meta-analysis. PLoS One. 2019;14:e0223185.
42. de Jonghe B, Lacherade J-C, Sharshar T, Outin H. Intensive care unit-acquired weakness: risk factors and prevention. Crit Care Med. 2009;37:S309–15.
43. Cooney RN, Maish GO 3rd, Gilpin T, Shumate ML, Lang CH, Vary TC. Mechanism of IL-1 induced inhibition of protein synthesis in skeletal muscle. Shock. 1999;11:235–41.
44. Li YP, Reid MB. NF-kappaB mediates the protein loss induced by TNF-alpha in differentiated skeletal muscle myotubes. Am J Physiol Regul Integr Comp Physiol. 2000;279:R1165–70.
45. Keller CW, Schmidt J, Lünemann JD. Immune and myodegenerative pathomechanisms in inclusion body myositis. Ann Clin Transl Neurol. 2017;4:422–45.
46. Dodig D, Tarnopolsky MA, Margeta M, Gordon K, Fritzler MJ, Lu JQ. COVID-19-associated critical illness myopathy with direct viral effects. Ann Neurol. 2022;91:568–74.
47. Hashem MD, Nelliot A, Needham DM. Early mobilization and rehabilitation in the ICU: moving back to the future. Respir Care. 2016;61:971–9.
48. Wang J, Ren D, Liu Y, Wang Y, Zhang B, Xiao Q. Effects of early mobilization on the prognosis of critically ill patients: a systematic review and meta-analysis. Int J Nurs Stud. 2020;110:103708.

49. Hashem MD, Parker AM, Needham DM. Early mobilization and rehabilitation of patients who are critically ill. Chest. 2016;150:722–31.
50. Camargo Pires-Neto R, Fogaça Kawaguchi YM, et al. Very early passive cycling exercise in mechanically ventilated critically ill patients: physiological and safety aspects—a case series. PLoS One. 2013;8:e74182.
51. Wollersheim T, Grunow JJ, Carbon NM, et al. Muscle wasting and function after muscle activation and early protocol-based physiotherapy: an explorative trial. J Cachexia Sarcopenia Muscle. 2019;10:734–47.
52. Patel BK, Pohlman AS, Hall JB, Kress JP. Impact of early mobilization on glycemic control and ICU-acquired weakness in critically ill patients who are mechanically ventilated. Chest. 2014;146:583–9.
53. Nelke C, Dziewas R, Minnerup J, Meuth SG, Ruck T. Skeletal muscle as potential central link between sarcopenia and immune senescence. EBioMedicine. 2019;49:381–8.
54. Coelho-Junior HJ, Picca A, Calvani R, Uchida MC, Marzetti E. If my muscle could talk: myokines as a biomarker of frailty. Exp Gerontol. 2019;127:110715.
55. Burtin C, Clerckx B, Robbeets C, et al. Early exercise in critically ill patients enhances short-term functional recovery. Crit Care Med. 2009;37:2499–505.

# Part XIII

# Ethical Issues

# Rethinking the Role of Palliative Care in the ICU

# 40

M. S. F. Chong and V. Metaxa

## 40.1 Introduction

Being critically ill is a highly stressful experience for patients and their families, as they are often exposed to a multitude of intensive care interventions, whilst experiencing the existential fear of death in an alien environment. Despite continuing medical advances, mortality in the intensive care unit (ICU) remains significant, at approximately 16% worldwide [1]. Therefore, the transition from curative treatment to care that focuses primarily on comfort is an integral part of critical care, and ICU doctors and nurses should have the skills to recognize and help with this transition, as well as to manage distressing symptoms and support families around the end of life [2]. After decades of focusing mainly on technical advances and mortality figures, the importance of other outcome measures, such as preserved quality of life, the quality of care given to those dying, and the quality of human relationships involved in each death are slowly being recognized [3].

Concerns about delayed identification of dying, inadequate symptom management, and poor communication with families have been reported in the ICU, negatively influencing patient comfort, family trust, and satisfaction [4, 5]. The application of palliative care values in ICU practice has been proposed as an answer to these concerns, a holistic approach, and a way of improving the quality of care given to critically ill patients and their families [6]. Nonetheless, the integration of palliative care in the ICU has not been without barriers, not least because the interventions that constitute palliative care in the critical care setting and the outcomes that should be measured remain nebulous [7]. Furthermore, there is significant

M. S. F. Chong
Department of Critical Care, Kingston Hospital NHS Foundation Trust, London, UK

V. Metaxa (✉)
Department of Critical Care, King's College Hospital NHS Foundation Trust, London, UK
e-mail: victoria.metaxa@nhs.net



J.-L. Vincent (ed.), *Annual Update in Intensive Care and Emergency Medicine 2023*, Annual Update in Intensive Care and Emergency Medicine,
https://doi.org/10.1007/978-3-031-23005-9_40

variation in the advanced integration of palliative care across hospitals in the world, with only 20 countries achieving this globally (8.5%) [8].

In this chapter, we will discuss the definition, barriers, and models of palliative care services in the ICU. We will explore primary palliative care skills with which all ICU clinicians should be familiar, as well as indications for advanced specialty palliative care referral. Last, we will identify gaps in current knowledge and propose an agenda for future research.

## 40.2 Definition

Palliative care is an active and holistic approach for patients with terminal illness and their families, from the point of diagnosis or recognition, through to death and beyond. The word 'palliative' is derived from Latin *palliare* meaning 'to cloak'. Pain, dyspnea, and emotional stresses are eased while death approaches from serious illness. The aim is to maximize the quality of life not only by effective symptom management, but also by psychological and spiritual support of the affected patients and those close to them. It requires a multidisciplinary approach, from which the expertise of general physicians, oncologists, surgeons, nursing staff, physiotherapists and religious advisors are pooled and utilized.

Palliative care is linked with the modern hospice movement and Dame Cicely Sunders, who founded St Christopher's Hospice in London in 1967 [9]. She developed a modern approach to the care of the dying, drawing attention to the end-of-life care needs of patients with advanced malignant disease. She introduced the idea of 'total pain', which included the physical, emotional, social, and spiritual dimensions of distress. Palliative care was first recognized as a separate medical specialty in the UK in 1987, dedicated to relieving suffering and improving quality of life for patients with life-limiting illness. Access to palliative care has grown globally, however, this specialist care is not ubiquitous throughout the world [8].

The meaning of palliative care has evolved over time. The term originally referred to the care of patients with terminal diseases, which in the early days predominantly meant cancer. It now refers to the care of patients with serious, life-limiting, usually chronic illnesses, whether or not they are imminently dying. The World Health Organization (WHO) defines palliative care as "an approach that improves the quality of life of patients and their families who are facing problems associated with life-threatening illness. It prevents and relieves suffering through the early identification, correct assessment and treatment of pain and other problems, whether physical, psychosocial or spiritual" [10]. Palliative care medicine is applied as early as possible to patients with active, progressive, far advanced disease, for whom the prognosis is limited and the focus of care is on quality of life rather than the prolongation of death.

## 40.3 Barriers to Palliative Care in the ICU

In the ICU, death often occurs after an acute life-threatening illness or an exacerbation of chronic life-limiting illness. The majority of these deaths occur after there is a decision to withdraw or withhold treatment [11]. Frequently, treatment withdrawal in critical care is associated with ethical issues that can make the process challenging and is subject to great variability between individual physicians, departments, and geographical areas [12]. The supportive net offered by palliative care could be a valuable resource in the management of terminally ill patients in the ICU, an essential component of comprehensive care, regardless of age, diagnosis, or prognosis [2]. Despite these assertions, there are ongoing challenges for optimal integration of palliative care in ICU settings, due to both individual and organizational factors.

Some of the key barriers for this integration are associated with the acute nature of critical illness and the historical link between palliative services and imminent death. It is frequent for patients and families to have unrealistic expectations regarding ICU outcomes and express concerns that incorporation of palliative care will hasten death [13]. The conflation of palliative with end-of-life care is long-lasting and tantamount to the misconception that palliative and critical care are mutually exclusive or sequential rather than being complementary and concurrent approaches.

The most prominent ICU clinician-related barriers to primary palliative care are linked with the insufficient training invested in relevant communication skills for palliative care conversations. Relaying the transition from curative to comfort care to the patient and their family requires communication and relational training, which when lacking, can make this process challenging [14]. Organizational factors, such as inadequate staffing levels and/or high patient acuity result in competing demands on clinicians' time, who tend to prioritize interventions for patients likely to recover, rather than communication about, education around, and management of a dying patient [15, 16]. In specialist settings, such as surgical or oncological ICUs, challenges may arise from the special relationship formed between primary physicians and 'their' patients. The strong sense of personal responsibility for patient outcomes and the emotional attachment that is formed lead to difficulty in communication with patients and families about poor outcomes, and sometimes conflict with intensive care physicians about goals of care [17, 18].

On a global scale, there is a recognized insufficient access to palliative care, as only 14% of people who need palliative care currently receive it worldwide [9]. According to a WHO survey, funding for palliative care was available in 68% of countries and only 40% of countries reported that the services reached at least half of patients in need. Some health system policies do not integrate palliative care services into the structure and financing of national healthcare systems at all levels of care. Many people in low- and middle-income countries do not have sufficient access to opioid analgesics for the relief of pain and respiratory distress [19].

## 40.4 Models of Palliative Care

There are two main ways by which palliative care could be integrated into the ICU. First is the consultative model, which focuses on increasing the involvement of specialist palliative care consultants in the care of ICU patients and their families, as external consultants. Many initiatives using this model identify triggering criteria as indications for palliative care referral, such as baseline patient characteristics (age, functional dependence, length of stay) or clinical diagnosis (global cerebral ischemia, post-cardiac arrest, severe brain injury) [20]. Following the referral, a palliative care consultant and often an advanced practice nurse provide a comprehensive ICU palliative care consultation. The second approach, the integrative model, attempts to embed palliative care principles and interventions into usual ICU care, delivered by the critical care team as part of their daily practice for all patients and families facing critical illness. A combination of the two approaches is described as a mixed model.

The choice between the two models depends on the culture of individual ICUs and whether they are receptive to external consultation, but also on the availability of the palliative care team. In order to provide comprehensive care, the specialist palliative care team should have adequate staffing levels for 24/7 provision, understanding of the unique nature of ICU patients and their families, and possess skills to address them. Their expertise and substantial resources, as well as the continuity that they may provide in the care of the patient discharged from the ICU are invaluable. On the other hand, the integrative model requires the endorsement of its value by all critical care stakeholders, a continuous commitment to education and training, as well as incorporation of palliative care-related data into the unit's performance indicators. However, the very nature of ICU care includes the majority of palliative care values and critical care staff take pride in delivering the same kind of holistic care. Integration will ensure that optimal palliative care is delivered alongside active treatment by personnel that already care for the patient and their family, and understand the complicated environment of critical care.

Models to enhance palliative care involvement in the ICU, either with an integrative or a consultative approach, may not be mutually exclusive but rather allow variable degrees of overlap. Furthermore, while the delivery of palliative care for patients with critical illness has been associated with improvement in ICU and hospital metrics, the effectiveness of either palliative care model on outcome measures has been variable and difficult to demonstrate consistently [21]. In a recent systematic review, the consultative model appeared to have a more significant impact on reducing ICU length of stay and was associated with a greater number of decisions for limitations of life-sustaining treatment and do-not-attempt cardiopulmonary resuscitation (CPR) orders; however, nurse satisfaction appeared greater after integrative interventions [7]. Given the inherent challenges in each approach, a sustainable mode of delivery requires a mixed model, in which primary palliative care is delivered by the ICU team with concurrent, appropriate use of the consultative model, and palliative care consultants are reserved for patients at highest risk of having unmet or long-term palliative care needs [22].

## 40.5 Primary (Generalist) Palliative Care

Primary palliative care is provided by clinicians who have not undergone specialty training in palliative care but provide front-line care to patients. The core competencies in palliative care should be a component of the armamentarium of any intensivist, just as knowledge in cardiology, neurology, or microbiology is. The key palliative care interventions, which all ICU clinicians should demonstrate competency in, are: (1) communication skills, (2) ethical decision-making (including conflict management and redirecting goals of care), (3) symptom management, (4) advance care planning, and (5) bereavement care.

Communication skills are an essential component of critical care practice and extend beyond simple information exchange, as the majority of ICU patients are unable to participate in direct conversation. Critical care staff often require the involvement of the patient's family and/or friends to understand their values and wishes, especially around the end of life. Inadequate communication with physicians is frequently observed and leads to feelings of dissatisfaction, anxiety, and depression for families, as well as increased risk of conflict and burnout for clinicians [5]. Critical care providers should prepare meetings with families as they would organize any other invasive medical task, verifying the most important data and ensuring that their own values do not interfere in the relationship with patient's relatives [23]. Structured approaches to family conferences, such as the use of the VALUE mnemonic (Table 40.1), are recommended by international societies, as a guide for effective and empathetic family communication [24]. Given the evidence demonstrating the importance patients and families place on high-quality communication in the ICU, it is intuitive to assume that well-trained clinicians would improve the quality of communication in the critical care setting. Evidence confirms that training programs significantly improved clinician-reported communication skills and comfort with family communication, although no specific program was proven superior. The joint guidelines for family-centered care from a number of Critical Care Societies recommend that ICU clinicians receive relevant communication training as one element of critical care training [24].

Ethical decision-making is an unavoidable part of the critical care environment, where challenging life and death situations are frequent and involve multiple stakeholders (doctors, nurses, patients, and families). Withholding and withdrawing life-sustaining treatment account for the majority of deaths in the ICU, so many ethical dilemmas arise from disagreements around redirecting the goals of care. The risks

**Table 40.1** VALUE: a 5-step mnemonic to improve communication with families in ICU

| | |
|---|---|
| V | Value comments made by the family |
| A | Acknowledge family emotions |
| L | Listen |
| U | Understand the patient as a person |
| E | Elicit family questions |

Designed by University of Washington End-of-Life Care Research Program at Harborview Medical Center and benefits of intensive care interventions should always be individualized to each patient, taking into account their pre-morbid state, the acuity of the presenting situation and, most importantly, their views on quality of life. Decisions should be made by the multidisciplinary ICU team, together with patients and families, aiming to establish a partnership and achieve consensus. Individuals in environments characterized by poor interdisciplinary interactions and poor ethical decision-making climates demonstrate higher levels of burnout and low morale, whereas patient outcomes and treatment decisions may be compromised [25]. Unfortunately, while interprofessional decision-making improves the patient and family experience, and reduces the risk of intractable conflict and burnout, it is often suboptimal [26, 27]. Conflicts surrounding end-of-life decisions may occur for a variety of reasons, including ethno-cultural differences, personal biases, and organizational characteristics of critical care [27]. Lack of knowledge or education in health ethics is a common cause of ethical dilemmas and conflict occurring in the ICU. Problems arising from knowledge deficits could decrease considerably if professionals receive training in recognizing the emerging moral dilemmas and obtain competencies in ethical deliberation and decision-making.

Symptom management involves treating a wide range of symptoms that accompany advanced progressive disease, aiming to improve not only the quality of life for patients receiving multiple interventions, but also the quality of their death. Specific symptoms ICU clinicians should be able to manage around the end of life include pain, agitation, respiratory distress, and delirium. Regarding pain management interventions, most guidelines recommend the use of opioids and benzodiazepines for symptom relief, with morphine and midazolam being the most commonly used medications [28]. In the ICU setting, intravenous infusions and bolus doses are recommended, with the alternative of using subcutaneous medications, if intravenous access is not available. The doses used are generally higher than those recommended in guidelines and progressively increase before the withdrawal of life-sustaining treatment [28]. Concerns around maximal doses and the contribution of analgo-sedation in shortening a patient's life have not been supported by the literature and should not hinder attempts to alleviate symptoms during end-of-life care [29]. Non-physical symptoms should be recognized and addressed, with specific focus on the psychological, spiritual, and existential aspects of critical illness. Spirituality, which includes religious and existential care, has been recognized as an essential domain of palliative care and access to appropriate spiritual care, such as specific cultural or religious rituals, should be facilitated where possible. Existential suffering has been described as the morbid suffering relating to loss of hope, futility, remorse, and fear of death [30]; specialist palliative care consultation should be sought promptly when the limits of the critical care specialist's experience have been reached [29].

Advance care planning offers people the opportunity to discuss their future care and support, including medical treatment, while they have the capacity to do so. It has been proposed as a way to promote self-determination in situations where the individual has lost decision-making capacity and cannot make important life and death decisions. Advance care plans have significant theoretical advantages, as they allow patients to refuse future therapies and plan their future care, ensuring that the treatments they receive are consistent with their values and wishes. In the critical setting, they have the potential to assist intensivists in their decision-making, especially as many patients have impaired level of consciousness near the end of life. Despite the conceptual advantages, advance decision planning can be problematic in the ICU setting, as the acute nature of the injury and the speed of deterioration often preclude meaningful discussions [31]. However, ICU physicians can still be involved in other forms of forward planning, either when reviewing patients on the wards as part of the outreach team or by communicating the risks and benefits of future care options, and educating families about the anticipated clinical course of the illness [32].

Bereavement care is essential for supporting families through the death of a loved one and it is a natural part of critical care nursing in particular [33]. Evidence suggests that primary discrete bereavement support interventions (e.g., a personal memento, a handwritten condolence letter, a post-death storytelling meeting, research participation, and use of an ICU diary) were all well accepted by the bereaved families [34]. These relatively simple interventions could become part of standard ICU practice following a patient's death, theoretically improving family experience after an often life-changing event. However, the appropriateness and effectiveness of different bereavement interventions have not been investigated extensively in the critical care setting. Although bereavement support is acknowledged as an important aspect of end-of-life care in the ICU, provision is variable, and literature suggests that outcomes may not always be beneficial [35]. In view of these disparities, exploratory research to test the effectiveness of different bereavement interventions is urgently needed. In the meantime, every ICU should aim to embed culturally appropriate, basic bereavement care in their practice, identify families at risk of complicated grief, and refer them to more specialist bereavement services if required.

## 40.6 Specialist (Secondary) Palliative Care

Specialty palliative care consultation is provided by qualified, subspecialty-trained palliative care clinicians, whose role has moved beyond the narrow scope of providing symptom management around the end of life, towards more holistic care at any stage of a life-limiting condition. Their skills range from managing refractory physical symptoms to conducting complex family meetings and/or navigating through spiritual or existential distress [36]. Their extensive training may prove valuable when there are communication issues between the team and with patients and families. Specialty palliative care involvement has been shown to help with discussion around limitation of life-sustaining treatments, do-not-attempt CPR orders, and hospice referrals by facilitating in depth discussion on goals of care at end of life [37]. Early referral to the specialist palliative care team may also maintain continuity of care after discharge from critical care, by enabling medication transition from ICU to ward settings and providing ongoing support for patients and families until either death or hospital discharge, with appropriate handover to community services. The palliative care team can also co-ordinate discussions regarding the preferred place of care with the patient or family, with the ability to facilitate admission to specialist palliative care units or even home if appropriate.

Despite estimates that a large subset of ICU patients could benefit from palliative care, the integration of specialist palliative care in the ICU has been extremely variable, with evidence, mainly from North America, suggesting a decrease in ICU admissions and reduced ICU length of stay [38], but minimal data from the rest of the world. Several barriers have been identified hindering the involvement of the specialist team in daily ICU practice, including insufficient staff education about what palliative care specialist may add to patient care and the insufficient numbers of specialists to take on all aspects of palliative care in ICU [36]. In many hospitals, there is resistance to involving palliative care early by intensive care teams and/or specialty teams, as it is perceived as a sign of giving up and associated with end-of-life care. Specialist teams are often contacted after the decision to withdrawal treatment has been made, leading to a very sequential model of care, which risks fragmentation in patient care during a very stressful period. Last, the availability of trained palliative care clinicians is far from the norm in Europe, Asia, and Africa, where overall the development and acceptance of the palliative care discipline is much less than in North America [7].

In an attempt to increase the involvement of specialty palliative care consultations, recent efforts have focused on the use of screening criteria or triggers to prompt automated specialty palliative care consultation [39, 40]. Proposed triggers include predicted length of ICU stay >5 days, risk of death >25%, or potentially irreversible functional change precluding eventual return to home [20]. Palliative care involvement has also been advocated for patients over 80 years of age, with active stage 4 malignancy, post-cardiac arrest, or intracerebral bleed requiring mechanical ventilation. Despite being intuitive, these triggers have demonstrated good specificity but low sensitivity for predicting 6-month mortality [41]. Newer triggers, such as sepsis, metastatic and non-metastatic cancer, and weight loss at ICU admission have been proposed. However, the absence of an accepted definition of 'palliative care needs' and the lack of consensus regarding the best outcomes for the various trigger criteria render the identification of patients who may benefit from specialist palliative care input difficult.

## 40.7 Future Research

Integrating palliative care into critical care is advocated as a way to mitigate physical and psychological burdens for patients and their families. Despite recent studies that support this positive association, the evidence remains limited and unevenly distributed globally. Limitations have already been identified in the definition of what distinguishes primary palliative care (skills that all clinicians should have) from specialist palliative care (skills for managing more complex and difficult cases), which ICU interventions are also palliative care ones, and what are the appropriate outcomes to measure the effectiveness of these interventions [7]. Initial attempts should focus on clarifying which basic elements of critical care fall under the umbrella of palliative care and test interventions to increase their acceptance by ICU clinicians. A second step should be a clear research agenda on ICU-based palliative care interventions, maybe focusing on areas that have shown positive results (such as multi-faceted educational projects) [7]. Last, a consensus on which outcomes have the greatest value to measure in the ICU setting, targeting the specific needs of the critical care patients, their families, and the staff is necessary. Larger studies in populations with diverse cultural and social differences will assess whether the use of palliative care in the ICU is not only beneficial in high income countries but globally.

## 40.8 Conclusion

Critical care-based palliative care is a holistic approach to caring for critically ill patients. It focuses on improving the quality of dying and death by anticipating, preventing, and treating physical, psychological, spiritual, and existential suffering. It encompasses clear and sensitive communication with families, shared decision-making based on patients' values and symptom management around the end of life. This can be delivered by the ICU staff or specialist healthcare professionals, via a consultative or integrative model of palliative care. Critical care clinicians should be competent in primary palliative care skills, whereas specialist palliative care expertise can contribute when required, with good interdisciplinary collaboration. Such a mixed model will empower ICU staff in the day-to-day practice and help overcome the important barriers, such as insufficient palliative care specialist numbers and intensivist hesitancy. The clarification of what constitutes ICU-delivered palliative care interventions, the identification and measurement of clinically important outcomes, as well as attempts to identify a palliative care model that could be applicable worldwide constitute items for future research and education.

## References

1. Vincent JL, Marshall JC, Namendys-Silva SA, et al. Assessment of the worldwide burden of critical illness: the intensive care over nations (ICON) audit. Lancet Respir Med. 2014;2:380–6.
2. Edwards JD, Voigt LP, Nelson JE. Ten key points about ICU palliative care. Intensive Care Med. 2017;43:83–5.
3. Dunstan GR. Hard questions in intensive care. Anaesthesia. 1985;40:479–82.
4. Puntillo KA, Arai S, Cohen NH, et al. Symptoms experience by intensive care unit patients at high risk of dying. Crit Care Med. 2010;38:2155–60.
5. Azoulay E, Chevret S, Leleu G, et al. Half the families of intensive care unit patients experience inadequate communication with physicians. Crit Care Med. 2000;28:3044–9.
6. Kavalieratos D, Corbelli J, Zhang D, et al. Association between palliative care and patient and caregiver outcomes: a systematic review and meta-analysis. JAMA. 2016;316:2104–14.
7. Metaxa V, Anagnostou D, Vlachos S, et al. Palliative care interventions in intensive care unit patients. Intensive Care Med. 2021;47:1415–25.

8. Lynch T, Connor S, Clark D, et al. Mapping levels of palliative care development: a global update. J Pain Symptom Manage. 2013;45:109–1106.
9. Baines M. From pioneer days to implementation: lessons to be learnt. Eur J Palliat Care. 2011;18:223–7.
10. World Health Organization. Palliative care. Available at: https://www.who.int/news-room/fact-sheets/detail/palliative-care. Accessed 14 Jul 2022.
11. Sprung CL, Cohen SL, Sjokvist P, et al. End-of-life practices in European Intensive Care Units: The Ethicus Study. JAMA. 2003;290:790–7.
12. Mark NM, Rayner SG, Lee NJ, et al. Global variability in withholding and withdrawal of life sustaining treatment in the intensive care unit: a systematic review. Intensive Care Med. 2015;41:1572–85.
13. Aslakson RA, Curtis JR, Nelson JE. The changing role of palliative care in the ICU. Crit Care Med. 2014;42:2418–28.
14. Lamiani G, Mistraletti G, Moreschi C, Andrighi E, Vegni E. Cultivating empathy and soft skills among intensive care residents: effects of a mandatory, simulation-based, experiential training. Ann Transplant. 2021;26:e931147.
15. Baker M, Luce J, Bosslet GT. Integration of palliative care services in the intensive care unit: a roadmap for overcoming barriers. Clin Chest Med. 2015;36:441–8.
16. Fassier T, Lautrette A, Ciroldi M, et al. Care at the end of life in critically ill patients: the European perspective. Curr Opin Crit Care. 2005;11:616–23.
17. Deeg HJ. Treatment ethics, quality of life and health economics in the management of hematopoietic malignancies in older patients. Bone Marrow Transplant. 2015;50:1145–9.
18. Olson TJP, Brasel KJ, Redmann AJ, et al. Surgeon-reported conflict with intensivists about postoperative goals of care. JAMA Surg. 2013;148:29–35.
19. World Health Organization. Assessing national capacity for the prevention and control of non-communicable diseases: report of the 2019 global survey. Available at: https://www.who.int/publications/i/item/9789240002319. Accessed 17 Nov 2022.
20. Nelson JE, Bassett R, Boss RD, et al. Models for structuring a clinical initiative to enhance palliative care in the intensive care unit: a report from the IPAL-ICU Project (Improving Palliative Care in the ICU). Crit Care Med. 2010;38:1765–72.
21. Aslakson R, Cheng J, Vollenweider D, et al. Evidence-based palliative care in the intensive care unit: a systematic review of interventions. J Palliat Med. 2014;17:219–35.
22. Hua M, Wunsch H. Integrating palliative care in the ICU. Curr Opin Crit Care. 2014;20:673–80.
23. Curtis JR, Patrick DL, Shannon SE, Treece PD, Engelberg RA, Rubenfeld GD. The family conference as a focus to improve communication about end-of-life care in the intensive care unit: opportunities for improvement. Crit Care Med. 2001;29:N26–33.
24. Davidson JE, Aslakson RA, Long AC, et al. Guidelines for family-centered care in the neonatal, pediatric, and adult ICU. Crit Care Med. 2017;45:103–28.
25. Benoit DD, Jensen HI, Malmgren J, et al. DISPROPRICUS study group of the Ethics Section of the European Society of Intensive Care Medicine: Outcome in patients perceived as receiving excessive care across different ethical climates: a prospective study in 68 intensive care units in Europe and the USA. Intensive Care Med. 2018;44:1039–49.
26. Curtis JR, Vincent JL. Ethics and end-of-life care for adults in the intensive care unit. Lancet. 2010;375:1347–53.
27. Michalsen A, Long AC, DeKeyser GF, et al. Interprofessional shared decision-making in the ICU: a systematic review and recommendations from an expert panel. Crit Care Med. 2019;47:1258–66.
28. Laserna A, Durán-Crane A, López-Olivo MA, et al. Pain management during the withholding and withdrawal of life support in critically ill patients at the end-of-life: a systematic review and meta-analysis. Intensive Care Med. 2020;46:1671–82.
29. Durán-Crane A, Laserna A, López-Olivo MA, et al. Clinical practice guidelines and consensus statements about pain management in critically ill end-of-life patients: a systematic review. Crit Care Med. 2019;47:1619–26.

30. Bruce A, Scheiber R, Petrovskaya O, Boston P. Longing for ground in a ground (less) world: a qualitative inquiry of existential suffering. BMC Nurs. 2011;10:2.
31. Horn R. "I don't need my patients' opinion to withdraw treatment": patient preferences at the end-of-life and physician attitudes towards advance directives in England and France. Med Health Care Philos. 2014;17:425–35.
32. Pattison N, O'Gara G, Wigmore T. Negotiating transitions: involvement of critical care outreach teams in end-of-life decision making. Am J Crit Care. 2015;24:232–40.
33. Egerod I, Kaldan G, Albarran J, et al. Elements of intensive care bereavement follow-up services: a European survey. Nurs Crit Care. 2019;24:201–8.
34. Efstathiou N, Walker W, Metcalfe A, et al. The state of bereavement support in adult intensive care: a systematic review and narrative synthesis. J Crit Care. 2019;50:177–87.
35. Pattison NA, White C, Lone NI. Bereavement in critical care: a narrative review and practice exploration of current provision of support services and future challenges. J Intensive Care Soc. 2021;22:349–56.
36. Quill TE, Abernethy AP. Generalist plus specialist palliative care - creating a more sustainable model. N Engl J Med. 2013;368:1173–5.
37. Zalenski RJ, Jones SS, Courage C, et al. Impact of palliative care screening and consultation in the ICU: a multihospital quality improvement project. J Pain Symptom Manage. 2017;53:5–12.e13.
38. Khandelwal N, Kross EK, Engelberg RA, et al. Estimating the effect of palliative care interventions and advance care planning on ICU utilization: a systemic review. Crit Care Med. 2015;43:1102–11.
39. Hua MS, Li G, Blinderman CD, et al. Estimates for the need for palliative care consultation across united states intensive care units using a trigger-based model. Am J Respir Crit Care Med. 2014;189:428–36.
40. Secunda K, Krolikowski KA, Savage MF, Kruser JM. Evaluation of automated specialty palliative care in the intensive care unit: a retrospective cohort study. PLoS One. 2021;16:e0255989.
41. Hua MS, Ma X, Li G, et al. Derivation of data-driven triggers for palliative care consultation in critically ill patients. J Crit Care. 2018;46:79–83.

# Index




J.-L. Vincent (ed.), *Annual Update in Intensive Care and Emergency Medicine 2023*, Annual Update in Intensive Care and Emergency Medicine,
https://doi.org/10.1007/978-3-031-23005-9